Headache and head pain

DIAGNOSIS AND TREATMENT

Headache and head pain

DIAGNOSIS AND TREATMENT

ROBERT E. RYAN, Sr., M.S.(Otolaryngology), M.D., F.A.C.S.

Professor of Otolaryngology, St. Louis University School of Medicine;
Past President, American Association for the Study of Headache;
Diplomate, American Board of Otolaryngology;
Director, Ryan Headache Center, St. Louis, Missouri;
Chief, Department of Otolaryngology,
St. John's Mercy Medical Center,
St. Louis, Missouri

ROBERT E. RYAN, Jr., M.D.

Associate Director, Ryan Headache Center, St. Louis, Missouri;
Associate Otolaryngologist, St. John's Mercy Medical Center,
St. Louis, Missouri; formerly Fellow, Mayo Clinic,
Rochester, Minnesota

with 30 illustrations including five in three colors

The C. V. Mosby Company

Saint Louis   1978

616.047
H432

The C. V. Mosby Company
11830 Westline Industrial Drive, St. Louis, Missouri 63141

Library of Congress Cataloging in Publication Data

Main entry under title:

Headache and head pain.

    Earlier ed. by R. E. Ryan published under title:
Headache, diagnosis and treatment.
    Includes index.
    1. Headache. I. Ryan, Robert Emmett. II. Ryan,
Robert Emmett, 1946-   [DNLM: 1. Headache—
Diagnosis. 2. Headache—Therapy. WL342 H432]
RB128.R9 1978   616'.047   78-8973
ISBN 0-8016-4242-6

CB/CB/B 9 8 7 6 5 4 3 2 1

To
C. F. R.
and
L. M. R.

Contributors

J. D. Carroll, M.D., F.R.C.P., F.R.C.P.E.

Reader in Clinical Neurology,
University of Surrey,
Guildford, Surrey, England;
Consultant Neurologist,
Regional Neurological Unit,
Royal Surrey County Hospital,
Guildford, Surrey, England

Seymour Diamond, M.D.

Clinical Assistant Professor, Neurology,
The Chicago Medical School;
Director, Diamond Headache Clinic, Ltd.,
Chicago, Illinois

Edward J. Hempstead, D.D.S., F.A.C.D., F.A.G.D.

St. John's Mercy Medical Center;
Oral Surgery Associate,
DePaul Community Health Center,
St. Louis, Missouri

Robert S. Kunkel, M.D.

Staff Physician,
Department of Internal Medicine,
Cleveland Clinic Foundation,
Cleveland, Ohio

Ninan T. Mathew, M.D., F.R.C.P.(C)

Clinical Associate Professor of Neurology,
University of Texas School of Medicine;
Clinical Assistant Professor of Neurology,
Baylor College of Medicine,
Houston, Texas

Edgard Raffaelli, Jr., M.D.

President, Brazilian Headache Society,
São Paulo, Brazil

Walter R. Stafford, M.D., F.A.C.S.

Clinical Professor and Acting Chairman,
Department of Ophthalmology,
St. Louis University,
St. Louis, Missouri

Preface

Since the publication of *Headache* many years ago, there has been an abundance of research. This research, of course, has been primarily in the field of vascular headache, especially the migraine type of headache problem. This research has been directly concerned with etiology and treatment. All of the newer concepts concerning headache are presented, whether they be theoretical or factual. All of the pertinent material contained in the senior author's previous headache books that is still up-to-date is also included in this publication.

In this book, we attempt to discuss as many of the various forms of headache and head pain as possible. The various forms of pathologic conditions producing headache are also mentioned and discussed. The amount of discussion, of course, varies in proportion to the importance and frequency of the type of headache. We have even tried to include some conditions producing headache that are somewhat rare but nevertheless frequently mentioned in the medical literature. This seems justifiable if this is to be a complete book on headache and head pain.

The etiology of some forms of vascular headache still remains unknown in spite of the fact that continuous research is taking place on this form of headache. All of the various theories of this aspect of vascular headache are presented. All of the recommended types of treatment for the various forms of vascular headache are presented. This is true in both the symptomatic and the prophylactic forms of treatment. Some of these forms of treatment we recommend and some forms we do not. However, to be fair to the reader, all are presented.

The usual symptomatology of the various forms of headache is thoroughly presented. However, it should be borne in mind that atypical cases are always to be found in any type of chronic headache problem.

Headache is naturally one of the most common complaints with which the average practicing physician is confronted. This is true in many fields of medicine such as otolaryngology, ophthalmology, internal medicine, family practice, neurology, psychiatry, dentistry, and many other specialties.

Both the physician and the patient are much more aware of the problem of chronic headache than they were some 20 years ago. They both desire to solve the problem.

One of the best ways to help to solve a

chronic headache problem is to take a careful, thorough, good history of the problem. This is especially true in the case of vascular headaches. Because of this, history taking has been thoroughly discussed.

The importance of the examination of patients is also outlined. This includes all of the various radiologic and laboratory tests that may be required in some forms of headache problems.

Cerebral blood flow and the physiologic basis of head pain are also mentioned, outlining the various areas in the head that are either sensitive or insensitive to pain.

A headache problem can be simple to solve or can be quite complex, requiring much time and effort. Naturally, some of these problems cannot be solved completely. However, both the physician and the patient must remember that each case requires "essence of patience and tincture of time."

It is our sincere hope that we have discussed headache in this book in an appealing fashion and in a manner interesting to all members of the medical profession, regardless of their special field of interest.

Robert E. Ryan, Sr.
Robert E. Ryan, Jr.

Acknowledgments

We have been extremely fortunate to have several outstanding authorities in the field of headache as contributors in the preparation of this book.

Desmond Carroll, one of the outstanding neurologists of Europe, has made an outstanding presentation of ophthalmoplegic migraine, a subject to which he has devoted years of research.

Seymour Diamond of Chicago has provided an excellent description of biofeedback and its use in the field of headache. This is probably one of his chief interests in headache therapy, a subject on which he is a well-known authority.

Edward Hempstead has outlined dental headache very completely.

Robert Kunkel, of the Cleveland Clinic, has presented the chapter on headache associated with systemic diseases. His presentation is thorough and complete, and we are very fortunate to have it as a portion of this book.

Ninan Mathew, of Baylor University, has covered headache of neurologic etiology.

This outstanding neurologist has indeed made a valuable contribution to this book.

Edgard Raffaelli, Jr., the president of the Brazilian Headache Society, has presented the limbic system for us. Ed is one of the outstanding authorities on this subject and he has made an excellent presentation for us.

The head of the ophthalmology department of St. Louis University School of Medicine, Walter Stafford, has done an excellent job on the chapter dealing with headache of ophthalmologic origin.

To these men we are ever grateful for the excellent material they have given us for this presentation. We hope that you, the reader, will enjoy their efforts as much as we have.

We also wish to thank Miss Karen Pirino and Mrs. Mildred Winn, the librarians of St. John's Mercy Medical Center, who gave us so much help with the presentation of this book.

Robert E. Ryan, Sr.
Robert E. Ryan, Jr.

Contents

Headache and head pain
DIAGNOSIS AND TREATMENT

Introduction

Pain is a complaint of patients encountered in any form of clinical medical practice. The term "pain" is not easily defined. In ancient Greek writings pain is spoken of as a punishment or penalty. Aristotle spoke of pain as a quality of the soul, a state of feeling that was the opposite of pleasure. Headache is a form of pain. The medical term for headache, cephalalgia, is from the Greek meaning a condition of head pain.

Probably the most common complaint of the medical patient today, or certainly one of the most common, is headache. The problem of treating patients suffering from recurring headaches is commonly encountered in almost every type of medical practice.

Headache may be mild or severe, organic or functional. It may be of psychogenic origin, the symptom of serious illness, or something between these two extremes. Regardless of its classification, every chronic headache requires a thorough evaluation, accurate diagnosis, and prompt treatment.

Headaches have been found to antedate history. In ancient civilizations, as far back as the prehistoric Indian tribes of America and the Egyptians, there is evidence that people suffered the excruciating pains of headache. In many ancient writings, we can find that these prehistoric people had devised numerous methods of cure and various odd types of treatment.

In a random survey made by Louisiana State University School of medicine, it was found that 64.8% of the people questioned had headache problems of one type or another.[1] Other estimates of the number of people in the United States suffering from headache at one time or another are as high as 90%. It seems safe to say that most people suffer from headache at some point in their lives; it is rare to find a person who has never experienced a headache on some occasion.

Though headache frequently occurs in organic disease, the vast majority of headaches encountered are benign. Nevertheless, organic disease must be ruled out in each patient.

Headache in itself is not a disease; it is merely a symptom of a disease. Headache drives the patient to see a physician in an effort to obtain relief from pain.

In the United States, headache ranks high as a source of revenue for manufacturers of patent and proprietary headache remedies. Television, radio, and newspaper advertisements for these drugs have made Americans "headache conscious."

In diagnosing the average headache prob-

1

lem, the physician must rely on a good case history; occasionally diagnostic tests will be required to establish a difficult diagnosis.

The frequency and severity of the headache attacks determine the extent to which the headache problem will incapacitate the patient. Because of this incapacitation, the headache problem is important economically and socially. Headache is a frequent reason for absenteeism at work, and it tends to lower the individual's efficiency while at work.

Because there are innumerable types of headache, diagnosis often presents a seemingly insurmountable problem. Many people attach little significance to the common headache. This is true in cases where the headache attacks are mild, transitory, and infrequent. When headache attacks become frequent or severe, the individual should seek medical attention by a competent physician.

As a general rule, pain acts as a warning signal or an indicator that something is not acting as it should, either within the orga-nism or in the relationship of the organism to its environment. This is also true in the case of head pain. The exact significance of this warning should be evaluated. However, because so many different physical, emotional, and environmental factors may produce a headache attack, evaluation may not be easy.

Clinical and pharmacologic research in the past 15 years has given the practicing physician a great deal of aid in the field of headache therapy. As pointed out by Graham,[2] the knowledge of headache mechanisms acquired during the past 25 years has surpassed that accrued over the preceding 2,500 years. Studies in headache are moving forward and justify the attention of all physicians who wish to deal successfully with this most common of painful human experiences.

REFERENCES

1. Ogden, H. D.: The treatment of allergic headache, Ann. Allergy **9:**673, 1951.
2. Graham, J. R.: Profiles in headache, Med. Sci., pp. 647-675, Nov. 25, 1960.

CHAPTER 1

Mechanisms of head pain

THE PHYSIOLOGIC BASIS OF HEAD PAIN

The pain in the ordinary type of headache, and also in most other types of headache, is generally of intracranial origin. It may be correctly stated that pain in the head may originate in one of three anatomic structures:

1. The tissues covering the cranium
2. The cranial periosteum
3. Certain intracranial structures

These intracranial structures sensitive to pain include (Figs. 1-1 to 1-4):

1. Trigeminal nerve
2. Glossopharyngeal nerve
3. Vagus nerve
4. The first three cervical nerves
5. The cerebral arteries
6. The dural arteries
7. Parts of the dura at the base of the brain
8. The great venous sinuses and their venous tributaries from the surface of the brain

Because the intracranial vessels are under nervous control, the production of headache through a reflex action that may be initiated from various parts of the body and in an excitable or an emotional state is readily understood on the basis of a vascular nature.

Observations of conscious patients during intracranial procedures have established that the cortical gray matter of the brain and the dura mater are insensitive to pain.[1] Because of the sensitivity of the pial and dural vessels, it is believed that the majority of headaches are vascular in nature. The pain in these cases is due to vasodilation and the excitation of the sensory nerve endings that are situated either on the wall of the blood vessel itself or in its immediate neighborhood. It is further thought that vasoconstriction occurs first; this is followed by a period of vasodilation and then congestion in the pia mater. Because of the initial vasoconstriction and the local anemia which results, there may also be edema and a resulting rise in the intracranial pressure (Fig. 1-5).

The areas which are generally insensitive to pain (Fig. 1-6) are:

1. The cranium
2. The brain itself
3. Most of the dura
4. The pia-arachnoid
5. The choroid plexus
6. The ependymal linings of the ventricles

Sudden changes in the intraventricular pressure, whether in the form of a rise or a fall, are likely to cause attacks of headache. This may be true even if there are no significant changes in the general intracranial

3

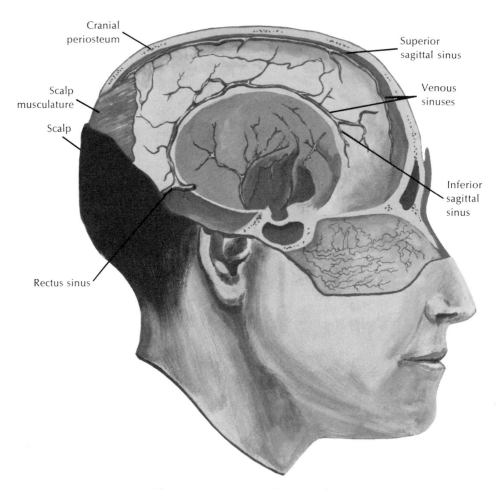

Fig. 1-1. Structures sensitive to pain.

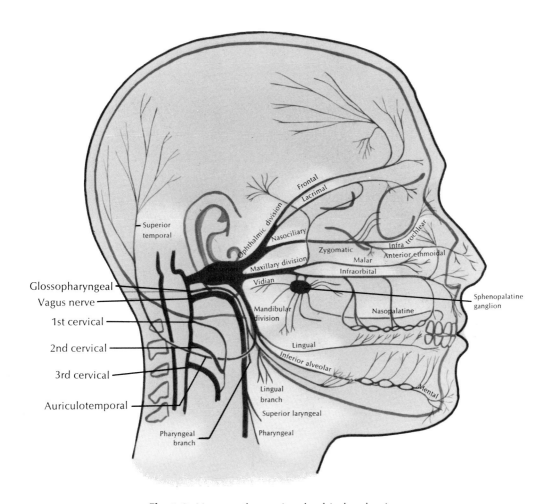

Fig. 1-2. Nerve pathways involved in head pain.

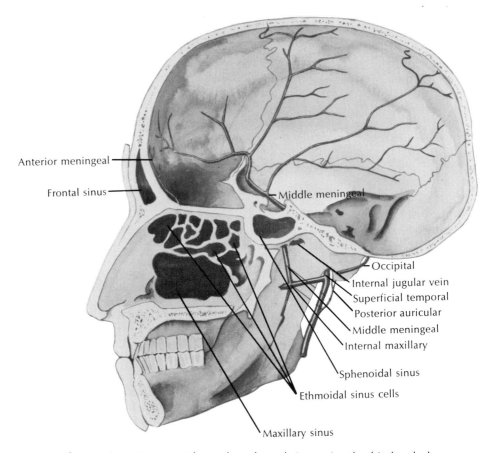

Anterior meningeal

Frontal sinus

Middle meningeal

Occipital

Internal jugular vein

Superficial temporal

Posterior auricular

Middle meningeal

Internal maxillary

Sphenoidal sinus

Ethmoidal sinus cells

Maxillary sinus

Fig. 1-3. Some intracranial vessels and nasal sinuses involved in headache.

pressure. Lowering the pressure within the third ventricle and the optic thalami forming the ventricular walls may also cause headache. This may result from withdrawing cerebrospinal fluid as is done in a spinal puncture.

The most common extracranial sources of headache are the pericranial muscles and the extracranial arteries (Fig. 1-7). Irritation of one or both of these either by vascular compression or constriction with resultant ischemia or by muscle contraction by traction in pain receptors in the involved area will result in pain. The severity of this pain is directly proportional to the force of the contraction of the musculature involved. Distention of the extracranial arteries will produce pain along the course of the artery or arteries involved. This distention is in-

creased with each systolic ejection of blood, which in turn produces a pulsating or throbbing type of pain.

Headache is often a signal that something is wrong. If the headache does not appear until the patient is elderly, such conditions as temporal arteritis, glaucoma, or generalized vascular insufficiency must be considered. If the patient presents a history of convulsions, hemiparesis, or hemianesthesia of unexplained origin along with the symptom of headache, angiomatous malformations may be suspected. Basilar artery insufficiency may be suspected if the headache is severe, throbbing, located in the occipital area, and aggravated by changes in the patient's posture. Headache accompanying a sudden onset of paralysis of any of the cranial nerves along with vi-

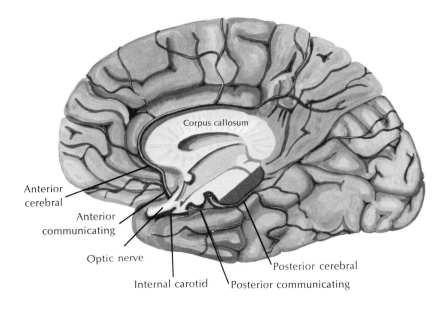

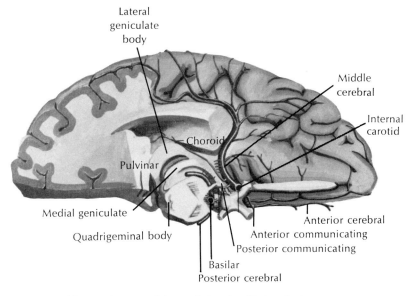

Fig. 1-4. Intracranial vessels involved in headache.

sual field defects may be indicative of an aneurysm. Headache that is pulsating, intense, and of short duration accompanied by tachycardia, pallor, nausea, vomiting, and excessive perspiration may make the physician suspicious of a pheochromocytoma.

Headache may arise from pathologic anomalies of the nasal passages, nasal sinuses, the ear, the throat (including the larynx or the pharynx), or the cervical spine. Headache may also result from a neuralgia of the nerves of the scalp or from nasal sinus disease. Headache may occur as part of the symptomatology of a great variety of disease states, such as we find in nephritic ar-

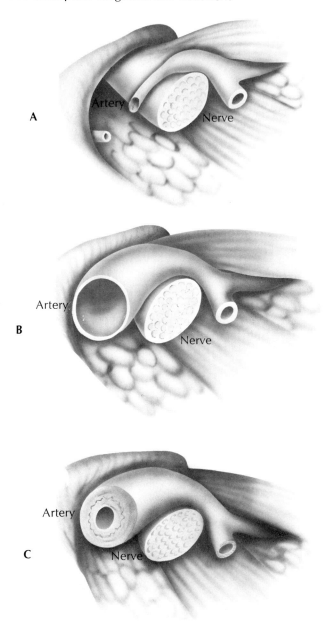

Fig. 1-5. A, Vasoconstrictive phase. **B,** Vasodilatory phase. **C,** Vascular edema phase.

terial hypertension and many other conditions of a toxic nature.

Headache that may occur in such intracranial conditions as tumor, abscesses, or hemorrhage is usually the result of a general rise in the intracranial pressure; however, this type of head pain may also be due to the irritations of sensitive nerve endings in the immediate neighborhood of the lesion. It is entirely possible that the vasomotor reactions involving the intracerebral vessels or variations in the pressure within the ventricular system may be factors in the production of head pain.

"Pain arising from the stimulation of the sensitive intracranial structures above the

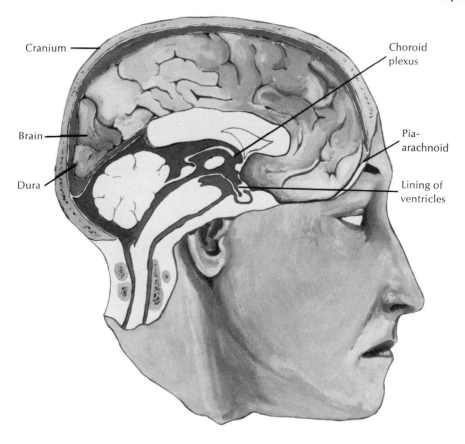

Cranium

Brain

Dura

Choroid plexus

Pia-arachnoid

Lining of ventricles

Fig. 1-6. Structures insensitive to pain.

tentorium cerebelli is felt anterior to a vertical plane passing between the ears and is transmitted by the trigeminal nerve. Pain arising from the stimulation of intracranial structures below the tentorium cerebelli is felt posteriorly to this plane and is transmitted by the glossopharyngeal nerve, the vagus nerve, and the first three cervical nerves." This fact has been brought out by Horton.[3]

Any sudden or severe headache that occurs with an uneventful onset should be investigated thoroughly by the physician. This is true also in cases of headache associated with such symptoms as fever, convulsions, mental confusion, or loss of consciousness. Posttraumatic headaches following a blow to the head should also be studied thoroughly. Any chronic daily or frequent headache is abnormal, as is a re-

curring headache problem in children or in older patients who had previously been free of headache.

In a comparative study of the pulse waves of normal vessels and headache patients' vessels, Tunis and Wolff[4] found that there was relative vasoconstriction even during headache-free intervals in those patients afflicted with chronic headache. They further found that concurrent constriction of nutrient arteries and increased muscle contraction can result in headache.

Headache may result from the radiation of pain from the extracranial branches of the trigeminal nerve to its intracranial terminations. It is also reasonable to assume that certain toxic substances may, in some instances, induce headache through a direct action on the blood vessels.

All of these facts are important when the

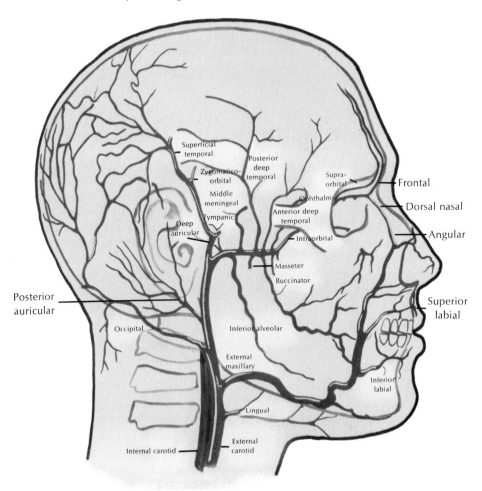

Fig. 1-7. Extracranial vessels involved in headache.

physiologic basis of head pain is being considered. They will, in no small way, often help the physician who is trying to diagnose a difficult headache problem. These factors are often helpful to distinguish between a psychologic and an organic or pathologic headache problem.

Regardless of the age of the patient, headache that interferes with the routine living habits of the patient should be taken seriously by both the patient and the physician, because it indicates that something is wrong. The patient takes the problem seriously or he would not seek the advice of the physician. It is therefore up to the physician

to diagnose the cause and institute proper treatment regardless of the pathophysiology of the case.

CEREBRAL BLOOD FLOW

During the past few years there have been several articles in the medical literature concerning the cerebral blood flow in vascular headaches. One of the first reports concerning the cerebral blood in patients during a migraine attack was made by O'Brien.[5] In this report the patient breathed a mixture of XE-133 and air for a period of 5 minutes on a closed circuit system. (When using the inhalation technique it is difficult, if not impossible, to avoid contamination from the external carotid system. This technique also requires roughly 20 or so minutes for completion and it is therefore difficult to study a migraine patient through the various phases of the attacks due to the rapid changes which take place.) O'Brien found a mean decrease of 20% in cerebral blood flow during the migraine attack, with no asymmetry between hemispheres even if the headache were unilateral.

In still another report O'Brien[6] found a reduction of the blood flow of 23% in the prodromal stage (aura) with no difference in the hemispheres. He also found an 8% increase in flow during the actual headache. He concluded that the reduction in the blood flow may have been underestimated during the prodromal stage. O'Brien[7] noted that the blood flow was marked, bilateral, and not limited to the small area of cortex directly related to the symptoms.

Skinhoj has also done a considerable amount of research in the field of cerebral blood flow using intracarotid XE-133 infusion. Skinhoj and Paulson[8] studied the cerebral blood flow in a migraine patient and found a 67% reduction of flow in the prodromal stage. They concluded that certain parts of the brain become anoxic during the prodromal period. Olesen and Skinhoj[9] found that no change in cerebral blood flow was produced by adrenaline, noradrenaline, angiotensin, or serotonin. They found histamine to cause only a slight increase in cerebral blood flow following intracarotid infusion.

In still another study on cerebral blood flow using the XE-133 intracarotid injection method, Skinhoj[10] found a marked reduction in flow in four patients during the prodromal phase and in six migraine patients during the actual headache phase. At times the flow was low enough to be critical for brain oxygenation. During the actual headache phase there was a hyperfusion (increased flow). These patients also had an intracerebral lactate acidosis, indicating a subclinical cerebral hypoxia.

In reporting at the London Migraine Symposium in 1976 on cerebral blood flow, Hachinski and associates[11] presented evidence that the flow diminished during the prodromal stages and increased above normal during the actual headache phase. They theorized that cerebral blood flow changes may be focal and may occur in areas of the cerebral circulation not measured with the intracarotid XE-133 technique. Mathew and co-workers[12] also found the cerebral blood flow to vary with the clinical phase of the vascular headache. They found the blood flow to decrease during the prodromal phase and they found a cortical hyperfusion during the headache phase. In addition, they found the cerebral blood flow to be normal during the headache phase of muscle contraction and psychogenic headache. They measured the cerebral blood flow with the intraarterial radioisotope technique and a gamma camera.

Saurugg and Schnaberth[13] made measurements of the isotopic cerebral blood flow in migraine patients. They found the cerebral blood flow to be normal in these patients between attacks.

Janzen and associates[14] studied the injection of contrast media into the cerebral blood vessels in normal patients. They found these patients to have an immediate transient constriction of the vessels followed by a dilation. They state that this is due to the irritating effect of the contrast medium employed. They further point out that in migraine there seems to be a delayed reaction, which they believe to be due to a decreased permeability of the blood-brain barrier.

Norris, Hachinski, and Cooper,[15] in studying the changes in the cerebral blood flow during a migraine attack, found a decrease in flow during the prodromal phase, a rise above normal during the actual headache phase, and a persistence of the elevated flow following intramuscular injection of 0.5 mg of ergotamine tartrate.

All of these studies seem to agree that during the prodromal stage of migraine there is a decrease in the cerebral blood flow. How this is produced is still uncertain. However, this decrease may be sufficient to impair the required oxygenation of the brain itself. Skinhoj[10] has found certain biochemical changes similar to those seen in cerebral hypoxia in the cerebral spinal fluid of migraine patients. Welch and co-workers[16] make similar statements.

The increase in cerebral blood flow which seems to be the constant finding in all of these reports may well be a compensatory response to the cerebral hypoxia present during the prodromal stage.

REFERENCES

1. Horton, B. T., and Macy, D., Jr.: Treatment of headache, Med. Clin. North Am. **30:**811, 1946.
2. Best, C. H., and Taylor, N. B.: The physiological basis of medical practice, ed. 2, Baltimore, 1939, The Williams & Wilkins Co.
3. Horton, B. T.: Headache; clinical varieties and therapeutic suggestions, Med. Clin. North Am. **33:**973, 1949.
4. Tunis, M. M., and Wolff, H. G.: Studies on headache, Arch. Neurol. **71:**425, 1954.
5. O'Brien, M. D.: Cerebral cortex perfusion roles in migraine, Lancet **1:**1036, 1967.
6. O'Brien, M. D.: Cerebral blood changes in migraine, Headache **10:**139, 1971.
7. O'Brien, M. D.: The relationship between aura symptoms and cerebral blood flow changes in the prodrome of migraine, Proceedings of the International Headache Symposium, Elsinore, Denmark, May 16-18, 1971, American Association for the Study of Headache and Danish Migraine Society, pp. 141-143.
8. Skinhoj, E., and Paulson, O.: Changes in focal cerebral blood flow within the internal carotid system during migraine attack, Acta Neurol. Scand. **43:**254, 1970.
9. Olesen, J., and Skinhoj, E.: The influence of certain vasoactive amines on the regional cerebral blood flow in man, Proceedings of the International Headache Symposium, Elsinore, Denmark, May 16-18, 1971, American Association for the Study of Headache and Danish Migraine Society, pp. 145-152.
10. Skinhoj, E.: Hemodynamic studies within the brain during migraine, Arch. Neurol. **29:**207, 1973.
11. Hachinski, V. C., Norris, J. W., Cooper, and Edmeads, J. G.: Migraine and the cerebral circulation, International Migraine Symposium, London, Sept., 1976.
12. Mathew, N. T., Hrastnik, F., and Meyer, J. S.: Regional cerebral blood flow in the diagnosis of vascular headache, Headache **15:**252, 1976.
13. Saurugg, D., and Schnaberth, G.: Cerebral blood flow (isotope studies) and acid base balance in the CSF in migraine, Munch. Med. Wochenschr. **117:**1511, 1975.
14. Janzen, R., Tanzer, A., Zschocke, S. T., and Dieckmann, H.: Post-angiographic delayed reactions involving the cerebral blood vessels in migraine sufferers, Z. Neurol. **201:**24, 1972.
15. Norris, J. W., Hachinski, V. C., and Cooper, P. W.: Changes in cerebral blood flow during a migraine attack, Br. Med. J. **3:**676, 1975.
16. Welch, K. M. A., Chabi, E., and Nell, J. H.: Biochemical comparison of migraine and stroke, Headache **16:**160, 1976.

CHAPTER 2

Patient evaluation

DIFFERENTIAL DIAGNOSIS OF HEAD PAIN

The problem of differential diagnosis of headaches is often a very complicated one. The symptoms and the complaints of the patient are often colored by the patient's subjective reactions, and this will, in turn, merely add to the difficulty of classifying each individual headache problem. The classification of the type of headache that is present in an individual is based on the site of the pain, the source of the pain, its character, the frequency and duration of the attacks, and the nature of any associated manifestations.

An important item in obtaining the proper diagnosis for a headache patient is to observe the patient's general behavior when he is giving his headache "story." In other words, when the patient is complaining of head pain, does he act as though he actually has an organic disorder or does he act as though it might be psychogenic in nature? This point is often easy to decide by merely observing the patient's behavior. The patient's expressions while he is describing his symptoms or the expressions he exhibits while he claims to be having an attack are of utmost importance. If a patient with a psychogenic problem claims to be having head pain, quite often he does not express pain at all, nor does he have a painful expression on his face while he is having an attack. He is not inhibited either at work, sleep, or play by the headache attacks. The exact opposite is true with a true organic type of headache problem.

The headache patient should be permitted to describe his symptoms in his own words. The physician should not try to put words in the patient's mouth. The physician should not say, for example, "Your headache is not a sick headache, is it?" This may sway the patient's opinion one way or another and may lead the patient to give the wrong answer. The correct way to ask such a question would be, "Is your headache a sick headache?" This will leave the answer entirely up to the patient.

The physician must determine whether there is any element of nervous tension present. If there is such a problem, it must be treated along with the headache problem, for if both are not attacked the desired results will not be obtained in the treatment program.[1,2]

Chronic, long-existing headache which is present as the only symptom in the patient's history is usually less dangerous than is a headache that occurs with an uneventful onset and that is a relatively new symptom to a patient who has never had a headache problem before.

If there is a history of trauma in the etiology of the headache problem, and if the headache begins more or less immediately after the trauma occurs, it is generally less dangerous a form of headache than the one that has its onset a considerable length of time following the trauma. This is true regardless of the length of time the headache persists. The headache with a short duration is usually less serious than one that persists for several days or longer.

Headache which is accompanied by other symptoms such as drowsiness, personality changes, aphasia, convulsions, vertigo, memory distortions, nystagmus, ataxia, and papilledema may also indicate a serious etiology. Correct diagnosis is essential in such cases. These additional symptoms could indicate an intracranial tumor.

Sudden, severe headache associated with vomiting and stupor along with ptosis of the eyelid, a stiff neck, and fundus hemorrhages may indicate a subarachnoid hemorrhage of a minor nature. These headaches may last up to a week and the patient may recover. Blood in the spinal fluid should make the physician suspicious of a minor subarachnoid hemorrhage. If a second hemorrhage should occur the patient may have major neurologic symptoms or the attack could even be fatal. In these cases recurrences are common and the death rate is quite high.

Frequently recurring headaches may indicate a serious underlying disease or severe psychologic disturbance. These cases should therefore be thoroughly investigated by the physician. Cerebrovascular aneurysms, angioma, or malformations of the cerebral arteries are often the cause of recurring throbbing headaches. These headaches are usually on the same side, have a rather sudden onset, and rapidly become intense.

Psychogenic headaches are often seen in patients who have no organic involvement of the nervous system. These headaches tend to be unremitting and may be of varying duration.

Hypertension should also be considered as a cause of headache, but the blood pressure has to be extremely high both systolically and diastolically to produce headache. A low-grade hypertension in a patient will generally not produce a headache problem. Should it occur, this type of headache is usually in the occipital area of the head and is usually increased or started by any form of straining. It is commonly present in the morning on arising and is of the pulsating type.

Some chronic headache problems may require special tests in order to establish the correct diagnosis. This list of special procedures could include a neurologic examination, sinus x-ray, skull x-rays, cervical spine x-rays, electroencephalogram, brain scan, blood tests, or funduscopic examination.

A general physical examination of the headache patient is helpful in the differential diagnosis, and its results should be carefully examined. The clinical history of the headache patient is one of the most important items—in fact, probably the most important single item—in the differential diagnosis of the headache problem. Both of these topics are discussed later in this chapter.

Many physicians have undoubtedly listened on numerous occasions to patients complain of their headaches. These complaints may be of real head pain, or they may be emotional. Too frequently the physician may take the easy way out and merely give the patient a prescription calling for aspirin or some preparation of that nature. This is done in cases where not enough thought has been devoted to the problem. In such cases, it is not too long before the patient returns to the physician still suffering from the head pain; however, by this time there may perhaps be additional emotional problems. On this second visit, if the condition is still taken too lightly, the physician will merely prescribe another analgesic stronger than the first one, such as aspirin with codeine or an APC preparation. When the patient finds that this is not producing the results he desires, he will become rather upset and in most cases will probably decide to seek the advice of another physician. Other physicians, however, will undoubtedly have no better results if they employ the same methods as the first one and take the problem too lightly.

The headache patient must be observed thoroughly, and in order to do this he will have to be seen on more than one occasion. It may frequently be necessary to observe the patient intermittently for weeks or even longer in order to classify the headache correctly. On all of the patient's visits to the physician, the clinical notes made by the physician should be carefully and immediately recorded. The physician should not rely on memory and dictate notes 24 hours later.

In difficult and severe cases of headache, it may often be necessary to constantly observe the patient during the performance of diagnostic tests or during the execution of the treatment program prescribed.

Cephalalgia may arise from intracranial, pericranial, or extracranial conditions. Many headaches may occur independent of any specific disease, while still others may occur as a constant symptom of a particular disease. This should be remembered in diagnosing such conditions.

The age of the patient must be considered in every headache problem. If the patient is elderly, such things as temporal arteritis, hypertension, cervical arthritis, and occlusive vascular disease must be considered in the diagnosis of the case. Morris[3] points out that in establishing a diagnosis of the chronic headache problem, the history should contain not only an acute or attack profile but also a lifetime health profile.

It is extremely important in diagnosing headache problems to remember that the combination of several forms of headache may occur. Such a condition is referred to as a mixed type of headache. In such a condition both types of headache should be treated independently but simultaneously.

King[4] states that in diagnosing headache problems he believes "that severe headaches are probably the main symptom of a definite clinical entity which necessarily must be treated with specific agents."

Chambers[5] believes that the diagnosis of any headache problem can be facilitated if the patient can be examined while he has a headache. The physician will find an otoscope, ophthalmoscope, nasopharyngoscope, and an educated finger to be of help in solving the average headache problem; a thermometer, reflex hammer, tuning fork, pin, and blood pressure apparatus are also helpful.

The physician who focuses attention chiefly on the results of the patient's physical examination and laboratory tests will all too often miss the diagnosis.

HISTORY TAKING

In order to give the proper treatment to any headache patient, a correct diagnosis must be made. One of the most important single factors in obtaining this correct diagnosis is the taking of a thorough, complete history. No headache problem may be completely classified unless this is done. This case history should be very detailed, and it will usually yield information which will permit the physician to classify the headache and to select the proper treatment. This should be the first step in the management of any headache problem.

The history may often be long and involved. If this is the case it will not be possible to take the complete history at one session. Leading questions should then be employed to help simplify the task. As the patient is discussing his headache problem, the physician should attempt to analyze the patient's personality and general make-up. These factors may be an intrinsic part of the causative agents in some headache patients.

If patients have headaches that are severe enough and recurrent enough to cause them to seek the advice of a physician, they should be thoroughly investigated to rule out organic disease. This is true in spite of the fact that the incidence of organic disease is rather low in patients who have recurring chronic headache problems. Early and correct diagnosis will save these patients from a great deal of pain, which in many cases is quite severe. It will save them from many useless procedures, and occasionally it may even save their lives. This diagnosis depends a great deal on the obtaining of a good thorough history from the patients. Most physicians who deal with headache problems agree that before the proper treatment can be given, the proper diagnosis or classification of the headache must be made.[1-4]

As stated before, headache is one of the most common symptoms seen in the practice of medicine today, but the physician often fails to suspect just what is wrong. As a result, the correct diagnosis is not made. One of the big difficulties is that many headache patients usually fail to tell their story properly. They may not tell of the typical headache attacks but merely some of the side effects or secondary manifestations, such as abdominal distress, vertigo, fatigue, or the many illnesses they have experienced in their lifetime. Often patients may believe that their headaches are beyond help because of some past experience. This will also make the history taking somewhat more difficult. Some patients will tell their headache stories in such a vague fashion that no one could possibly make a diagnosis from their story. This is indeed unfortunate, because quite often the diagnosis of some headaches can be made from a complete history alone. This is especially true in a case where the laboratory tests, x-ray studies, and the general physical examination are all negative. The patient will naturally emphasize the elements of his headache which are most important in his mind. In most cases, however, he probably will need help in recalling episodes of lesser importance.

Description of illness

The patient should be encouraged to describe his illness to the best of his recollection. On many occasions his description of the pain will indicate that he is suffering from more than one type of headache. In such a case, he will have a so-called mixed headache and should be treated accordingly.

In taking a history in a headache case, the physician should let the patient give a full description of the case, in his own words.

Physical signs are very seldom present in a patient who complains of a chronic headache problem. This makes the case history of the case even more important in establishing the correct diagnosis.

The physician should be prepared to listen to the patient's responses to questions before asking any further questions. In doing this, each answer given by the patient can be evaluated independently and thoroughly.

It is of primary importance to understand from the very start just what the patient means by the word "headache." Very often a person will state that he has a headache and then, when he is asked to describe this condition, the physician is surprised to learn that no actual head pain exists at all. Some patients complain of what they call headache, but, when questioned about their meaning of the word, they give quite a variety of conditions, none of which is actually head pain. Among the conditions that have been called headache are loss of memory, a generalized "woozy" or foggy feeling, loss of balance, a tight feeling in the scalp, a burning sensation in the musculature of the neck or shoulders, stiffness of the neck, and many other complaints of this sort. Understanding what the patient means by the word "headache" should be one of the first things to develop in the taking of a proper headache history.

Often a patient's description of his headache attacks is so characteristic that it will provide clues toward the diagnosis of the problem.

Any family history of headache is extremely significant, especially in cases of migraine. It is essential to delve into this aspect rather thoroughly in many cases. Quite often the headache will skip a generation in some families.

First attack

The patient should be asked when the first headache attack occurred and then should recall the events in their proper sequence when giving the physician the history of his headache problem. In most cases, he will need some help from the physician in doing this. He should be told to go back to the very beginning and take each subsequent episode in the proper sequence in which it actually occurred. This will take considerable thought on the part of the patient and, as stated before, more than one session is often required in taking a complete case history of a difficult headache problem.

Onset time

The onset time of the headache should be investigated. This may often provide the clue for the classification of the headache.[3] Onset time is of utmost significance in such types of headache as histaminic cephalalgia, which usually occurs at night during the early sleeping hours.[8] Tension headache also tends to occur at night or during the relaxing phase following the actual tension phase.[9] In many cases of hypertensive headache, the head pain will begin in the early morning hours and often will tend to disappear after the patient has been up and about for a short time. From these facts it is not too difficult to see why the onset time is significant.

Frequency

The frequency of the attacks must be investigated. Do they occur every day, a few times a week, once a month, or irregularly? Some cases of headache, such as histaminic cephalalgia, occur at rather lengthy intervals, whereas some others occur several times a month or more. Migraine, for example, is definitely associated with the menstrual periods, but quite often patients will experience headaches several times between periods. Some headaches show a seasonal element. Some—in fact many—headache patients have their attacks at irregular intervals. This is especially true in the case of the tension type of headache; however, whether the attacks have an irregular pattern or a definite, set routine does not matter. What actually does matter is that the facts be known by the physician.

Intensity

The intensity of the pain should be discussed. Is the pain severe in nature, or is it just a mild type of head pain that can be endured but is very annoying? As example of these two extremes would be histaminic cephalalgia and the head pain that may be the result of constipation. To our knowledge, there is no head pain so severe as that found in histaminic cephalalgia. The pain experienced from the toxic effect of constipation, however, is milder in nature.

The physician must never take the patient's description of the severity of the pain too lightly. It is important to observe the patient's facial expressions when he is describing the severity of the pain. We firmly believe that, regardless of where the pain is located, in the head or in the feet, the average patient cannot smile when describing its severity. He will tend to have a frown on his face, as if to say, "I hope I never get it again." This is a good fact for the physician trying to rule out a psychogenic headache problem to bear in mind.

Character of pain

There are many different types of head pain. In the migraine we find a throbbing type of head pain. In tension headache, the patient will often describe his head pain as a feeling of band-like sensations about the head or pressure within the head or scalp. The histaminic cephalalgia patient, on the other hand, will complain of a burning, excruciating, severe type of pain. The patient with myalgia of the head will present a tender type of pain with soreness in the muscular tissue in the areas involved. From these few examples one can see that different types of headache present different characteristics of pain. Knowing the character of the head pain is thus important in making the correct classification of the headache problem.

Associated manifestations are important in helping to identify the type of headache the patient presents, especially in cases in which the type of pain and other factors have no definite characteristics. Perhaps the patient is sensitive to sudden temperature change. An example of this is myalgia of the head. A patient can have a headache precipitated by air conditioning, drafts, fans, and cold, wintry weather.

Duration

The duration of the attacks is a matter which should be discussed. Is the attack of short duration, lasting merely a matter of minutes (as is the case in the histamine type of headache), or is it much longer, lasting several hours or several days (as in migraine cases)? Is pain constant during the attacks or intermittent? Will the pain attack continue over one stretch of time or will it start and then have periods of remission and periods of pain intermingled?

Type of onset and termination

What type of onset and termination do the attacks have? Do the attacks begin suddenly, reach their maximum intensity immediately, and then terminate in the same abrupt manner? This type of onset and termination is seen in the vascular histamine type of head pain. There are, however, head pains that start gradually, slowly build up in intensity to a peak, then slowly become less severe and gradually terminate. A typical example of this gradual type is the pain characteristically seen in myalgia of the head.

Location

The location of the painful areas should be noted, though this actually does not indicate anything as far as the seriousness of

the problem is concerned. Is the pain bilateral, unilateral, or generalized throughout the entire head? If we suspect that the pain results from sinusitis, what sinuses are involved? A maxillary sinusitis will produce a pain in the areas of the cheeks, either bilateral or unilateral, depending on whether one or both maxillary sinuses are involved. The other nasal sinuses likewise will have their painful areas in certain definite locations in the head. A tension headache may be a generalized type of headache. On the other hand, the histamine type of head pain is always unilateral. It can alternate between sides but it is never on both sides at the same time. However, usually the typical histaminic cephalalgia patient has painful area always on the same side. The pain in myalgia of the head characteristically starts on one side of the head and migrates to the other. In doing this, the pain may vanish from the original site, or it may stay in the original area and spread along the migratory tract involved. Either condition is quite commonly found in this type of head pain. From these various examples, it is easy to see why the location of the head pain is of such importance in taking a headache case history.

Time of attack

When does the headache attack begin? Is its onset time associated with any certain time of the day, week, or month? A headache which is present each morning on awakening or one that awakens the patient at night should be investigated.

Age

The age of the patient should also be taken into consideration. Certain disease entities such as temporal arteritis, hypertension, and depression are seldom found in children but are common in older age groups.

Cause of onset

The cause of the onset of the attacks of head pain should be investigated, since it often is of help in correctly classifying a headache case. Is there any definite thing that the patient associates with the headache's etiology? Is there anything that the patient says definitely will bring on an attack? Some common conditions that headache patients often will consider as the cause of their headache attacks are fatigue, worry, overwork, and mental or emotional upsets. Quite commonly in migraine cases we find the patient associating attacks with her menstrual periods. Migraine attacks may just precede the menstrual periods or may be during the period itself. In many cases of myalgia of the head, patients associate the cause of the onset of the pain with severe or sudden temperature change, drafts, air conditioning, and the like. Of course, in sinusitis the onset of head pain is associated with nasal and upper respiratory infection. The tension headache sufferer and the migraine-tension type can associate the development of the attack with such factors as mental fatigue and overwork.

Nasal pathology or symptoms

Does the patient routinely experience any nasal obstruction or discharge with the attacks? If there is discharge, is it watery or thick? If it is thick, is it mucoid or purulent? These are important questions, especially if we are suspicious of sinusitis as being the cause of the headache. Does the patient experience difficulty in breathing through the nose while he has the headache? In histaminic cephalalgia, one of the cardinal symptoms is nasal congestion and obstruction in the nasal passage on the same side as the head pain. This is present only during the short period of the headache attack. The patient should be asked if the nasal obstruction or discharge is bilateral or unilateral. The question of rhinorrhea is important primarily because 90% of the people with a headache problem think it results from a sinusitis condition. Because the patient has this in mind, it has to be ruled out. This is especially true in cases in which there may be a psychogenic cause. If the patient be-

lieves the condition is due to sinusitis, it is often very difficult to convince him that it is not. If a patient states that he has sinusitis, the physician should not take this for granted. A large percentage of the patients who claim to have sinusitis actually have a head pain from some other condition which has nothing whatsoever to do with sinusitis.

It was this sinusitis element that first aroused our interest in the field of headache. In starting to take a history of a patient, the natural first question to ask the patient is, "What is your trouble?" Many would answer such a question by stating, "I have sinus trouble." When this was the answer, the next question would be, "Why do you say you have sinus trouble?" The answer would invariably be, "Because I have such terrible headaches." In investigating cases of this type, it was interesting to see how many actually had sinusitis headaches and how many actually had conditions having nothing to do with the nasal sinuses. Many of these individuals really had such conditions as migraine, myalgia of the head, or histaminic cephalalgia, and some even had a psychogenic type of head pain.

Ophthalmic conditions

The eyes should be investigated in taking a good case history of a headache problem. Does the patient notice during the headache attack that he has any abnormalities with the eyes? Is there any conjunctivitis during the headache attack? In a typical case of histaminic cephalalgia, the patient will usually notice a conjunctivitis and a lacrimation of the eye on the same side as the head pain.

Is the head pain associated in any way with reading? Does it often come on following the reading of the daily newspaper or watching television? This would lead one to suspect some refractive error, and the eyes should be examined to see whether the patient may need glasses or, if he already wears them, needs a change in the lens prescription. This is quite common in headache and should not be overlooked. The headache produced by this type of refractive error is usually not severe.

The patient should be asked about photophobia, the condition in which the bright reflection from a light or the sun makes the head pain more severe. This is commonly seen in cases of migraine. When a person is having a migraine attack, he usually prefers to be in a dark room. He will generally state that if he looks into a bright object such as a light his head pain is greatly magnified.

Scotoma should also be investigated. The patient should be asked if he has any visual disturbance preceding or during the attack. This may be manifested in such forms as spots before the eyes, contraction of the visual field, blind spots, scotomas, or temporary hemianopia. The scotomatous condition is quite frequently seen in migraine and is rather characteristic. It presents itself as a point of light appearing in the field of vision, generally toward one side. It gradually enlarges and becomes zigzag, glimmering, and even colored. The visual disturbances are usually present for only a few moments in most cases of migraine. If such a condition is present, we can certainly rule out many types of headache. Therefore, it is very important to ask the patient during the taking of the history, "Do you have any visual disturbances during your headache attacks?"

Tenderness

Another point to bring up in taking the proper history of a headache patient is tenderness. Does the painful area of the head feel tender when touched or when pressure is applied? Patients with myalgia of the head will state that if the pain is in a certain location the same area is tender to the slightest touch. In cases of sinusitis, it is quite common to observe that the painful areas are tender to pressure, and if pressure is exerted over the area involved the pain will be much more noticeable and more severe. This is definitely not the case in the majority of other types of headache and is therefore

a point worth mentioning in connection with history taking.

Gastrointestinal conditions

One other factor that should be considered in the case history is the gastrointestinal symptoms. This is especially important in cases of migraine. The patient should always be questioned about nausea and vomiting with the headache attacks. If present, when do they occur? Do they occur at the onset, during the height of the attack, or near the termination of the actual pain? Most migraine headache patients experience nausea with their attacks and some experience vomiting, but the percentage with vomiting is not nearly so large as that with nausea.

In medicine, we are told that there are two expressions which we should not use, "always" and "never." In other words, things should not be stated as being 100%. However, contrary to this rule, we have never seen a true classic case of migraine in which the patient would not reply in the affirmative when asked, "Do you have a sick headache?" Sick headache is indeed a true characteristic of migraine. This is not true in most other types of head pain; therefore, when the nausea and vomiting are present and the patient claims to have a "sick headache," the physician may be helped in diagnosing the case.

Other factors

As mentioned previously, the patient's expressions and behavior should be observed while he is telling his story. Thorough observation at this point is exceptionally helpful in most cases, especially if the cause is functional.

The sleeping habits of the patient should be noted. Does his headache interrupt his normal sleeping pattern? Does the headache tend to have its onset while the patient sleeps? Does the patient have dreams that wake him at night and does he then awaken with a headache? Does the patient have an inability to fall asleep? These questions should be asked for they may indicate certain types of headache patterns. The psychogenic headache patient never has his sleep disturbed by his headaches. The histaminic cephalalgia (cluster headache) patient usually awakens during the night with a severe headache. The depression headache patient usually has difficulty in falling asleep.

Is the headache in any way associated with the patient's occupation, school work, etc.? If some people do not enjoy their work or school, they will tend to have a ''Monday morning headache.'' This, of course, is psychogenic. However, some occupations may cause organic types of headache such as myalgia or muscle tension headache.

Is the headache in any way associated with the weather? Is it seasonal? This is an associated manifestation of some forms of headache such as myalgia.

Are the headaches associated with any hormonal factors such as oral contraceptives or menstruation? Are the patients free from headache while pregnant? These conditions are often seen in migraine patients.

The treatment program that the patient has followed in the past is also helpful in establishing the proper diagnosis. What medications have and have not helped? The physician should make sure when the patient is giving this part of the history that the drugs were taken in the proper dosage and at the proper time.

The history is extremely important in each individual chronic headache problem. It will provide the correct diagnosis in most cases. Once the correct diagnosis has been established, the proper treatment program, both symptomatic and prophylactic, can be instigated.

SUMMARY

1. What the patient means by ''headache''
2. Family history
3. When the headache first occurred
4. Onset time
5. Frequency
6. Intensity
7. Character
8. Duration
9. Cause of onset
10. Location
11. Scotomas
12. Photophobia
13. Vomiting
14. Nausea
15. Sick headache
16. Rhinorrhea
17. Lacrimation
18. Nasal discharge
19. Termination
20. Any tenderness
21. Any nervous tension
22. Any associated manifestations
23. Full description, in patient's own words
24. Observation of patient's expressions
25. Observation of patient's behavior
26. Age of patient
27. Any sleep disturbance
28. Associated with weather—seasonal
29. Past treatment: effective and noneffective

EXAMINATION OF THE HEADACHE PATIENT
Examination of ears, nose, and throat

After the history has been taken, the next logical step toward the correct diagnosis should be the examination of the patient. A complete examination of the ears, nose, and throat should be made. If anything found in this routine examination appears in any way to be significant, it should be rechecked by a competent otolaryngologist. The examination of the nasal passages is important to rule out any pathology of the nose or nasal sinuses. The condition of the nasal septum should be observed. Is it in midline or deviated to one side? Are there any septal deformities, such as spurs? If the septum is deviated or if there are spurs present, do they in any way contact the lateral wall of the nasal passage? Quite often, pressure by the septum against the lateral nasal wall superiorly or posteriorly in the area of the sphenopalatine ganglion will produce head pain. If this is the case, the condition is much more pronounced when the patient has some form of nasal congestion that will cause the turbinate tissue to become engorged and increase this pressure.

Examination of the nasopharynx is also needed. On occasions pressure from nasopharyngeal tumors will produce head pain.

In some cases the chief concern of the patients was a head pain in the area of the ear. On examination, it was found that the patient had a growth in the laryngeal area. In most of these cases the growth proved, on microscopic section, to be carcinoma. Although this is not a common cause of head pain by any means, it certainly shows that it is justifiable to perform a laryngoscopic examination.

There are many cases in which we find chronic suppurative otitis media producing head pain. This type of condition should be handled by a competent otologist, since the majority of such cases that have reached this far-advanced stage usually will not respond to the medical form of treatment and, in the final analysis, require a surgical procedure to correct the pathologic condition present. The pain encountered in most of these cases is in the nature of a pressure type of head pain and may be due to the enlargement of a mass of cholesteatoma. The pain produced by chronic suppurative otitis media may also be an indication of possible intracranial complications resulting from the primary ear condition. These conditions are naturally very serious and should be handled accordingly. It is not fair to the patient to pass off any type of chronically discharging ear too lightly, since it could eventually lead to serious trouble.

After a routine examination of the ears, nose, and throat has been made, if there is a suspicion of sinusitis, sinus x-rays should be ordered to clinch the diagnosis. The same is true in cases where the physician is suspicious of ear pathology; an x-ray of the mastoids is justifiable.

Examination of the eyes

If the physician thinks that the head pain may result from some refractory error, the patient should consult an ophthalmologist for a refractory examination. It is quite common to find cases in which eyestrain produces headaches. Astigmatism is a common cause of head pain, as are hyperopia, myopia, and presbyopia. These conditions need to be ruled out.

General physical examination and laboratory tests

A general physical examination and routine laboratory tests are frequently helpful in diagnosing a case of headache. Frequently head pain is caused by hypertension, anemia, leukemia, or other blood dyscrasias, such as polycythemia or anoxemia. Blood examination will help to rule out such things if they are suspected.

Many infectious diseases can produce headache as one of their symptoms. In such cases, a general physical examination plus routine laboratory studies proves to be helpful. If some condition requiring some special form of laboratory procedure is thought to be the possible cause of a headache problem, the procedure should be undertaken without hesitation. For example, if the physician suspects a cervical arthritis or rupture of cervical disc, an x-ray of the cervical area of the spine is in order as part of the examination of the patient.

Many genitourinary conditions and gynecologic conditions can produce head pain as a symptom. If this is the case, a genitourinary or a gynecologic examination may be useful. Eclampsia produces head pain, as does nephritis. In such conditions the history of the patient would point toward the etiology.

If the head pain is thought to be caused by traumatic head injury, x-rays of the skull will identify such conditions as skull fracture (but not concussions), which are frequently found.

The blood pressure should be checked in all headache patients. Hypertension is quite frequently found to be the cause of some headaches that have had many forms of treatment, but to no avail. The headache problem could have been solved by merely remembering to check the blood pressure.

Neurologic examination

In some headache cases, a neurologic examination may be required, especially when all previous examinations have been negative. All cases thought to be psychogenic should have some form of neurologic examination. However, no headache should be called a psychogenic headache until all forms of pathology have been ruled out.

Before making a meticulous neurologic examination of the systems, a rapid check of the patient may reveal a number of important points. Some abnormal attitudes may be discovered, or abnormal postures or deformities may be noted.

The gait of the patient should be observed by having the patient walk without assistance. In observing the patient's walk, the examiner should look for any spasticity or unsteadiness. If the gait is abnormal in any way, it should be charted in the examination notes. The hysteric gait has no definite characteristics and is rather bizarre and nondescript.

Coordination can be checked by means of the Romberg test. Pointing and past-pointing tests may also help. Coordination of skilled acts should also be tested.

Such things as tremor should be looked for. If tremor is present, its location, rate, amplitude, and rhythm should be observed. Any other abnormal involuntary or spontaneous movements, such as fibrillations, choreic movements, athetosis, spasms, dystonic movements, or convulsive spastic movements, should be noted.

The reflexes—both deep and superficial—should be checked in all neurologic examinations. Under the heading of deep reflexes are included the biceps, triceps, jaw-jerk, pectoral, radial, ulnar, patellar, suprapatellar, Achilles (ankle-jerk), and leg flexion reflexes. Ankle clonus should also be checked. As for the superficial reflexes, those tested should include the palmar, abdominal, epigastric, suprapubic, cremasteric, gluteal, anal, and plantar. Pathologic reflexes to be considered are the Babinski toe sign, the Oppenheim toe maneuver, and the Chaddock, Schaffer, and Rossolimo signs.

Normally, all of the reflexes—both deep and superficial—can be elicted and are equal on both sides. If these reflexes are naturally hypoactive or hyperactive, they should be equally so on both sides. It is when these reflexes are unequal that they become significant of some pathologic disturbance. There is also significance attached to a condition in which there is a discrepancy between the deep and the superficial reflexes. If pathologic reflexes can be demonstrated in addition, then a definite lesion can be inferred, but not the nature of this lesion.

There are also a number associated reflexes that may be elicited, such as tonic neck reflexes, Brudzinski's sign, Hoover's sign, Kernig's sign, and several others. If a definition or description of any of these reflexes is desired, a neurology book should be consulted.

In a general neurologic examination, the condition of the patient's muscular system should be observed. The status of the nervous system should be checked. Is the nerve tender, hyperirritable, or hypoirritable? Examination of the sensory system may also be included. Generally speaking, this is the most tedious and most difficult part of a neurologic examination. Because of this, it is frequently the most unreliable part.

Special examination of the cranial nerves may be included. In headache patients, the most important of these is the optic nerve. The examination of the optic nerve embraces visual acuity, fields of vision, and the fundus examination. Of these, the fundus examination is the most important as far as the subject of headaches is concerned. If there are defects in the various fields, they may precede any ophthalmoscopic changes, or they may also persist in the absence of ophthalmoscopic changes. Scotomas precede optic atrophy in some conditions, such as retrobulbar optic neuritis or early multiple sclerosis.

The fundus examination is important if there is any suspicion that there might be intracranial involvement causing the headache. Every fundus examination should include inspection of the optic nerve disc, the retina, especially the macular region, and the blood vessels. Each eye is examined and the two eyes should be compared. The color of the disc should be noted, as well as its margins. The condition of the blood vessels should be observed.

If there is any supicion of subarachnoid hemorrhage, meningitis, or many other types of disease, a spinal fluid examination is helpful. It necessitates the procedure of a spinal puncture to withdraw the spinal fluid. The pressure of the fluid should be observed when doing the spinal tap. This, of course, is not necessary in all cases of headache, but it does help in making the proper diagnosis in some cases. The use of spinal puncture for diagnostic purposes should be done with care and caution. The patient should be relaxed, the correct size needle should be used, the fluid should be examined for cells, and the protein content should be established.

Radiologic examination

Radiologic examinations of the skull, directing attention to possible erosions, calcifications, or shift of the pineal gland, may be helpful in establishing diagnosis of certain headache problems. Besides all of these measures, there are other procedures available that may be helpful in diagnosing the case and that might be included in the examination.

The electroencephalogram (EEG) may help the physician diagnose cortical tumors. Another test that may be used is echoencephalography. This technique detects supratentorial space-occupying lesions through a lateral shift of the M-echo elicited from the third ventricle.

Pneumoencephalography, another proce-

dure which may be helpful, involves air injections into the ventricles, the subarachnoid space, or cerebellomedullary cistern to detect abnormalities. Ventriculography is another diagnostic aid in chronic headache problems in which intracranial mass lesions are suspected.

Cerebral angiography is a method of radiographically investigating the distribution of the cerebral arterial supply. The radiographs are taken immediately after injection of a solution opaque to x-rays is made into the common carotid artery. The brain scan (brain scintigraphy) has been used for the past 20 years or so. It is very helpful in the diagnosis of neurological disorders and intracranial neoplasms. This type of test is roughly 85% effective in screening patients with suspected intracranial neoplasms.

Computerized axial tomography (CAT scan) of the head is another radiographic procedure used to detect intracranial neoplasms and neurologic disorders such as brain tumors, cerebral atrophy, cerebral infarcts, and hydrocephalus without the use of any contrast agents or radioactive material. Its diagnostic error is relatively low, usually less than 5%. This procedure uses the EMI brain scanner. This machine makes it possible to analyze the depths of the brain without any discomfort or danger to the patient. It permits analysis of the variations in x-ray absorption through multiple sections of brain substance.

The EMI scanner is actually an x-ray unit in the true sense of the word. The machine examines the head in a series of brain slices from the base of the skull to its vertex. The patient's head is placed into a "cap" that projects into a water-containing box, and the patient is told to be absolutely still. Photons are passed through the skull in a narrow beam to sensitive crystal detectors. The transmission of these x-ray photons can be measured and analyzed by a computer that demonstrates the internal structure of the brain. An average study involves 28,000 absorption values, which are analyzed by density. The average test requires only 30 to 45 minutes for completion and is fast, accurate, and safe to use.

Gammaencephalography is another procedure offering high diagnostic accuracy in routine screening of brain lesions. This is not an expensive procedure nor does it require numerous personnel. Isotope encephalography is a method of examination that detects the excessive uptake by a tumor or other brain lesion of a radiographically detectable radioactive substance. A positive finding is highly significant; a negative one does not, however, exclude the possibility of a tumor. This procedure is quite valuable in the detection of multiple metastases.

Sonoencephalography uses ultrasound to provide information about the intracranial contents. It is useful for the detection of displacement of midline structures by such things as space-occupying lesions.

Another new procedure that indirectly might help in diagnosing vascular headache problems is thermography. The body temperature is determined and its variation from the normal physiologic state is measured. This provides the physician with a photographic map of the patient and permits the assessment of blood flow in headache patients. This is especially useful in histaminic cephalalgia (cluster headache), since many of these patients will have a facial thermogram containing multiple spotted areas of dense coolness in the supraorbital region of the headache side. These areas are supplied by the extracranial branches of the internal carotid artery and by the external carotid artery. This is not seen as routinely in cases of migraine regardless of the type (common, classic, or a variant).

SUMMARY

1. General physical
2. Routine laboratory tests
3. Eyes
4. Ears
5. Nose
6. Throat
7. Neurologic
8. Skull x-rays
9. Sinus x-rays
10. Blood pressure

If certain organic lesions are suspected, special diagnostic tests may be indicated.

1. Electroencephalogram (EEG)
2. Ventriculogram
3. Pneumoencephalogram
4. Angiogram
5. Brain scan
6. EMI scan
7. Gammaencephalogram
8. Isotope encephalogram
9. Thermogram

REFERENCES

1. Ryan, R. E.: A new agent for the treatment of migraine and histaminic cephalalgia, J. Missouri Med. Assoc. **48**:963, 1951.
2. Ryan, R. E.: Treatment of headache, J. Missouri Med. Assoc. **48**:106, 1951.
3. Morris, R. W.: The nature and treatment of headache, Pharm. Index, pp. 6-12, Dec. 1974.
4. King, G. S.: Headaches and their treatment, N. Y. State J. Med. **51**:255, 1951.
5. Chambers, W. R.: Experiences in severe intractable headaches, South. Med. J. **47**:741, 1954.
6. Ayash, J. J.: Headache and head pain, Lancet **69**:389, 1949.
7. Friedman, A. P.: Current therapy, Philadelphia, 1950, W. B. Saunders Co., p. 563.
8. Horton, B. T.: Symposium: head and face pain; Medicine, Trans. Am. Acad. Ophthalmol. Otolaryngol. **49**:22, 1944.
9. Ryan, R. E.: Fiorinal for symptomatic treatment of nonvascular headache, Med. Times **80**:291, 1952.

CHAPTER 3

Headache therapy

OBJECTIVES

Diagnosis of the cause of the headache and the correction of its underlying pathologic process are the chief concerns of the physician. However, the physician must undertake to provide the patient with symptomatic treatment even while the case is being evaluated.

The physician must understand the personality of the patient and also should be aware of any physiologic condition that may be associated with the headache problem. This will aid in establishing the correct treatment program. It will also aid in the physician-patient relationship, and in any successful pharmacologic treatment program the physician-patient relationship has to be a good one. Naturally, proper headache treatment depends upon the etiology of the problem.

The history of medicine is replete with the discovery of new products that have continually added to the physician's armamentarium solutions to long-existing therapeutic problems. Too frequently we find in the medical literature reports of a new preparation that is claimed to produce remarkable results in one form of headache problem or another. On further investigation, it is found that the new preparation is not so remarkable as the initial report

indicated and is of very little value. It is rather common to find an article describing excellent results obtained with a drug in treating headaches, either symptomatically or prophylactically, and then never see another report of any type on the subject. Most of these preparations have been found to be either of a questionable value, or, at best, they will appear to help only an occasional patient. However, this is not always the case. During the past several years many new headache preparations have been researched and many of these are now on the open drug marked and are helpful in a large percentage of cases. Examples include Cafergot,[1] Fiorinal,[2] and the suppository preparation known as Cafergot-PB.[3]

Because of the complexity of most headache problems, the typical headache patient and the physician will receive in an optimistic fashion every new drug or new type of gadget introduced on the market as a sure cure for headaches. In an extremely large percentage of cases of these "sure cures" there are nothing but disappointing end results. There are usually no "short cuts" in the treatment of a real headache problem, and most preparations on the open drug market are useless if used without the advice of a competent physician.

26

Because of the many recent advances in the understanding of the etiology of various forms of chronic headache, the physician has many more agents to employ effectively in their treatment. Because of this the patient is now able to treat his headache problem and abort most of the acute attacks, and he is also able to reduce both the frequency of the attacks and the severity of the pain, or even avoid the attacks completely. This may be considered to be controlling the headache problem and relieving the patient's fear of future attacks.

The objectives of all types of headache treatment should be twofold:
1. Alleviate the pain of the headache attack. This may be called the symptomatic type of headache treatment.
2. Prevent any subsequent headache attacks from taking place. This is the prophylactic type of headache treatment.

Johnson[4] states that headaches of intracranial origin can be caused by anoxia, emotion, fever, sepsis, nitrites, lumbar puncture, alcohol hangover, constipation, subarachnoid hemorrhage, brain tumor, and irritation of the fifth, ninth, tenth, or upper three cervical nerves. He concludes his article: "It is probable, for some time to come, the symptomatic treatment of headache will depend upon aspirin, sedation and sympathy—augmented, when necessary, with codeine." Not only do we disagree with this statement, but we fear it would be extremely dangerous to combat any chronic headache problem in this manner.

It is the physician's responsibility to recognize the stimulus producing the physiologic reaction that is responsible for the patient's head pain. In turn, the patient should be advised to avoid the stimulus, if at all possible. If the cause is organic, it should be eliminated. If it is a physical factor or a situation causing nervous tension, the patient should be instructed to avoid it. If this stimulus cannot be completely avoided (if it fits into the patient's general living conditions at home or into his working conditions), the patient must be instructed how to minimize its effects. In some cases, this is done by helping the patient obtain a better understanding of his abilities and limitations.

The objectives of all headache treatment should include the alteration of all pain mechanisms. This may require drug therapy, psychologic reassurance, or in some cases surgical procedures (for example, sinusitis type of headache).

In the symptomatic type of headache treatment, the pain should be dulled or aborted by the administration of drugs. The type of medication used depends on the type of headache. Headache varies so widely in severity that a corresponding wide variety of drugs are used for a proper treatment program. The treatment program does not actually begin when the physician institutes pharmacotherapy, psychotherapy, or whatever is needed in each particular case. It actually begins when the patient initially consults the physician, for diagnosis has to be made before treatment can be started. A history of the case must be accurately taken to establish the diagnosis, so the history taking is actually the first step in the treatment program.

The physician should fully discuss the case with the patient, explaining all of the ramifications of the problem. The explanation of the problem is usually appreciated, for most of these patients are desperate for help. Following this explanation to the patient, the actual therapy program should be started.

Analgesics and sedatives of a mild nature may be useful in the initial stages of drug therapy, but, on the whole, they have decided limitations. Vasodilating or vasoconstricting drugs may alter the mechanism or abort the pain and thus be helpful in the symptomatic form of treatment of certain vascular types of head pain.

Habit-forming drugs such as morphine and codeine have *absolutely no place* in the treatment of chronic headache problems. If they are used, the best result one can expect will be the creation of a new problem, one that will be far more difficult to handle than the initial headache problem.

If some form of systemic condition is present in the case, these conditions must be treated concurrently. Examples of this are hypertension, thyroid abnormalities, and hypoglycemia.

Headache may be the result of multiple factors and processes. If this is the case, all factors or processes should be treated independently and simultaneously. The treatment program, therefore, depends on the etiology of the case.

Many forms of headache are extremely difficult to treat. An example is the post-traumatic headache resulting from an accident in which a legal suit is involved. Generally, the only successful form of treatment in a case such as this is the settling of the lawsuit.

No treatment program will be successful unless the correct diagnosis has been made. No case of histaminic cephalalgia (cluster headache) can be treated with drugs and procedures that are ordinarily used for acute nasal sinusitis (such as antibiotics and analgesics). On the other hand, no case of acute nasal sinusitis will respond to the treatment program used for histaminic cephalalgia (such as vasodilatory drugs and ergotamine). This shows the importance of the correct diagnosis in the treatment program.

Therefore, in summation, it may be said that all headache problems should be treated both symptomatically and prophylactically, and the treatment should be directed toward the permanent relief of the headache in each case. If this is accomplished, both the patient and the physician will be very grateful.

DRUGS
Analgesics

Analgesics are small, heterogeneous group of compounds chiefly employed for the symptomatic relief of pain. Most of these drugs also have an antipyretic effect.

The analgesic group of drugs acts by raising the pain threshold through depression of the pain centers located within the thalamus. The chief use of analgesics is in the control of pain associated with certain forms of neuralgias, myalgias, and cephalalgias. The analgesics are not of sufficient strength to be of value when the pain is too severe. Actually this group of drugs is far less effective for relieving pain than are such drugs as morphine, meperidine, or codeine; their chief advantage is that they are not narcotic.

An advantage of the analgesics is that they do not dull any of the special senses or the consciousness of the patient, nor do they reduce the patient's motor activity.

Increasing the dosage of one of the analgesic drugs will increase its duration of action. However increasing the dosage will not produce any greater relief of the pain, because the analgesics have a maximum effect, or limit, beyond which there is little or no additional increase in the pain threshold. If various analgesics are combined, their effect in relieving pain is not any greater, since the ultimate threshold is no greater than that of the strongest component in the combination used. However, if submaximal doses of several analgesics are combined, a maximum effect in relieving pain may be produced with a minimizing of the side effects of each analgesic.

The analgesic drugs do not potentiate the hypnotic action of the barbiturates, nor do the barbiturates potentiate the action of the analgesics.

The most useful of the analgesic group of drugs in the field of symptomatic relief of headache are the antipyretic coal tar derivatives. In this group are such drugs as acetylsalicylic acid and acetophenetidin.

SALICYLATES

The most frequently used analgesics in relieving the symptoms of headache are the salicylates. However, the salicylates are valuable only in cases in which the headache attacks are of a moderate severity. The salicylates are also useful in alleviating the pain of certain forms of neuralgia and myalgic conditions.

Acetylsalicylic acid was one of the earliest drugs to be synthesized. Despite this, many facts about this drug are still unknown to medical science. The actual mechanism of the analgesic action of acetylsalicylic acid is still essentially unknown, even though extensive research has been carried on for many years.

There are some minor side reactions that occur when acetylsalicylic acid is used over prolonged period. However, the salicylates seem to be the least noxious of all the popular drugs of this type. The toxic symptoms of salicylism consists of headache, vertigo, tinnitus, subnormal hearing, dimness of vision, mental confusion, sweating, thirst, nausea, vomiting, diarrhea, and an increase in the pulse rate and respiratory rate. When used in large doses the salicylates will reduce the blood prothrombin. They also increase the urinary excretion of uric acid. Recovery from these symptoms is usually very rapid if the administration of the salicylates is stopped.

The upper intestinal tract absorbs salicylates much faster than does the lower intestinal tract, but regardless of the route of administration (oral or rectal), the salicylates are absorbed more rapidly than most other drugs. Blood levels appear to be proportionate to the dosage of the drug. There is no selective distribution in the body; salicylate is found in all of the tissues and the fluids of the body, but the level is just as high in the blood as it is any place in the body.

The salicylates are excreted mainly through the urine, with a small amount excreted by sweat and saliva. This excretion usually begins within a few hours after administration of the drug, and is usually complete within 24 hours.

Idiosyncrasy to salicylates usually will present itself in the form of a skin rash or anaphylactic-like reactions. The rash may be erythematous, pruritic, eczematoid, des-

quamative, or urticarial. Most patients who develop a rash from prolonged use of salicylates are usually found to have a history of some form of allergy.

Much research has been done concerning the addition of so-called buffering agents to acetysalicylic acid. The buffered forms of aspirin are claimed to bring about quicker relief from headache attacks than the non-buffered forms. However, no statistical difference has been found in the time required to give relief, the duration of the relief obtained, or the degree of the relief; nor is it possible to tell any difference in gastrointestinal tolerance.[5,6] Other investigators have found that the plasma levels attained by both forms are the same. It is therefore likely that antacids serve no useful purpose as additives to plain acetylsalicylic acid. Examples of these buffered analgesics are Bufferin and Ascriptin.

There has been much discussion within the past several years concerning kidney damage from the abusive use of analgesic drugs. In a study of 138 cases, Segaert and associates[7] found that the preparations containing acetophenetidin were the only ones that caused any kidney damage, and this was in the form of interstitial nephritis. In another study Prescott[8] found that acetophenetidin was associated with an increased urinary excretion of tubular cells and red blood cells, but not leukocytes. This probably indicates necrosis of cells and a toxic effect on the epithelium.

Clausen and Harvald[9] believe that the concept that long-term abuse of analgesics may cause a chronic interstitial nephritis with renal failure is now generally accepted. Usually these patients have taken mixed analgesics containing acetophenetidin, acetylsalicylic acid, and acetanilid. Of these acetophenetidin has been thought to be the nephrotoxic agent. Most patients who are acetophenetidin abusers are chronic headache patients. While the incidence of side effects from this drug is rather low, they may be very serious and may lead to severe complications for the patient.

Aspirin itself can produce gastritis and even gastrointestinal bleeding. It may also produce clotting abnormalities by decreasing blood platelets, which leads to hypoprothrombinemia.

In studying renal irritation produced by aspirin Scott, Denman, and Dorling[10] found that aspirin administered in therapeutic doses causes a transient increase in urine cell count, which can be misconstrued as renal disease. These cells are derived from the renal tubules and possibly from a considerable length of the nephron. Sustained salicylate therapy apparently does not cause chronic renal damage.

The actual analgesic effects of acetylsalicylic acid are not fully understood. However, it probably acts centrally, perhaps subcortically, in an unknown manner. It may also have actions on the peripheral nervous system and appears to dampen chemoreceptors for pain, at least from the viscera.

ACETOPHENETIDIN

Acetophenetidin (phenacetin) is another effective analgesic, but it produces more side effects than the salicylates and therefore its usage is not as widespread. Its mode of action is the same as that of the salicylates. It is rapidly absorbed from the intestinal tract and is conjugated in the body with glucuronic acid and sulfuric acid, in which form it is rapidly excreted in the urine. When combined with other analgesic drugs, the action is somewhat smoother and more efficient. The dosage of each drug is reduced and therefore the combination is far less toxic.

OTHER ANALGESICS

Other analgesics with antipyretic actions are antipyrine, aminopyrine, colchicine, cinchophen, and veocinchophen. These drugs, however, are not used as frequently as acetylsalicylic acid or acetophenetidin.

Besides plain acetylsalicylic acid, other popular analgesic preparations on the drug market are Empirin Compound, Anacin, Bufferin, Fiorinal, propoxyphene (Darvon), pentazocine (Talwin), ibuprophen (Motrin), Minotal, and Phrenilin.

Empirin Compound is a combination of acetylsalicylic acid, caffeine, and acetophenetidin. Anacin is a similar combination, whereas Bufferin contains aspirin in a buffered form.

Fiorinal is composed of caffeine, acetylsalicylic acid, and acetophenetidin, like Empirin, with the addition of allylbarbituric acid (Sandoptal).

Phrenilin is composed of acetaminophen, sodium butabarbital, and caffeine. It seems to be helpful in alleviating the pain of tension headache and it also helps to reduce tension-anxiety states.

Minotal contains acetaminophen and sodium butabarbital. It is helpful in the relief of tension headache in selected patients.

Phenaphen is another combination analgesic. It consists of phenobarbital, acetophenetidin, and aspirin.

Synolgas is composed of promethazine, aspirin, acetophenetidin, and caffeine. It is helpful in selected cases of tension headache.

Motrin is used chiefly for rheumatoid arthritis but it has been used experimentally in cases of tension headache and has been found to be as effective as aspirin but not any more effective. This study was on a double-blind basis with a crossover with Motrin, aspirin, and placebo. Both aspirin and Motrin proved to be more effective than placebo, but Motrin and aspirin seemed to be about equally effective.

Some believe that propoxyphene (Darvon) does not possess any more analgesic relief than does placebo. We agree, as far as vascular headaches are concerned. This drug does not produce any better results in these cases than does simple aspirin, and it is a great deal more expensive than aspirin. Propoxyphene has very little addictive potential when it is taken orally, but it can occur in some cases. This drug is practically completely demethylated in the body and becomes ineffective within 24 hours. Overdosage can cause central nervous system depression.

We do not recommend the use of pentazocine (Talwin) in vascular headaches or any of the headaches generally encountered.

The selection of one of these preparations is a matter of individual choice; one will work better on one patient, while another will prove to be superior with another. The patient should inform the physician which product seems to produce the best results—that is, which is the quickest to relieve the headache while producing the least amount of side effects.

Ergotamine tartrate*

Ergot is a fungus that attacks grains and other grasses in almost every part of the world. It is obtained commercially from infected rye. Its use in the treatment of headaches was recommended as early as 1898. In 1921, the alkaloid ergotamine tartrate was developed, and it is now one of the most widely used drugs in the field of vascular headache. In fact, it would be safe to say that frequently this drug is overused.

Ergotamine tartrate was actually the first preparation on the drug market that seemed to give patients relief from the headache of their migraine attack.

Mode of action. This drug is a very potent vasoconstrictor that tends to restore the cerebrovascular system to its normal tone. The effect of ergotamine tartrate depends on its ability to prolong vasoconstrictor action, apparently acting directly on the smooth muscles of the blood vessels, and not as an antagonist to the sympathetics.

In a study of ergotamine tartrate, Berde[11] found that one of the ways in which ergot influences vascular tone may be by increasing output of noradrenaline while reducing its reuptake. This fact may be important in the treatment of migraine.

Hilton and Zilkhak,[12] when studying the

effects of ergotamine tartrate on the blood platelets aggregation responses of migraine patients, found that it appears that the reduced platelet aggregation rates resulted from ergotamine occupying serotonin receptor sites on the platelet membrane. The serotonin uptake sites on platelets and drug interaction with them may resemble uptake sites and drug interaction on other body surfaces, such as vessel walls or neuronal membranes.

The aggregation responses of the blood platelets in migraine patients was also studied by Hilton and Cummings[13]; in this study findings similar to those of Hilton and Zilkhak were reported. Hilton and Cummings stated that the aggregation responses were significantly inhibited by ergotamine, especially in patients taking large doses. There may possibly be a similar response at neuronal and vascular sites, and this may contribute to the relief of migraine.

In a study on the mode of action of ergotamine in canine and human arteries, Muller-Schweinitzer[14] found that in arterial vascular smooth muscle ergotamine behaves as a noncompetitive antagonist, with considerable stimulating activity when tested against serotonin. Moreover it could be demonstrated that ergotamine, in contrast to its alpha-adrenergic blocking activity in peripheral vascular smooth muscle, did not change responses to noradrenaline in basilar arteries. Both the vasoconstrictor activity and the lack of noradrenaline antagonism in basilar arteries might contribute to the therapeutic efficacy of ergotamine in migrainous attacks.

Saxena and Vlaam-Schluter[15] studied the role of some biogenic substances in migraine and the relevant mechanism in antimigraine action of ergotamine in animals. They found that ergotamine caused an enormous decrease in carotid blood flow with no, or only slight, elevation of arterial blood pressure, suggesting that the vasoconstrictor effect in carotid vascular bed may be selective. The drug also reversed the vasoconstriction induced by serotonin

---

*Other aspects of ergotamine tartrate are discussed under treatment in migraine Chapter 4.

into a vasodilator response. No specific effect of the drug was demonstrated on the responses to noradrenaline, histamine, or bradykinin. Reflex pressor response to reduction of pressure in the carotid sinus was antagonized by ergotamine, demonstrating its vasomotor depressor effect. Such effect was produced in doses higher than those needed to cause carotid vasoconstriction.

Regional hemodynamic investigation confirmed a relatively selective vasoconstrictor action of ergotamine on the carotid vascular bed. The vasoconstrictor effect decreased in the following order: common carotid bed, internal carotid bed, femoral bed, superior mesenteric bed, renal bed, vertebral bed, coronary bed.

Based on the pharmacologic interactions between the effects of ergotamine and several biogenic vasoactive substances, it was concluded that selective carotid vasoconstriction appears to be a most important mechanism underlying the excellent therapeutic value of ergotamine in migraine headaches.

Route of administration and dosage. The first preparation to offer any real help for the migraine patient was ergotamine tartrate, known as Gynergen. It acts best when administered at the first symptom of an attack. Most physicians believe that it requires 30 to 45 minutes for the effects of ergotamine to become manifested. The best average dosage seems to be 0.5 mg subcutaneously or intravenously. The average oral dose is 5 mg. The oral form is less effective than the injectable form, and it cannot be used in cases of severe nausea. Even if the patient keeps the preparation down, absorption through the stomach is much slower than normal during or following severe nausea.

Side effects. The main side effects of ergotamine tartrate are nausea or vomiting. These occur in the majority of the cases after the injectable form has been used and are less common after the oral form has been used. Occasionally there is paresthesia; cramps in the arms and legs

can occur. Physicians know that any preparation of ergot can produce gangrene, but this is extremely rare.

Ergotamine tartrate is not habit-forming, but some patients will develop a tolerance to large doses of the ergot alkaloids. It is contraindicated in septic states, coronary diseases, any obliterative vascular diseases, or cardiac conditions.

Friedman[16] reported that the addition of caffeine seems to have improved the efficacy of ergotamine. The dosage of ergotamine can be reduced, there are fewer side effects, and the rapidity of action is increased. The effectiveness of caffeine is probably based on its cerebrovasoconstrictor action and psychic stimulation. Possibly it aids in increasing the rapidity of the absorption of ergot. In addition toxicity studies have shown that caffeine reduces the possibility of side effects of the ergotamine tartrate.[17]

Ergotamine tartrate should not be used when peripheral vascular disease is present or in patients who have known hypertension or coronary heart disease. Patients with impaired hepatic function should not receive ergotamine tartrate because this drug is detoxified in the liver. Other contraindications are impaired renal function, pregnancy, and sepsis. Patients with any hypersensitivity to the drug should not receive it. Ergotamine tartrate cannot be used without careful observation of the patient. In fact, every patient on ergot therapy for headaches should be carefully watched for toxic manifestations, and the pulses of the hands and feet should be periodically checked. At the first indication of toxicity, the drug should be stopped, and measures to produce vasodilation should be initiated.

There are reports of so-called ergotism in the medical literature. Most of these indicate that the drug was not correctly used or was used in cases where it was contraindicated.

In reviewing the literature, Chaqual and Cartier[18] found that epidemics of poisoning with grain infected with *Claviceps purpurea* have been widespread. In the eleventh century one such epidemic ravaged the Dauphine, a province of France. During the Crusades the dauphinois brought home from Egypt the body of a hermit found in the desert near Thebes and reburied it in the church of Motte-aux-Bois. The story was that Jesus had appeared to this hermit and had promised him fame. This so-called St. Antoine-le-Viennois was celebrated for his help in the cure of ergotism, then called "mal des ardents" or "disease of fire." The saint is depicted with a small cross of unusual pattern, a bell, a pig, the symbol of a hermit, and several small flames representing the holy fire of the disease. Monasteries were established for the treatment of ergotism, which was looked on as a divine punishment. It was not until the eighteenth century that German and French researchers discovered its cause.

Bollinger and Preter[19] present five cases in which the patients developed intermittent claudication, paresthesia, and weakness in one or more extremities after brief or prolonged use of an ergot alkaloid. These patients were found to have spastic stenosis of the arteries in the affected extremities, which was caused by the use of a nonhydrated ergot alkaloid. One patient had been taking an oral preparation, while in the others rectal administration of ergotamine tartrate had triggered the disorder. Three patients gave a history of using ergot alkaloids for many years, while in the other two the vascular symptoms developed between 3 and 15 days after ergot therapy was started. Arteriography revealed segmental areas of stenosis in the brachial, superficial femoral, or popliteal arteries. Treatment consisted of discontinuing the ergot alkaloid and administering diazepam by a slow drip, as well as xanthinol niacinate and eupaverin. Four patients recovered completely. The fifth patient showed no regression of the ischemic manifestations during a follow-up period of 7 months. In conclusion they state that

ergotamine preparations have an alpha-adrenolytic effect but, on the other hand, constrict the smooth musculature of the blood vessels. Some patients develop reversible disorders of blood flow, even after relatively small doses of ergotamine, so an individual hypersensitivity may be the cause. Severe side effects of ergotamine medication are rare; their incidence is estimated to be 0.01% of all patients.

McLoughlin and Sanders[20] state that the beneficial action of ergot in migraine is traditionally thought to result from specific vasoconstrictor effect on the extracerebral blood vessels, which are dilated and pulsate during a migrainous attack. The main toxic side effects are caused by its alpha-adrenergic blocking activity, causing peripheral vasoconstriction. The incidence of ergotamine toxicity, reported as 0.01%, may be one of three types; acute toxicity from the brief administration of small doses, resembling an allergic condition; acute poisoning from the brief administration of very high doses; and chronic poisoning from the prolonged administration of therapeutic doses. They say that this iatrogenic condition is completely preventable if ergotamine is used judiciously in the treatment of migraine and not prescribed continuously over long periods.

Brinc and Hjeltnes,[21] in a study of ergotamine as a cause of arterial insufficiency, observe that severe side effects from the ergot alkaloids occur with a frequency of 0.01%, as the result of their vasoconstrictor effect. The most common of these side effects is arterial insufficiency, which may cause gangrene of the upper or, more often, lower extremities. The less severe side effects of ergotamine tartrate are often overlooked; these include nausea, diarrhea, thirst, pruritus, vertigo, muscular cramps on exertion or even at rest, paresthesia, cold skin, and reduced pulsation. These symptoms should always be carefully looked for in patients known to be taking this drug. Brinc and Hjeltnes point out that headaches can occur in the form of a rebound reaction, with recurrent attacks on the day following medication with ergotamine tartrate.

The treatment of ergotism consists primarily in withdrawal of the drug. The administration of vasodilators such as papaverine, nicotinic acid, nitrites, and sympathetic blocking have been used with variable success.

The prescribing of ergotamine tartrate requires specific indications and a review of the contraindications and possible side effects. Regular follow-up is necessary. Ergotamine tartrate medication should be reported whenever patients undergo roentgenologic investigation, to avoid the erroneous diagnosis of arteriosclerotic arterial insufficiency.

Imrie[22] describes two cases of arterial spasm associated with oral ergotamine therapy. In both cases, the major organic pathology was at first suspected, but withdrawal of ergotamine resulted in both clinical and arteriographic improvement.

Reus[23] presents a case of ergotism resulting from the use of rectal suppositories containing 2 mg of ergotamine tartrate for 1 year. The patient was a migraine victim who complained of severe intermittent claudication. Translumbar aortography showed a normal aorta and normal common iliac arteries. The arteries of the pelvis and in the periphery of the legs however, were strikingly narrow. A typical sign was the hair-thin appearance of the vessels in the adductor canal. Ergotamine was stopped, and the patient was treated with isoxsuprin by intravenous infusion and with anticoagulants. After 1 week the patient was back to normal.

Carliner and associates[24] report a case of peripheral vascular ischemia of all four extremities successfully treated with an intravenous infusion of sodium nitroprusside, a vasodilator. The patient had been using rectal suppositories containing 2 mg of ergotamine tartrate. The patient completely recovered following the infusion. Sodium nitroprusside has a rapid effect and cessation of action, allowing precise titration of dose, and it can be administered for prolonged periods. The authors suggest that ergotamine-induced vasospasm should be treated initially with intravenous administration of fluids, anticoagulants (preferably heparin), and a vasodilator such as sodium nitroprusside. Only if these are unsuccessful should other, less firmly based approaches be utilized, such as sympathetic blockage, sympathectomy, and periarterial stripping.

A case of ergotism with arteriographic demonstration of bilateral axillary artery involvement has been reported. The physician should be alert to the possibility of ergotism in cases of peripheral arterial insufficiency.[25]

In discussing the overuse of ergotamine tartrate in fifty-two cases, Horton and Peters[26] say that they did not encounter toxic reactions from ergotamine tartrate in a single case of classic migraine. This is because classic migraine does not and cannot occur daily. It is the daily headache that eventually leads to the excessive use of this drug. Migraine-tension headaches, however, may occur daily. It is the tension phase of the migraine syndrome that brings on the daily headache. They further state that the daily use of the drug makes the patient more and more dependent on it for relief of pain. As the vasoconstricting effect of the drug on the carotid arterial tree begins to wear off, a rebound phenomenon occurs—a withdrawal headache begins, and more ergotamine tartrate is taken to combat the withdrawal headache. A vicious cycle develops, and it takes more and more ergotamine tartrate to produce the desired effect. Thus vasospastic phenomena may develop, usually in the extremities, and may be accompanied by peripheral neuropathy.

When frequent doses of ergotamine tartrate have been used over a long period, withdrawal headache is common. This headache is thought to result from rebound vascular dilation, not unlike the headache experienced with caffeine withdrawal or during the administration of indomethacin.

In this regard, Andersson[27] made a study of forty-four patients, of whom thirty-three had a history of migraine, who were given ergotamine preparations. Within 6 months, these patients were taking the drug daily and concomitantly developed chronic daily headaches. The majority also had signs of mild chronic ergotism characterized by nausea, vomiting, and mild peripheral circulatory insufficiency. When ergotamine was stopped, withdrawal symptoms developed with exacerbation of daily headaches. The majority of these patients were able to discontinue the daily use of ergotamine and the pattern of headache changed, diminishing or disappearing entirely. Andersson concluded that ergotamine should be used intermittently and for a few days each month only. If more frequent medication is indicated, other drugs should be employed for which tolerance or dependence does not develop.

Roswell, Neylan, and Wilkinson[28] also report on ergotamine-induced headache. They say that although 80% of patients with migraine are said to respond to ergotamine initially, tolerance to ergotamine accompanied by an increased incidence of headache is reported with growing frequency. They emphasize that regular administration of ergotamine is associated with tolerance, an increased frequency of headaches, and withdrawal headaches.

Friedman and von Storch[29] have found that there is some danger in using ergot preparations in the treatment of migraine. In some patients the use of ergotamine relieves the headache attack for which it is administered, but at the same time it leads to an increased frequency of these headaches. They believe that this is caused by the development of tolerance by these patients to the ergotamine tartrate.

Wolfson and Graham[30] have reported in detail a case in which a patient developed a tolerance to large doses of ergot alkaloids. This is something that has been noticed with other drugs, so it is entirely possible that this could happen with ergot. We see it frequently with antibiotics and antihistamines,

so it seems to be a factor for considerable interest and investigation with the ergot preparations.

Spasm of the musculature of the blood vessel walls is the chief symptom of ergotism. Ergot is therefore contraindicated in patients with Raynaud's disease, thromboarteritis obliterans, arteriosclerosis, coronary insufficiency, and liver or spleen damage. The best treatment of this condition is prophylactic by careful control of the amount of ergot taken by the patient. However, if it has already occurred, symptomatic treatment may require alpha-sympathetic blockers or anticoagulants or fibrinolytic agents. Of course, ergot withdrawal is an absolute necessity.

Heparin

Treatment of migraine with heparin is based on the assumption that heparin increases the number of basophils and the amount of uroheparin (heparin excreted in the urine). It also lowers the level of low-density lipoproteins. This in turn reduces the severity and frequency of the attacks.

Studies of basophils and heparin have been made by Thonnard-Neumann[31-33] (see pp. 86-89). Briefly, they showed that during an attack of migraine there were more basophilic leukocytes found in the blood from the earlobe on the affected side than there were from the earlobe on the nonaffected side (headache-free side). This suggests that basophils take part in the spontaneous termination of an attack of migraine by the release of their heparin content, thus causing deficiency of heparin.

In another study Neumann[34] administered heparin to migraine patients either by intravenous injection or by aerosol inhalations. He found that after repeated administrations of heparin, that the basophilic leukocytes and also the uroheparin levels were at a normal level. This level remained normal when the therapy was discontinued for a period up to 14 months.

Neumann believes that the aerosol administration of heparin was more effective than was the intravenous route. The aerosol treatment reduced the migraine headache index 86%, whereas the intravenous form showed about 75% improvement. It is believed that better results were obtained with the aerosol route of administration than with the intravenous route because injected heparin is rapidly bound to proteins and lipoproteins; 25% is taken up by the liver, only 2% goes to the lungs. Aerosol heparin, on the other hand, is in a free state when it reaches the alveoli. There it encounters a vast bed of capillaries through which it reaches the arterial circulation. The lungs receive the entire cardiac output, and with it a number of bioactive substances from the gastrointestinal tract via the liver. Lung heparin is, therefore, in a strategic position to interact with vasoactive compounds. The lungs also contain an abundance of cells that can accommodate heparin—epithelial and endothelial cells, macrophages, mast cells, and basophil-like cells. The strongly ionic groups of the heparin molecule will allow it to accumulate in these cells at higher concentrations than in the extracellular space and to serve as a large storage deposit from which heparin can be released into the arterial circulation, where it can interact with vasoactive mediators. The aerosol heparin was given at weekly intervals in individual doses varying from 2500 to 5000 units of heparin. The average intravenous dosage was 5000 units. No side effects were observed with the use of either intravenous or aerosol heparin.

Neumann contends that heparin prevents migraine attacks by its ability to interact with various vasoactive mediators either by binding them directly, by competing with them for tissue-binding sites, or by stimulating or inhibiting enzyme activity.

Histamine

Histamine is formed by the decarboxylation of the essential amino acid, histidine. It is present in varying concentrations in almost every part of the body. It was initially prepared as a pure synthetic product in 1907. Histamine apparently plays an important part in anaphylactic and allergic reactions. However, its specific role has not definitely been proved.

When administered parenterally, histamine is rapidly absorbed. It seems to be totally ineffective when it is given orally.

Histamine apparently has some action on almost all tissues, but its principal effects seem to be contraction of smooth muscle, and dilation and increased permeability of the capillaries, and increased secretion of various glands. The reaction of histamine is of short duration, indicating that it is rapidly destroyed or inactivated. This may possibly be caused by deamination with subsequent oxidation.

It is believed that localized vasodilation, altered capillary permeability, and resulting edema provoked by the local release of histamine or histamine-like substances are the common denominator of allergic diseases and of some diseases not now fully recognized as being allergic in nature.

When histamine is administered intravenously, cutaneous vasodilation is observed. This begins with the face and the neck, and gradually spreads over the upper extremities and thorax. This vasodilation varies with the rate of administration, but usually it is more marked in redheads and in blondes than it is in brunettes. There is also a slight lowering of the blood pressure, but this is usually insignificant and not noticed by the average patient. There is, however, usually a definite increase in the skin surface temperature; this is most pronounced in the head and neck regions. The heart rate also increases slightly when histamine is administered intravenously, and there is some dilation of the coronary arteries. It has no effects on electrocardiograms, however. These changes disappear and the values return to normal levels shortly after completion of the infusion.

Histamine causes a greater increase in the blood flow to the central nervous system than any other drug known. It will cause an almost immediate dilation of vessels of the cerebral cortex when it is administered intravenously. Histamine is a normal direct stimulus for the secretion of gastric juice, and other nervous and humoral stimuli may activate this histamine mechanism.

Histamine will cause an increase in the oxygen consumption that is roughly proportional to the rate at which the drug is administered. This can be demonstrated by comparing samples of venous blood obtained before and after intravenous histamine administration. The oxygen content of the venous blood also increases when histamine is administered intravenously.

Free histamine is continuously produced in the tissues at variable rates, which might be an indication that it functions physiologically as a regulator of the microcirculation.

Histamine is one of the substances within the body that is released from the tissues during injury or inflammatory reactions. In the blood, histamine resides in the basophil cells. Some histamine is actually stored in the mast cells of the tissues, and it is believed to be freed from these mast cells by various conditions that may cause an expulsion of granules followed by a release of histamine from the heparin-protein portion of the granule.

Drinking alcohol may precipitate an attack of various forms of vascular headache and flushing of the skin, possibly because some of these alcoholic beverages contain histamine. This assumption is based on the fact that when an excessive amount of histamine is given to a histaminic cephalalgia or a migraine patient, a headache will be brought on. Large amounts of histamine are found in red wines and sherries. Lesser amounts are found in the white wines, port, and beer. However, bourbon, scotch, and brandy contain no histamine.

Histamine has been a form of prophylactic therapy for migraine and histaminic cephalalgia for many years, and in numerous cases it is very satisfactory. Because effects of histamine therapy are of short duration, it is not surprising that continuous intravenous therapy, to the limit of the patient's capacity, proves to be more effective in producing tolerance than do repeated subcutaneous injections, which result in only a brief exposure to the action of the histamine preparation.

Histamine has been found to be of value in Meniere's syndrome, urticaria, sudden nerve deafness, multiple sclerosis, retrobulbar neuritis, temporal arteritis, vasomotor rhinitis, asthma, photophobia, corneal ulcer, and peripheral vascular disturbances.

Histamine in saline supplies 1.1 mg of histamine diphosphate (0.4 mg histamine base) per 100 ml in 0.9% sodium chloride solution. This is referred to as Horton's formula. It is sterile, nonpyrogenic, and stable.

Histamine may be given intravenously on an ambulatory basis, in the office or hospital, and the patient may return to work after completion of the administration. To prevent a possible excess of gastric acidity, a meal should be eaten prior to the infusion. Otherwise, an oral antacid may be required. Regardless, a slow rate of injection must be initially observed and, if this is tolerated, the rate may be increased gradually to a point that will just barely produce a mild flush or full sensation in the head.

Maximum vasodilation should be obtained, but the administration rate should be kept below a level that will cause discomfort to the patient. Therefore, histamine has to be used wisely by one who is well acquainted with the drug and its reactions on the patient. Too much of the preparation is just as useless as too little.

Reactions may occur during intravenous administration of histamine. The patient should therefore be closely watched for signs of too rapid injection or of intolerance to histamine itself. The usual manifestations, if this should occur, are a generalized sensation of warmth, a fall in the blood pressure, a sensation of fainting, a severe headache, an acute allergic phenomenon, or bronchoconstriction. If any of these symptoms do occur during histamine intravenous therapy, the rate of the injection should be either decreased or discontinued. Occasionally an injection of a 1:1000 solution of epinephrine may be required.

Histamine has been used in many patients with known peptic ulcer without producing any bad effects, in spite of the fact that it can possibly increase gastric acidity.

The antihistaminic drugs, by blocking specific histamine effects, actively interfere with and modify typical allergic and anaphylactic processes. In the allergic reaction, histamine is probably not the primary factor involved, but it is the chemical released secondarily to some disruptive process within the cell.

Histamine may be a final common pathway for a variety of physiologic mechanisms that lead to the excitation of the gastric secretory cells.

One difficulty with studies on histamine is that the physiologic effects observed in experimental animals do not always occur in human beings.

In order to understand the clinical use of histamine, it is necessary to appreciate its physiologic effects in humans. It is a substance that can be isolated from practically every human tissue except the central nervous system. It is found in the peripheral sensory nerves but not in the peripheral motor nerves. Histamine is a normal constituent of human blood, and it is found chiefly in the granular leukocytes. The exact manner in which histamine is held in the granular leukocytes of the blood and in the fixed cells of the body is not known, but the rapidity with which it can be liberated strongly suggests that it is not permanently bound to the cellular protoplasm. The presence of this substance in the granular leukocytes and in the fixed cells does not give rise to clinical signs and symptoms until it is released in its free form.

The concentration of histamine in the human blood is said to be approximately 4 μg per 100 ml. The range in a normal person is perhaps 2 to 7.5 μg per 100 mg of blood. Although the concentration of histamine remains constant in the blood of normal persons, it tends to fluctuate markedly in people affected with allergic disturbances.

An intradermal injection of histamine produces dilation of those capillaries in direct contact with the drug, a diffuse flare caused by dilation of the surrounding arterioles resulting from local axon reflexes, and an area of edema. However, there is no convincing evidence than an intracutaneous injection of histamine can be used to determine whether a person is histamine-sensitive or histamine-insensitive.

Histamine causes the liberation of epinephrine from the medullary portion of the suprarenal gland. This can be demonstrated in cases of pheochromocytoma and can be used as a test for this condition. A rise in the blood pressure results from excessive release of epinephrine. The action of histamine on the cortex of the suprarenal gland can probably be measured indirectly by the response of the eosinophils in the blood. The cortical discharge of steroids in humans occurs very promptly following the administration of histamine.

With almost all of the other various forms of prophylactic treatment of migraine and histaminic cephalalgia, there are many various side effects. In the case of histamine, however, this is not true. We have never observed any unwanted side reaction from the administration of histamine itself. However, reactions can result from faulty technique when the drug is used by someone not experienced with it and with the precautions that should be exercised.

Some patients might be hypersensitive to histamine; therefore, great care must be given to the initial use of the drug with each individual patient. The headache patient who can obtain relief prophylactically by the use of the correct amount of histamine can also have a headache attack precipitated by an overdose of the drug. Therefore, careful, precise dosage adjustment is necessary to obtain the desired results and to prevent the possibility of bringing on an attack of the headache.

Histamine is not a cureall drug, but it is a useful drug, especially in the treatment of certain forms of vascular headache.

Opiates

The opiates are actually part of the analgesic group. They are used for the relief of severe pain and for their sedative effects. However, they are seldom used in the treatment of chronic headache because they are addicting in nature. When treating a chronic headache problem we never give a patient a habit-forming drug; such a drug can cause a greater problem than the headache—namely, drug addiction.

Among the most commonly used of the opiate group of analgesic drugs are codeine, morphine, and meperidine (Demerol).

CODEINE

Codeine is much less potent than the other two, but it is rather effective in relieving pain or severe headaches. This drug is usually used in the form of codeine phosphate or codeine sulfate, and it may be given to the patient by mouth or by injection. It is absorbed from the intestinal tract and excreted largely in the urine.

Codeine has a depressing action on the respiratory center, but this action is not nearly as prominent as the same action of morphine. Other side effects produced by codeine are nausea, vomiting, constipation, and miosis.

Codeine is considerably more potent than any of the antipyretic type of analgesics. However, it is only about one fourth as potent as morphine. It is not nearly as addictive as morphine. In fact, it is less addictive than any of the other opiates. In situations in which morphine is contraindicated for various reasons, codeine can be used with fair effectiveness in the control of pain. Codeine produces relatively little euphoria and is therefore less desirable to the potential addict than such drugs as morphine.

Combinations of codeine with some mild form of analgesic agent are commonly used to relieve pain refractory to the analgesic agent alone. Such combinations relieve pain with doses of codeine that are ineffective when given alone. Codeine is perhaps most frequently prescribed for the type of headache associated with the common cold, acute sinusitis, or other infectious conditions. It is also used frequently in cases of posttraumatic headache. In such cases codeine alone or in combination may be indicated when less potent analgesics fail. Codeine is also used in cases of intracranial aneurysm, cerebrovascular accidents, or certain cases of neuritis.

We have never found codeine or any of the opiates to be of much value in cases of vascular headache such as migraine or histaminic cephalalgia. For this reason, plus the danger of any habit formation, we never prescribe codeine in any case of vascular headache.

MORPHINE

Morphine is an effective drug for severe pain. It acts on the pain centers in the optic thalami. Continuous dull pain is relieved more readily than is sharp intermittent pain. Larger doses of morphine are required to relieve existing pain than when used after medication has taken effect.

In the presence of severe pain, analgesia is obtained before the pain threshold has reached its maximum. This is due to the alteration in the pattern of the pain reaction.

Morphine also tends to lessen the patient's anxiety and fear; while still aware of the existing pain, the patient seems to tolerate it better after administration of morphine. Morphine produces euphoria, muscular relaxation, freedom from anxiety, lethargy, dimness of vision, apathy, loss of concentration, and loss of sleep. It may also slow respirations, constrict the pupils, and cause mental depression, constipation, nausea, and vomiting.

Morphine is well absorbed from the gastrointestinal tract and the subcutaneous tissue. It is not absorbed by the intact skin but will pass through mucous membranes. It is eliminated primarily by the kidneys by glomerular filtration; a portion is excreted unchanged via other routes, such as the liver and lungs. Morphine should not be used in cases of chronic vascular headache such as migraine and histaminic cephalalgia.

MEPERIDINE (DEMEROL)

Meperidine is a synthetic preparation with analgesic properties that are less effective than morphine but more effective than codeine.

Meperidine produces a mild sedative effect when used in ordinary therapeutic doses. Occasionally euphoria is produced, and the possibility of addiction is always present. The most common side effect is vertigo; other side effects include profuse sweating, nausea, vomiting, and occasionally respiratory depression.

Meperidine is absorbed readily and usually it is hydrolyzed by the liver and kidneys and excreted in the urine.

OTHER DRUGS

Other drugs belonging to the opiate group of analgesics are heroin, methadone, and dihydromorphinone (Dilaudid). However, these drugs are not as widely used as codeine, morphine, and meperidine in cases of headache.

The opiates may be employed in acute headaches but they have no place whatsoever in the field of chronic headache problems. This point cannot be stressed too strongly.

Tranquilizers and antidepressants

There are many drugs available today to combat anxiety, which is often a factor in the etiology of migraine.

Anxiety may be defined as an unpleasant mood of tension and apprehension. It is very closely associated with fear. Anxiety is a state of tension in which the individual is afraid but does not know what he fears. Like fear, severe anxiety has prominent autonomic effects. Fear, however, is an emotion that is sharply focused on immediate dangers. Anxiety is usually imposed by the anticipation of future dangers, distress, or difficulties. People and their troubles vary; some individuals are frequently anxious over seemingly trivial matters, others are unaffected by the same experiences.

Anxiety is usually the result of an accumulation of repressed, presumably dangerous, impulses that threaten to break into consciousness. Usually as a child the individual repressed these impulses because he was afraid of them and because he felt incapable of expressing them appropriately. As long as he represses them he can continue to avoid facing them. If the strength of the accumulated impulses increases past the individual's capacity to repress, he must either face them, find new ways to control them, or disguise their expressions.[35] Activities that arouse anxiety are avoided and those that diminish it are sustained. Anxiety may spur people to perform difficult tasks in a simple, skillful manner. Still, anxiety may be a hindrance, as some well-prepared students demonstrate when facing a critical examination.

Anxiety is a medical problem when it is excessive, inappropriate, or without obvious cause. Chronic anxiety may be punctuated by or may begin with an acute attack, but it may be a steady and distressingly prolonged disturbance of mood. The individual is "on edge" and tense. He may also have a feeling of hopelessness or sadness along with the anxiety. The intellectual powers are diminished, and there is considerable difficulty in concentrating and thinking clearly. Common precipitants of anxiety in daily life are circumstances of conflict in which an action is demanded but the correct action may be rather difficult to discern.

The manifestations of anxiety fall into three groups. First are the inner feelings of tension, apprehension, and dread that form the anxious mood itself. Second are disturbances of the intellectual power of the anxious individual. Third are the autonomic, visceral, and endocrine changes.[36]

The treatment of anxiety varies with the cause and the severity of the anxiety. Many individuals who are merely mildly anxious may be helped by a sympathetic physician who is willing to listen carefully to the patient's difficulties and be able to offer some support, assistance, or advice. Individuals having a more severe form of anxiety will require stronger treatment of a pharmacologic type. The sedatives and hypnotics have been the preferred agents for the relief of anxiety in the past. This group of drugs had many shortcomings (such as addiction), so a newer group of drugs has been developed for use in these cases.

It is rather difficult to actually evaluate the effects of any drug in the treatment of the state of anxiety because it is almost impossible to measure the condition correctly. It is natural for the physician to assume that the patient is suffering from anxiety if he complains of an inability to sleep, is apprehensive about the future, or describes either real or imaginary threats to life or security. Such a verbal account actually constitutes in itself a very obvious state of anxiety. Other conditions that could denote anxiety are a peptic ulcer, ulcerative colitis, nervous mannerisms, changes in facial expression, or even asthma.

Some authorities also consider such things as drug addiction evidence of anxiety. It seems, however, that this would actually involve much more than anxiety; it is actually a complex behavior problem.

OLDER ANTIANXIETY DRUGS

The sedative-hypnotic drugs are frequently classified as barbiturates and nonbarbiturates. This classification is based on chemical structure, and other than this it serves no direct purpose.

The barbiturates are regarded as being general depressants. They depress a wide range of cellular functions in many vital organ systems such as the activity of nerve tissue, skeletal muscle, smooth muscle, and cardiac muscle. The barbiturates resemble each other with respect to their differential action on various functions.

The effects of the barbiturates on the metabolism of the brain have been the subject of a large volume of research. There is a decrease in the energy-yielding reactions in the brain. Cerebral oxygen uptake, lactic acid production, and heat production are diminished.[37]

The barbiturates have some degree of local anesthetic action. There is an increase in the threshold of electrical stimulus to the peripheral nerves and a slowing of the conduction velocity.[38]

The effects of the barbiturates on the electrical properties of cell membranes and on the transmembrane ion flux show a decrease in the amplitude and rate of rise of the action potential when muscle is bathed in solutions of barbiturates.[39]

It is generally believed that the synapse is the site of action of the hypnotic group of drugs. In fact transmission across neuronal and neuroeffector junctions is far more susceptible to interference by the barbiturates than is conduction along nerve or muscle fibers. Barbiturates selectively depress transmission in sympathetic ganglia in concentrations that are without detection on nerve conductions, neuroeffector junctions, cardiomuscular muscle, or smooth muscle.[40]

The tendency of barbiturates to act selectively on synapses suggests that activity transmitted through polysynaptic pathways should be susceptible to barbiturate depression.[41]

The barbiturates are potent respiratory depressants, affecting both the drive to respiration and the mechanisms responsible for the rhythmic character of respiratory movements.[42] In oral form the barbiturates do not produce significant cardiovascular effects, except for a slight decrease in the blood pressure and in the heart rate. This is minimal, and only to the same degree as one normally finds during normal sleep.[43]

The oxybarbiturates tend to decrease the

tone of the gastrointestinal musculature and the amplitude of rhythmic conditions. This is partially peripheral and partially central in action, depending on the dosage used. Gastric secretions may be slightly decreased by the barbiturates.[44]

In the therapeutic dose range, the barbiturates do not impair normal hepatic function unless the individual is hypersensitive to the drug.[45]

NEWER ANTIANXIETY DRUGS

There is a newer group of drugs used in the treatment of anxiety states, called (minor) tranquilizers. This group of drugs has somewhat supplanted the hypnotic and sedative group of drugs.

Tranquilizers have the ability to calm hyperactive agitated individuals without causing any marked confusion, drowsiness, or disorientation. Unlike the sedative-hypnotics, the tranquilizers do not produce sleep. The tranquilizers, on the whole, seem to be of more benefit to severely agitated individuals than the sedative-hypnotic agents.

Tranquilizers should not be used in cases of anxiety without sufficient cause. This group of drugs is a highly potent group that exerts its action on the central nervous system. These drugs should not be used by a physician who does not have a thorough knowledge of the drug's action, side effects, and contraindications. These drugs, although believed to be nonhabit-forming, are very potent. The patient using them should be under the routine supervision of the physician, so that if any side effects occur the use of the drugs should be immediately discontinued.

The prescription of tranquilizers in antianxiety states is greatly abused. They are used too often to attempt to change the attitudes and the emotions of many patients. Many patients receiving these extremely potent drugs actually do not require them. What they need is a sympathetic, understanding physician. If the physician would spend a little time with these anxious patients and discuss their problems with them, many would not require this potent type of therapy.

Nevertheless, tranquilizers are used; if used correctly, they are generally successful as an antianxiety agent.

PHENOTHIAZINE DERIVATIVES

The phenothiazine derivatives are classified as major tranquilizers. They not only act on the central nervous system but also exert significant effects on organ systems throughout the body.

These drugs produce a considerable degree of sedation when given initially. They produce psychomotor slowing, emotional quieting, and indifference. This has been described as the neuroleptic syndrome.[46]

The phenothiazine derivatives appear to bring about changes at all levels of the cerebrospinal axis. Large doses result in an electroencephalogram (EEG) characteristic of drowsiness.[47]

The actions of these drugs in the cardiovascular system are complex because they produce a direct effect on the heart and blood vessels and also indirect effects through actions on the central nervous system and autonomic reflexes.[48] These drugs produce hypotension, a direct depressive action on the heart, an increase in coronary blood flow, and rapid heartbeat.

The phenothiazine derivatives may produce a diuretic effect either because of the depressant action on the secretion of the antidiuretic hormone, inhibition of reabsorption of water and electrolytes by a direct action on the renal tubules, or both.[49]

These drugs are most useful in the treatment of conditions marked by psychomotor activity. They often tend to rapidly reduce the psychotic patient's panic, fear, anxiety, and hostility. Relatively small doses are required to suppress anxiety. However, because of the severe side effects that may occur, may physicians prefer to avoid their use and to employ a minor tranquilizer.

The first successful type of tranquilizer to be widely used was chlorpromazine

(Thorazine), a phenothiazine derivative. This drug has side effects that result from secondary actions on the central and autonomic nervous systems and others that are merely allergic in nature.

Chlorpromazine may produce drowsiness, dry mouth, nasal congestion, constipation, or amenorrhea.[50] Reports of agranulocytosis[51] and jaundice are found in the literature, as are reports of extrapyramidal reactions closely resembling a parkinsonian syndrome.[52]

PROPANEDIOL DERIVATIVES

The derivatives comprise another group of drugs used by the physician for the treatment of anxiety. The most widely used drug of this group, and one of the most widely used drugs in the treatment of anxiety, is meprobamate (Equanil).

Meprobamate is clearly different from the phenothiazine derivatives. It is actually a derivative of mephenesin, a skeletal muscle relaxant. Meprobamate itself has some skeletal relaxant effects.

Meprobamate is considered a minor tranquilizer and is advocated mainly for the suppression of the less severe manifestations of anxiety and tension. This drug helps to control mild to moderate degrees of emotional upset in individuals who react adversely to environmental stress.[53]

Side effects of meprobamate consist of the production of a hypotensive effect. This is more pronounced when the drug is used in elderly individuals. Overdosage may produce a loss of consciousness, shock, respiratory depression, and even death. Urticaria or even erythematous rash may appear with the use of this drug. Some blood abnormalities, including agranulocytosis, anemia, and leukopenia, have also been found with the use of this drug, but they are rare.

Meprobamate is used in a great variety of conditions involving anxiety. The drug appears to have its greatest effect in treating anxious neurotic patients by increasing their ability to concentrate and by decreasing their destructiveness.[54] Meprobamate has been found to be useful in the treatment of some psychotic patients who manifest anxiety.[55] This drug does not appear to be useful in the treatment of hallucinations and delusions.

BENZODIAZEPINE DERIVATIVES

Another minor tranquilizer used in the treatment of anxiety is chlordiazepoxide (Librium).[56] This preparation, a benzodiazepine derivative, is probably one of the most widely used drugs in America today.

Differences in the behavioral effects caused by the benzodiazepine compounds and meprobamate and the barbiturates have been demonstrated in experimental animals.[57]

Chlordiazepoxide blocks electroencephalographic changes aroused from stimulation of the brainstem reticular formation. It depresses the duration of electrical after discharge in the limbic system, including the septal region, the amygdala, and the hippocampus.[58]

This drug also relaxes the skeletal muscles, which makes it especially useful in cases where anxiety and tension tend to intensify symptoms. It actually has no effect on the muscle spasm, which is of a purely organic nature.[59]

The most common side effects of this drug are drowsiness and lethargy; these are found primarily in elderly individuals. Chlordiazepoxide has a slight depressing effect on the respiration, blood pressure, the pulse rate.[60] Some individuals receiving this drug become excited and have a heightened sense of well-being. Other side effects are skin rash, nausea, decreased libido, stimulation of the appetite, and on rare occasions agranulocytosis. Poisoning with this drug is very rare.

Another minor tranquilizer that is used very successfully as an antianxiety drug is diazepam (Valium). This drug is closely related to chlordiazepoxide and is successful in suppressing the manifestations of anxiety and tension.

The most common adverse side effects of diazepam are drowsiness, vertigo, fatigue, and ataxia. Occasionally nausea, blurred vision, hypotension, skin rash, slurred speech, constipation, impaired memory, and tremor are seen.

Diazepam has a direct action on the central nervous system and exerts peripheral effects on the cholinergic, adrenergic, and tryptominergic systems. It is apparently nonsedative in its ability to impair discriminative conditioned avoidance responses.[61] Diazepam is also advocated as a centrally acting muscle relaxant. It abolishes spastic rigidity.[59] In this respect it is similar to chlordiazepoxide. Like other central nervous system depressants diazepam has been associated with withdrawal symptoms if it is abruptly stopped after prolonged usage at high dosage levels. It should not be used in patients having psychotic tendencies underlying their anxiety.

Patients using this drug should avoid alcohol and any occupation requiring mental alertness. It should be used cautiously in elderly patients and in patients with hepatic problems or impaired renal functions. It should also be avoided in patients with glaucoma.

Diazepam is one of the most widely used antianxiety agents on the drug market today. It is very useful in dealing with anxiety reactions stemming from stressful circumstances or whenever somatic complaints are concomitants of emotional factors. It is also useful in cases of psychoneurotic states manifested by anxiety or tension. Because of its side effects it should be used only on the advice and supervision of a physician who is aware of these side effects. It is a potent minor tranquilizer and should be handled with respect both by the physician and by the patient.

TRICYCLIC COMPOUNDS

Another small group of drugs, the tricyclic compounds, may be helpful in the treatment of anxiety state accompanying depression. Depressed states tend to vary in severity and the use of antidepressant drugs must be individualized accordingly. The tricyclic compounds fall under the general heading of antidepressant drugs.

These drugs are not as widely used as the barbiturates and the tranquilizers, but in some instances they may be of benefit. Only a few of these tricyclic compounds used in anxiety states associated with depression will be discussed.

Amitriptyline (Elavil) is an antidepressant that also produces some tranquilizing effects. It may be used to relieve depressive reactions and anxiety that accompany chronic illness. The tranquilizing component to its action is particularly useful in the management of depressed phases of anxiety and manic depressive states and in the treatment of involutional melancholia.[62]

Some patients using this drug respond quickly (within 1 week), while others may take as long as 5 or 6 weeks. Amitriptyline acts on the central nervous system to relieve mental depression. It is not a monoamine oxidase inhibitor. This drug slows the spontaneous electrical activity of the central nervous system.[63]

The side effects of this preparation include drowsiness, vertigo, nausea, hypotension, tremor, weakness, headache, heartburn, and incoordination. Numbness and tingling of the limbs, including possible peripheral neuropathy, have been reported occasionally,[64] and rarely agranulocytosis has been reported.[65]

Close supervision on the part of the physician is required in cases where this drug is employed at any high dosage level or for any prolonged period of time.

This drug should not be used with or for at least 2 weeks after discontinuing the use of a monoamine oxidase inhibitor. Because of its atropine-like activity it should be used cautiously in patients with glaucoma, urinary retention, epilepsy, and possible suicidal tendencies.

Triavil, a combination of amitriptyline (Elavil) and perphenazine (Trilafon), is another tranquilizer-antidepressant. It is used with patients who have a moderate to severe anxiety and a depressed mood, patients with depression and severe anxiety, and patients with depression and anxiety in association with chronic disease.[66]

This drug is contraindicated in cases of central nervous system depression resulting from drugs, bone marrow depression, urinary retention, pregnancy, and glaucoma.

It should not be given in conjunction with or for 2 weeks after the withdrawal of a monoamine oxidase inhibitor.

Summary

The most commonly prescribed drugs for the handling of anxiety states by the practicing physician have been described. Naturally there are many other drugs used for this purpose, but all of these cannot be dealt with in a book of this nature.

Anxiety is a very common condition for the physician to come into contact with today. It is far more common than it was 20 or even 10 years ago, because the stress and the strain of normal everyday life have gradually increased. There is every indication that the future will lead to an even greater increase in the stress factor that plays such a prominent part in the etiology of their condition. It is generally believed that medical science has been able to keep pace with this increased amount of stress and strain by discovering new and more powerful drugs to combat them. Drug research will have to continue until the ideal drug or drugs are found.

All of the drugs mentioned produce some of the desired effects in some people. Some people respond better to one drug than another. It is therefore a matter of selectivity. The patient should be given the drug that seems best suited. If it does not work well enough, another drug should be tried until optimum desired results are obtained. To obtain the optimum results, both the physician and the patient must be satisfied.

Unfortunately, all of the drugs mentioned have some side effects. Naturally it is the desire of those doing any type of drug research to discover an agent that will produce the desired results and will have no undesirable side effects. Perhaps a drug of this type will someday be found to treat anxiety. It is this hope that supplies the energy and the desire to all those involved in drug research, be it chemical or clinical. To achieve this the physician must employ "essence of patience and tincture of time."

BIOFEEDBACK AND ITS APPLICATION TO HEADACHE
SEYMOUR DIAMOND

In the past, the scientific study of behavior has generally been concerned with the physical aspects of biologic organisms. The primary subject of this research has, of course, been human beings, whose behavior is undoubtedly the most complex, least understood, and truly the most interesting. In attempting to comprehend the unique quality of the intricate interior life and the subjective world of experience, feelings, moods, and thoughts of humans, the objective world of observable phenomena has been used as a standard. The behavioral scientist has been confined to the study of only those external and internal events that we are capable of measuring and whose existence is assured by virtue of their physical reality. Hence, the bulk of scientific data concerning behavior has been obtained by observations of individuals interacting with the external environment.

In this endeavor to understand our role in the external environment, we have lost touch with a very important concept, that of self. In many Eastern cultures, achievement of self-awareness has long been of primary importance and is directly related to the act of physiologic self-discipline. To yogis, Zen masters, and other practitioners of spiritual disciplines, physical self-awareness and control are merely the worldly resources available to every person that can be employed in the achievement of spiritual awareness. Many spend entire lifetimes in controlled discipline of the mind, searching for the spiritual awareness of total harmony with the all and nothing of the universe.

In Western cultures these practices have always been looked on as curious and exotic and surely of no relevance to our own existence. Control over autonomic functions, for example, has been looked on only with curiosity. The most notable skeptics, without a doubt, have been members of the scientific community, whose calculating and logical outlook on the world has generally been in complete disharmony to these ancient rituals. Only recently have scientists attempted to really understand the biologic basis for these practices and to apply them to already existing scientific principles. To the surprise and disbelief of many, such research has led to the development of a new and exciting technique known as biofeedback, which enables us to relate to our interior self in a manner not previously possible in Western culture.

It is difficult to conceive in this disposable age of plastics, frozen foods, supersonic jets, and the like, where "time is of the essence," that we could possibly find the time to attain any sense of self-awareness. And yet, it is this very time that is calling on something more within ourselves to cope with the tensions and anxieties affecting a large portion of society. There are those who have learned to adequately cope with these pressures of daily life, and many who have not. This inability to cope is manifested in a variety of psychologic and physiologic problems to which modern medicine does not always have the answer. Herein lies the importance of biofeedback. It helps us get back in touch with ourselves and, being a mechanical device, it does so in a manner that fits well into the framework of our society. It is only when we get back in touch with ourselves that we will be better able to cope with the pressures of daily life. This will ultimately lead to a much saner and healthier existence.

Biofeedback is thus a technique that combines modern electric technology with ancient Eastern practices and modern psychology. Complex electric devices are used to carefully monitor various bodily functions such as heart rate, muscle tension, blood pressure, temperature, and brain wave activity, functions of which we are generally unaware. Norbert Weiner, the mathematician, coined the word "feedback" and defined it as a method of controlling the system by reinserting into it the results of those past performances. Biofeedback, then, is a special case where the system is a biologic system and where the feedback is artificially mediated by mechanical detection amplification and display instrumentation rather than being present as an inborn feedback loop within the biologic system. Simply, biofeedback is a method of teaching a person to control a previously unused or involuntary controlled function of the body through the use of instrumentation. Most frequently it is used to control the autonomic nervous system and thus functions such as heartbeat, blood pressure, and blood flow, but it can also be used to teach a person control over all previously unused portions of the motor nervous system. The basic principle behind these techniques goes back to the Russian scientist, Ivan Pavlov, and his conditioned reflex discovery (Fig. 3-1). From this came the theory of operant conditioning, which is the basis for instrumental learning or biofeedback technique (Fig. 3-2). Instrumental learning provides the conditioned stimulus, along with an opportunity to respond in various ways. The correct response is then reinforced or rewarded. After several reinforcements, the stimulus serves as a signal for the subject to perform the learned response. Sometimes all that is needed for successful conditioning of humans is the knowledge of their accomplishments.

Working at almost the same time as Pavlov, Johannes Schultz,[67] in Germany, developed a mind-body training system called autogenic training. In Schultz's system, the patient directed himself, repeating a series of phrases to help him relax (these will be described in detail later). The role of the physician was purely as a teacher. This technique thus came into the realm of self-regulation. These procedures are remarkably like yoga, where the disciple chants a series of mantras to help him achieve inner

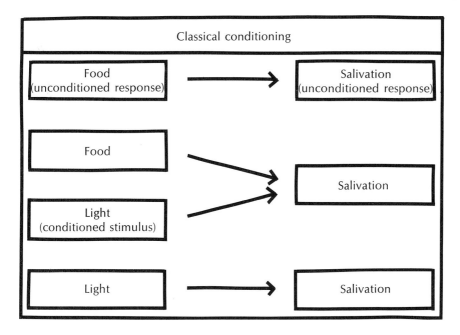

Fig. 3-1. Classical conditioning starts with an unconditioned stimulus. The conditioned stimulus that it is paired with comes to act as a substitute in producing the unconditioned response. (From Diamond, S., and Dalessio, D. J.: The practicing physician's approach to headache, ed. 2, Baltimore, 1978, The Williams and Wilkins Co.)

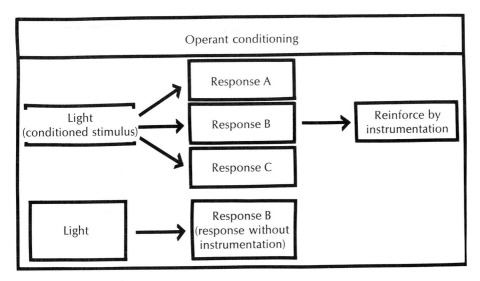

Fig. 3-2. In instrumental learning, a conditioned stimulus is presented along with an opportunity to respond in various ways. The correct response is reinforced. After several reinforcements the stimulus serves as a signal to perform the learned response. Humans usually do not need reinforcement such as food; the feedback of achievement is sufficient reward. (From Diamond, S., and Dalessio, D. J.: The practicing physician's approach to headache, ed. 2, Baltimore, 1978, The Williams and Wilkins Co.)

discipline. And in yoga, too, the master is merely a teacher, showing the disciple the way, but never insisting or intruding. It is interesting that in the early 1930s, when Schultz was doing his work, Edmond Jacobson, of the University of Chicago, developed his technique of progressive relaxation, which was very similar to Schultz's methodology. Both Jacobson's[68] and Schultz's techniques suffered because of the long and arduous period of training necessary to achieve results. They never gained great popularity because of these difficulties.

These concepts formed the basis for the work of Dr. Joe Kamiya[69] at the University of Chicago. In 1962, he published a report describing experiments in which people learned both to estimate the amount of alpha or beta brain waves they were producing and to turn their brain alpha rhythm on at will. A computer connected to the electroencephalograph (EEG) turned a sound signal on whenever alpha waves appeared in the individuals' EEG recordings, and they soon learned to keep the tone on or off at will, though they could not explain how they did it. Some described a feeling of well-being and tranquility associated with these waves. These experiments were the first to suggest that biofeedback techniques could promote self-control over internal physiologic events by enabling the individual to discover and reproduce mental events that in turn have predictable effect on a specific visceral function.

Although our interest is in headache, and the use of biofeedback in headache has been established, it would be most apropos to discuss other possible applications of biofeedback in medicine.

The possible potential of these techniques is manifested by the myriad of research being carried on in various medical centers throughout the United States. At the Menninger Foundation, Dr. Elmer Green[70] is training volunteers to produce theta waves while fully conscious. His volunteers learn to induce hypnagogic-like images from their preconscious while fully awake. Perhaps eventually psychiatrists will be able to monitor their patients' brain wave patterns during free association. Thus, the EEG may substantiate the depth of association.

Dr. Maurice B. Sternman,[71] working at the VA Hospital in Sepulveda, California, has discovered a previously unrecognized EEG rhythm localized over the sensorimotor cortex. He calls this the sensorimotor rhythm 12 to 14 hertz (cycles per second). This rhythm occurs only when the subject is completely quiet and motionless. Dr. Sternman's work with cats has shown that the animals can be taught to produce the rhythm at will. The animals can even learn to resist the convulsions generally associated with injections of hydrazine compounds.

At the Bedford, Massachusetts, VA Hospital, Dr. Thomas Mulholland[72] is studying children with attentional disorders. These children are allowed to watch as much television as they want, but the set turns off when brain waves produce alpha rhythms. Thus, to keep the television program on, the child's brain has to be alert and attentive, producing beta rhythms.

At the University of Wisconsin, Madison, Dr. Francis M. Forster[73] and his associates have reported some success in treating epilepsy in one patient who developed seizures induced by photic stimulation. The patient watched flickers of light at frequencies close to the critical rate. A computer analyzed changes in electric activity of the patient's brain waves. When these waves became seizure-like in frequency, the computer turned off the light and began a series of auditory clicks, attempting to disrupt the seizure pattern.

At Rockefeller University, New York City, Dr. Neal Miller[74] and his associates have demonstrated that many autonomic responses can be induced in animals by reward learning (also known as instrumental or operant conditioning). To rule out the possibility that the autonomic responses were controlled by skeletal muscles under voluntary control, curare was administered and breathing was maintained by artificial means. Animals showing the response the investigators wanted to elicit (such as fast heart rate or high blood pressure) were rewarded or reinforced. The reward was electric stimulation of the pleasure centers in the hypothalamus. In this way, Dr. Miller and his group taught their animals to increase or decrease blood pressure and heart rate, to produce localized blood flow to an ear, and to vary urinary secretions or gastric and intestinal contractions. The Miller team has also been successful in controlling blood pressure in humans for a temporary period with biofeedback technique.

These examples represent only a portion of the various ways in which biofeedback has been applied. It would appear that we have only begun to scratch the surface of developing the far-reaching potential that biofeedback has in its applications to medicine.

To date, the most solidly established clinical application of biofeedback has been in the treatment of particular forms of headache. Until recently, the treatment of headache has relied primarily on drug-related therapy. In many cases, this is not a satisfactory form of treatment since some drugs can create a physical dependence and in themselves can be as incapacitating as the headaches. However, many patients can only be helped by drug therapy, and many patients may need a combination of drug therapy with biofeedback to solve their problem. Biofeedback is not the messiah of headache treatments but a useful adjunct in the carefully selected patient. It allows for treatment of headaches and either eliminates or limits the use of drugs in these specific patients. However, biofeedback training cannot be applied to all types of headache, and in many cases the only, and therefore, the best, treatment is still drug-related therapy.

The idea of using a combination of biofeedback and autogenic training to alleviate the problems of migraine headache patients was first suggested by Dr. Elmer Green[75] of the Menninger Foundation. One of the volunteers who was in a training program to learn control of brain waves and to reduce electromyographic potential in the forearm muscle structure and to increase blood flow in the hand was fortuitously discovered to be able to abort a migraine headache by raising the temperature of her hand. This unexpected discovery led to the development of the "hot-hand theory" of Sargent, Green, and Walters for treating migraine headaches.

Work by Green and his staff had shown that local peripheral temperature is directly related to the blood flow in that area, as measured by a photoplethysmograph. In the treatment of the patient mentioned, it was noted that the increase of blood flow to the hand was accompanied by a spontaneous remission of the migraine headache. In this innovative case, the woman achieved a voluntary elevation in hand temperature of 10° F in approximately 2 minutes. With this initial success, the researchers attempted to further test this technique on two other volunteers. These results, though not conclusive, were sufficiently encouraging to conduct controlled studies.

Sargent used the autogenic training phrases of Schultz in training patients to raise hand temperature.[76] The idea stemmed from previous reports by Schultz which had shown that, in some cases, individuals were able to alleviate migraine attacks while performing the autogenic training exercises. The combination of autogenic training with biofeedback training appears to be a credible association, and we are indeed indebted to the researchers of the Menninger Foundation for devising this combination, since this method has proved to be quite successful in our own clinical work.

At approximately the same time that the Menninger Foundation was making its discovery, a similar breakthrough was made for muscle contraction (or tension) headaches by a group of researchers from the University of Colorado Medical Center. In 1969, Budzynski, Stoyva, and Adler[77] described a technique for producing deep muscle relaxation by means of an informational feedback system in which the person hears a tone with a frequency proportional to the electromyographic (EMG) level of the muscle being monitored. This new technique was originally applied to patients with tension headache. Five volunteers, solicited by advertisements in the newspaper, were used in the initial study. With this biofeedback training and relaxation method the patient not only learned to produce low frontalis EMG levels but also showed substantial subsequent reduction of headache frequency. Ensuing work with a larger number of patients at the University of Colorado Medical Center confirmed these initial systematic observations, as did our own work at the Diamond Headache Clinic.

Autogenic-biofeedback training, as it has since been called, solicits the patient's direct involvement in treatment and therefore delegates much of the responsibility for the control of headaches to the patient. This is a breakaway from the traditional physician patient relationship, in which the physician has total control of the therapy. It is a return to a holistic form of medicine in which the patient plays an integral role in treatment. Through biofeedback training the patient first develops a new internal awareness to the manner in which he responds subjectively to situational or external stimuli. This expanded awareness includes a concrete sense of physiologic responses to such stimuli. It is thus our goal, using biofeedback training, to help patients reach this individual realization and to apply it to the next stage of the learning process, that is, acquisition of voluntary control over physiologic functions that have demonstrable effect on headache problems.

To start with, the correct choice of biofeedback modality is vital in promoting an appropriate response from the patient. In treating a patient with vascular headaches, there are two methods of choice. We have found that temperature training is the preferred method where the patient exhibits the "classic" migraine symptoms. These people first get a warning preheadache and can, therefore, best utilize the vascular control skills learned through temperature training at the first warning signs. This will frequently abort or at least diminish the severity of the subsequent attack. However, our work has shown that patients do better when they receive EMG feedback in addition to temperature feedback, because EMG feedback teaches them relaxation techniques (Fig. 3-3). Stress can provoke migraine.

On the other hand, patients who exhibit nonclassic migraines or a mixed diagnosis of vascular and muscle contraction headache are best treated with a combination of temperature training and EMG feedback training. In those patients with exclusively muscle contraction headache, EMG training is the preferred choice of treatment. At our clinic most patients receive both the temperature and EMG feedback training, since many migraine headaches appear to have a psychogenic component and vice versa.

The following will present a review of the techniques employed in both forms of biofeedback training. The proper training of these techniques is essential if the full potential benefits of biofeedback therapy are to be realized. The conventions that will be discussed here have emerged from our extensive experience with a great many headache patients. They are basically designed to teach the patient to develop new voluntary physiologic control skills that have proved to be effective in reducing both the frequency and the severity of headaches. In general, our findings at the Diamond Headache Clinic have confirmed the work of past researchers.

The general temperature control training procedures employed at the Diamond Headache Clinic focus primarily on the pa-

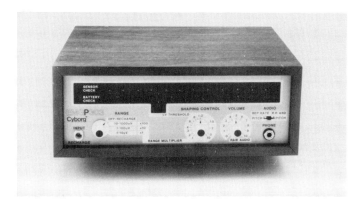

Fig. 3-3. Electromyographic training machine. (Courtesy Cyborg Corp.)

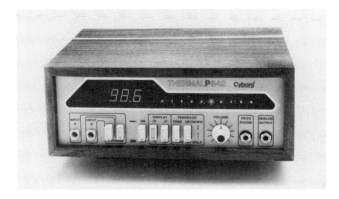

Fig. 3-4. Thermo training biofeedback machine. (Courtesy Cyborg Corp.)

tient's capacity to increase finger and hand temperature. These procedures, though always carried out with the specific needs of the particular patient in mind, can be generally outlined.

As a rule, 4 to 5 weeks of intensive biofeedback training with follow-up biofeedback practice at gradually decreasing intervals and regular practice of the new learned responses with out biofeedback, to maximize in vivo transference, prove sufficient. The therapist must, however, be prepared to alter scheduling in cases where this rather brief sequence does not yield the expected results. Local patients are seen twice weekly in the first month for biofeedback treatments. If the patient is from out of town, we endeavor to arrange twice daily sessions for the first 2 weeks.

During office visits, the patient sits in a quiet, dimly lighted room in a reclining chair. The room is furnished in a comfortable, relaxing style, with a decor quite different from the traditional clinical setting. In addition, the room is kept moderately warm, to facilitate temperature training. This warm, pleasant, comfortable ambience, free from external distractions, has proved to be very important, particularly at early stages of the skill learning process where patient relaxation and concentration are both essential.

For home practice (described in detail later) similar environmental conditions are highly recommended. In general, the patient should endeavor to practice temperature control exercises in a quiet, warm room. This may sometimes be difficult to achieve as, for example, in the case of a parent with young children or a busy businessperson. A suggestion we often make is to practice in the bathroom or wait until the children are outside or sleeping.

The initial training itself consists of three elements: (1) a temperature biofeedback signal supplied by the monitor (Fig. 3-4); (2) patient exercises, which are first done while receiving biofeedback, and (3) careful record-keeping to identify problem areas and chart progress. At the start of each session the patient's hand temperature is determined and recorded. When the session concludes similar data are noted, with special attention to any change, as well as the patient's subjective assessment of mood change and relaxation achieved during the session.

During the last week of intensive training, patients are progressively weaned from the biofeedback monitor. This is accomplished by altering the home exercise sequence by instructing the patient to practice twice a day with biofeedback instruments (temperature trainer) and twice daily without it. This process is essential, since the ultimate goal of the training program is to develop new patient control skills that do not depend on biofeedback machines. In this context, biofeedback itself is only a temporary facilitating mechanism, a therapeutic tool, which, when the task is completed, should be laid aside. This concept should be made clear to the patient.

After the intensive training period of 4 to 5 weeks, follow-up visits are indicated. These will generally decrease, with most patients requiring only a few reinforcement sessions. Out-of-town patients are generally seen monthly for 3 to 6 months. If, for whatever reason, the patient's condition regresses, an increase of follow-up visits and additional months of home use biofeedback trainers may be considered necessary.

As previously indicated, each patient undergoing temperature training is given an inventory of autogenic phrases adopted from the well-known work of Johannes Schultz. The phrases which we use are autosuggestive, focusing on feelings of warmth and relaxation. The following phrases are among those we generally use with headache patients:

I feel quite quiet. . . . I am beginning to feel quite relaxed. . . . My ankles, my knees, and my hips feel heavy, relaxed, and comfortable. . . . My solar plexus and the whole central portion of my body feel relaxed and quiet. . . . My hands, my arms, and my shoulders feel heavy, relaxed, and comfortable. . . . My neck, my jaws, and my forehead feel relaxed, they feel comfortable and smooth. . . . My whole body feels quiet, heavy, comfortable, and relaxed. . . . I am quite relaxed. . . . My arms and hands are heavy and warm. . . . I feel quite quiet. . . . My whole body is relaxed, and my hands are warm and relaxed and warm, my hands are warm, warmth is flowing into my hands, they are warm, warm.

In addition to using these autogenic phrases, patients are advised to focus on warm images, for example, putting their hands in a hot tub of water, sitting on a hot beach or by a fire. They are told to focus on a relaxing image, like being on a rubber mattress in a pool with the sunlight streaming down on their hands. One patient was very successful when she thought of gardening, a hobby she found relaxing, and also imagined the sunlight warming her back. If focusing on warm images does not help, the patients consider sensations in their fingers, that is, tingling or pulsating. This proved beneficial to a patient who imagined slamming his finger with a hammer. He could consistently elevate his temperature 10° to 15° F by doing this. Listening to a tape of the autogenic phrases, while using the monitor, is very helpful. Success at training has been particularly demonstrated when patients listen to their own voices reading the phrases, since they sometimes tend to resist training when listening to a tape in the clinician's voice.

As indicated, hand temperature control learning is substantially enhanced by diligent home practice. All of our patients are given detailed instructions to accomplish this. We provide a temperature biofeedback monitor on a rental basis during at least the first 4 weeks of biofeedback therapy as an integral part of the home training program. In addition, depending on the case, taped exercise instructions to be used in conjunction with biofeedback may be given for practicing at home.

Besides providing the patient with instantaneous biofeedback of hand temperature performance during these initial practice sessions, the home biofeedback trainer also provides helpful inducement for practice. The importance of maintaining patient motivation cannot be overemphasized. This is something to which both the physician and the clinician must pay great attention during the entire program.

Patients are instructed to use their home trainer twice daily, from 10 to 15 minutes for each session. They are also encouraged to employ it with their emerging control skills whenever preheadache warnings occur or at the time of headache onset. The importance of regular, twice daily practice must be stressed. The patient is told repeatedly that in this way he builds the very self-control skills that decrease the chances for experiencing a headache. Home practice sessions should be scheduled 3 to 4 hours apart, since the hands can get only so warm, and the purpose of the home training is to generalized the effect of the temperature increase control. Since many patients experience early awakening from headaches or wake up in the morning with a headache already present, they are also instructed to practice immediately before bedtime.

Each patient with a temperature feedback monitor at home is instructed to record what occurs during all practice sessions in a daily diary. The first item to be checked is the degree of warmth the patient feels in the hands before the training sessions. If the patient is aware of the hands being quite warm before starting to practice, he should not be discouraged by a small increase in temperature during the session, since he

began in a state of substantial vasodilation. At the end of each session, the patient is asked to judge the degree of relaxation. Has his mood changed during the session? Many patients will complain of tension following the session, since he has concentrated, perhaps too much, while on the trainer. The patient is also asked to record the exact amount of change in the hand temperature during the session in degrees.

After the first week of training, the patient is told to record the speed at which he achieves warmth. This is most important, since the patient may only need a 2° to 3° change in temperature to successfully abort a migraine. If this can be accomplished in 1 or 2 minutes, the patient may be able to effectively use his new skill at the first signs of a headache. During the second week the patient should try to elevate the hand temperature 1° in 1 minute. The following week the goal should be increased to 1½° and should continue to increase thereafter, assuming, of course, that the first goal has been achieved.

The patient's chart is reviewed on subsequent clinical visits to note progress with the trainer and to check on the daily practice sessions. Home practice sessions are conducted in essentially the same manner as clinical sessions, that is, in addition to the biofeedback, the patient also uses the autogenic phrases previously mentioned. The patient is either provided with a list of the autogenic phrases or a tape, either in the clinician's or the patient's voice.

Until now, the techniques that have been described are those commonly employed in the treatment of adults with vascular headaches. Comprehensive studies in both the United States and Scandinavia have shown that migraines are also observed in children, with an occurrence rate of apparently 5%. In treating children with migraine headaches, it has been the plan of our clinic to use a minimal amount of drug therapy. It is our hope that if a headache problem is diagnosed and treated at an early age, many of these children will not, as adults, develop the accompanying depression and drug habituation that are so prevalent in older patients with chronic headache problems. Autogenic training combined with biofeedback is, therefore, the optimal therapy for our younger patients at the clinic.

The basic procedures utilized for children in the clinic are essentially the same as those previously described. The importance of daily practice at home is explained, and it is stressed that the child is in control of his own practicing. We explain to the child that he alone is responsible for his therapy and if he does not wish to practice, it is his decision. We do not want him to practice because of parental urgings. The home sessions are as described for adults. The child is also asked to keep a daily record of the sessions. During follow-up visits, these records are discussed with the patient, not with the parents. The therapist is then able to determine whether or not the child is practicing as he should.

In general, we have found that children acquire the necessary skills much faster and more easily than do adults. It is analogous to the comparative ease with which children learn a new language. They are generally fascinated with the equipment and are better able to focus all of their energies in the direction of acquiring the desired skills. This overall willingness to participate in the therapy is demonstrated in our results with children. A far superior success rate is indicated as compared to that of adults. This is to be expected. In addition to their willingness, they also have fewer responsibilities and pressures facing them in their daily lives. These basic differences between children and adults have also given us an indication of some of the basic psychologic problems affecting the success rate in our adult patients.

Whatever the age, patients suffering from vascular headaches receive both temperature and electromyographic feedback training. Following each in-clinic temperature training session, an electromyographic session is administered. The use of the EMG

feedback trainer is done exclusively in the office. Twenty-minute sessions are conducted in a dark, quiet room, usually immediately following the temperature session. The patient remains in a reclining position (Fig. 3-3). He is told that we are monitoring frontalis muscle activity and that if facial, shoulder, and/or neck muscles are tense, a high pitched tone is produced. He is then instructed to decrease the tone by relaxing. It is suggested that he focus on relaxation of the entire body while receiving biofeedback. Electrodes are placed on each temple and a set of stereoheadphones is used to minimize external noise and distraction. There are variable sensitivities on the monitor so that, as the patient reduces tension at one level, the monitor will be reset to the next higher sensitivity. With each level, decreasing the tone becomes more challenging.

As with temperature training, we utilize instructions to assist the patient in discovering how to relax the frontalis muscle and the other target muscle groups just described. It is first suggested to the patient that he learn to identify certain tensor points in his face, neck, and shoulder areas while the monitor is giving biofeedback signals. Certain progressive relaxation exercises adopted from the work of Joseph Wolpe are given to the patient to help him identify these points. The following are some of the key instructions we give:

Let all your muscles go loose and heavy. . . . Just settle settle back quietly and comfortably. . . . Wrinkle up your forehead now, wrinkle it up tight; now smooth it out. . . . Picture your entire forehead and scalp becoming smoother, as the relaxation increases and spreads. . . . Now frown and crease your brow; study the tension. . . . Let go of the tension again, smooth out your forehead once more. . . . Now, close your eyes tighter and tighter; feel the tension. . . . Now relax your eyes. . . . Keep your eyes closed, gently, comfortably, and notice the relaxation. . . . Now clench your jaws, bite your teeth together, study the tension throughout your jaws. . . . Relax your jaws now; let your lips part slightly; appreciate the relaxation. . . . Now press your tongue hard against the roof of your mouth; look for the tension. . . . Now let your tongue return to a comfortable and relaxed position. . . . Now press your lips together, tighter and tighter. . . . Now relax your lips; notice the contrast between tension and relaxation. . . . Feel the relaxation all over your face, all over your forehead and scalp, eyes, jaws, lips, tongue, and your neck muscles. . . . Press your head back as far as it can go and feel the tension in your neck. . . . Roll it to the right and feel the tension shift. . . . Now roll it to the left. . . . Straighten your head and bring it forward and press your chin against your chest. . . . Now let your head return to a comfortable relaxed position. . . . Study the relaxation. . . . Let the relaxation develop. . . . Now shrug your shoulders tight, right up. . . . Hold the tension, hold it. . . . Now drop your shoulders and feel the relaxation; neck and shoulders relaxed. . . . Shrug your shoulders again and move them around. Bring your shoulders up, forward and back. . . . Now let them relax and feel the relaxation.

These exercises are to be practiced at home, twice daily, although, as already mentioned, they are to be done without biofeedback instrumentation. If the patient is also receiving temperature biofeedback training, he is told to practice the EMG exercises after the temperature training. There is a tendency for the hands to become warmer during progressive relaxation training; therefore, to do these exercises before working with temperature biofeedback would tend to diminish the effect of focused hand-warming procedures. As with temperature control, many patients have noted a decrease in the severity of their headaches when they practice the progressive relaxation exercises at the first symptoms.

In the clinic, patients do not go through progressive relaxation exercises while on the monitor. Instead, when receiving biofeedback they are told to stay as quiet as possible and to keep their eyes closed. Warnings are given to the patient that sudden eye movement, swallowing, and taking a deep breath will tend to increase the tone,

but it should decrease quickly. Since many patients are found to be teeth grinders or have an excess of tension in the jaws, we suggest that they open their mouths slightly while on the monitor, keeping their lower jaw loose and limp. If this decreases the tone, they are to practice this exercise several times during the day.

Another suggestion is to move the head forward so that the chin rests on the chest. If this process decreases the sound of the biofeedback signal, the patient has tension in the neck. This is often observed in patients with muscle contraction headache. The patient may be more successful in training if not in a reclining position. Pressure on the neck may be alleviated if the patient sits upright in a straight-back chair.

At home, the patient continues to practice progressive relaxation. We preferred that he record these exercises on tape. Home use of the exercises and clinical sessions on the EMG monitor assist the patient in recognizing stress points. In addition to teeth grinding, patients often identify jaw clenching, tightening of the forehead, wrinkling of the brow, obvious tension in the neck, and tightening of the shoulders as common stress points. By learning to relax these points under times of stress, at the first symptoms of headaches, and at bedtime, patients have noticed a reduction in the severity of their headaches. They are told to do exercises immediately before bedtime to avoid early awakening with headaches.

Patients make two or three clinic visits per week during the first month, with the visits gradually decreasing from then on. Again, intensive training is given to out-of-town patients twice daily. Regression in training pattern or increased stress in their home or working situation would probably necessitate an increase in visits. To record the progress of patients, a daily chart (Fig. 3-5) is kept, noting frequency, severity, and duration of headaches. If there has been a pattern in the patient's progress with biofeedback, the first step has been to decrease

HEADACHE CALENDAR

PATIENT'S NAME: _____

DATE STARTED: _____

DATE	TIME	SEVERITY OF HEADACHE	MEDICATION FOR PAIN	DOSE	RELIEF

1. Record all headaches:
   SEVERE   -- Incapacitating, unable to carry on with every-day duties
   MODERATE -- Annoying but not incapacitating
   MILD   -- Able to carry on with normal duties
   NONE   -- Free from headache

2. Record any medication taken for headache and the amount taken.

3. Record relief from headache pain:
   COMPLETE   -- Free from pain
   ALMOST COMPLETE -- Pain present but not disturbing patient
   MODERATE   -- Has discomfort but not as severe as prior to
                                        taking medication
   SLIGHT   -- Minimal improvement of questionable significance
   NONE   -- No relief

4. Time: A.M., P.M., or NITE

Fig. 3-5. Headache calendar.

the severity of the headaches themselves. This probably results from the EMG training. We hypothesize that if patients relax at the time of a headache and do not tense obvious stress points, the headaches are not as severe. If patients are diligent in practicing the temperature and EMG exercises, they will notice a decrease in the frequency of their headaches. Often, the more severe headache, the migraine, will occur on rare occasions, but many patients will complain that their milder headaches become more frequent. What seems to be happening, in reality, is that the migraine has masked the muscle contraction headache, and when the severe type disappears, the milder form draws more attention. When the patient has mastered hand temperature control, he is usually able to abort migraine headaches. If the patient warms his hands at the first symptoms of a headache, he is usually able to stop it. In many cases, all symptoms will then disappear.

The role of the therapist or the technician is a focal one in the training program, and it must be emphasized. On the first visit the therapist explains the goals of biofeedback training. This is extremely important for establishing the correct cognitive orientation of the patient. The therapist also instructs the patient in the use of the temperature or the EMG trainer. At this visit, a one-to-one relationship is established between therapist and patient.

On follow-up visits, the therapist should report any problems to the physician. This is extremely important to keep in close touch with the patient's progress. The therapist also plays a key role by encouraging the patient, emphasizing and praising all progress, and helping to stimulate motivation. This is a key part in any effective therapy program.

Goals are not generalized, with the training continued on an individual basis. External factors affecting training are identified. For example, patients may be told that warm hands presession may result in a small increase on the temperature monitor. The patients are assisted in recognizing stress points and any patterns in headaches and in reviewing and redesigning biofeedback techniques. All of these functions require careful diligent attention from the therapist. Obviously, the attitude of the therapist can affect the patient's success. A relaxed manner is necessary with patients along with confidence in the use of various instruments. Flexibility in the various

techniques will help in each patient's therapy. Firmness is also required with the patients in stressing home practice and in maintaining high motivational levels.

Despite substantial success with our clinical biofeedback program, I must admit that our expectations have not been fully achieved. Two problems intrude more frequently than we would like. First, too many patients become lax in their daily practice. Again, encouragement is vital with each patient, whether it involves noting progress on a monitor or advising the patient of certain factors that may be detrimental. The therapist must provide the patient with clear, reasonable guidelines. Second, some patients who perform well in the clinic do not exhibit full carryover of their nascent skills to in vivo situations. This may be caused by the fact that, in the clinic, the patient is removed from the normal environment and has not been trained to cope with it as well as if he had received the therapy at home.

This same sort of rationale can be used to explain the differential success we have noted in our out-of-town patients. As explained earlier, our out-of-town patients receive a more intensive form of biofeedback therapy than the routine therapy given to our local patients. We have observed a marked contrast between patients' success during training and follow-up visits. These patients experienced a restful 2 weeks during their initial training period. Problems at work and home were ignored, since they were on a "therapeutic vacation." On their return home, they were faced with the same environment. They returned to the clinic with reports of no change in their headaches and decreasing abilities on the temperature trainer. The patients also became lax in practicing their autogenic exercises. Their activity at home greatly differed from the rigid practice schedule they maintained while at the clinic. Thus, even though the more intensive form of therapy is excellent for learning biofeedback training, there is a major problem in incorporating this training into everyday life, which is the ultimate goal of the treatment. The optimal solution would be to make biofeedback therapy more readily available in various clinics around the country. It is my hope that this will occur as the apparent benefits of biofeedback training in the treatment of headache are realized.

In summary, I have been impressed with the effectiveness of biofeedback despite the fact that originally I had serious reservations toward its usefulness with headache patients. Long-term retrospective analysis of our results have shown biofeedback as a valuable tool in helping difficult headache problems. As a learning technique it has proved of help to me with a great number of my most difficult patients.

ACUPUNCTURE

Probably one of the most controversial subjects to appear in the field of medicine in the past 10 or more years is acupuncture. Much has appeared in the literature claiming good results with the use of acupuncture in the field of anesthesia and analgesia. However, an equal number of articles can be found disproving the use of acupuncture for either or both of these two purposes. Still another large group of investigators will conclude that they are not sure of its value. So, for this reason, the role of acupuncture in anesthesia or analgesia is quite controversial.

Acupuncture is claimed by some investigators to be a successful form of prophylactic treatment of migraine. Most experts in the headache field, however, do not consider acupuncture to be effective for this type of treatment.

The exact origin of acupuncture is not known, but it is believed that it started in China during the Stone Age. Actually the early needles used in acupuncture were made of bone, bamboo, or stone. It was not until about 12 B.C. that bronze needles were tried. Iron was initially tried about the year 6 B.C. At one time or another needles made of gold and of silver were used. According to Chinese literature Pien Chueh, a rather

famous Chinese physician who lived around 5 B.C., is called the "Father of Acupuncture."

In order to understand acupuncture, the so-called meridian concept must be known. According to the Chinese theories, the chi flows from organ to organ and to all parts of the body through a network of subcutaneous channels called ching-lo or meridians. The ching are the larger of the two and run vertically. The lo are smaller and run horizontally, they are actually branches of the ching. Thus the ching-lo connects all the organs and various forms of tissue of the body structure. It is the ching-lo, according to the Chinese, that regulates all body functions and pathology. There are twelve principle meridian periods, and their pathways alternate from one meridian to another, each meridian period being 2 hours; so the circulation through the entire twelve meridians requires 24 hours for completion.

In relation to the theory of meridians, Lee[78] believes that the head is an area where three yang meridians anastomose to each other. Each meridian has its own pathway that occupies a certain area on the head. The yang equilibrium meridian is located on the front part of the head; the yang minimum meridian is on the lateral side, while the yang maximum meridian occupies the parietal and occipital area of the head. Vertex headache represents ailments of the conception vessel and "foot yin" equilibrium meridian or liver meridian. Headaches are known as referred pain, which may have intracranial origin. Experimentally, pain caused by intracranial stimulation is referred to a certain area of the head. Stimulation of pain receptors in the intracranial vault above the tentorium, including the upper surface of the tentorium itself, causes referred headache anterior to the ear, which is called frontal headache. Pain impulse from subtentorium causes is termed "occipital headache." This theory of meridians is quite acceptable for its close interrelationship with the different innervation of areas on the head.

Lee states that headache can also be classified by external and internal origin. The external causes consist of any alteration of the external environment related to the physiology and pathophysiology of the human body. The internal causes consist of headaches resulting usually from liver, spleen, and renal diseases, but they may be caused by imbalance of chi and blood. This type of headache is more likely to result from migraine, hypertension, neurasthenia, sinusitis, cerebral concussion, and diseases caused by intoxication. Headaches of internal cause may be put into four categories: (1) "excess of liver fire," (2) deficiency of kidneys, (3) phlegm obstruction, and (4) deficiency of blood and chi.

The Chinese theory of medicine is based on the flow through the body of the life energy (called chi) and blood. The blood nourishes the chi, which enters the body at birth and leaves at death. This comes from the Taoist Chinese philosophies. Further, the Taoist theory of universal opposites is present throughout nature, yin being the negative and yang being the positive in all concepts. It is between this yin and yang that the major body organs are divided. The yin (negative) group of organs is comprised of the liver, spleen, lungs, heart, kidneys, and tissues covering these organs. The yang (positive) group of organs is composed of the stomach, gallbladder, urinary bladder, small and large intestines, and the body cavity containing these organs. The negative or yin group of organs belong to the tsang or solid organs. Their function is to protect and maintain the body. The positive or yang group belong to the fu or hollow organs, and their function is to receive, digest, and excrete food. Together they both regulate the body functions. We thus have the tsang-fu concept.

According to Chinese medical theories the etiology of any disease is divided into either internal or external causes. The internal causes are generated from within the body. The external causes include

changes in the external environment and related physiology and pathology. Together these are called Hsieh-chi or devil energy.

The Chinese use four principal methods for diagnosis: (1) "wun" or inquiry (history), (2) "wang" or examination, (3) "wen" or hearing, and (4) "chieh" or pulse diagnosis.

Kim[79] advocates acupuncture in the treatment of migraine. He says that acupuncture triggers a series of local events, liberating histamine, serotonin, bradykinin, and prostaglandins, which alter the permeability of cell membranes. The products of tissue injury in turn initiate a chain of events leading to increased secretion of corticosteroids via a corticotrophin-releasing factor and corticotrophin (ACTH). The corticosteroids exert an antiinflammatory effect, which stabilizes the cranial blood vessels to the action of vasoactive substances in the blood. These effects will be provoked locally by any type of tissue damage and are not specific for acupuncture injury. Kim believes that acupuncture leads to a specific release of corticosteroids or that specific steroids are produced by stimulation of the major acupuncture points. He believes that acupuncture stimulation produces local vasoconstriction, which may produce a specific vasoconstriction of the cerebral vessels or a similar effect via the autonomic nervous system, thereby relieving the headache.

Kajdos[80] also discusses the use of acupuncture in the role of prophylactic treatment of headache. He states that for the purpose of acupuncture most cases of migraine can be classified into three groups by palpation of the radial pulses. These groups are named after the pulses most affected—kidney, stomach, and gallbladder migraines. The "kidney type" of migraine consists of a dull prodromal pain within and between the eyes and an urge to urinate. Changes in the weather are activating factors. The patient may show "an inclination to edema." Following these prodromal features, the pain often starts abruptly, mostly behind the eyes. The "gallbladder type" of migraine has characteristically prodromal symptoms of nausea and flatulence. The headache is unilateral. In the "stomach type" of migraine prodromal symptoms of yawning, anorexia, and dull epigastric pain occur. The headache is confined to both temporal areas and the forehead.

Kajdos presents a series of 309 patients (209 women and 100 men) who were treated for headaches of various types using these techniques. Of these, 136 (44%) responded very well to treatment: after eight to ten sessions the headaches disappeared completely (or almost completely). Another 128 patients (42%) showed considerable improvement but were not completely headache-free. Forty-five (14%) showed no improvement.

Bischko[81] finds that the therapy of acupuncture for migraine is very individual and quite complex, but he claims the rate of effectiveness to be high.

Pontinen and Salmela[82] say that the response during acute attacks differs from that of prophylactic interval treatment. Needling of local tender points provides a poor and short effect. During an acute attack it is sometimes necessary to start needling from the symptomless side to avoid aggravation of symptoms. The interval treatment can be based on standard schemes including both local and segmental or distal points. At the beginning the patients were treated once weekly. The treatment schedule was then changed because some patients not reacting to therapy given at weekly intervals responded well when treated at shorter intervals of two to three sessions during the first week. The needling is then repeated once monthly. Patients not responding to standardized therapy are asked to return during an acute attack in order to find the most effective points. Their schedule is then based on these points.

Johannsson and associates[83] conducted a double-blind study using acupuncture in chronic tension headache. The patients were randomized in two groups. One group of eighteen patients was treated with traditional acupuncture combined with electroacupuncture, according to the acupuncturist's judgment. The other group, consisting of fifteen patients, was treated with placebo acupuncture, that is, the needles were placed some centimeters from the traditional acupuncture points. The patients were informed that two different acupuncture methods would be used but they did not know by which method they were treated. Each patient was given ten treatments distributed over two periods. Each period consisted of five treatments given during 1 week. The interval between the periods of treatment was 4 weeks. The patients recorded their headaches for about 60 days after the first treatment was given. Good results were noted among the patients who were treated with traditional acupuncture. A corresponding overrepresentation of less good results was noted among the patients treated with placebo acupuncture.

Subjective improvement was experienced by ten of eighteen patients in the group treated with traditional acupuncture and by seven of fifteen patients treated with placebo acupuncture. The consumption of analgesics was not significantly different between the two groups. No significant difference regarding the different psychologic variables was observed between patients with traditional acupuncture and placebo acupuncture or between improved and unimproved patients. Johannsson and coworkers concluded that the comparison between traditional acupuncture and pacebo acupuncture for treatment of chronic tension headache revealed significantly better results when traditional acupuncture was used. No connection could be demonstrated between the effect of treatment and suggestibility.

Okazaki and co-workers[84] advocate Ryodoraku therapy for migraine headache relief. This stands for good electroconductive lineage system. Age or sex of the patients does not affect the outcome of the treatment. Within a treatment category, longer duration of symptoms appeared to give poorer results. The number of treatments and the number of points treated showed a direct positive relationship to good subjective responses. The three patients treated by general regulating point therapy alone had uniformly poor results. General regulating points and reactive electropermeable point treatment also yielded good to excellent responses. The group with the most extensive therapy showed a preponderance of excellent results. Usually, the patients who reported good or excellent results were able to decrease their analgesic intakes significantly.

In the study fifteen out of twenty patients showed good to excellent responses to the therapy. Since all of the patients did not respond to conventional medical remedies, the results obtained suggests that Ryodoraku therapy is a worthwhile technique to try on migraine headaches. It also appears that a combination of the therapies, such as general regulating points and reactive electropermeable points, produce better effects. although placebo effect cannot be entirely ruled out.

Lee and associates[85] performed 979 acupuncture treatments in 261 patients with chronic pain. A substantial number of patients stated that they had relief immediately following a series of four acupuncture treatments. It did not matter whether the needles were placed in the traditional meridian locations or in arbitrary fixed control points. Four weeks following treatment, 65% of the patients reported little or no reduction in the intensity of their pain, 17% reported a 50% reduction, and 18% at least a 75% reduction.

Cheng[86] studied the use of acupuncture in headache problems. Thirty-three patients were treated by acupuncture using body loci, ear points, and electrical stimulation. Sixteen patients suffered from migraines, twelve from tension headaches, two from cluster headaches, one from vascular head-

aches, and two patients from headaches whose etiology was uncertain. The patients received from three to sixteen treatments. Of the thirty-three patients, five had only three treatments and ten had five or fewer. Eighteen patients had good results—no headache at all. Twelve patients had fair results; that is, they sometimes had headaches, but they could be controlled with a few repetitions of treatment or by analgesics at a lesser dosage than they were taking at the beginning of treatments. Three patients had no response at all or poor results; however, these discontinued treatment before it could be evaluated whether they were actually absolute no-response cases. Of the thirty-three patients, two had a good response after only two treatments; four had a good response after ten treatments. However, most of the patients had a good response after six to eight treatments. A course of treatment usually required ten to fourteen visits before definitive evaluation of the results could be made.

Lee and co-workers[87] believe that neither the mechanism of chronic pain nor the mechanism of acupuncture is fully understood. Thus, treating chronic pain with acupuncture is analogous to a blind person riding a blind horse. Yet there are numerous testimonials of acupuncture therapy relieving the pain of low back discomfort, arthritis, neuralgia, and headache. Of the 533 patients treated, all had been treated previously with drugs and many had been treated surgically. When pain persisted, patients sought acupuncture as an alternative to conventional modes of therapy. While 52% of patients reported at least 75% relief of pain immediately after their last acupuncture treatment, pain returned to many. However, 4 weeks later, 19.3% of patients still had excellent pain relief. These researchers question whether the results of their study represented the results of acupuncture or the results of counterstimulation. They point out that their study was not designed to offer an explanation of the mechanism by which the patients obtained pain relief. However, they did attempt to study the placebo effect by placing needles in other than the traditional meridians. This portion of their study suggests that electric stimulation at traditional meridians was unimportant. However, if the effectiveness of therapy results from counterstimulation, this, too, would be produced by the electric stimulation of the needles in the arbitrary control points. Thus, it was impossible for them to separate a placebo effect from this mechanism.

Leung and associates[88] tested acupuncture in neuralgia of the head and neck, migraine, and trigeminal neuraglia; they report 45% of the patients either had partial or complete relief from the painful attacks.

Chiu and Derrick[89] believe that while some cases of headache may be relieved by acupuncture, continued observation of the patient is essential to detect new disorders totally unrelated to the original condition.

Laitinen[90] studied the use of acupuncture in thirty-nine migraine patients. The acupuncture technique involved needling the acupuncture locus B1-2 in the medial corner of the eyebrow to achieve relief of pain. Locus L1-4, situated dorsally between the first and second metacarpal bones, was also needled to achieve "balance" in the mascular tonus of the head. Each needle was manipulated at 5-minute intervals for 20 minutes. No electric stimulation was used. Laitinen concluded that all patients showed initial improvement, but only five patients were improved after 6 months. He points out that the study does not exclude the possibility that the results may be caused by the power of suggestion.

The possible explanation of the mode of action of acupuncture is actually still a mystery. The traditional Chinese theory presents no scientific evidence. Hypnosis, autosuggestion, and cultural background may play some role. The magnetic theory states that the meridians are the lines of force around a magnet, and acupuncture induces all electric discharge of the condenser and intervenes in the magnetic force. Believers in the humoral theory state that pinprick releases cortisone, histamine, or catecholamine. Neutral theory is more likely the basis for acupuncture, although we do not know all the pain mechanisms.

Acupuncture may be of benefit in the field of headache therapy; however, as yet, it has not been successfully found to produce good enough results to warrant its inclusion in the physician's armamentarium for this condition.

REFERENCES

1. Horton, B. T., Ryan, R. E., and Reynolds. J. L.: Clinical observations on the use of E.C.-110, a new agent for the treatment of headache, Proc. Staff Meet. Mayo Clin. **23:**105, 1948.
2. Ryan, R. E.: Fiorinal for symptomatic treatment of nonvascular headache, Med. Times **80:**291, 1952.
3. Ryan, R. E.: A new agent for the treatment of migraine and histaminic cephalalgia, J. Missouri Med. Assoc. **48:**963, 1951.
4. Johnson, A. S.: headaches of medical practice, N. Engl. J. Med. **252:**101, 1955.
5. Cronk, G. A.: Laboratory and clinical studies with buffered and nonbuffered acetysalicylic acid, N. Engl. J. Med. **258:**219, 1958.
6. Batterman, R. C.: Comparison of buffered and unbuffered acetylsalicylic acid, N. Engl. J. Med. **258:**213, 1958.
7. Segaert, M., Michielsen, P., Verberckmoes, R., and Vandenbroucke, J.: Abuse of phenacetin-containing preparations, Acad. Ziekenh St. Rafael, Leuven T. Geneesk. **26**(18):891, 1970.
8. Prescott, L. F.: Analgesic drugs and renal damage, Lancet **2:**91, 1965.
9. Clausen, E., and Harvald, B.: Nephrotoxicity of analgesics, Acta Med. Scand. **170:**469, 1961.
10. Scott, J. T., Denman, A. M., and Dorling, J.: Renal irritation caused by salicylates, Lancet **1:** 344, 1963.
11. Berde, B.: Some new vascular and biochemical aspects of the mechanism of action of ergot compounds, Headache **11**(4):139, 1972.
12. Hilton, B. P., and Zilkhak, J.: Effects of ergotamine and methysergide of blood platelet aggregation responses of migrainous subjects, J. Neurol. Neurosurg. Psychiat. **37**(5):593, 1974.
13. Hilton, B. P., and Cummings, J. N.: Hydroxytryptamine levels and platelet aggregation responses in subjects with acute migraine headache, J. Neurol. Neurosurg. Psychiat. **35**(4):505, 1972.
14. Muller-Schweinitzer, E.: Comparative studies on the mode of action of ergotamine in canine and human arteries. In Headache—new vistas, Florence, Italy, 1977, Biomedical Press, p. 75.
15. Saxena, P. R., and Vlaam-Schluter, G. M.: Role of

some biogenic substances in migraine and relevant mechanism in antimigraine action of ergotamine—studies in an experimental model for migraine, Headache **13**:143, 1974.

16. Friedman, A. P.: Review of the headache problem, Am. Pract. **1**:948, 1950.

17. Ryan, R. E.: Cafergot for relief of headache—a further study, J. Missouri Med. Assoc. **47**:107, 1950.

18. Chaqual, M., and Cartier, P.: Ergotism: case report: "mal des ardents," Union Med. Can. **103**(1): 85, 1974.

19. Bollinger, A., and Preter, B.: Spasm of limb arteries due to ergotamine tartrate, Deutsch. Med. Wochenschr. **98**:825-829, 1973.

20. McLoughlin, M. G., and Sanders, R. J.: Ergotism causing peripheral vascular ischemia, Rocky Mt. Med. J. **69**(2):45, 1972.

21. Brinc, L., and Hjeltnes, J.: Ergotamine as a cause of arterial insufficiency, Tidsskr. Nor. Laegeforen. **94**(28):1906, 1974.

22. Imrie, C. W.: Arterial spasm associated with oral ergotamine therapy, Br. J. Clin. Pract. **27**(12):457, 1973.

23. Reus, H. D.: Angiography in a case of ergotism, Herz. Kreislauf **5**(12):510, 1973.

24. Carliner, N. H., Denune, D. P., Finch, C. S., Jr., and Goldberg, L. I.: J.A.M.A. **227**(3):308, 1974.

25. Kramer, R. A., Hecker, S. P., and Lewis, B. I.: Ergotism: report of a case studied arteriographically, Radiology **84**:308, 1965.

26. Horton, B. T., and Peters, G. A.: Clinical manifestations of excessive use of ergotamine preparations and management of withdrawal effect: report of 52 cases, Headache **2**:214, 1963.

27. Andersson, P. G.: Ergotamine, Headache **15**:118, 1975.

28. Roswell, A. R., Neylan, C., and Wilkinson, M.: Ergotamine-induced headaches in migrainous patients, Headache **13**(2):65, 1973.

29. Friedman, A. P., and von Storch, T. J. C.: Ergotamine tolerance in patients with migraine, J.A.M.A. **157**:881, 1955.

30. Wolfson, W. Q., and Graham, J. R.: Development of tolerance to ergot alkaloids in a patient with unusually severe migraine, N. Engl. J. Med. **241**: 296, 1949.

31. Thonnard-Neumann, E., and Taylor, W. L.: The basophilic leukocyte and migraine, Headache **8**: 98, 1968.

32. Thonnard-Neumann, E.: Some interrelationships of vasoactive substances and basophilic leukocytes in migraine headaches, Headache **9**:130, 1969.

33. Thonnard-Neumann, E.: Heparin in migraine headache, Headache **13**:49, 1973.

34. Thonnard-Neumann, E.: Migraine therapy with heparin: pathophysiologic basis, Headache **16**: 284, 1977.

35. Aldrich, C. K.: Psychiatry for the family physi-

cian, New York, 1955, McGraw-Hill Book Co., p. 143.

36. Buson, P. B., and McDermott, W.: Textbook of medicine, Philadelphia, 1967, W. B. Saunders Co., p. 1450.

37. Quatsil, J. H.: Respiration in the central nervous system, Phys. Rev. **19**:135, 1939.

38. Heinbecker, P., and Bartly, S. H.: Action of ether and nembutal on the nervous system, J. Neurophysiol. **3**:219, 1940.

39. Thesleff, S.: The effect of anesthetic agents on skeletal muscle membranes, Acta Physiol. Scand. **37**:335, 1956.

40. Exley, K. A.: Depression of autonomic ganglia by barbiturates, Br. J. Pharmacol. Chemother. **9**:170, 1954.

41. Wikler, A.: Effects of morphine, Nembutal, ether, and eserine on the neuron and multi-neuron reflexes, Proc. Soc. Biol. Med. **58**:193, 1945.

42. Dejours, P.: Chemoreflexes in breathing, Physiol. Rev., pp. 86-102, 1962.

43. Price, H. L., and others: Effect of sodium thiopental on circulatory response to positive pressure inflation of lungs, J. Appl. Physiol. **4**:629, 1952.

44. Rosenblum, M. J., and Cummins, A. J.: The effect of sleep and of amytal on the motor activity of the human sigmoid colon, Gastroenterology **27**:445, 1954.

45. Sessions, J. T., Jr., and others: The effect of barbiturates in patients with liver disease, J. Clin. Invest. **33**:1116, 1954.

46. Delay, J., and Dericker, P.: Utilization of psychiatric therapy of the phenothiazines central elective action, Ann. Med. Physiol. **110**:112, 1952.

47. Link, M.: Significance of EEG pattern changes in physiopharmacology, Electroencephalogr. Clin. Neurophysiol. **11**:398, 1959.

48. Dobskin, A. B., and others: Physiological effects of chlorpromazine, Anesthesia **9**:157, 1954.

49. Gaunt, R., and others: Interactions of drugs with endocrines, Ann. Rev. Pharmacol. **3**:109, 1963.

50. Lehmann, H. E.: Use and abuse of phenothiazines, Appl. Ther. **5**:1057, 1963.

51. Hollister, L. E.: Allergy to chlorpromazine manifested by jaundice, Am. J. Med. **23**:870, 1957.

52. Ayd, F. J., Jr.: A critical appraisal of chlordiazepoxide, J. Neurophyschiatr. **3**:177, 1962.

53. Bulla, J. D., and others: Further controlled studies of meprobamate, Am. Pract. Dig. Treat. **10**:1961, 1959.

54. Uhr, L., and others: Behavioral effects of chronic administration of psychoactive drugs to anxious patients, Psychopharmacologia **1**:150, 1959.

55. Hollister, L. E., and others: Meprobamate in chronic psychiatric patients, Ann. N.Y. Acad. Sci. **67**:789, 1957.

56. Randall, L. O., and others: Pharmacology of methaminodiazepoxide, Dir. Nerv. System, **27**:7, 1961.

57. Cook, L., and Kelleher, R. T.: Effects of drugs

on behavior, Ann. Rev. Pharmacol. **3**:205, 1963.

58. Domino, E. F.: Human pharmacology of tranquilizer drugs, Clin. Pharmacol. Ther. **3**:599, 1962.

59. Payne, R. W., and others: Diazepam, meprobamate, and placebo in musculo-skeletal disorders, J.A.M.A. **88**:229, 1964.

60. Zbiden, G., and others: Experimental and clinical toxicology of chlordiazepoxide, Toxicol. Appl. Pharmacol. **3**: 619, 1961.

61. Randall, L. O., and others: Pharmacological and clinical studies of Valium, a new agent of the benzodiazepine class, Curr. Ther. Rev. **3**: 405, 1961.

62. Dorfman, F.: Clinical experience with amitriptyline, Psychosomatics **1**:153, 1960.

63. Baisa, J. A., and Saunders, J. C.: Amitriptyline, and new antidepressant, Am. J. Psychiatr. **117**: 739, 1967.

64. Ayd, F. J., Jr.: Toxic somatic and psychopathologic reactions to antidepressant drugs, J. Neuropsychiatr. **2**:119, 1961.

65. Gault, J. E.: Agranulocytosis due to amitriptyline, Lancet **2**:44, 1963.

66. Coffee, E. J.: Combined amitriptyline and perphenazine in combined depression and anxiety, J. Med. Assoc. Georgia **53**:107, 1964.

67. Schultz, J. H., and Luthe, W.: Autogenic training: a physiologic approach in psychotherapy, New York, 1959, Grune & Stratton, Inc.

68. Jacobson, E.: You must relax, New York, 1934, McGraw-Hill Book Co.

69. Kamiya, J.: Conditioned discrimination of the EEG alpha rhythm in humans, paper presented at the meeting of the Western Psychological Association, San Francisco, April, 1962.

70. Green, E.: The varieties of healing experience: exploring psychic phenomena in healing, a transcript from the Interdisciplinary Symposium of October 30, 1971.

71. Sterman, M. B., Lopresti, R. W., and Fairchild, M. D.: Electroencephalographic and behavior studies of monomethylhydrozine toxicity in the cat, Ann. N.Y. Acad. Sci. **26**:407-408, 1969.

72. Mulholland, T.: The automatic control of visual displays by the attention of the human viewers, Proceedings of 1969 Conference on Visual Literacy, New York, 1970, Pitman.

73. Forster, M., Booker, H., and Ansel, S.: Computer automation of the conditioning therapy of stroboscopic induced seizures, Trans. Am. Neurol. Assoc. **91**:232-233, 1966.

74. Banuazzizi, A., and Miller, N.: Instrumental learning by curarized rats of a specific visceral response, intestinal or cardiac, J. Comp. Physiol. Psychol. **68**:1-7, 1968.

75. Sargent, J., Green, E. E., and Walters, E. D.: The use of autogenic feedback training in a pilot study of migraine and tension headaches, Headache **12**:120-124, 1972.

76. Wolpe, J., and Lazarus, A. A.: Behavior therapy techniques, New York, 1966, Pergamon Press.

77. Budzynski, T. H., Stoyva, J., and Adler, C. S.: Feedback induced muscle relaxation: application to tension headache, Behav. Ther. Exper. Psychiatry **1**:1970.

78. Lee, G. T. C.: Treatment of headache employing acupuncture, Am. J. Chin. Med. **2**:341, 1974.

79. Kim, S. S.: Acupuncture: mode of action in migraine headache, Am. J. Acupunct. **3**:108, 1975.

80. Kajdos, V.: The acupuncture treatment of headaches, Am. J. Acupunct. **3**:34, 1975.

81. Bischko, J.: Akupunktur bei Kopfschmerzen, Migraine Symposium, Innsbruck, Austria, May, 1974, p. 272.

82. Pontinen, P. J., and Salmela, T. M.: Acupuncture treatment of migraine, Scandinavian Migraine Symposium, 1969.

83. Johannsson, V., Kosic, S., Lindahl, O., Lindwall, L., Link, H., and Astrom, J.: Acupuncture and chronic tension headache, a "double blind trial," Bergen Migraine Symposium, June, 1975, pp. 42-44.

84. Okazaki, K., Sadove, M. S., Kim, S. I., Lee, M. H., and Cheng, D.: Ryodoraku therapy for migraine headache, Am. J. Chin. Med. **3**:61, 1975.

85. Lee, P. K., Andersen, T. W., Modell, J. H., and Saga, S. A.: Treatment of chronic pain with acupuncture, J.A.M.A. **232**:1113, 1975.

86. Cheng, A. C. K.: The treatment of headaches employing acupuncture, Am. J. Chin. Med. **3**:181, 1975.

87. Lee, P. K. Y., Modell, J. H., Andersen, T. W., and Saga, S. A.: Incidence of prolonged pain relief following acupuncture, Anesth. Analg. **53**:229, 1976.

88. Leung, S. J., Fan, C., and Seehzer, P. H.: Acupuncture therapeutics, Anesth. Analg. **53**:942, 1974.

89. Chiu, W. J., and Derrick, W. S.: Acupuncture indication, techniques, and preliminary clinical result, Texas Med. **71**:66, 1975.

90. Laitinen, J.: Acupuncture for migraine prophylaxis: a prospective clinical study with six months' follow-up, Am. J. Chin. Med. **3**:271, 1975.

SUGGESTED READINGS

Appenzeller, O.: Pathogenesis and treatment of headache, New York, 1976, Spectrum Publications, Inc.

Biofeedback in action, Medical World News, March 19, 1973.

Bonica, J. J., and Fordyce, W. F.: Operant conditioning for chronic pain. In Bonica, J. J., Procacci, P., and Pagni, C. A., editors: Recent advances on pain, pathophysiology and clinical aspects, Springfield, Ill., 1974, Charles C Thomas, Publisher.

Brown, B. B.: New mind, new body—biofeedback: new directors for the mind, New York, 1974, Harper & Row, Publishers.

Diamond, S.: Biofeedback—new and promising, Consultant **15:**2, 1975.

Diamond, S.: Biofeedback therapy with electronic teaching aids, Patient Care, August, 1975.

Diamond, S., and Dalessio, D. J.: The practicing physician's approach to headache, Baltimore, 1973, The Williams & Wilkins Co.

Diamond, S., and Franklin, M.: Intensive biofeedback therapy in the treatment of headache, presented at 6th Annual Meeting of Biofeedback Research Society, February, 1975.

Diamond, S., and Franklin, M.: Biofeedback—choice of treatment in childhood migraine, presented at 7th Annual Meeting of Biofeedback Research Society, February, 1976.

Diamond, S., and Franklin, M.: Autogenic training and biofeedback techniques in the treatment of chronic headache problems, Proceedings of Third World Congress of International Congress of Psychosomatic Medicine, 1977.

Diamond, S., and Franklin, M.: Autogenic training with biofeedback in the treatment of children with migraine, Proceedings of Third World Congress of International Congress of Psychosomatic Medicine, 1977.

Medina, J. L., Diamond, S., and Franklin, M. A.: Biofeedback therapy for migraine, Headache **16**(3): 115-118, 1976.

Wickramasekera, I.: Electromyographic feedback training and tension headache: preliminary observations, Am. J. Clin. Hypnosis **15,** October, 1972.

CHAPTER 4

Vascular headaches: migraine

Migraine was initially described in the first century A.D. by Aretaeus of Cappadocia. In spite of the early description of migraine, the exact etiology and pathophysiology of the condition still remain unknown. However, within the past 20 years a great amount of investigational research has been done on this subject.

Probably one of the most common types of vascular headaches is migraine. Certainly more has been written about migraine than any other type of vascular head pain. Migraine is a disease of the civilized and is of a periodic nature. Many consider this condition to be far more prominent in the intellectual type of personality. It has been estimated that migraine is found in 8% to 12% of all the patients seen in general practice.

For years the complexity of symptoms in migraine has been known, and many physicians have spent their lives investigating this problem. Today, though the exact cause of migraine is still unknown, the mechanism that produces the head pain, which is its major symptom, has been determined. The preheadache scotomas and probably speech disorders, paresthesias, and confusion result from vasoconstriction of branches of the internal carotid arteries. The headache results from the distention of arteries, chiefly of the branches of the external carotid, and the traction exerted on the pain-sensitive structures surrounding these vessels. This pain is due to the pressure, and tension is then transmitted to consciousness by way of the fifth (trigeminal), ninth (glossopharyngeal), and tenth (vagus) cranial nerves and the upper three cervical nerves. The intramural and perimural edema of the dilated arteries helps to intensify the severity of the headache.

Sustained dilation may give rise to changes in the arterial walls and render them less responsive to treatment.

The vasoconstriction phase of migraine occurs in the early stages of the attack. The actual cause of this vasoconstriction is not known. When this occurs, disturbances in vision, mood, and sensorium are often noted. These symptoms are unpleasant but usually do not cause much discomfort to the patient. This vasoconstriction phase is then followed by a rather persistent arterial dilation that is associated with the throbbing and pulsating type of head pain seen in migraine.

Later in the attack, the walls of the affected cranial arteries become thickened. Because of edema, these arteries become rather rigid and pipe-like. At this stage, the pain changes into a steady ache, in place of the throbbing, pulsating type of pain originally present. This severe type of pain in

66

the cerebral area may possibly be followed by contractions of the skeletal muscles of the head and neck. This shows that another component is added to the picture. The pain produced by the contractions of the skeletal muscles of the neck and head often outlasts the original vascular pain. Quite frequently migraine patients will note that their severe head pain will finally terminate but that they have tenderness and soreness of the neck and back of the neck that may linger for several hours and that are greatly relieved by heat and massage.

Headache is the most common symptom of migraine and certainly its most distressing feature. Migraine is definitely a symptom complex in which various pathological processes initiate a final common mechanism. It is a condition that is closely simulated by other disorders of known etiology, and frequently its diagnosis may be one of exclusion. The history of each patient must be carefully considered as an individual entity.

In checking over any group of histories taken from migrainous patients, one inevitably concludes that the primary etiologic factor in migraine is not the same in all patients. Any sizable group of patients may be divided into several smaller groups, each showing a predominant type of pathology different from the other. Usually, one will find multiple contributory factors in each case.

Migraine is a symptom complex resulting from a cranial vascular dysfunction in part dependent on a hereditary factor initiated by various pathologic processes and complicated by the influence of multiple secondary abnormalities.

Migraine is one of the common diseases seen in medicine today, but the physician often fails to suspect what is wrong. As a result, the correct diagnosis is not made. The trouble often is that the migraine patient usually fails to tell his story properly. Quite often he may not say much about the headache but may dwell primarily on the gastrointestinal symptoms, such as nausea

or vomiting, or the distress and general fatigue that may follow the attack. Quite often this is the case because the patient has been led to believe that the headache phase of the condition is beyond medical help. Some people do not stress the headache phase of migraine because they are ashamed to complain of a headache; they concentrate on the other symptoms because of this false sense of modesty. These patients may therefore tell a story so vague, without even mentioning the headache attacks, that no physician could possibly make a diagnosis of migraine from their history. This is very unfortunate because the history of the patient is the most important factor in every case of migraine, insofar as making a diagnosis is concerned.

One of the main difficulties besetting the physician treating headache patients is the task of carefully separating a maze of symptoms and complaints into various clinical entities. This division is a necessity because no headache can be properly treated if it has not been properly diagnosed.

Migraine is the most common type of vascular headache known. Because of this, in any discussion of chronic headache, the subject of migraine will always be brought to the forefront.

Migraine is well known for its gastrointestinal symptoms and its pronounced systemic symptoms. It is especially familiar to the ophthalmologist because of its ocular manifestations. While the headache is only a part of the widespread systemic disturbance, it is the most prominent feature of the migraine attack. Because of this feature, the syndrome is known as migraine headache.

As a rule, migraine sufferers have a superiority complex. They are of a most ambitious, meticulous, hard-working class to whom no task is insurmountable; they pay strict attention to every minute detail of their appointed tasks. These people, even when experiencing the severe pain of their attacks, will try to carry out their usual daily work with the same detail and perfection that they exhibit when free from headache.

Most migraine patients are optimists. By this we mean they all have the hope that they will soon discover the cause and the cure of their attacks. Migraine patients are often what we refer to as perfectionists. Many of these people have a psychologic problem in connection with this perfectionist attitude. Many are unable to reach the perfection in their work that their nature demands. Some suffer from a lack of appreciation or approval by others. About the only cure for most of these perfectionists psychologically is for them to realize that perfection in their case is actually unattainable.

Each migraine patient has his own formula for obtaining relief; some patients use diet, others exercise, still others rest. Some are heat-conscious and with the approach of a headache attack they will pack their heads in hot, wet towels or electric heating pads. On the other hand, there are those who do the same thing with ice. Others have much more fantastic regimes which they go through with their attacks.

Some of these patients will tell the physician taking their case history that their headaches are so severe that they will commit suicide if something is not done to relieve them. Actually, however, this is not too much of a problem, because during the actual headache attack the patient is entirely too sick to make the necessary effort and when the patient is free from the attack he feels absolutely fine and healthy and does not think of such things as self-destruction. So, for these reasons, suicide is usually not a part of the picture of the average migraine case; but naturally, it may occur on rare occasions.

Most migraine patients have consulted several physicians about their attacks and most of them are rather discouraged with the results of their medical treatment. Many of them have received treatment that was valueless and generally worse than useless. However, their general optimistic outlook keeps them looking for something new and keeps their hopes alive.

ETIOLOGY

During the past 10 to 15 years there have been many papers presented in the medical literature concerning the etiology of migraine. Some of these theories are that migraine is caused by hormones and oral contraceptives, diet, tyramine, phenylethylamine, serotonin, amines, basophilic leukocytes and mast cells, genetics (family history), and prostaglandins. All of these theories will be fully discussed. Besides these factors, there are older theories, many of which no longer seem to be substantial. One theory that seems to fit into this category is the allergic theory.

Ostfeld and associates[1] report that localized edema accompanying vasodilation during vascular headache of the migraine type increases the severity of the headache. This local edema is due to the intracapillary pressure shift caused by vasodilation and is associated with a lowering of the deep pain thresholds. A substance apparently exists in the local fluid accumulation that damages tissue and lowers pain thresholds. They claim further that the nonlocalized edema associated with migraine appears during periods of increased alertness and driving activity and can be induced, in patients subject to the migraine type of headache, without inducing the headache itself. This can be abolished without preventing headache. Diffuse edema is not usually related to the migraine mechanism.

The generally accepted theory today is that of vasodilation of the branches of the external carotid arteries with the dural and cerebral arteries participating to a minor degree. The preheadache scotomas have been shown to be due to the vasoconstriction of the branches of the internal carotid artery, with resultant anoxia and distortion of occipital cortical function.[2] It is further believed that other symptoms, such as confusion, are also due to cerebrovascular constriction. The muscular tenderness of the scalp and neck results from the sustained contraction of the cervical and scalp muscles due to the underlying tension and the initial pain itself.[3]

All migraine patients have in common an excessive lability and hyperreactivity of the vascular system.

In regard to the etiology of migraine, King[4] states that the primary location of pain has been found to be in the sympathetic nerves accompanying the external head branches of the external carotid arteries. This theory has been brought forth by extensive research. In these research experiments, these branches of the external carotid have been found to become dilated, locally, through a lack of nerve control. It is the dilation of these arteries that is believed to be the factor producing pain in their accompanying vasomotor nerves. The local dilation or distention of these arteries is entirely dependent on conditions that react on the sympathetic nervous system and constitute the condition known as migraine.

There is also a theory concerned with the amount of fluid contained in the body tissue. Some have maintained that the pain is the result of an excess of fluid in the body tissues, which in turn raises the tension in the arteries. On the other hand, there are those who contend that the amount of fluid in the body tissues is diminished and that this results in the concentration of toxins in the bloodstream to the point where the system reacts with pain. These theories on the whole are generally discarded today.

Allergy

The claim that migraine is an allergic disease has been based on the facts that (1) migraine is found in many patients with allergic disturbances such as hay fever or asthma, (2) some observers have found that a large proportion of patients with migraine have positive skin reactions to some allergens, (3) some observers have cured migraine by prescribing a restricted diet, (4) recurring, sudden, unexplained attacks are typical of other manifestations of al-

lergy, and (5) some observers have found eosinophilia in several patients with migraine. None of these seems pertinent enough to classify migraine as an allergic disease. Most headache experts believe that migraine has absolutely nothing to do with allergy. Although an occasional patient might be allergic and also have migraine, such patients are relatively rare. It would seem, therefore, that it is a disservice to the migrainous patient to label him as allergic.

Hormones and oral contraceptives
HORMONES

The hormonal theory has always been one of the leading theories of the etiology of migraine. However, since the advent of "the pill," more interest has been aroused in regard to this theory than every before.

That migraine is predominantly seen in women (about 80% of the cases, conservatively) is a fact. That most, but not all, of these women patients most commonly associate their headaches with their menstrual period is also a fact. Most women will state that they can expect a headache just before, during, or at the end of their menstrual period. Many patients will complain that they also experience a headache attack commonly in the middle of their menstrual cycle. This tends to make one think that these attacks at the middle of their cycle are associated with ovulation.

The majority of the female patients who suffer from migraine notice that they are headache-free during pregnancy. This is especially true during the last 6 months of pregnancy. There are some patients, however, who find that their headaches are more severe during pregnancy. This, however, is rare and not the general rule of thumb. Either way, hormonal change is thought of as the etiologic factor.

Many patients who have had hysterectomies but who still have their ovaries experience headaches every 28 or 30 days or so, and they frequently state to their physician that they suspect that this period represents the time when they would be having their periods.

A small percentage of migraine patients tend to have fewer headaches after they have passed menopause. This is not common, but it does occur. It also points to the hormone theory of the etiology of migraine.

Peters[5] states that migraine is frequently associated with menstrual periods and often diminished after menopause, but that it may begin or be accentuated at that time. Dalsgaard-Nielsen and associates[6] noted that boys and girls aged 7 to 13 years had a similar incidence of migraine, but after the age of 13, the girls had a higher prevalence and more severe headaches than the boys. This fact suggests that the hereditary factors predisposing to migraine may have a similar sex distribution but that the hormonal changes associated with menstruation seem to increase the headache susceptibility in females.

The fact that migraine in women tends to occur at times of hormonal change, the menarche, before or during menstruation, at ovulation, or at menopause was pointed out by Greene and Dalton.[7,8]

Menstrual headaches of the migraine type tend to increase with age and parity, but many tend to improve after the natural menopause. At the same time tension, depression, and body swelling (fluid retention) affect many women before, during, or after menstruation, but depression is more common in older women.[9]

Epstein and co-workers[10] point out that a menstrual periodicity of attack has been widely held to occur in some women with migraine, although it has been shown that maintenance of the plasma progesterone levels did not delay the expected attacks in women with premenstrually linked migraine. Menstruation itself was delayed. The attacks, however, were also delayed if the estradiol levels were raised above physiologic levels. They concluded that no specific hormonal changes are associated with the occurrence of an attack of migraine.

In another study of the effect of estrogen on migraine Somerville[11] made some interesting observations. The purpose of his study was to determine how long a patient needs to be exposed to high levels of circulating estrogen before estrogen withdrawal produces migraine, and whether the premenstrual administration of estrogen can prevent estrogen withdrawal migraine. Daily blood samples were collected between 8 and 9 A.M. The plasma progesterone and estradiol levels were measured by means of competitive protein-binding methods. Somerville concluded that several days of exposure to high estrogen levels are required to provoke migraine on estrogen withdrawal. Prophylaxis by way of premenstrual estrogen administration is ineffective.

Another interesting study of the menstrual cycle and headache was made by Kashiwagi and associates.[12] They found that no one type of headache seems more likely to be exacerbated in relation to the menstrual cycle. The association between hysteria and vascular, combined vascular-muscle contraction, and unclassifiable headache on the one hand and between hysteria and reported exacerbation of headache in relation to the menstrual cycle may lead one to an erroneous impression linking vascular headache particularly to menstrual cycle changes in severity or frequency. No association was found between headache type and premenstrual exacerbation or exacerbation at any time in the menstrual cycle.

Similar findings are reported by Dalton,[13] who also stated that no relationship seems to exist between type of headache and premenstrual exacerbation. She concluded that all types of headache may occur more frequently at some time of the menstrual cycle.

ORAL CONTRACEPTIVES

As stated previously, the use of "the pill" stimulated interest in the hormonal phase of the etiology of migraine headache. Oral contraceptives have been used extensively since the early 1960's. There has been a considerable amount of interest in the influence they have in the incidence of migraine in the female patient. The migraine type of headache in users of oral contraceptives is actually a side effect of this form of medication.

In an attempt to minimize unwanted side effects, researchers have tested a large number of synthetic estrogen and progestogen doses and combinations. The two estrogens used are ethinyl estradiol and 17α-ethinylestradiol 3-methyl ether (mestranol). These inhibit ovulation by blocking the release of follicle-stimulating hormone and have an anabolic effect.

The progestogens used are either the 19 nortestosterone derivatives or the 17α-hydroxyprogesterone derivatives. These compounds all have varying degrees of potency as far as ovulation inhibition is concerned. All block the release of the luteinizing hormone and produce progestational, estrogenic, antiestrogenic, androgenic, glucocorticoid, and anabolic effects.

Because of the risk of thrombosis, oral contraceptives containing more than 50 μg of estrogen should not normally be prescribed. If the dose of progestogen were increased, when combined with a constant dose of estrogen, peak incidences of breakthrough bleeding, effects on the veins (including thrombosis), headaches, and depression occurred. Gain in weight and aggression were most likely with those oral contraceptives which had a high incidence of vascular effects (both venous and arteriolar).[14]

Progestogenic pills containing higher doses of estrogen had a low incidence of headaches and depression. This type produced a pseudodecidual response in the endometrium and was the one most similar to the hormone balance of pregnancy, which normally produces a feeling of well-being.[15]

Endometrial biopsies provide a good method for determining the hormone balance. In a normal cycle, the levels of estrogen and progesterone are found to be continuously changing and thus producing ovulation and menstruation.

Most of the oral contraceptives used at the present time are predominately progestogenic with a low amount of estrogen. With this type of compound, the growth phase is short and there is a prolonged secretory phase with a thin atrophic endometrium. The glands have a strong MAO activity for most of the cycle and the arterioles and the sinusoids are relatively prominent compared with the stroma and the glands. Thus, the oral contraceptives produce an effect somewhat like a prolonged premenstrual phase, and it is at this time in the normal cycle that women are most likely to experience headache and mood changes.

Synthetic estrogens and estrogen-progesterone combinations raise the blood levels of adrenal glucocorticoids, which in turn increases the activity of the enzyme tryptophan oxygenase. This increase in enzyol activity shunts tryptophan away from the serotonin pathway, with a subsequent lessening in the availability of this amine in the brain, resulting in clinical depression.[16]

Headaches were found to be related to the development of endometrial arterioles.[17] The changes leading up to the late secretory phase seem important. Somerville[18] has found that headaches occur when there is a fall in estrogen before menstruation, but the fall of estrogen at ovulation, while occasionally causing headaches, does not do this regularly. Thus, perhaps the postovulatory progesterone rise sensitizes the vessels to respond to the premenstrual fall in estrogens. With oral contraceptives Somerville found that various combinations of the same estrogen and progestogen produced a peak headache incidence when the dose of either estrogen or progestogen was increased. Further increase in dose resulted in a decrease in the incidence of headache.

There appear to be many mechanisms

that can increase the susceptibility to headache and the changes in mood in women. It is essential to be aware of the importance of oral contraceptives in altering the natural history of migraine. Oral contraceptive studies have highlighted the close interrelationship of many apparently diverse symptoms to the migraine syndrome. At present, progesterone and progestogens are used to treat menstrual migraine and premenstrual tension, while estrogens are recommended for menopausal flushing, headaches, and depression.

Some women have unusually dramatic reactions to basically normal hormone changes such as parturition and menstruation. The most sensitive women will get immediate headache attacks regardless of the dosage or type of oral contraceptive, while the least sensitive may have no overt symptoms.

In a study on the relationship of headache frequency to hormonal use in migraine, Kudrow[19] states that the increase of migraine attacks in women taking the contraceptive pill and the relationship between migraine and the menstrual cycle (menstrual migraine) indicates that intrinsic and extrinsic changes in estrogens may be involved in such headaches. Kudrow attempts to relate extrinsic changes in the body estrogens to the frequency of headache in a group of migrainous patients.

Patients (average age: 35 years) with migrainous headaches were divided into four groups: group A—women using estrogen-containing oral contraceptives; group B—women using supplemental or replacement estrogen preparations other than oral contraceptives; group C—women using no hormone preparations; and group D—male subjects with migraine. He concluded that nearly half the women whose headaches began after starting oral contraceptives may not be genetically migrainous subjects, implying that estrogens alter vasomotor stability. A direct or indirect effect of estrogens on the cranial blood vessels has not yet been described.

Carroll[20] believes that there is a significant incidence of headache in women taking oral contraceptives. Such headaches may be migrainous or depressive in nature. The pattern of preexisting migraine can be affected by the continued use of these preparations. Lessening of the frequency and severity of migrainous attacks can occur when the patient is changed from a preparation containing a relatively high dose of estrogen to one devoid of estrogenic and androgenic effects. Carroll states that the risk of a permanent neurologic deficit following an attack of migraine is slightly enhanced in patients who are taking oral contraceptives, and particularly when they are of relatively high estrogenic content. It seems advisable, therefore, to discontinue this form of contraception when migraine becomes very much more frequent and severe, and especially when focal features are added to the attacks.

Thromboses and permanent damage to the central nervous system could develop with these agents, particularly when there is a tendency to migraine. The risk of a stroke in young women using oral contraceptives seems to be enhanced by the presence of a migrainous history.

From a clinical standpoint there actually seems to be little doubt that oral contraceptives can increase not only the frequency but also the severity of a migraine attack. The increase in the severity of the attack occurs most often on the days when the patient is not taking the pill, and it would seem that it is the contraceptive pills with the higher estrogen content that are most likely to alter the pattern of the headache attacks. Oral contraceptives may actually precipitate typical migrainous headaches in those who have been previously headache-free. In the patients whose migraine attacks are aggravated, the possibility exists that the attack itself could produce a permanent structural lesion in the nervous system.

Such deficits, a rare complication of migraine, include visual field defects, particularly hemianopia, lesions of the retina and brainstem, and cranial nerve palsies. The effects of oral contraceptives, however, are not always to the disadvantage to the patient, for they may actually alleviate the migraine syndrome in some individuals. When the patient is changed from a contraceptive with a high estrogen content to one devoid of estrogenic or androgenic effects, she may experience improvement in the pattern of the migraine.[21]

In a study designed to ascertain the relationship, if any, between the use of oral contraceptives and headaches, Diddle and associates[22] found that of the 103 treated women in whom headache was a main complaint, thirty-three had suffered from migraine and forty-four from tension headaches, while twenty-six had experienced no headaches before treatment. Of the 103 women, 101 obtained relief by stopping treatment. In twenty-one treatment was discontinued; the other eighty-two complained less when reassured that headache was not a dangerous symptom and they continued the treatment. No relationship was found between the frequency and severity of the headaches and the duration of treatment. The headache usually developed shortly after withholding treatment. When water retention occurred, diuretics were ineffective in relieving the headache. The incidence of headache was approximately the same whatever the type of contraceptive drug used, although there was a suggestion that headache, particularly premenstrual headache, was more frequent with the combined type than the sequential. Larger doses produced headache more frequently than smaller doses.

Desrosiers[23] states that all authors agree that oral contraceptives have increased the frequency of migraine headaches, either by stimulating predisposing factors or by triggering additional attacks in those already affected by this disease. The general rule would appear to be that the mechanism is related to the withdrawal of the contraceptive. Continuous therapy does not provoke an attack, pregnancy most often prevents migraine, and a minority of patients are relieved of their migraine symptoms with contraceptives.

Dalton[24] states that to ascertain the effect of oral contraceptives on migraine, an analysis was made of self-administered questionnaires from 886 nonpregnant migraine sufferers aged 15 to 45 years (241 pill-takers, 290 ex-takers, and 355 non-takers), together with a 3-month record of migraine attacks in 416 women covering 1,239 menstruations. Migraine was worse in 34% of takers and 60% of ex-takers. On stopping oral contraceptives 39% of ex-takers improved. During menstruation 35% of attacks occurred in takers, 32% in ex-takers, and 27% in non-takers. A significant increase in migraine at midcycle was most marked among those whose migraine increased on "the pill" and those with severe attacks.

Another study on headache and the use of the oral contraceptives was made by Cohn-Larsson and Lundberg.[25] They presented their findings at a headache symposium of the Scandinavian Migraine Society in 1969. In a trial consisting of 1,676 women taking combined, sequential, or low-dose progestogen oral contraceptives, the frequency of headaches was studied. The mean pretreatment frequency of migraine was 13.5% and of unspecific headaches 5.3%. In subjects with migraine there was a significant decrease of symptoms during the treatment, while no significant changes were observed among those with unspecific headaches. Of the women without pretreatment headaches, 10.3% experienced headaches during treatment.

Carroll and Grant[26] studied the effect of oral contraceptives on the blood vessels and migraine. They found that a small proportion of women reported a change in the nature of their migrainous episodes in the period following the start of the contraceptive medication. While 12% of the patients reported improvement, 49% complained of a deterioration in their condition. Contraceptives with a high content of estrogen were found to carry a particular risk in this respect. The findings showed that the combination of progesterone and estrogen, which most often gave rise to episodes of headache, also gave the highest incidence of proliferation of the endometrial arterioles.

The pathologic findings led to the conclusion that the changes in the endometrial vessels paralleled the vascular changes in other parts of the body. Consequently, endometrial biopsy may be useful in the assessment of the vascular reaction to oral contraceptives.

Other important effects of oral contraceptives were observed in the form of a dilation of the uterine sinusoids and an increase in the density of the stroma around the walls of the blood vessels. A relationship appears to exist between the changes in the veins of the leg and those occurring in other parts of the body under the influence of oral contraceptives. Carroll and Grant concluded that the frequency of migrainous and depressive headache has increased in women taking oral contraceptives.

Psychologic factors must be considered when the incidence of headache associated with the use of oral contraceptives is concerned. Oral contraceptives may increase both the frequency and the intensity of established migraine, and they sometimes also precipitate vasomotor or depressive headaches. The incidence of headache appears to depend on the estrogen-progestogen ratio, since the high estrogen preparation is less well tolerated than the low estrogen one.

Pluvinage,[27] in a study on migraine, headache, and oral contraceptives, points out that when oral contraceptives are responsible for the headache, a change of the preparation not only reduces the incidence of the side effects but may indeed prove to be an effective prophylactic treatment of both migraine and common headache.

Psychologic factors play an important role in the incidence of headache associated with oral contraceptives; such factors include the educational background, social class, religious beliefs, psychologic status, and sexual life of the patient. Assessment of these facts is an important part of clinical management and psychotherapy, perhaps augmented by psychotropic medication, may be required.

It has been shown in many reports that the use of oral contraceptives causes headaches and migraine in those who did not previously suffer from them or increases the frequency and severity in those who previously suffered. Estimates on the frequency of headaches in patients taking oral contraceptives vary from 0.2% to 60%, depending on the proportion and type of estrogen and progestogen used in the preparation.

There are many factors that seem to cause an increase in headache attacks among migraine patients taking oral contraceptives. The incidence of attacks is greater when the patient is beyond 30 years of age or the menstrual cycle is longer than the usual 28 to 30 days. Patients who experience relief of their migraine attacks during the last trimester of pregnancy also seem to have an increase in their migraine attacks when taking oral contraceptives. Patients who notice that the onset of their migraine attacks began after pregnancy usually have an increase in their attacks while taking oral contraceptives. Women who associate their migraine with menstruation also are troubled in this respect with the oral contraceptives. Parity is another influencing factor.

Cohn-Larsson and Lundberg[28] in a study on headache and the oral contraceptives observed the frequency of the attacks, the age of the patients, the family history, and whether patients had pretreatment or not. The occurrence of migraine was shown to increase with age. From a study of the frequency of headache before treatment, this increase was calculated to be 0.8% per year between the ages of 16 and 40 years; for all types of headache the increase was 0.85% per year. Of the group 226 women (13.5%) had pretreatment migraine, 88 (5.2%) had other headaches, and 1,362 women (81.3%) had experienced no headache before treatment. Of the women with no pretreatment headache, 10.3% developed headaches when taking oral contraceptives (the expected frequency was 1.14%). Those with a positive family history showed a greater tendency to develop headache, but the type of drug taken had little effect.

Of the women with pretreatment migraine there was a decrease of symptoms during treatment. There was no significant change in the group with nonspecific pretreatment headaches. The results also showed that a significant number of women with migraine experience a decrease or disappearance of their symptoms when taking a combined type of oral contraceptive.

More serious complications than increased migraine attacks have also been reported in the literature on more than one occasion. Gardner, Hornstein, and ven den Noort[29] state that cerebral infarction of varying severity can result in these cases. They found that patients with simple migraine also run some risk in taking these medications unless they have done so for a considerable period of time without ill effect. There are, however, many patients who develop the prodrome who never go on to the more severe phases, usually because they discontinue the medication with or without medical advice. Since we have been aware of this syndrome, we have seen many additional patients whose cerebral migraine was becoming more intense and more focal while they were taking oral contraceptives. Presumably they were able to avoid lasting neurologic deficit by withdrawing from medication before the ischemia became critical.

Pendl and co-workers[30] observed acute cerebrovascular episodes in women taking oral contraceptives. In their study during a 3-year period, twenty-seven cases of cerebrovascular accidents associated with oral contraceptives were seen. The clinical manifestations were as follows: hemiplegia or hemiparesis, eight cases; hemihypesthesia, one case; complicated migraine with hemihypesthesia, three cases; complicated migraine with hemiparesis, one case; migraine, five cases; headache, one case; convulsive seizures, three cases; subarachnoid hemorrhage, two cases; death from sinus thrombosis, one case; and death due to occlusion of the middle cerebral artery, one case.

The risk of a thromboembolic accident in women taking "the pill" is about twice as high as that in comparable women not using oral contraceptives.

In conclusion it can be said that all migraine patients do not react the same to the use of the oral contraceptives. There are actually three distinct groups. One group is made up of those whose migraine headaches are aggravated by oral contraceptives and whose headaches are either more frequent or more severe, or both. Another group consists of those patients who experience no effect in regard to their migraine from the use of oral contraceptives. A third group (a very small one) consists of those patients who actually notice that they have fewer headaches and that their headaches are less severe when they take the oral contraceptives. Most women fit into groups one and two.

This represents what we found in a crossover study with patients first taking oral contraceptives and then stopping their use.[30a]

Diet

It has long been thought that there is a genetic relationship between migraine and the familiar allergic diseases. Many people have suggested that the ingestion of specific foods causes headaches of the migraine type in susceptible patients. There have been various reports in the literature on the subject of migraine headache in patients with recurrent headaches who were free of symptoms as long as certain foods were excluded from their diet. In some cases the choice of food to be eliminated was based on skin tests; some certain foods found to be frequent causes were arbitrarily excluded; and in other cases the final regimen was arrived at after a series of test trials.

The chief proponents of the allergic method have reported good results in the majority of their patients with headaches. Vaughan[31] estimated that the method was successful in 50% of cases. Rowe[32] reported that 87% of his patients who cooperated in the program received beneficial results after refraining from eating certain foods. These studies have met with some criticism in the past because they were done by specialists in allergic diseases. Since their practice included a predominance of patients with other allergic diseases, and they were consulted by patients who already suspected that their headaches might have an allergic basis, their series were presumably somewhat weighted with definitely or possibly allergic persons. Wolff[33] criticized the observations of these workers, stating that the studies were not adequately controlled and that the relief resulted from suggestion and a sense of security inspired by the confidence of the physician. Wolff reported a few cases when foods believed to have been proved causes of allergic headaches were administered without the patients' knowledge and they failed to produce symptoms.

A small minority of patients who give a typical history of migraine headaches believe that certain foods will precipitate their attacks. Some reports say that as many as 30% of migraine sufferers relate the onset of some of their attacks to the eating of these foods. The foods most commonly implicated are chocolate, alcohol, milk and milk products, cheese, fish, beans, citrus foods, pork, onions, wheat, and nuts. Chocolate is said to be cited by 75% of dietary migraine sufferers. Dark chocolate has been found to be more potent than milk chocolate.

TYRAMINE

Some, but not all, of the foods mentioned as suspected migraine precipitants contain a substance called tyramine. This is a naturally occurring sympathomimetic amine that acts directly on the blood vessels and also causes the release of norepinephrine. This is relevant since migraine is recognized as being a vascular disorder in which the onset of an attack is accompanied by a change in the size of the blood vessels.

Tyramine has been found to be present in certain cheeses, dairy products, smoked fish, and some alcoholic drinks. Like 5-hydroxytryptamine, dopamine, and epinephrine, it undergoes oxidative deamination in the body by the enzyme monoamine oxidase. Tyramine liberates endogenous aromatic amines from sympathetic nerve endings and serotonin from blood platelets.

Other vasoactive amines, namely dopamine and octopamine, have been found in beans and citrus fruits respectively. Port, chianti, and other red wines and some other alcoholic drinks contain histamine, which is also a vasoactive amine.

Possible mechanisms of action. There have been several reasons postulated as to the possible mechanisms by which tyramine might play a role in the precipitation of migraine attacks.

Migraine frequently occurs as a familial disorder, with a positive family history to be found in as many as 60% of chronic migraine sufferers in some studies. It has been believed that because of this fact there might be an inborn area of metabolism in some migraine sufferers due to a genetic enzyme deficiency of monoamine oxidase. Such a deficiency might occasionally lead to increased amine levels in the bloodstream. Another possible explanation of some attacks of migraine may be that certain people have a particularly sensitive, localized vascular response to circulating amines such as tyramine.

Using a direct chromatography method, Hannington[34] was able to discover the deficiency of tyramine sulfate. From this evidence she postulated that in dietary migraine the patients suffer from a deficiency in the enzyme responsible for the sulfate conjugation of tyramine and in this group we may be dealing with an inborn area of metabolism. Hannington does go on to point out the deficiency in this metabolic pathway does not necessarily mean that this deficit is the cause of the headache. She says that it is possible that the extra HPAA produced in the amine oxidase pathway is highly toxic and may cause a headache. In other words tyramine itself may not necessarily be responsible for the headache; it may merely act by its ability to release catecholamines or other pharmacologically active agents.

Sandler and others[35] have shown that these dietary migraine sufferers have a defect in amine inactivation that allows sufficient free tyramine to enter the bloodstream and initiate further sequence of events with headache as an end result. They believe that amine liberation is one of the essential events in the process leading to a migrainous attack. Although this inability to inactivate an oral tyramine load may be one triggering event leading to amine liberation in susceptible individuals, they believe that other amine-liberating sequences are probably of equal or greater importance. They say that the demonstration of abnormal catecholamine liberation in tyramine-sensitive migraine does not necessarily mean that the headache is a consequence of that liberation, but that it is equally possible that tyramine ingestion results in the release of some secondary factor responsible for the further train of events.

Blackwell and Mabbitt[36] have reported that several patients being treated with monoamine oxidase inhibitors occasionally develop severe headaches after eating cheeses and a few other foods. They have shown that these headaches result from the absorption of tyramine from the cheese, owing to the inhibition of monoamine oxidase, the enzyme responsible for the breakdown of tyramine in the intestine.

Alcohol is constantly mentioned by patients as a dietary precipitant of migraine attacks. It has been postulated that alcohol facilitates the absorption of tyramine and that circulating tyramine may be a factor in the headache associated with the drinking of alcohol. This would be consistent with the theory of Sandler that those patients who respond to tyramine with a headache absorb an abnormally high load of tyramine from the gut, and it is this high level of circulating tyramine and its inadequate excretion that causes the headache.

Metabolic pathways of tyramine metabolism. The general metabolism of the aromatic amines is known to be via oxidative deamination to the corresponding phenolic acids. Thus tyramine yields p-hydroxyphenylacetic acid. d-Hydroxyphenolic amines also undergo methylation at the 3 position before oxidation such that the corresponding 3-methoxy, 4-hydroxyphenolic acids are formed and excreted; methylation of simple 4-hydroxyphenols is not usually absorbed and it is not known whether tyramine would undergo such a reaction. Conjugation is another pathway which has been previously overlooked. Smith and associates[37] have shown that this is an alternative but important pathway for both the amines and their corresponding acids, as appreciable levels of compounds have now been found in the urine of both patients and normal controls.

Clinical studies

Hannington's study. ''As tyramine is the chief pressor amine that has been investigated in relation to reactions occurring in patients taking monoamine oxidase inhibitors, it seems reasonable to investigate the possible role of tyramine in precipitating migrainous headaches." This work was carried out by Hannington.[34]

She selected thirty-two patients, seventeen who suspected dietary causes for their migraine and fifteen who did not suspect that certain foods precipitated their migraine attacks. These patients were told that various capsules would be given to them and they were then to fill out a questionnaire to be completed and returned shortly after taking the capsule. They were identical capsules; some actually contained 100 mg of tyramine hydrochloride; similar capsules containing 100 mg of lactose were used as a control in these patients. "This is roughly equivalent to the amount of tyramine that could be found in 3½ ounces of cheese rich in tyramine." Hannington's results seem to show "that there is a high incidence of headaches after the patients in the dietary migraine group took the oral tyramine. Every one of the patients in that group developed a headache on at least one occasion after 100 mg of tyramine. . . . In patients where subsequent doses of 100 mg failed to produce a headache the dose was increased to 125 mg and on most occasions a headache occurred." In the seventeen patients who were believed to have headache caused by certain food substances, nine had no effect when taking the tyramine in one of the trials and in forty instances headaches were precipitated. When they were given the lactose capsules there were twenty-four episodes where no headache was produced and there were two episodes where a migraine attack was produced. In the fifteen nondietary migraine patients tyramine provoked no headache on thirty different occasions and produced a migraine attack twice. In this same group lactose was given fourteen times with no effect and in three instances it produced a migraine attack.

Hannington concluded that in certain patients oral tyramine can induce a typical migraine headache. Headaches were similar to the usual attacks experienced by these patients.

Ryan's study. In Ryan's study[38] seventy-five known chronic migraine sufferers were selected and questioned regarding any family history of migraine attacks, whether any drugs were being taken by the patient at that time, and whether any of these patients had ever noted an association between the onset of their headaches and the consumption of any particular foods. They were questioned specifically about foods that had been implicated in dietary migraine in previous studies. Each patient received two identical appearing capsules marked A and B. They were then told that ingestion of either one or both of these capsules might produce symptoms of a migraine attack. The patients were instructed to take capsule A on their next headache-free morning and then to observe themselves for the next 24 hours. They were then told to take capsule B in a similar manner on their next headache-free morning. Each patient was given a form to fill out regarding the response to each capsule. This was a double-blind study with each patient receiving 125 mg of tyramine hydrochloride in one capsule and a placebo in the second identical appearing capsule.

After the initial study was completed the results were analyzed. The patients were categorized as being: 1, dietary-positive by history; 2, alcohol-positive by history; and 3, dietary-negative by history. The results were then classified according to the patients' history and as to whether they were tyramine-negative after the ingestion of their capsule. After this first trial was completed, and because of the results obtained in this trial, it was decided to conduct a second trial using the same group of patients, this time giving certain selected patients 125 mg of tyramine hydrochloride while giving others 250 mg of tyramine hydrochloride. Again all patients received a second identical appearing capsule containing a placebo. Another alteration in the second stage of the trial, again because of the results obtained in the initial trial, was that the patients were told that this time they were being given a different capsule in an effort to prevent the development of a headache throughout that day. The dosage of tyramine selected for each patient was based on the response in the first study. All patients who had a positive alcohol history and all patients with a positive dietary history who did not respond to the tyramine in the first trial received 250 mg of tyramine hydrochloride in the second trial. The results from this study were then recorded and analyzed.

Group 1 patients were those who had a positive dietary history. This consisted of twenty-seven patients. In this group in the initial study, ten were tyramine-positive and placebo-negative, nine were tyramine-positive and placebo-positive, five were tyramine-negative and placebo-positive, and three were tyramine-negative and placebo-negative. Group 2 patients consisted of those who had a positive alcohol history. This consisted of thirteen patients of whom one was tyramine-positive and placebo-negative, one was tyramine-positive and placebo-positive, six were tyramine-negative and placebo-positive, and five were tyramine-negative and placebo-negative. Group 3 patients were those who believed that there was no dietary cause for their headache. This consisted of thirty-five patients of whom three were tyramine-positive and placebo-negative, seven were tyramine-positive and placebo-positive, five were tyramine-negative and placebo-positive, and twenty were tyramine-negative and placebo-negative.

In the second stage of the study the groups were kept intact and the results from each group were separated into two groups of patients, one group receiving 125 mg of tyramine and one group receiving 250 mg of tyramine.

In the group 1 patients fifteen received 125 mg of tyramine and of these two were tyramine-positive and placebo-negative, eight were tyramine-positive and placebo-positive, three were tyramine-negative and placebo-positive, and two were tyramine-

negative and placebo-negative. Twelve patients received 250 mg of tyramine and two of these were tyramine-positive and placebo-negative, one was tyramine-positive and placebo-positive, two were tyramine-negative and placebo-positive, and seven were tyramine-negative and placebo-negative.

All thirteen patients in group 2 received 250 mg of tyramine. Of these none was tyramine-positive and placebo-negative, two were tyramine-positive and placebo-positive, two were tyramine-negative and placebo-positive, and nine were tyramine-negative and placebo-negative. In group 3 there were thirty-five patients, and all received 125 mg of tyramine. Of these one was tyramine-positive and placebo-negative, six were tyramine-positive and placebo-positive, five were tyramine-negative and placebo-positive, and twenty-three were tyramine-negative and placebo-negative.

In group 1 patients, fifty-four sets of samples were given to twenty-seven different patients and there were twenty-nine tyramine-positive responses to 125 mg and three positive responses to 250 mg of tyramine compared to twenty-four positive responses to the placebo. In group 2 patients thirteen sets of samples of 125 mg and thirteen sets of samples of 250 mg of tyramine were given. There were two positive responses to 125 mg and two responses to 250 mg of tyramine. There were eleven positive responses to the placebo group. In group 3 patients seventy sets of samples were given to thirty-five different patients. In this group there were seventeen tyramine-positive responses and thirty-three positive responses to the placebo.

Another interesting finding is the reproducibility of results in each patient in the two studies. In all categories combined, of the twenty-seven patients who were tyramine-positive in the first trial, only fifteen had a positive response in the second trial. In the initial study there were thirty-three positive responses to the placebo, while in the second study only twenty-six patients responded to the placebo.

In all groups combined there were more patients responding with a headache to the placebo than to the tyramine. Also there were only fifteen patients who had a positive response to tyramine in both trials. In the second trial there were seven fewer patients responding to the placebo. This led to the belief that the power of suggestion played a role in the etiology of migraine to a greater extent than the tyramine did.

Forsythe's study. Forsythe[39] studied the effect of tyramine in children with migraine. Sixty-one children with migraine were selected for his studies. Fourteen boys and two girls were aged 4 to 9 and the rest were 10 to 14. Identical capsules containing either 100 mg of tyramine or 100 mg of lactose and labeled 1 and 2 were given to the patients with instructions to take capsule 1 between 4 and 6 P.M. and capsule 2, 48 hours later. Twelve children developed a headache within 48 hours of ingesting the tyramine. Ten children developed a headache 48 hours after ingesting the placebo, and four children developed a headache within 48 hours of ingesting both capsules. Thirty-three children were unaffected by either capsule. Of twelve children affected by tyramine six had been given the tyramine first and six a placebo first.

Five children developed a headache within 48 hours of tyramine ingestion, eleven developed a headache after placebo ingestion, and four developed a headache after tyramine and placebo ingestion. In a second trial conducted by Forsythe eighteen children were unaffected in this study. In this trial children with more frequent migrainous attacks often showed a tendency to headaches following ingestion of placebo, thus suggesting that the efforts to avoid spontaneous migraine coinciding with placebo ingestion were successful. He concluded that tyramine is probably not an important etiologic factor in the migraine of childhood.

Moffetta's study. Moffetta[40] studied the effect that chocolate had on a group of twenty-five volunteer migrainous subjects who had observed that headaches regularly occurred after the ingestion of small amounts of cocoa products. This was done using a double-blind placebo control method.

He concluded two studies. In the first all subjects were sent two samples, the second 2 weeks after the first. One sample contained chocolate and the other a placebo of synthetic fat. Both samples had the same texture. Forty-eight hours after eating the sample each subject filled out a questionnaire indicating whether he had experienced a headache and if so, whether it resembled a usual migraine. Study 2 was similar to the previous study, but only fifteen of the subjects took part.

In study 1 fifteen headaches occurred in fifty subject sessions, eight after chocolate and five after placebo. One subject had headache after both chocolate and placebo and eleven had no headaches after either sample. In study 2 ten headaches occurred in thirty subject sessions, five after chocolate only, three after placebo only. One subject had a headache after both and six had no headache after either sample. Only five of the fifteen subjects who participated in both studies responded consistently. Of the twenty-five subjects used in the chocolate study more than half reported cheese also caused their migraine attacks.

From the results of his study Moffetta suggested that chocolate on its own is rarely a precipitant of migraine.

Osvald-Cernes' study. Osvald-Cernes[41] studied the effects of tyramine in producing migraine attacks in sixty patients with chronic migraines. Of these patients twenty-four suffered from classic migraine and thirty-six from common migraine. Twenty-six of the patients considered their migraine to be precipitated by some particular foods, thirty-four patients did not. The patients were tested with 100 mg of tyramine in a double-blind crossover method.

Two thirds of the patients in group 2 did

not get any headache at all. Four got a headache from placebo, five from tyramine, and two after both tyramine and placebo. Half of the patients in group 1 did not get any headache at all. Four got a headache from placebo only, three from tyramine only, and six from both tyramine and placebo.

Since the purpose of his study was to find out the connection between dietary migraine and tyramine, Osvald-Cernes later retested those nine patients in group 1 who got a headache from tyramine only or both tyramine and placebo. Only eight patients finished this study, and they were given three capsules of tyramine each to be taken at three different occasions. Therefore there were twenty-four total capsules given. There was no reaction at all on twenty of these capsules. Four of the patients responded with a slight headache on one capsule each; three of these four patients were from the group that earlier had gotten a headache from both tyramine and placebo, and they considered themselves to get a headache very often (meaning twice daily one or two times a week). Osvald-Cernes concluded from these findings that this amount of tyramine did not act as a precipitating factor in dietary migraine.

Shaw's study. Shaw[42] wished to examine changes in fat metabolism during migraine attacks. Those patients with a history of migraine after eating cheese were selected, as it has been reported that attacks in such patients were due to sensitivity to tyramine. He reported the findings in nine patients who had this history of dietary migraine. All patients said that they had attacks after ingestion of cheese and therefore avoided it. In one investigation patients received 200 mg of tyramine in a capsule orally; in the second, which was used as a control, six received placebo. The patients were unaware of which capsule they were receiving.

None of the patients reported a headache in the 48 hours following ingestion of tyramine, although two reported a typical migraine headache after taking a placebo.

From the results of his findings Shaw concluded that in patients with dietary migraine there was no evidence of tyramine absorption and no evidence that tyramine precipitated their attacks. Therefore tyramine did not appear implicated in the provocation of dietary migraine in his patients.

PHENYLETHYLAMINE

The foods cited most commonly by migraine sufferers as precipitants of their attacks were chocolate, dairy products (especially cheese), citrus fruits, and alcoholic drinks. These have been listed in the order of frequency with which they are mentioned by roughly one out of three migraine sufferers who link the eating of certain foods with the onset of some of their attacks.

Chocolate is most commonly cited as a cause of dietary migraines. Chocolate, however, contains little or no tyramine. An analysis of this substance has been done to identify the headache-precipitating factor in chocolate. It was thought that chocolate contained one or more vasoactive amines like tyramine. Initial testing in six reliable dietary migrainous subjects using samples of chocolate from which the total amine content had been removed confirmed that the amine content of chocolate contains the headache-precipitating fraction.[43] When a vasoactive amine, phenylethylamine, was identified in chocolate, further clinical testing was undertaken. This demonstrated that 3 mg of phenylethylamine, the average amount found in 2-ounce bars of chocolate, precipitates headaches in selected subjects.[43]

Many cheeses and some red wines also contain this compound. Sandler[44] conducted a study designed to determine whether oral phenylethylamine alone can provoke migrainous attacks in susceptible subjects. A capsule containing lactose was sent to forty-six migraine sufferers whose headaches were normally provoked by chocolate. Twenty-four hours after taking the capsule the subjects completed and returned a questionnaire. A further capsule with similar appearance, but containing 3 mg of phenylethylamine, was then sent out together with another questionnaire. The patients were not aware of the contents of either capsule.

Three men and thiry-three women completed the trial. Six of the thirty-six patients developed headaches after ingesting the lactose capsule, while eighteen of the thirty-six were affected after ingesting phenylethylamine. Two patients developed headaches after both capsules. One had a mild headache on both occasions but vomited only after phenylethylamine. It was concluded that a cause-and-effect relationship existed between the ingestion of phenylethylamine and migraine headache in certain patients.

Sandler states that it is of interest to note that phenylethylamine appears to be somewhat more effective than tyramine in its ability to release vasoactive substances from the perfused lung preparation. Phenylethylamine, which does not possess hydroxyl groups, cannot be conjugated as a sulfate, unlike most other biologically active monoamines, including tyramine. Its predominate inactivation pathway is likely to be one of oxidative deamination by monoamine oxidase.

McCulloch[45] used phenylethylamine to study the cerebral circulation. Phenylethylamine was administered to six animals and it produced a significant reduction in cerebral blood flow. Cerebral capillary and endothelial cells are known to contain large concentrations of monoamine oxidase. He postulated that the monoamine oxidase deficits which are thought to occur in migraine sufferers are reflected in tissue other than platelets, for example, the enzymic component of the blood-brain barrier. This might provide an explanation as to why cerebral vessels in migraine patients are more sensitive to phenylethylamine than those in normal patients. He believed that this characterization of the cerebral vascular response to phenylethylamine provided further support for the implication of phenylethylamine as a pathogenesis for migraine.

CONCLUSION

There does seem to be much evidence that certain vasoactive amines may precipitate or at least play a role in precipitating migraine attacks. However, from the results published at the present date there does not seem to be sufficient evidence to state that tyramine is the precipitating cause, since there are many more reports and many more patients in whom the tyramine was thought to be able to produce a headache where it did not, and where actually the placebo produced a greater number of headaches. On the subject of phenylethylamine sufficient investigation has not been carried out to this point to be able to categorically state that ingestion of oral loads of tyramine will precipitate migraine attacks in these patients. Further investigation needs to be done in this field.

Serotonin

The serotonin theory for the etiology of migraine has been prominent for several years. Serotonin is also referred to in the medical literature as 5-HT or 5-hydroxytryptamine.

Most of the serotonin found in the blood is bound to the platelets, specifically the granules (often called the dense bodies). This can be observed by using the electron microscope. During a migraine attack the serotonin level in the blood platelets shows a sharp decrease, often as much as 40%. It was shown by Hilton and Cumings[46] that the blood platelets of the patient with migraine can be distinguished from the platelets of the nonmigrainous patient (control patient) by the aggregation responses of the platelets to serotonin.

Most of the headache experts supporting the serotonin theory of the etiology of migraine point out that during a migraine attack there is also an increase in urinary excretion of 5-HIAA (5-hydroxyindoleacetic acid), which is the main catabolite of serotonin. This was pointed out by Sicuteri and associates.[47] The serotonin level in the cerebrospinal fluid does not change during migraine attacks.

In studying the blood platelets with the electron microscope, Grammeltvedt, Hovig, and Sjaastad[48] found that the mean number of dense bodies in the migraine patients was slightly lower than that in the control group. There was no significant difference in the number of dense bodies in the platelets examined during or between attacks in the patients with migraine. Serotonin-induced changes in the shape of the platelets in patients during their attacks were not found, nor did they find any attack-induced alterations in other organelles within the platelets.

It has been shown that the injection of reserpine can cause migraine[49] and also a decrease of serotonin from the platelets.[50] However, it also causes a depletion of serotonin and other amines from storage sites within the central nervous system. So the question arises: is the migraine-provoking effect of reserpine due to its effect in the platelets or not?

There have been many studies that have implicated the role of serotonin in attacks of migraine. This serotonin theory has raised the possibility of pain being provoked by an altered concentration at the cerebral level. If the concentration is reduced sufficiently, it is possible that a central supersensitivity is induced similar to that produced by denervation at the vascular level. Sicuteri[51] believes that it is possible that some painful syndromes represent a cerebral 5-HT deficiency and that sufferers from recurrent headaches may have a disorder of cerebral 5-HT metabolism with a latent (free period) or manifest (attack) deficiency of brainstem 5-HT. Daily chronic headaches may represent a permanent deficiency with a secondary supersensitivity toward 5-HT. He believes that the antiserotonin drugs which are prophylactic against migraine could

have a control antagonist mechanism if supersensitivity is more important.

Sicuteri[47] further advances the theory that continuous painful stimuli from the periphery are prevented from reaching the perceptive area by the inhibitory function of thalamic structures and that 5-HT is the inhibitor mediator. When the cerebral 5-HT is depleted, these impulses are no longer inhibited, which results in the pain of the attack. This pain from 5-HT depletion may represent a chemical approach to the mechanism of central pain in the thalamic syndrome. He concludes that if one accepts that central pain derives from a deficiency of 5-HT, then antiserotonin drugs may act by protecting the hypersensitive receptors to 5-HT or by taking the place of the missing 5-HT by acting as a false transmitter.

Sjaastad[52] states that in view of other possible actions of reserpine, one cannot be certain that the influence on platelet serotonin is the crucial factor in the reserpine-like migrainous headache. He further believes that studies of the effect of reserpine on migraine cannot be taken as evidence that any causal relationship exits between platelet serotonin and the development of attacks. He believes that the benefit from intravenously administered serotonin is unlikely to be due to the replacement of lost intracellular serotonin. However, since serotonin does not cross the blood-brain barrier, its action is likely to be explicable in terms of its pharmacologic action on the cardiovascular system, rather than centrally.

In studying the effects of reserpine and chlorpromazine on serotonin uptake of platelets from migrainous and control patients, Hilton[53] suggests a possible explanation of the difference in findings between the aggregation response and the 5-HT uptake is that there are two receptors—one is equivalent to the D receptor of smooth muscle and provides a model for vascular 5-HT receptors, and another one is concerned with 5-HT transport across the membrane. In migrainous subjects, the former 5-HT receptors are not as readily occupied as in the control subjects. A defect in constrictor sites would make blood vessels more liable to dilate in response to the documented fall in 5-HT levels at the onset of an attack of migraine.

Hale[54] concluded that ascending 5-HT neurons do not seem to play any important role in central modulation of pain. Thus if 5-Ht is an important factor in migraine, this is probably not due to changes in pain sensitivity secondary to functional changes in ascending 5-HT neurons.

An outstanding study of the role of humoral mediators in migraine headache was presented by Fanchamps,[55-57] who has contributed as much or more than anyone in this aspect of headache research. He states that arterial distention is not sufficient to explain the origin of the pain experienced by the migraine patient. To give rise to an acute migrainous pain, there must also be an associated lowered pain threshold of the receptors situated in the walls of the affected vessels. A number of humoral factors intervene in the chain of events that culminates in migraine headache, such as plasmakinin, serotonin, and histamine. Fanchamps says that at the start of the attacks the blood platelets release serotonin. At the same time the mast cells in the affected area release histamine and proteolytic enzymes that split plasmakininogens to form plasmakinins. Free serotonin and histamine increase the capillary permeability and thus favor transudation of plasmakinin into the vessel walls and the perivascular tissues. The combined effect of serotonin and plasmakinin on the vessel wall receptors reduces the pain threshold. On the other hand, the bulk of the released serotonin is excreted in the urine as 5-HIAA, and the plasma serotonin thus falls. Serotonin has a constricting effect on the extracranial arteries and a dilating effect on the capillaries. The fall in the plasma level induces hypotonia of these arteries and capillary constriction. This results in a passive distention of the arterial walls. The

two factors necessary for the production of pain are therefore both present; namely, a lowering of the pain threshold and vascular distention.

Deshmukh and Harper[58] did a study on the effect of serotonin on the cerebral and extracerebral blood flow circulation when it was infused in anesthetized baboons. They concluded that the differential action of serotonin on cerebral and extracerebral circulations could produce the preheadache phase of migraine associated with cerebral vasoconstriction and the headache phase due to extracerebral vasodilation, in accordance with the classic migraine theory.

In another study of blood serotonin concentrations in patients with migraine, Tretyakova and Fets[59] used an ultraviolet absorption method to determine the total blood serotonin content. The mean blood serotonin level between attacks with migrainous subjects was not significantly above the level in the controls. In the prodromal period, however, it rose to three times the normal level but then fell, so that at the time of maximum severity of the attack it was much lower, although still above normal.

At the start of an attack the blood contained increased concentrations of serotonin as well as another substance of similar chemical nature. This substance could not be identified, but it was not 5-hydroxyindoleacetic acid. They concluded that migraine is thus preceded by high blood levels of serotonin together with another, as yet unidentified, substance, which is presumed to originate from changes in the central structures of the autonomic nervous system. The serotonin enters the bloodstream in larger concentrations because of increased vascular permeability and there becomes inactivated or bound by platelets, so that its concentration falls.

In another study on serotonin and platelet aggregation, Hilton and Cumings[60] collected blood from patients with both classic and common migraine. Collections of blood were made during the actual migraine attack and when the patients were headache-free. The platelet aggregation responses were studied and the serotonin was estimated. The results were compared with control patients and it was concluded that the migraine patients, both between attacks (while headache-free) and during attacks, showed lower mean blood serotonin levels than the control patients.

In still another study of serotonin levels in the whole blood during the migraine attacks and between attacks, Rydzewski[61] made fluorimetric estimations of total 5-HT in blood of migrainous patients during an untreated migraine attack. Total blood 5-HT dropped during a migraine attack to about 68% of its former level, returning to preheadache values by the time the pain ceased. Mean values for total blood serotonin were 65.1 at the beginning of a migraine attack, 57.9 at the peak, 61.0 at the end, and 91.2 in the headache-free period. No correlation between the intensity of the headache and the concentration of 5-HT during a migraine attack was found.

Hardebo and Evinsson[62] studied the mechanical action of serotonin and the effect of related inhibitors in intracranial and extracranial vessels. They studied the vasomotor effects of various concentrations of serotonin in vitro simultaneously on intracranial (middle cerebral) and extracranial (external maxillary and lingual) arteries of chronically sympathectomized cats. The effect of 5-HT was at first analyzed in relaxed vessels. They found that 5-HT contracted both types of arteries in a dose-dependent manner. The alpha-adrenergic receptor antagonist phentolamine did not inhibit the response in a way that could be expected for a substance with solely alpha-agonistic properties. The contractile action of 5-HT in intracranial arteries, on the other hand, could not be antagonized by methysergide in this manner. Instead, the maximum contractile effect of 5-HT was reduced. The constriction in extracranial arteries was inhibited in a competitive way by methysergide.

As stated previously not all headache experts accept the serotonin theory of the etiology of migraine. Somerville[63] found that there was no significant difference in levels of either platelet-bound or free serotonin in jugular compared to forearm blood, either between or during headaches. During migraine, however, there was pronounced fall in platelet serotonin observed, but this was not accompanied by any rise in the free levels of serotonin, which, if anything, tended to decline. Somerville concluded that serotonin liberated from platelets during migraine is either metabolized rapidly or bound to other structures such as erythrocytes with such rapidity that no rise in its free level in plasma occurs. The question of whether the fall in platelet serotonin is related directly to the vasodilation of migraine must be examined more critically.

Somerville's study does not support the view that platelet loss of serotonin is due to "damage" to platelets passing through the functionally abnormal scalp circulation which exists at the time of the migraine headache.

While the serotonin theory of the etiology of migraine is very popular, it is all theoretical, and not all headache experts consider it to be positive.

Kinins, catecholamines, and monoamine oxidase

There are many factors thought to be involved in the etiology of migraine. One group commonly referred to in this respect is the kinins.

The kinins are peptides formed by the enzymatic action of kallikrein on the alpha-globulin plasma substrate kininogen. The kinins cause vasodilation and increased permeability of the small blood vessels.

Bradykinin is the best known of the kinin group. When bradykinin is injected intravenously, systemic hypotonia results along with cutaneous vasodilation and headache. If the injections are of sufficient quantity, this headache may be of the migraine type. In the painful area, there is found to be an accumulation of enzymes which produce a peptide called neurokinin. This peptide causes local vasodilation and inflammation.

The catecholamines, especially noradrenaline, may also take part in the pathophysiology of migraine. A local release of noradrenaline will produce ischemia, which in turn causes release of other vasoactive agents. It is also believed that the metabolism of the catecholamines is indirectly associated with the headache brought on by tyramine in susceptible individuals.

Monoamine oxidase is also frequently referred to when the etiology of migraine is discussed.

Migraine patients have decreased platelet monoamine oxidase activity. There seems to be a genetic enzymatic defect on metabolism of the monoamines and other vasoneuroactive substances.

Monoamine oxidase is normally found in the granular portion of most parenchymal tissues of human beings. These tissues deaminate several amines such as serotonin, tyramine, tryptamine, and dopamine.

It is entirely possible that the inhibition of monoamine oxidase during migraine attacks could bring about an increase in activity of vasoneuroactive agents. These in turn would produce their effects locally in the microcirculation, such as the adventitia of the large vessels.

Basophilic leukocytes

Another theory concerning the etiology of migraine deals with the basophilic leukocytes. A tremendous amount of work in this field was done by Ernst Thonnard-Neumann.[64,65] This gentleman has pioneered most of the work in the medical literature concerning the basophilic leukocyte and migraine, so most of what is said here is based on his fine work.

Sicuteri[66] states that the mast cells have a direct or indirect importance in the storing and releasing of some active substances. When the mast cells of the head are stimulated by the injection of a histamine liberator into the carotid arteries, vasodilation, edema, pain, and the clinical features of migraine occur. Sicuteri concluded that migraine pathogenesis involves microvaso-

active substances such as those in the mast cells. The mast cells are abundant in all loose connective tissue and are especially great in number around blood vessels. In the blood, the basophilic granulocyte plays the part of the mast cell in the tissue. Both the basophil and the mast cell contain histamine and heparin, and there is, therefore, a close relationship of these two types of cells.

In a study on the basophilic leukocyte and migraine:

Blood samples were taken from both ear lobes of nine migraine and nine non-migrainous patients during one-sided headaches. Such samples were also taken from migraine after attacks. For the migraine group, chamber counts of leukocytic composition showed: (a) significantly more basophils on the affected than the unaffected side during attacks but no significant between-sides difference afterward; (b) significant but complementary during-versus-after differences for each side—on the affected side, more basophils during attacks than after and, on the unaffected, fewer basophils during attacks than after; (c) no significant difference in total white cell counts in any comparison. For the non-migraine group, no significant difference was found for either basophil or white cell counts. Differential basophil counts of stained smears from migraine-patient samples indicated significantly more metamyelocytes on the affected side during attacks than (a) on the unaffected side during attack or (b) on its own (previously affected) side after.*

In this study Thonnard-Neumann[64] found:

results for total basophils and basophilic metamyelocytes showed significantly more of both going to the affected side than the unaffected during, but not after, migraine attacks. Also, the sum of total basophils over sides remained about constant whether or not a headache was disturbing the balance between them . . . . By contrast, the onset of migraine raised the sum of metamyelocytes. . . about twice as much as total basophils. This suggests that the number of mature basophils decreased accordingly during attack. . . . *

It is believed that one difference between the basophils found in the blood and those that are found in the tissues is that the basophils in the blood are less active.[67] The basophils are believed to possess mobility.

*From Thonnard-Neumann, E., and Taylor, W. L.: The basophilic leukocyte and migraine, Headache **8:**98-107, 1968.

and it is thought that they "perform a temporary function that is later taken over by the mast cells because of their greater supply of humoral substances."[68]

In his study on basophilic leukocytes and migraine Thonnard-Neumann suggests

that basophils assist the local mast cells throughout the attack. Basophils were being delivered at an increased rate to the affected cranial region from shortly after the onset of a headache until at least 24 hours thereafter. Sicuteri's[66] finding—that the number of local tissue mast cells decreased during attack—suggests that the assistance of the basophil was needed.*

He concludes:

The total amount of available histamine present at any particular time and site seems to be the sum of local free and mast-cell-bound histamine plus what is brought in by basophils. . . . The results of this study indicate that the onset of a migraine attack is associated, on the affected side, with a rise in the number of basophils . . . . However, the basophils (like the mast cells) also contain heparin, so it also is being brought to the affected side at an increased rate during attack. The heparin is in a bond with histamine and both are attached to the cell's granules.*

In 1969 Ernst Thonnard-Neumann won the Wolff Award from the American Association for the Study of Headache for his paper entitled, "Some Interrelationships of Vasoactive Substances and Basophilic Leukocytes in Migraine Headache."[65] The following paragraphs are taken from this excellent paper.

The implication of tissue mast cells in the pathophysiology of migraine was demonstrated by Sicuteri.[66] He found in biopsy specimens taken from the temple region of patients during migraine attacks that the number of mast cells was reduced and that the remaining cells had suffered a partial loss of their granules. The granules of tissue mast cells contain heparin and histamine. Counterparts of the mast cell in the tissue are the basophilic leukocytes in the blood.[67] Like mast cells, the basophils contain heparin and histamine. This suggests a close functional relationship between the two cell systems.

This writer, together with W. L. Taylor,[67] recently investigated the distribution of blood basophils in the extracerebral cranial circulation of migraine patients. In blood samples taken from both ear lobes during an

attack of one-sided migraine headache, they found more basophils on the affected than on the unaffected side of the head. The difference in the counts between the sides disappeared when the headache had subsided. No difference between sides was found in the blood of patients who suffered from one-sided headaches of other than migraine origin. The total white cell count did not show this bias . . . .

The use of basophilic leukocytes offers several advantages over that of tissue mast cells. Cell counts can be made with a great degree of accuracy and cell morphology is less distorted in blood smears than in tissue sections. Furthermore, the discomfort caused the patient when obtaining specimens is very slight, allowing samples to be taken frequently and at short intervals.

The studies were made in female patients who suffered from frequent attacks of migraine headache. A comparable group of female subjects who were free from migraine served as controls. The numbers of basophilic leukocytes (B.L.) per cubic millimeter of blood and per hundred white cells were counted. . . . Migraine patients and non-migraine controls received single injections of heparin, histamine, serotonin, norepinephrine, tyramine, and reserpine. Reserpine was given intramuscularly; the other agents were given by intravenous injection. Blood samples were obtained before challenge and 30 minutes, four hours, and 24 hours after challenge. Since maximum response to challenge occurred at different times for different substances, those intervals were chosen for evaluation at which the majority of subjects showed maximum changes. Migraine patients received the injections on migraine-free days.*

In migraine patients, serotonin and norepinephrine produced significant rises in the number of basophilic leukocytes over pretreatment levels. Heparin, histamine, tyramine, and reserpine caused reductions in basophil values which were significantly below levels before challenge. In the control subjects the injection of heparin, serotonin, and tyramine caused no significant alterations in the basophil counts. After histamine and reserpine a significant drop and after norepinephrine a significant rise occurred. When the changes in basophil levels which the agents had caused in migraine patients were compared with those in the control subjects, significant differences in the response of the basophilic leukocytes of the two populations were found for all chal-

*From Thonnard-Neumann, E., and Taylor, W. L.: The basophilic leukocyte and migraine, Headache **8**:98-107, 1968.

*From Thonnard-Newmann, E.: Some interrelationships of vasoactive substances and basophilic leukocytes in migraine headache, Headache **9**:130-140, 1969.

lenging agents with the exception of histamine. Histamine caused in migraine and nonmigraine subjects a similar drop in basophil levels.

The morphology of B.L. was studied during and after attacks of migraine headache in blood smears stained with Wright-Giemsa solution. Blood was taken from both ear lobes and from the affected temple region during one-sided headaches and after the attacks had subsided. B.L. were examined for cell size and cell shape, position of the nucleus, and cytoplasmic contents. Cell age was determined. . . . Basophils were also examined for number and size of granules and the appearance of fused granules and of stained or empty vacuoles. Also noted was the prevalence of ruptured cells with scattered granular contents. Similar morphologic studies were made . . . after challenge with the chemical mediators. . . .

In blood smears made during migraine attacks, basophils were observed which contained very few granules. In some cells granules were replaced by vacuoles. The cells did not appear damaged; in particular, there was no increase in the proportion of ruptured cells. Degranulated basophils were most frequently seen in smears taken from areas near the site of the headache, such as the temple region, or the ear lobe on the affected side. After migraine attacks had subsided, only few of these cells were found. No difference in basophil morphology was apparent if the attacks had subsided spontaneously or after ergotamine tartrate therapy. . . .

Some moderate changes in basophil morphology were seen in blood smears which had been obtained after challenge when changes in total basophil numbers were at their peak. After histamine, some degranulated basophils were seen; after tyramine and reserpine, basophils appeared in which granules were displaced by clear vacuoles. Norepinephrine caused some fusion of granules and degranulation. Heparin was the only compound after which an increase in basophils with coarse granules was observed.

In a previous study[64] it was found that during one-sided attacks of migraine headache more basophils went to the affected side than to the unaffected side of the head. In the present investigation it was observed that more degranulated basophils appeared in samples from the affected temple region or the ear lobe on the side of the headache than from places further removed, i.e., the other earlobe or a finger. The combined findings suggest that the B.L. participate in the migraine process through the contents of their storage granules. The undamaged appearance of the cells indicates that during the migraine attack the release of chemical mediators stored in basophils is not accompanied by cell destruction. This degranulation process should, therefore, be sharply distinguished from the violent disruption of B.L. with shattering of granules in the general circulation of laboratory animals caused by

their exposure to chemical agents. . . . The phenomenon of basophil degranulation close to the site of the headache supports previous evidence that it is in the microcirculation and the tissues where the major changes in basophil activity take place.[67]

The disappearance of basophilic granules can either mean that they and their soluble contents have been released through the cell membrane or that the cell has taken up humoral compounds and during this process granules have been lysed inside the cell.[64]

Histamine occurs in tissue mast cells and B.L. together with heparin in a loose bond.[67] . . .

When degranulation occurs, histamine probably is released first from the granules and is followed by heparin.[70] Riley[71] considers the main task of histamine from mast cells to be the preparation of other tissue cells for the uptake of heparin. Usually little of the heparin which has been liberated from mast cells seems to reach the circulation. But Sicuteri's findings[72] of hypocoagulative changes in the blood of migraine patients toward the end of an attack indicate that physiologically active heparin has been set free. He observed changes in the thrombelastrogram which were similar to those seen after the injection of heparin. It would seem reasonable to assume that the blood basophils were the source of that heparin.

Heparin caused a significant drop in the number of basophils of all but one of the migraine patients within one-half hour after the injection. In the control population there was a random response to heparin. . . .

. . . In the studies here, the outstanding change in the basophils of heparin-treated migraine patients was an increase in cells with coarse granules. . . . The lesser degree of intracellular changes after heparin in the B.L. of migraine patients, as compared with normal subjects, would seem to indicate that the basophils of migraine patients already possessed before challenge a near-capacity load of endogenous heparin. This apparent reluctance of basophils of migraine patients to accept more heparin, together with the rapid decrease in absolute basophil numbers after the injection of heparin, may be part of a hemostatic process which is accelerated by repeated attacks of migraine.

Histamine was the only compound tested which caused changes in basophil response of migraine patients which were similar to those of the control subjects. . . .

The significant rise of basophil values in migraine patients produced by serotonin contrasts with the nonsignificant changes which this bioamine caused in the controls. The findings may be taken as additional evidence of the implication of serotonin in migraine.[73] Australian researchers[74] have recently reported that serotonin plasma levels of migraine patients were increased shortly before and reduced during an attack. In spite of a number of animal and in vitro studies on the interactions between serotonin, histamine, and heparin, our knowledge of their in vivo interrelationships in man is scant. . . .

. . . During one-sided attacks of migraine headaches, more degranulated basophils were found in blood samples from the temple region and the ear lobe on the headache side than in places further removed, i.e., the other ear lobe or a finger.

In order to study the role basophilic leukocytes may play in the pathophysiology of migraine headache, their response to challenge with various chemical mediators was determined in a group of female patients who suffered from frequent attacks of migraine. Heparin and histamine, which are hemoral constituents of basophilic leukocytes, caused, when injected, a drop in basophil levels. The injection of tyramine or reserpine also produced a reduction in basophil values, whereas after serotonin or norepinephrine the counts rose. The changes from prechallenge levels were significant for each group.

The response to the same chemical agents in a group of female subjects who were free from migraine was significantly different from that of the migraine patients for each mediator with the exception of histamine. After histamine a similar reduction in basophil values was found in both populations.

Migraine prophylaxis with methysergide or medroxyprogesterone caused a significant reduction in the total number of basophils, the proportion of basophilic metamyelocytes, and of degranulated basophils.

When serotonin or reserpine was given after four weeks of migraine prophylaxis with either drug, a reversal of the previous effects of serotonin and reserpine on the number of basophils was observed.

The same reversal was found when heparin was given one-half hour before the injection of serotonin or reserpine.*

Not all headache researchers agree with Thonnard-Neumann. At a headache symposium in Elsinore, Denmark, in 1971, Appenzeller and Scott[75] questioned that the reported changes in basophilic leukocyte counts observed during the migraine attack on the side of the headache were merely a reflection of the change in the caliber of the vessels on the side of the pain.

Degranulation of basophil leukocytes has been reported during the attack of migraine.[65] Appenzeller's studies, however, do not support this interpretation. He did not observe degranulation of basophils even though the number of basophilic leukocytes was increased to levels comparable to those found during hemicrania. He did not, however, induce headache, and the stimulus

---

*From Thonnard-Neumann, E.: Some interrelationships of vasoactive substances and basophilic leukocytes in migraine headache, Headache **9:**130-140, 1969.

might not have been sufficiently prolonged for degranulation to occur.

Appenzeller's studies in controls and migraine patients do not support the view that basophils are related to the pain of migraine.

Genetics

For all practical purposes a positive family history might well be considered in discussing the etiology of migraine. Migraine is perhaps the only form of headache which presents a family history as part of its symptomatology. We would estimate that about 50% of the patients afflicted with migraine have a family history of this headache. There is no other form of headache problem which presents any percentage of family history at all. Certainly other forms of headache such as histaminic cephalalgia, myalgia, muscle contraction headache, nasal sinusitis, or any others do not have a family history background. This is indeed an interesting fact and an important one.

In a study on migraine in families, Barolin and Sperlich[76] made some interesting observations. They found that in 450 cases of migraine seen over a period of 11 years, a family history of the disease was observed in 22% of the cases. Genealogic trees are given for eight of these families to illustrate the incidence of migraine, or any other form of cerebral attack, and the nature of the EEG tracing, whether normal or of the migraine type. Familial similarities were found especially in regard to the EEG; more than one third of the patients had abnormal EEG tracings. They found that the most common linkage of migrainous subjects within a family was mother to daughter. The mother was more often affected than the father; female relatives were more often affected than the male ones. It was rare for the disease to skip a generation. Chromosomal analysis of two families gave normal results. They concluded that the only difference that could be found between migrainous patients with a family history and those without one concerned the age of onset: 50% of cases starting before puberty had a family history, as opposed to only 5% of those developing after the age of 35 years.

A genetic predisposition to migraine does not always result in the development of the disease; this may depend on other factors. In women, sex hormones may play a role as a predisposing factor.

Young and Barth[77] report on a family in which migraine was present in four successive generations. In this family, migraine was present as an autosomal dominant with the hemiplegic and common forms of migraine phenotypic variants of the same disease.

In a study on the influence of hormones on headache in women Grant and associates[78] found that the hereditary aspect of migraine may depend on inheriting a particular immune pattern which might cause a special sensitivity to hormone effects on blood vessels. This might account for the suppression of menstrual migraine by cortisone or large doses of progesterone. Deficiency of progesterone is not likely to be responsible for the premenstrual syndrome, as the period following menstruation is usually the time which is most often free from symptoms and at this part of the cycle there are very low levels of progesterone. Unfortunately, the most reactive women are also the most sensitive to the side effects of drugs or hormones given to treat migraine. We are still awaiting a satisfactory answer to this problem.

Espin Herrero and Barcia Marino[79] made a review of the genetic factor involved in the etiology of migraine. They found that familial migraine occurred in 62.7% of the patients studied. A study of the family histories indicated that the genetic factors involved are multiple alleles with various degrees of penetration, possibly caused by errors of amine metabolism, cerebrovascular malformations, vasolability, neuroautonomic debility, and personality.

Most authorities agree that a hereditary factor is present in the development of migraine. Among homozygous twins both are affected in 50% of cases of migraine; in heterozygous twins this occurs in only 10% of the cases.

Ziegler and co-workers[80] found that the presence of familial aggregations and the dubious evidence as to twin concordance would seem to strengthen the possibility that a common environment, or at least a common environment affecting certain individuals, may be the reason for the familial aggregation in migraine. They concluded that of all the many clinical features of headache studies, they did not find concordance in any that was significantly different in monozygotic versus dizygotic twins. It is, of course, still possible that among the large population of headache patients there are small groups with a genetically determined characteristic.

Migraine might well be considered a heterogeneous condition with some still unidentified inherited predisposing factors that require interaction with environment to produce symptoms.

Barraquer-Bordas and associates[81] suggest that migraine associated with paresis of the facial nerve has been reported only infrequently in the literature, particularly so during recent years. There is recurrent facial paralysis, often with alternation of sides, sometimes associated with paralysis of other cranial nerves and with brainstem lesions. The paralysis is sometimes purely over the lower part of the face, which might indicate a central origin. Hereditary familial occurrence is quite exceptional. The cases reported were in a family in which migraine has been transmitted through three consecutive generations, with the prosoplegic type appearing only in the third generation and affecting preferentially the female sex. They concluded that the mechanism involved is probably a segmental arterial constriction and compression of cranial nerves by the edematous arterial wall; the artery concerned is probably the internal auditory; and the compression occurs in the facial nerve canal. The familial character suggests a dominant autosomal transmission of an arterial, migraine-producing mechanism and of facial nerve vulnerability.

Heredity plays an important part in the production of migraine, as does the personality of the individual. Wolff and co-workers,[82] in a study of 119 migraine patients, found that 70% of them presented a family history of migraine headaches.

In migraine, it has been observed that the overwhelming majority of patients present common personality features which, though not pathognomonic of migraine or associated with migraine alone, are likely under certain conditions to call forth pernicious emotional reactions.[83] The predominant characteristics of this personality structure are childhood shyness, obedience, neatness, reliability, stubborn inflexibility in certain circumstances, adult perfectionism, ambitiousness, inelasticity, tension, resentment, and repetitiousness, but also efficiency, poise, and social grace. As a result of this personality pattern, the migraine patient is in constant tension, with resultant autonomic and vasomotor instability.

Friedman, von Storch, and Merritt[84] found a hereditary factor in 65% of these cases and also that women predominate by a ratio of two to one. They also found in their survey that migraine began before the age of 20 in 55% of their cases, that it was rare to find the initial attack occurring after the age of 40, and that the attack would occur less than once a week in about 60% of their cases.

Hirsch[85] believes that patients are afflicted with migraine because of (1) an inherited predisposition built in the individual and (2) a depletion of energy from any cause beyond the body's ability to spring back, which allows this predisposition to erupt. This theory would be hard to explain, as in extensive surveys it has been found that only 60% to 70% of such patients are found to have a family history of migraine.

Lippman[86] claims that migraine sufferers have an inherited chemical imbalance that makes them overly sensitive to physical and mental stimuli.

Dalsgaard-Nielsen[87] believes that there is a lacuna between our acquaintance with the clinical manifestations of migraine and our poor knowledge of its true nature. A variety of factors of external and/or internal ictogenic nature—psychogenic, vascular, neurologic, and histohumeral—cooperate to trigger the reaction, which is the headache. The pattern of the reaction seems based on genetic factors: a family history is obtainable in 89% of cases, and in 73% one or other parent is found to have migraine. Theories of heredity based on a gene with incomplete penetrance can be discarded; the inheritance pattern is probably multifactorial.

In conclusion it seems that there is definitely a strong tendency for migraine to occur in families, much more so than is found in any other form of headache. This does not mean, however, that people with a history of migraine in their families will develop other forms of headache. No, they merely have a great possibility of being afflicted with only migraine, as if that is not enough.

Prostaglandins

The prostaglandins are a unique group of cyclic fatty acids with vast and potent biologic effects involving almost every organ system in a variety of species, including the human. The immediate precursors of prostaglandin synthesis are essential, unsaturated, fatty acids. It is now believed that they are needed in the diet because they play a pivotal role in being converted to prostaglandins. The transformation of unsaturated fatty acids to prostaglandins is catalyzed by prostaglandin synthetase, an enzyme specifically inhibited by essential fatty acid analogues and a number of anti-inflammatory agents. A variety of physiologic stimuli will evoke release of prostaglandins. The significance of prostaglandin E or prostaglandin F release remains unclear, since these two groups of prostaglandins are extensively metabolized by the lung and thus cannot qualify as true circulating hormones. It is likely that prostaglandins are released into the venous circulation by many heterogeneous stimuli. It appears that release into the venous circulation reflects an increase in prostaglandin synthesis within a particular tissue or organ, leading to a functional change in that system, followed by a secondary overflow release of prostaglandin into the blood for eventual metabolism in the lung.

Interest in the role of prostaglandins in migraine has been great since the demonstration that prostaglandin E_1 (PGE_1) infusion into humans with no history of migraine could consistently cause migraine-like headaches with abdominal cramps and nausea. PGE_1 seems to be a potent extracranial vasodilator as a consequence to stealing blood from the intracranial territory. It has been believed that tyramine, serotonin, and phenylethylamine may be able to stimulate the release of prostaglandins from the lungs. Drugs known to inhibit prostaglandin synthesis have been reported to be effective in migraine patients.

Thus, current ideas on PGE_1 involvement could account for the vasodilator phase of a migraine attack, the nausea and abdominal disturbances, the supposed actions of tyramine, serotonin, and phenylethylamine in precipitation of migraine attacks, and the pain.

Prostaglandins have been found in every tissue in which they have been sought. They are manufactured by an enzyme complex known as prostaglandin synthetase. The most important substrates for prostaglandin synthetase are dihomo-γ-linolenic acid, the precursor of the one series of prostaglandins such as PGE_1, and arachidonic acid, the precursor of the two series such as PGE_2. The precursors are stored in the form of membrane phospholipids from which they are split and made available to the synthetase by phospholipase A_2. The synthetase system first converts the precursors to the endoperoxidases PGHS and PGGS, which are then changed to the major pros-

taglandins to the thromboxanes or to other relatively inactive end products.[88]

Intravenously injected prostaglandin E may provoke headache attacks sometimes indistinguishable from migraine,[89] with PGE_1 being more effective than the mildly active PGE_2.[90,91] The fact that an intravenous prostaglandin should give rise to a headache is at first surprising, because in some animal species over 95% of prostaglandin E_1, E_2, and $F_{2\alpha}$ is removed on the first pass through the lungs.[92] If these findings can be extrapolated to humans, then presumably the headache resulting from intravenous prostaglandin infusion is likely to stem from the action of minute concentrations only that have escaped inactivation and have gained access to the systemic circulation.

Alabaster[93] infused 5-hydroxytryptamine into the pulmonary artery of an experimental animal and noted the release of prostaglandins and of other less well-identified, pharmacologically active substances into the pulmonary vein. It was considered possible that a similar phenomenon occurs in human migraine; that in response to a suitable triggering agent, small concentrations of a prostaglandin or other active substance are released directly from the lungs into the systemic circulation to act on receptors in the cerebrovascular bed. Therefore, it was considered better to examine arterial blood in an attempt to identify the agent responsible for migraine.

Yamamoto[94] infused prostaglandins into the carotid arteries of dogs and the epicerebral vessels were observed by fluorescein angiography. The regional cerebral blood flow was monitored by lithium drift silicone detectors placed on the surface of the cortex to measure clearance. Infused PGE_1 constricted the epicerebral arteries to less than 700 μm in diameter and reduced regional blood flow by 42%. The addition of 0.08% alcohol blocked these changes. PGF_2 in twenty-five produced vasoconstriction of the smaller cerebral arteries only. A lesser but still significant reduction (35%)

occurred in the regional cerebral blood flow. The angiograms demonstrated a slower circulation time. Subsequent dissection showed that the circle of Willis in these dogs received a variable contribution of blood from the external as well as the internal carotid arteries. Welch[95] assessed the response of the cranial vasculature to prostaglandins by simultaneous measurement of internal and external carotid blood flow in the monkey. $PGF_{2\alpha}$ reduced flow in both external and internal carotid arteries due to a vasoconstrictor effect similar in degree to that of serotonin. High doses of $PGF_{1\alpha}$ had no effect on internal carotid flow and only a minimal vasoconstrictor effect on the external carotid artery.

In studies in which 200-ng doses of PGE_1 were injected into the carotid artery, in spite of unaltered cerebral profusion pressure and alveolar carbon dioxide, significant alteration in intercarotid flow occurred simultaneously with an increase in external carotid flow. This suggests a constrictor effect of PGE_1 on the internal carotid vasculature occurring simultaneously with dilation of the external carotid. When PGE_1 was infused solely into the internal carotid artery in the same group of animals, there followed no effect on the internal carotid flow. Welch postulated that this finding might be explained in two ways:

1. The first possibility accepts the fact that PGE_1 constricts cerebral vessels. When infused into the internal carotid artery at the time of external carotid artery clamping, PGE_1 might perfuse the extracranial tissues through newly opened collateral channels. Since PGE_1 dilates external carotid resistance channel vessels, resultant flow increase would be conducted by the common carotid artery and mask any decrease in internal carotid flow due to intracranial vasoconstriction. Such a possibility is considered unlikely from their finding, since tourniquet pressure was applied to extracranial tissues and arbors to prevent collateral channels.

2. The second possibility does not accept PGE_1 as a cerebral vasoconstricter. When PGE_1 is injected into the common carotid artery with the external carotid artery patent, a marked falling resistance of the external vascular bed occurs in all cases. This should reduce perfusion pressure in the carotid system by further accentuating pressure drip along the common carotid artery and effectively reducing cerebral perfusion pressure measured at the carotid bifurcation. Pressure drop in autoregulating vessels results in a flow decrease, which can also be disproportionately greater relative to such pressure fall which is a result of reduction in resistant vessel radius due to elastic recoil under reduced transmural pressure. Welch's experiments suggested that increased arterial levels of PGE_1 will cause extreme dilation of the external carotid vasculature and abolish cerebral autoregulation, resulting in redistribution or steal of blood from the internal carotid artery. The steal theory also affords explanation for a frequent observation that cerebral ischemic symptomatology persists during the headache phase of a migraine attack.

As a conclusion, Welch hypothesized that the characteristic flow change can be caused by a single agent that has a differential effect on external and internal carotid flow to simultaneously cause external carotid dilation with steal of blood from the internal carotid system.

Because of their hypothesized implication in the pathogenesis of migraine, Pickard[96] studied the effects of serotonin and $PGF_{2\alpha}$ and PGE_2 on the intracranial and extracranial vascular beds to see whether their actions are consistent with the circulatory changes in migraine. These compounds were administered by intracarotid infusion. The results of his studies showed that PGE_2 and $PGF_{2\alpha}$ significantly reduced both cerebral blood flow and the utilization rate of oxygen. Both serotonin and PGE_2 enormously constricted the ipsilateral internal carotid artery, as demonstrated by carotid angiography. When the blood-brain barrier was disrupted transiently with the hypertonic urea technique, both PGE_2 and serotonin considerably reduced both cerebral blood flow and the utilization rate of oxygen. In his study, both PGE_2 and serotonin also increased the external carotid artery blood flow and the temporalis blood flow enormously. In another study, Olesen[97] studied patients who underwent diagnostic arteriography. The cerebral blood flow was measured in sixteen smaller areas of the hemisphere by means of the intracarotid injection of a radioactive gas. First, a measurement was taken in the resting state. Then PGE_1 was infused into the internal carotid artery for 5 minutes. The infusion was stopped approximately 30 seconds to inject the tracer and draw blood samples, then it was resumed.

The results were consistent in these patients. All had a mild increase in cerebral blood flow averaging 11.2%. The flow increase was seen diffusely all over the hemisphere. During the PGE_1 infusion, the skin of the glabellar region and conjunctiva became red and infected. This area is supplied by a branch of the internal carotid artery.

Pennink[98] injected $PGF_{2\alpha}$ into the chiasmatic cisterns of anesthetized dogs via the optic foramen in an attempt to produce cerebral vasospasm. The occurrence of vasospasm was assessed by repeated arteriography using Hypaque 60%. The blood pressure of the circle of Willis was recorded with a pressure transducer inserted into the contralateral carotid artery which was occluded at its origin by a clamp. Six out of eighteen patients injected with blood alone developed vasospasm, compared with twelve out of thirteen injected with 4 ml of blood plus 20 ng/kg of $PGF_{2\alpha}$. The blood pressure of the circle of Willis fell during the injection, then rose again due to a rise in systemic blood pressure, then fell again. Injection of 2 ml of cerebrospinal fluid with 20 ng/kg $PGF_{2\alpha}$ produced vasospasm in all four dogs. PGE_1 failed to produce vasospasm in three dogs.

Pennink concluded that $PGF_{2\alpha}$ but not PGE_1 may induce cerebral vasospasm. He postulated that the F_2 type of prostaglandin known to be present in brain tissue is released by trauma or blood into the cerebrospinal fluid.

Anthony[99] studied the relationship of plasma PGE_2 in migrainous patients. Thirty patients with severe and frequent migraine attacks were admitted to the hospital for investigations. All interval therapy was suspended for 1 week before admission and no ergotamine or analgesic preparations were allowed for 2 days prior to admission. Once the headache developed in these patients, blood was collected almost quarter-hourly for the duration of the attack and for a further 1 to 2 days after it ended. Arteriovenous differences in plasma levels of PGE_1 were measured. Migrainous patients showed no difference in plasma levels between the preheadache, headache, and postheadache periods. Three patients showed a rise in plasma levels of more than 10% during headache, two showed a fall, and the remaining seven showed no change. PGE_1 levels in venous and arterial blood collected simultaneously showed no regular pattern of arteriovenous difference between normal subjects and those suffering from various neurologic diseases, migraine, or cluster headaches.

The half-life of prostaglandins in the blood is less than 30 seconds. At 1½ minutes after intravenous administration of PGE_2 to human subjects, only about 3% was present as natural PGE_2 in the blood, and more than 40% was recovered as the 15-ketodihydrometabolite. Therefore, Anthony believed that plasma levels of natural prostaglandins do not accurately reflect endogenous rates of formation, and results might be difficult to interpret. He believed that more reliable information could be obtained by estimation of an initial metabolite that has a relatively longer half-life and is not synthesized in the blood.

Again, with prostaglandins, we are in the same situation as we are with many other substances being studied in regard to their etiologic implication in migraine. As observed from the numerous articles and investigations being carried out, there seems to be some evidence of prostaglandin involvement in the precipitation of migraine attacks. However, the exact mechanism of action is not known, and further investigative work must be carried out to elucidate the exact mechanisms by which prostaglandin may play a role in the precipitation of migraine attacks.

Tryptophan

A good deal of interest has been paid for quite some time to tryptophan metabolism in migraine. Sicuteri has reported a good effect after tryptophan given during a migraine attack.[100] Increase of 5-HIAA in cerebrospinal fluid was found after tryptophan ingestion.

Fanciullacci[101] studied the plasma levels of tryptophan in migraine patients during acute attacks. He found that there is an increase of free tryptophan during a migraine attack but that tryptophan shows no significant difference from that of control subjects during a migraine-free period. The increase of free tryptophan during a migraine attack could be due to the fact that these patients fast during their attacks.

Szule-Kuberska conducted a study whereby she tried to follow tryptophan metabolism on both the nicotinic and the serotonin pathways. Twenty patients were included in this study, fifteen with common and five with classic migraine. Six blood samples were taken from each patient, the first in the morning while fasting, followed by five others at 2-hour intervals. Investigations of 12-hour serum tryptophan after the ingestion of 10 mg of *dl*-tryptophan metabolized in urine collected during 24 hours in and between migraine attacks were made. 5-HIAA levels in urine in and between migraine attacks were also measured.

In the majority of their cases, tryptophan curves in migraine attacks went down slowly, much more slowly than in control periods. They believed that this might suggest that the metabolism of tryptophan during migraine attack was diminished. In five cases, tryptophan curves were slightly higher during the attack of the headache than in the headache-free period. There is no other difference in tryptophan curves in and between migraine attacks. Normal tryptophan returned to the original level after 12 hours in all cases. Also, endogenous tryptophan level was remarkably lower just before an attack of migraine in only five cases.

In all fifteen cases, the level of tryptophan metabolized in urine during a migraine attack was significantly lower than in the headache-free period. No significant difference between the level of 5-HIAA in urine during migraine attacks and in headache-free periods could be found.

They concluded that the appearance of tryptophan curves seems to suggest that the absorption of tryptophan in migrainous patients is not being affected and is very similar to absorption in control periods. The metabolism of tryptophan during migraine attacks happens to be slightly diminished. It might be due to lesser activity of tryptophan pyrrolase. In regard to comparison of urine tryptophan-metabolized contents during migraine attacks with that of a headache-free period, the phenomenon of tryptophan disappearance might be noted. They postulated that tryptophan is probably metabolized in the process of platelet 5-HT restitution or processed in cerebral metabolism so slowly that it could not be observed, as there was only a collection of urine over 24 hours.

There is no conclusive evidence that tryptophan is involved in the precipitation of migraine attacks, but there does appear to be enough circumstantial evidence pointing to the fact that further studies need to be carried out.

Limbic system dysfunction

EDGARD RAFFAELLI, Jr.
The key to the understanding of the start of a migraine attack lies in the central nervous and central autonomic systems.
Friedman, 1969

In spite of being one of the most common nervous system dysfunctions afflicting mankind, migraine still is, owing to its complexity, one of the most difficult dysfunctions to treat. The global clinical picture of migraine (that is, which also emphasizes the importance of migraine equivalents) was hardly ever considered in the past. Today a considerable number of authors refer to such equivalents, mentioning not only transitory hemiparesis or hemiplegias, which are rather uncommon, but also other equivalents that are not so dramatic but are much more frequent, such as vertigo and crises of pseudoangina.

Nevertheless, the evolutive clinical picture of migraine started being considered but recently, and it is now clear that the study of the evolution of the dysfunction in an individual from infancy, as compared to the evolutive clinical picture of other migraineurs, gives a better understanding of the nervous phenomena involved.

Those authors who try to validate or invalidate epilepsy as being the etiologic basis for migraine draw statistics based on the convulsions that occurred to the patients in the group under study, or else they refer to EEG findings. Neither argument leads to a satisfactory conclusion, and the opinions on the subject are still divided, although the majority of authors do not accept a relationship between epilepsy and migraine. For this group, one of the most important arguments is that anticonvulsant drugs have little effect on migraine.

The EEG findings of migraineurs show a positivity varying from 10% to 70%, according to the author, and this fact alone is sufficient to show that no correlation can be established based on such findings. Since 20% of the electroencephalograms of epileptic individuals are normal, the EEG is not really a choice test in migraine. As a matter of fact, with the data available today, there is no particular test of an etiologic nature for chronic headache. What is available, though, is what has always been the most important weapon of the physician: the history of the patient.

The history of the migraineur generally starts in infancy. Frequent vomiting, crisis of pallor with sweating, sleep disturbances, and intestinal disturbances are common in the early phase. As the child grows, there are breath-holding spells on crying, motion sickness, leg pains that are mistaken for rheumatism or called "growth pains," short-lived headaches that start and end abruptly, faintings in church or in parades, asthmatic crises, nocturnal enuresis that occasionally goes on up to puberty or adult life, night terror or unreasonable fear, somnambulism, somniloquism, bruxism, and behavior disturbances, among the more common complaints.

The most important turnpoints in the life of the migraineur are puberty and/or menopause. It is during the more intense hormonal life that the headache sufferer presents symptoms more evidently. Epigastric pains, for instance, may occur in infancy, but they are found more frequently in puberty. The same may be said about flushing: it is a peculiarity of menopause, but sometimes it starts during puberty and even in infancy.

Generally speaking, before the thirtieth birthday the migraineur already has a well-developed picture of neurovisceral dysfunction, and headaches have already become a routine. Vertigo, which in infancy was represented by motion sickness, by this time is already well defined, as are crises of dyspnea, paroxysmal tachycardia, pseudoangina, and gastrointestinal and sleep disturbances. Nightmares, which are the probable substrate of night terror in infancy, become more evident now. Memory loss, which is a constant in this group of patients, is seldom found in infancy and puberty (during these two periods inattention and lack of concentration are more easily found); before 30, though, the majority of these patients complain of a faulty recent memory. Sexual disinterest (which is equivalent to coldness in women and impotence in men) generally starts in the decade from 20 to 30 in women and in the following decade in men. Labyrinthine disturbances usually become evident when the patient ceases having migraine attacks; such attacks are then substituted by labyrinthine crises. It is not uncommon, though, that a labyrinthine disorder be one of the first manifestations of the neurovisceral dysfunction. When this happens, the patient may not end up having attacks of migraine and the maximal manifestation of dysfunction continues to be the labyrinthine disturbances. Perhaps the earliest oto-neurologic sign is tinnitus, which is evident in many children.

One thing that makes the study of migraine extremely complicated and that sometimes makes the complaints of migraineurs hard to believe is that such complaints are not coincident with the clinical data obtained. For instance, the complaint of arterial blood pressure dropping is very common, but when the blood pressure is measured during the crisis or soon after it, it generally is normal. Although this complaint may seem irrelevant, it portrays a real situation. The headache sufferers, notably women, have sudden and short-lived drops in arterial blood pressure; in the future, though, such patients frequently develop a so-called emotional arterial hypertension. Sicuteri,[102] in 1971, showed that migraineurs have a highly significant depression in the monoamine oxidase activity of their platelets, which might explain the evolution to hypertension.

The first physician to write an autobiographic report on migraine was Charles Lepois, in 1714.[103] He believed that his attacks were brought about by alterations in climate, especially the appearance of west winds and rainstorms. In 1971, Sulman[104] studied the effect of the hot and dry desert wind, the Sharav of Israel, in 200 weather-sensitive patients, and he called it "irritation syndrome, due to hypothalamic serotonin hyperactivity or hyperproduction." Patients who suffered from the "serotonin irritation syndrome" developed migraine associated with nausea or vomiting, amblyopia, need for higher dioptric glasses, sleeplessness, irritability, tension, edema, palpitations or precordial pain, dyspnea, hot flushes with sweating or chills, allergic complaints such as vasomotor rhinitis, conjunctivitis, laryngitis, pharyngitis, tracheitis, increased activity of the intestines, polyuria or pollakiuria, and, in rare cases, even tremor, olfactophobia, phonophobia or photophobia. Sulman's findings explain why the migraine sufferer is ill adapted to sudden changes in climate: the problem is biochemical and not psychologic, as shown by the urinalysis he made, which showed an increase in the serotonin excretion as a reaction to the electrical charge of the "weather front" that arrives 1 or 2 days before the hot dry wind itself. It is worth mentioning that Sharav's migraine occurs also in pregnant women.

This digression over a single paper intends to show that the genesis of the symptomatology may occur because of an external stimulus that does not depend on the patient. As well as the sudden alteration in climate, other external stimuli that are habitually effective are noise, light, movement, foods, strong smells, and emotion. Internal stimuli are provided by visceral and glandular mechanisms and also by general metabolism, especially carbohydrate metabolism, which is a function of the autonomic nervous system.

The existence of a regulating nervous mechanism is fundamental to keep people functioning in a straight line, so that after having suffered external or internal stimuli with their consequent autonomic responses they may return to an equilibrium without evident damage. In the migraineur there is a dysfunction of this regulating mechanism, so that stimuli provoke exaggerated reactions that are longer lasting and more intense than should be expected. With the passing of time, the excitability threshold diminishes and stimuli have their potency relatively increased.

When one analyzes the complaints of a migraineur, one notices that his ailments are dysfunctions which are common to all human beings occasionally but which in him are more frequent, more intense, and more complicated. The following is the history of a male migraineur, 38 years old.

The patient's main complaint was daily dull headache, which started 1 hour after lunch, and attacks of vascular headache two or three times a week. Past history included nocturnal enuresis up to 12 years of age; habitual leg cramps since childhood, generally nocturnal, which increased recently; one episode of somnambulism at 6; asthmatic bronchitis from 6 to 12 years of age; frequent nocturnal leg pains in infancy, with blood tests for rheumatism repeatedly normal; night terror which ceased at 12; and frequent nightmares, since "as far as I can remember." He had infrequent sudden attacks of shivering without an obvious cause during his youth, which led to negative tests for malaria. Motion sickness had been evident since his early childhood. At 18 he started to have occasional attacks of rotatory vertigo, and sudden changes of position, especially standing up after crouching, made him dizzy. When he was 16 he had sudden attacks of epigastric pain for which he had x-rays of the stomach and duodenum that proved normal; pains ceased after a few months and were replaced by habitual pyrosis which still bothered him. From infancy he complained of difficulty in falling asleep and waking up; in spite of sleeping 9 hours per night, he frequently complained of feeling sleepy during the day. As a child and as an adolescent he did not feel well when he smelled wax, gasoline, and perfumes; as an adult often developed a migraine if he inhaled such smells for some time. As a child he sometimes felt his ear block suddenly, as if he were going down a mountain to the sea; this sensation became more or less frequent, and it was followed by tinnitus. From his adolescence, he had allergic rhinitis, which would get worse when he became sexually aroused. At age 35 there started a progressive fall in his memory capacity and his sexual potency.

Up to 19 years old he had occasional headaches; from this age onward, he had frequent dull headaches with a growing intensity and frequency. After 25, daily, well-characterized tension headache occurred, as did attacks of paroxysmal tachycardia and precordial pains, not justified and not explained by cardiologic examinations and by three electrocardiograms, and intestinal disturbances characterized by occasional bouts of diarrhea. At 29, he had his first attack of typical vascular headache. Since then, he has had attacks of migraine every fortnight, then every week, and then every 2 or 3 days.

This history is not an exception. When taking the history of a migraineur, if one asks for all details since childhood, one notices that the person has lots of dysfunctions, which even though common to all human beings, are more frequent and more intense in him than in "normal" subjects. This does not mean that all migraineurs have exactly the same dysfunctions; it only means that such dysfunctions are plentiful in these individuals. We know that such symptoms are parts of a single clinical picture, because they are complaints that are common to all migraineurs. As a matter of fact, such complaints are common to all human beings under stress, especially emotional stress. That leads to the conclusion that the migraineur has as a characteristic the faculty of answering in an exaggerated way to stimuli, whether internal, external, or emotional.

If briefly analyzed from a biochemical point of view, this history tells us that the patient has adrenergic, serotonic, histaminic, and cholinergic alternances: the attacks of tachycardia and the precordial pains may be caused by an adrenergic mechanism; somnolence, diarrhea, allergic bronchitis in infancy, and present allergic rhinitis speak in favor of a serotonin-histamine mechanism; the epigastric pains in the past and the present pyrosis suggest a cholinergic-histaminic mechanism. How to explain, though, with chemical mediators, the nightmares, the motion sickness, the vertigo, the difficulty to sleep and to rise, the dyssomnia, the memory impairment, the sexual disinterest? Migraineurs are not adrenergic, or cholinergic, or serotonic; they have an abnormal response to stimuli with a consequent abnormal liberation of mediators. From patient to patient or in the same patient, there may occur, according to different stimuli, a greater or smaller liberation of one mediator as related to the others.

If, instead of only thinking of chemical mediators, we try to explain the migraine patient's complaints in terms of neurophysiology, we have to think of several cerebral structures that would be responsible for such dysfunctions. Thus, we could ask: which regulating mechanism could explain the intergration of stimuli in terms of reactions from the cortex, from the autonomic nervous system from the thalamus, from the reticular system, from the hypothalamus, from the hippocampus?

In 1878, Broca[105] called "le grand lobe limbique" those structures that surround the brainstem and that lie beneath the cortical mantle. Papez[106] in 1937 called attention to these nervous structures and postulated that their role was the superior control of emotion. Thus were born the ideas and the studies for the configuration of the limbic system, whose function would be that of a computer that receives its data from internal and external stimuli, including emotion, hence regulating the psychologic and neurovegetative behavior of the individual.

There is a widespread tendency, both lay and medical, to blame the genesis of multiple complaints on emotional problems. As a matter of fact, when emotions act on the limbic system, they bring about visceral (functional) reactions: the organ itself is normal, but the chemical mediator stimulating it is being liberated in abnormal quantities and provoking its dysfunction. This end result, as we know, is not exclusive of emotion: other stimuli, like weather changes and alcohol, for instance, may cause the same type of reaction and with the same intensity.

In summary what have we got? The migraineur would be a patient with a limbic dysfunction, and therefore abnormally sensitive to internal and external stimuli, which cause in him, as an answer, a headache.[107-110] We could say, then, that the patient with a limbic dysfunction is a person who may respond to stimuli with a neuromuscular-vascular pain in the head. If we believe this affirmation, we can also say that the response may come from structures other than cranial vessels, nerves, or muscles and thus find an explanation for the attacks of paroxysmal tachycardia that occur in a normal heart. In these patients, the target organ would be the heart and not the cranial vessels. The same could be said about vestibular attacks: in such patients, the target organ would be the labyrinth.

With what we know today of the limbic system, it is impossible to prove that a limbic syndrome really exists, because the proof we have is circumstantial. Nevertheless, if we analyze the life of a female migraineur, the fact is that when her limbic system is activated for her hormonal periodic functions (menarche, menstruation, pregnancy, menopause), these are the occasions when the signs of a limbic dysfunction, positive or negative, are more evident. One of these signs is the sensitivity to odors that some pregnant women develop: smell is one of the functions of the limbic system (formerly called rhinencephalon), and the sharpening of this sense during pregnancy is a circumstantial proof that the activation of the limbic system may bring about a limbic dysfunction.

It is our opinion that in order to obtain a lasting effect in the treatment of headache, we have to treat not only the headache but the limbic symptoms as well. That is what the migraine specialist usually does, because, unlike the average physician, he or she believes in the complaints of the migraineur. When a diagnosis of "psychovegetative syndrome" is made to explain such complaints, the patient is treated with psychiatric drugs, instead of receiving the antichemical mediators that a neurologic diagnosis of "limbic syndrome" would entitle him to receive.

SYMPTOMATOLOGY

Headache, of course, is the most prominent symptom of migraine. This pain is of throbbing nature and rather periodic. It is hemicranial and usually persists for several hours or even for several days. The pain is rather severe and usually in the orbital, frontal, or temporal areas, but it may be localized to any site. Usually, preceding the actual headache attack the patient may notice some visual disorders such as scintillating scotomas, hemianopia, and blurred vision. Photophobia is also associated with migraine either in the prodromal phase or during the actual headache phase.

Schrire[111] says that retinal arterial spasm may occur in the early phases of migraine. When the spasm is severe the affected vessel may become occluded, leading to a permanent defect in the visual fields. He says of the known recorded cases of retinal artery occlusion in migraine, four involved the central artery of the retina, giving rise to severe uniocular blindness; four involved peripheral branches, producing sector field defects, and one possibly involved an intraneural branch of the central retinal artery, producing a central scotoma. Four cases showed no signs of local retinal or generalized arterial disease, and there was no indication of any possible source of the emboli. It is his conclusion that migraine should be considered as a possible cause in cases of retinal artery occlusion in which no cerebrovascular disease can be detected.

Olsen[112] suggest a new hypothesis to explain the scotoma in accordance with a concept of fluid dynamics, "inertial" ischemia. This hypothesis would explain the freqency of scotoma, which suggests a disturbance in the area supplied by only one posterior cerebral artery. It would also explain the rarity of permanent after-effects.

Scintillating scotoma can occur without the actual headache occurring. Aring[113] believes that this partial syndrome may be confused with transient ischemic attacks due to a reduction of arterial blood flow in the neck. This latter condition, however, may be accompanied by sudden transient blindness but not by hemianopic fortification spectra.

In describing scotomas with migraine, Alvarez[114] points out that men are more likely to see the zigzag line and women more likely to have atypical scotomas. Scotomas can appear before the actual headache. Some may have their scotomas mainly late in life, winding up with their headaches and nausea gone and only scotomas left. Alvarez believes that the entire brain is disturbed with a scotoma. There

may be a slight aphasia, with numbness, formication, pins and needles, muscle weakness, frequency of urination, or pain in the thorax or abdomen. For hours after a scotoma there may be sensitivity to light. Electroencephalograms performed during scintillating scotoma usually show nothing abnormal. Migrainous scotomas tend to change in character with age. Brilliant scotomas are seen in children.

As mentioned previously, migraine is more prominent in women and often associated with the menstrual period. These patients frequently have a family history of migraine, which is also an important symptom to note when taking the patient's history.

Very frequently, in fact in the majority of migraine patients, there is an element of nervous tension present. This is an important item to recognize and it must be treated along with the headache attacks. If tension is present and it is not treated properly, the general treatment program will not succeed.

The migraine patient has inherited a neurophysiologic system that for an unknown reason is susceptible to the deleterious effects of a variety of stresses. In many cases the patient also has a personality that in itself promotes the occurrence of stress. Therapeutic efforts should be directed toward correction of the abnormal of the cranial vessels during the acute attack, fortifying the sensitive vascular mechanism against future attack, and adjusting the patient to withstand the normal stresses that go with everyday life.

Patients have been described as overly conscientious and inclined to suppress normal aggression, but this is so in only about half the sufferers.

The most common symptom in migraine, next to the headache itself, is nausea. These patients universally claim their headaches to be "sick headaches." Many have vomiting; this will usually occur at the height of the attack and quite characteristically terminates their headache phase of the attack.

The average migraine patient will present a normal general physical examination, normal skull and sinus x-rays, normal neurologic and eye grounds, and normal electroencephalogram.

The day preceding the attack will find the migraine patient "on the top of the world." His life is fine, nothing is wrong, and no task is too great for him to tackle. Mentally, he is clear, sharp, and alert. His appetite and general health are normal. Later on in the day or the evening before an attack starts, he begins to feel mentally fatigued and weary. He has at this time a general letdown in his spirits. This he always attributes to an excessively hard day at the office or at work and believes that he is just tired out from it. He retires for the night, feeling utterly weary, and usually sleeps soundly the entire night. On awakening in the morning, at his usual hour, the patient either is confronted with the prodromal symptoms or the headache attack has fully developed. Most of these patients try to brace themselves and attempt to go through their daily routines in complete misery. This quite often requires superhuman efforts and energy, and in many cases it is almost impossible.

Unfortunately, the average migraine patient is not situated so that he can forego his day's work in order to effect an early termination of the attack or a reduction in the severity of the symptoms of the attack. Therefore, the patient becomes a slave to the circumstances and starts his daily toil with a resolve to "do or die." Being in a dull mental condition and in a physically weary condition that is almost insurmountable, this carrying on of the daily chores is next to impossible.

After he has passed through the automatic motions of doing his daily routine he returns to his home a wreck, physically and mentally, and goes to bed completely exhausted.

We find that emotional disturbances play an important part in migraine, especially in the previously mentioned perfectionist personality. These are usually seen in the form of depression and are rather pronounced.

The severity and frequency of the attacks are as variable as the clinical picture, making it difficult to assess the incidence of this disorder.

There are no distinctive clinical features on examination, nor any specific laboratory investigation to aid in the diagnosis of migraine. This may lead to a tendency to enlarge the boundaries of the disease so as to include other disorders within the definition.

Nick[115] believes that it is possible and useful to make a strict limitation as to what should be included in the diagnosis of migraine. The most important feature in setting these limits is the realization that migraine is a benign disorder which occurs in bouts that, while they may be disabling, are always self-limiting and regress completely.

Leaving aside certain cases of true epilepsy accompanied by headache, the slight hypersynchronous discharges seen in the electroencephalogram of many migraine patients are not characteristic of an epileptic constitution. Slight dysrhythmias may be found in some normal patients.

Alvarez[116] states that the migrainous constitution is frequently disclosed in childhood by episodes of motion sickness, cyclic vomiting, or the so-called bilious attacks. We have not personally been able to either confirm or deny this, since this would have to be handled by a pediatrician.

While migraine is more commonly seen in women, to say that true migraine occurs almost exclusively in women would be an overstatement. Some believe that the characteristic body build of a migraine patient constitutes a small, asthenic, delicately built woman. We find that the general body structure of the individual has nothing to do with migraine. Migraine is found in both sexes, in large and small, fat and lean, tall and short, young and old.

The age of the patient is not important. We have seen migraine in a child 5 years of age and in an adult in the sixties. Shea[117] states that if migraine attacks tend to occur for the first time beyond the age of 40 and are unilateral, they might possibly be the result of an aneurysm of the internal carotid artery. Williams[118] states that migraine usually starts before the second decade of life. Most migraine experts agree with this.

The head pain of the average migraine patient is not postural. By that we mean that the headache is not affected by the position of the body of the patient. Some receive relief by lying down, while others state that their headache is more severe if they recline. Exercise, however, will usually increase the pain.

Many female migraine patients notice that they become free from their attacks or that the attacks are of a much milder nature when they are pregnant. This is the general rule but not a universal one.

Briggs and Bellomo[119] believe that migraine may produce chest pain, palpitation, and fast pulse, either with or without head pain. The chest pain may simulate the pain in angina.

Ask-Upmark[120] found a rather frequent occurrence of inverted nipples among women in a family with a high prevalence of migraine. He also observed that migraine patients have very pronounced eyebrows.

Blair[121] describes thirty-six patients with both migraine and diabetes. Five patients lost their migraine completely or had a marked reduction in attack with the onset of control of diabetes. In four other patients nocturnal hypoglycemia precipitated migraine headaches. Of the remaining twenty-seven patients, six noted that fasting or missing a meal sometimes provoked attacks of migraine. A significant number of patients noted a reduction in frequency and severity of migraine after developing diabetes; but in twenty-one of the thirty-six patients diabetes in no way influenced migraine. He concludes that the blood sugar level is apparently the major and specific triggering mechanism of migraine in some patients.

Trauma is never thought of as being part of the history of the typical migraine patient. However, Barolin[122] examined a series of 450 patients with migraine over a period of 11 years to see whether their migraine could be traced to a previous trauma. Forty subjects, of whom twelve were children, were considered as possible cases of posttraumatic migraine.

Whiteley[123] made a study of 200 British physicians or their wives who regularly suffered migraine to see if such persons fall into a common personality pattern. No statistically significant physical, psychologic, or social traits were found.

DIAGNOSIS

If the physician knows the symptoms and signs of migraine, the diagnosis should not be too difficult. These, of course, are obtained in the history given by the patient. However, some patients give a history that is so confused, bizarre, and vague that no one could possibly make a diagnosis from it. This being the case, the only physician who is likely ever to guess what is really wrong with the patient will be the one who suspects from the patient's appearance, his mental and spiritual make-up, and his story that the patient is one with migraine and then goes ahead and digs out the typical history. This type of case may often require more than one session and may have to be done piecemeal.

The diagnosis of migraine is an important one, not only for the migraine condition itself but because so commonly the peculiarities of the nervous system and the whole body which go with this condition and underlie it can be explained. By this we mean all the hypersensitivity, the nervousness, tension, frailness, frequent complaints of illness, occasional spells of vertigo, nausea, vomiting, depression, and ophthalmic abnormalities (in the prodromal phase). Of course, the diagnosis helps determine the type of treatment, for without proper diagnosis there cannot be proper treatment.

From the symptoms and signs we can

gather that migraine is a paroxysmal, remissive syndrome. It may increase or it may decrease in severity. The autonomic and psychogenic aspects of puberty, the menstrual periods, the menopause, and the climacteric seem to have been neglected in the consideration of the migraine patient. Induction of the menopause for migraine is definitely not indicated.

There are a large number of infective, toxic, and metabolic diseases that give rise to headaches, but the majority cause no difficulty in differential diagnosis.

Nevertheless, difficulties in diagnosis can arise in the following conditions.

Histamine headaches. These headaches are unilateral, of sudden onset, and accompanied by flushing and lacrimation. They usually begin in the night, last up to 2 hours, and fade rapidly. Diagnosis is made on the history and the intense burning or boring quality of the pain.

Allergic headaches. These are associated with allergic rhinitis, which will be disclosed in the history.

Cerebral tumors. The headache may be intermittent and appear before abnormal physical signs are found, or before symptoms arise that would suggest an organic disease. These symptoms may consist of memory disorders, confusional states, and alteration of personality, which will eventually persist and become obvious.

Glaucoma. This is another cause of intermittent headache, and in some cases it has caused difficulty in differential diagnosis. During the attack glaucoma patients have a rise of intraocular tension with signs of congestion of the eye. This is generally seen in patients over the age of 40 years. Even if the visual fields are normal, as they will be in many early cases, it may be necessary for the intraocular tension to be measured on a number of occasions before the diagnosis is established.

Berry aneurysms. These may be suspected in ophthalmoplegic migraine. The decision as to whether arteriograms are indicated in such cases must be left to the neurologist. The presence of subarachnoid hemorrhages with a sudden intense severe pain and neck stiffness would suggest such as aneurysm.

Intracranial angiomas. These may be suspected if abnormal physical signs are found on examination of the nervous system. For example, finding skin angiomas must also make one suspect the presence of angiomas inside the skull.

Trigeminal neuralgia. Trigger areas are not to be found in migraine, but they are present in trigeminal neuralgia.

Posttraumatic headache. The history of trauma will differentiate traumatic headache from migraine.

Migraine and epilepsy

Since both migraine and epilepsy occur fairly frequently, it is not surprising that they will be found from time to time in the same patient.

There has been a great deal of discussion of the relationship between migraine and epilepsy. Some investigators believe that there is a connection between these two conditions. However, most headache authorities do not believe this. In our opinion migraine and epilepsy are two distinct conditions. It is true, certainly, that a patient with epilepsy may also have migraine, just as a patient with diabetes or asthma or any other condition may also have migraine.

In some cases of migraine electroencephalographic abnormalities may occur. This, however, is seen in only a relatively small percentage of patients. During the acute attack there may be reduced basal alpha activity.

In most migraine patients the electroencephalogram is normal. Some investigators claim abnormalities are found in migraine patients in the headache-free phase. However, the same abnormalities may be found in individuals who have never experienced a single attack of migraine.

Scollo-Lavizzari[123a] says that migraine may be called dysrhythmic and that the electroencephalographic findings in migraine are useful in excluding the presence of organic brain lesions or true epilepsy.

In 123 children with a diagnosis of migraine Jacobi and associates[123b] found the electroencephalogram to be normal in 48% of the cases. The abnormalities consisted of focal changes such as dysrhythmia of delta and theta waves and transient reductions of amplitude and frequency.

In 104 patients with migraine diffuse and local dysrhythmias were found in 72% of the tracings.[123c] They represent a transition stage between normal and abnormal electroencephalograms. Generalized bouts of dysrhythmia were recorded in more than 50% of adults and in 30% of children. Local changes occurred in fifteen adults and three children. Most were induced by hyperventilation. It is therefore suggested that dysrhythmia as an expression of increased irritability is due to a metabolic disturbance in different neuronal systems with temporary exacerbations affecting one or more systems. Hughes[123d] states that the most common electroencephalographic changes in migraine are long slow waves (three per second) in the occipital recordings of those patients with scintillation scotomas or neurologic deficits. About 40% of cases may show some abnormality. A very common finding is the persistence of cortical evoked responses to photic stimulation at higher frequencies than usual.

Barolin[124] says that about one-third of migraine patients have an abnormal electroencephalogram, but only about 4% of these patients have an electroencephalogram of an epileptic type.

Smyth and Winter[124a] found nearly half of 202 migraine patients had abnormal electroencephalograms. This was related to the length of history and the severity of the headaches.

Weil[124b] pointed out that between migrainous attacks, pronounced electroencephalographic activation during hyperventilation is the most reliable sign of dysrhythmic migraine. The major types of resting electroencephalographic patterns between attacks are (1) paroxysmal theta and delta patterns, usually with an amplitude of 50 to 200 μv, and (2) high-voltage spindles of 100 to 150 μv, occasionally with slow spikes interpolated. During an attack, electroencephalographic patterns frequently resemble tracings made during hyperventilation.

Barolin[124c] states that one should come to know certain abnormal electroencephalographic patterns in migraine and vascular headache and regard them as positive clues in a diagnostic procedure without deducing "masked epilepsy" too promptly. Especially marked in migraine patients is a strong response to hyperventilation. It can be regarded as an additional indication for vasolability and is characterized by dysrhythmia, as encountered relatively frequently in headache patients (sometimes clustered in the sense of Weil's paroxysmal dysrhythmia), and sometimes focal manifestations and spike discharges, which are also frequent in headache patients.

Towle[124d] found that in reviewing the characteristics of a group of electroencephalograms obtained over an 18-month period in forty-three patients with headaches, the main difference noted in comparison with fifty-eight normal control individuals was the greater prominence of the electroencephalographic hyperventilation response.

Dalsgaard-Nielsen,[125] in discussing the possibility of a relationship of migraine and epilepsy, points out that the occurrence in special personality types, the presence of precipitating factors, and the high incidence of dysrhythmia and heredity are typical of both migraine and epilepsy. He believes that these are not necessarily supportive evidence for a relationship between epilepsy and migraine. His investigations indicate that dysrhythmia in migraine may be due to vasoconstrictor cerebral disturbances.

After studying a series of 591 migrainous patients analyzed to establish whether any association exists between migraine and epilepsy, Ninck[125a] found that epilepsy is seen ten times more often among migraine patients than in a random population. He believes that patients suffering from both migraine and epilepsy do not form a unitary group and in only a few cases are both conditions due to the same organic disturbance. Most often the migraine appears to be the primary condition. Repeated spasm of the cerebral blood vessels leads to ischemic and hypoxic changes in the brain, mainly in the temporal region. The ischemic area then becomes epileptogenic, with pathologically increased ganglion cell discharges.

Discussing the relationship of migraine and epilepsy, Green and co-workers[125b] say that migraine may be either a precursor of epilepsy or a fortuitously associated condition; however, the fact that epilepsy can be provoked by vasospasm and cerebral anoxia suggests that migraine and epilepsy may have a common etiologic mechanism.

They found that abnormal electroencephalographic findings, such as a fourteen and six per second positive spike pattern, may be present in migraine in the absence of epilepsy. Dysrhythmia, which is present in 10% of the general population, occurs more often in both epileptic and migrainous subjects. These abnormalities may be intensified by hyperventilation in cases of migraine, although the electroencephalographic recording made during the attack differs basically from that found in epilepsy.

Lance and Anthony[125c] conducted a study of 500 patients with migraine and 100 with tension headache. Epilepsy was associated in 0.17% of those with migraine and in 2% of the others. The estimate for the general public is 0.5%. They concluded that no direct relationship existed between migraine and epilepsy.

In a study of 154 electroencephalograms of patients with migraine, Panzani[125d] found no significant relationship to exist between epileptic and migraine patients. He did, however, in this study find a definite relationship between asthma and epilepsy, which he says may be the result of a single mesodiencephalic lesion.

Basser[126] analyzed a series of 1,830 cases of migraine, paying special attention to those cases in which epilepsy was also present. All subjects were compared with a series of 548 patients suffering from tension headache. The incidence of epilepsy in the migraine group (5.9%) was found to be significantly higher than that in the tension headache group (1.1%).

Lees and Watkins[126a] believe that migraine and epilepsy are unassociated diseases which seldom coincide, or if so purely by chance. They state that the erroneous concept of relationship is based on the occasional loss of consciousness during migraine or the rare coexistence of migraine in epileptic patients. Unconsciousness in migraine usually is due to syncope or to the basilar form of the disease, which appears to produce functional disturbances in the brainstem reticular formation. Very few migraine patients show definite features of epilepsy during loss of consciousness; rigidity and incontinence may be accounted for by cerebral response to such vascular change as ischemia. In epileptic patients with coincidental history of migraine, the vascular headache may produce transient ischemia which precipitates a convulsive attack.

Savoldi and associates[126b] state that the electroencephalogram has definite limitations in studying migraine. They also believe that it is an important factor in investigating the relationship of migraine to epilepsy as far as the pathogenic mechanism is concerned.

The incidence of epilepsy in migrainous patients is higher than that which may be expected by chance. Conversely, there is a slightly higher incidence of migraine in epileptic persons than in control individuals.

In ten patients suffering from abdominal epilepsy, six children and four adults, Rios Mozo[126c] found no clear boundaries between abdominal migraine and abdominal epilepsy in children using clinical and electroencephalographic studies. Thus these types of conditions may be classified as abdominal migraine–epilepsy. In adults, the combination of abdominal migraine–epilepsy and hypotonic choledyskinesia is common and possesses a definite psychosomatic element.

Serratrice and associates[126d] believe that a clinical differentiation between migraine and epilepsy is often an artificial distinction and that the attacks may have a common mechanism. Three types of cases occur: a sequential form, in which a migraine attack is immediately followed by a seizure; an alternating form, in which epileptic crises are interspersed with migrainous attacks at varying intervals; and an involved form, in which it is impossible to distinguish the parts played by epilepsy and migraine respectively. They conclude that the frontier zones between migraine and epilepsy remain ill-defined, perhaps because these two conditions share a common physiopathologic mechanism.

Patients with vascular headache of the migrainous type have a higher incidence of electroencephalographic abnormalities than those examined without regard to classification of headache. Electroencephalographic abnormalities of patients with vascular migraine can be placed in two categories—focal and nonfocal.

After all of the investigations regarding this relationship of migraine and epilepsy, it appears that there are some who believe that such a relationship does exist. However, most authorities do not accept this theory. Naturally some migraine patients may also be epileptic and some epileptic individuals may also have migraine. However, to say that these two conditions are one and the same entity is purely theoretical, not factual.

Migraine patients may have some electroencephalographic abnormalities such as dysrhythmia, but this does not mean that they are are epileptic.

PROGNOSIS

The prognosis of migraine varies with the type of treatment employed and with its causal relationships. Thus, the prognosis depends not only on the disorder itself but often on the persistence of both the physician and the patient. They should not be discouraged if the results of one form of treatment are not as good as desired. Quite often the physician must experiment to find out what the migraine patient responds to best. Some patients receive benefit from certain preparations; others require other forms of treatment. This is especially true in the symptomatic phase of migraine treatment. Migraine is usually not fatal. The prognosis often depends on the physician's knowledge of migraine and of the patient and the patient's history. The prognosis often is improved by the patient's having complete confidence in the physician.

Complications due to migraine itself are rare; it might be said that most migraine cases never have complications. There have been a few cases reported in which hemianopia has become permanent after an especially severe attack. These were thought to be due to vascular thrombosis.

PROPHYLACTIC TREATMENT

Many migraine patients are ill-adjusted, rigid, repressed perfectionists, and they lack the average normal outlets of emotional life. However, merely employing psychotherapy alone will never bring about a cure in a case of migraine. The patient should be given emotional guidance. Most of these patients have common personality features. They are tense, striving individuals. Decreasing energy is coupled with increasing age, and failure to achieve perfection leads to deep-seated frustrations. These frustrations, when joined by hostility and resentments often carried over from childhood, may lead the individual to severe and frequent migraine attacks. The psychotherapy should consist chiefly of some good sound advice, along with emotional guidance. If the patient cannot remove the mental stimulus in his case, he must adapt himself so that he can minimize its effects. Of course, if there are any physical abnormalities found in the patient's general physical examination, they should be corrected. A general improvement in the patient's health will help in these cases also.

The patient will find that his attacks can

be prevented somewhat by his eliminating the elements of his daily life that cause him to live at continuous high tension. All migraine patients can, if they will, and they seldom do, control the frequency and severity of their attacks by curtailing every element that causes them to live at high speed and high nervous tension. High-pressure businessmen often complain of what they call the weekend type of migraine. This is due to absolute nervous relaxation from their high tension of the week's business worries and/or to the fact that there is a substitution of the nervous tension of business activities by the nervous tension of strenuous outdoor exercise such as golf, tennis, or other sports which may require not only physical exertion but also the same high degree of nervous tension as is required in their regular occupation.

During the past several years many new preparations have been brought forth in the investigative field of migraine prophylaxis. Some of these are now being marketed, but more are found on the European continent than in the United States due to the strict regulations of the Food and Drug Administration. Perhaps this strict form of regulation by the FDA is of benefit to the American migraine sufferer since it will prevent him from being subjected to drugs that may not be of any benefit to him or may be harmful to him. As is the case with the symptomatic form of drugs in migraine therapy a drug report will appear in the literature claiming dramatic results in the field of migraine prophylaxis but nothing further is heard about it after the initial report. This is usually due to the fact that further trials with these drugs prove it to be far less effective or not effective at all. We will present the preparations that are most widely used today both in the United States and elsewhere.

Methysergide (Sansert)

In the United States probably the most frequently used drug for the prophylaxis of migraine is methysergide, which is marketed under the name of Sansert. This is one of the few oral preparations that may be offered the patient in the United States for this purpose, because other drugs which are obtainable outside the United States (such as clonidine and BC-105) are not marketed due to FDA restrictions. While these other two drugs mentioned may not be quite as effective as Sansert, they certainly do not produce the dreadful side effects associated with the use of methysergide.

Methysergide maleate (1-methyl-D-lysergic acid butanolamide) was first suggested to be an effective agent in the treatment of migraine by Sicuteri[127] in 1959. Further observations were presented in 1960 by Friedman[127a] and by Graham,[127b] and again by Friedman in 1961.[127c]

Various theories have been advanced concerning the mechanism involved in which methysergide actually prevents headache. One theory is that the drug acts as a powerful serotonin antagonist and that it may act by neutralizing the effects of serotonin either in the blood vessels and in the tissues or in the central nervous system.[124,127-129]

Sicuteri and associates[130] further report on the 5-HT potentiation from methysergide. In one patient, after the local administration of a very small dose such as 10 mg, given acutely, the threshold effect of 5-HT was impressively enhanced, about ten to twenty times. An intense pain arose along the vein, and the test had to be interrupted. The pain persisted for an hour after the interruption and an analgesic was requested. 5-HT administered alone in a large amount in this patient provoked severe venospasm but not pain. The cause of this painful reaction is not known; however, this phenomenon resembles the painful reaction seen as a side effect in some patients after a few oral doses of methysergide.

Sicuteri and co-workers further suggest a possible method by which methysergide acts as an analgesic in migraine, by stating that it may work at the periphery (on cranial tissues and vessels) or at the center (on the nervous structures involved in cerebral assimilation of the pain). Another theory of the action of methysergide in migraine prophylaxis is that in some patients it has a vasoconstrictive action similar to that of ergotamine tartrate.[131,132]

Dalessio[128] theorized that it dampens the vasomotor responses of the hypothalamus. He further states[133] that in the prophylaxis of migraine, methysergide, a lysergic acid derivative, seems to exert its effects by modulating central vasomotor functions and by potentiating the vasoconstrictor responses of the cranial blood vessels to endogenous or exogenous catecholamines. The magnitude of cranial vascular responsivity is reduced, with subsequent reduction in the frequency and intensity of headaches. He concludes that the antiserotonin activity of methysergide may be associated with the ability of this substance to modulate central vasomotor functions and that serotonin functions as a strong, central, parasympathetic neurohormone in the integrated pattern seen in migraine.

There are others who believe that methysergide acts by antagonizing the inflammatory effects of neurokinin, which is a powerful bradykinin-like polypeptide.

Methysergide is generally characterized as an antiserotonin agent that acts on the D receptors present at several vascular and nonvascular sites.

Saxena,[134] however, found that this drug was not very effective in antagonizing the vasoconstrictor action of serotonin in the carotid vessels, the main target during the migraine attacks. The inhibition of serotonin-induced carotid vasoconstriction achieved with very high doses of methysergide could be secondary to carotid vasoconstriction, caused by the drug itself. Saxena concludes that it is strongly suggestive that the selective carotid vasoconstriction, but not peripheral antiserotonin or vasomotor depressant properties, is most relevant to the antimigraine action of the drug.

In still another study on methysergide and migraine Saxena[135] found that methysergide caused a slightly increased response

to noradrenaline and histamine, and ergotamine caused a strong enhancement of that response to bradykinin. He thus concluded that this cast doubt on the assumption that antimigraine drugs depend for their therapeutic effect on their antiserotonin action, a more likely explanation being a selective vasoconstriction produced in the external carotid bed. The noradrenaline-potentiating effect of methysergide probably also contributes to the therapeutic efficacy of antimigraine drugs.

Saxena has done a considerable amount of research in this field. He made another investigation on the possibility of selective vasoconstriction by methysergide.[136] In this investigation the arterial blood pressure, pulse rate, and blood flow were recorded in various arteries in anesthetized dogs. Methysergide reduced the blood flow in the carotid system but increased it in the femoral and vertebral arteries. No change was recorded in the renal or superior mesenteric arteries except that at higher doses a reduced mesenteric flow was present as well. The blood pressure was not significantly changed. Therefore methysergide seems to bring about an increase in the vascular resistance of the carotid territory, more marked in the internal carotid than the common carotid.

In studying the influence of methysergide on the storage of the biogenic amines, Owen and associates[137] found that in the isolated perfused spleen preparation of the cat methysergide exerted a dual dose-dependent effect on serotonin uptake. At 1 μg/minute methysergide enhanced the uptake of serotonin into storage sites; at 10 μg/minute it inhibited uptake. The enhancement of uptake observed at the lower methysergide dose level is thought to be its specific activity, whereas inhibition of uptake is probably characteristic of many members of the ergot alkaloid group at high dose levels. They found methysergide to produce a partial protective effect against the serotonin-depleting activity of reserpine in rats. Administration of methysergide 30 minutes before and 60 minutes after reserpine resulted in a dose-dependent reduction of serotonin depletion after reserpine. This protective influence of methysergide is speculated to contribute to its mechanism of action in migraine prophylaxis.

Hilton and Zilkha[138] studied the effect of methysergide on blood platelet aggregation in migraine patients. They found that migrainous patients, free from headache but receiving methysergide, showed significantly reduced rates of blood platelet aggregation induced by serotonin, compared with migrainous patients not receiving drug therapy or with nonmigrainous controls. There was no significant difference in the blood serotonin concentrations before or during drug treatment compared with controls. The fall in blood serotonin which occurred during the headache periods in migrainous patients not taking drugs was not observed during the headache periods of patients taking methysergide. The platelet aggregation rate of patients taking no drugs decreased, and the rate for patients taking methysergide remained the same compared with nonheadache periods. Platelet aggregation in response to serotonin depends on the availability of serotonin uptake sites; if the sites are occupied by a molecule of serotonin or an analogue, aggregation cannot take place. Thus it appears that the reduced platelet aggregation rates in this experiment were due to methysergide occupying serotonin receptor sites on the platelet membrane. They suggest that the serotonin uptake sites on platelets and drug interaction with them may resemble uptake sites and drug interaction on other body surfaces, such as vessel walls or neuronal membranes.

SIDE EFFECTS

Most of the reports in the medical literature concerning methysergide in the prophylaxis of migraine mention side effects. Some of these side effects can be very harmful to the patient while some are rather harmless. If the drug is discontinued soon enough most of these side effects will subside. However, if therapy is continued, they will not. It is generally agreed that methysergide should not be given either in a very large dosage schedule or for any great length of time.

Methysergide is closely related to LSD chemically. In this regard, Persyko[139] reported that content and sequential analysis of symptoms experienced and described by a patient following ingestion of a single tablet of methysergide. These symptoms appear to follow the pattern of reaction to LSD with three clearly discernible phases: initial, somatic; middle, neurotic; and terminal, psychotic. The "hallucinogenic" potential of methysergide appears to fall into a pattern of historical sequence, common to all drugs of dependence.

Lloyd-Smith and McNaughton[140] state that side effects were noted in 34.2% of patients and led to discontinuing the trial in 10.4%. Side effects promptly subsided when the drug was withdrawn. Methysergide appears to be a useful additional agent in the prevention of severe, frequently recurring migraine of common and cluster type. In the authors' small series it had little effect on headaches of combined tension and vascular type.

Lindeneg and Kok-Jensen[141] found pleurisy and pleural fibrosis developing with the use of methysergide in migraine patients. They describe four patients who developed pleurisy (bilateral in three) with disproportionately short breathing and persistent muscular pain during treatment with methysergide for 3 months to 2 years. In three a cardiac murmur was heard during treatment. After withdrawal of methysergide, two patients improved and the cardiac murmur disappeared. None of the patients had signs of retroperitoneal fibrosis. They conclude that there may be a causal connection between the pleural disorder and the methysergide treatment.

Friedman[142] says that in 20% to 40% of patients adverse side effects limit its usefulness while in 10% the side effects are intolerable. Pedersen and Moller[143] report that severe side effects necessitating withdrawal of the drug occurred in 7% of the patients. Other side effects were due primarily to insufficient circulation and could be reduced by individual dosage adjustment.

Daniell[144] reported on a case of methysergide treatment of migraine in which a side effect simulating Leriche's syndrome developed. This was a 36-year-old man who developed impotence and hip claudication while on methysergide maleate therapy. He had hyperuricemia and had recently received a sympathomimetic amine for weight reduction. Physical examination and oscillometric readings confirmed the presence of a generalized vasospastic reaction, which could not be modified by administration of sympathomimetic amines or adrenergic blocking agents. Discontinuation of methysergide maleate was followed by rapid disappearance of symptoms, abnormal physical findings, and abnormal oscillometric readings.

Utz and associates[145] point out the risk of retroperitoneal fibrosis when methysergide is used. They believe that after 1 year, continuous administration of methysergide maleate should be interrupted for 3 months and patients examined for retroperitoneal fibrosis by urinalysis, renal function tests, and excretory urography. If the drug is continued, examination should be repeated every 3 to 6 months. Retroperitoneal fibrosis developed in three patients with vasodilating headaches or migraine treated with methysergide for periods longer than 1 year. Causal relationship between drug and disease in unconfirmed, but administration to patients with known renal disease is probably inadvisable. Methysergide is contraindicated in those with peripheral vascular disease, serious hypertension, angina, coronary and hepatic insufficiency, and pregnancy.

Wagenknecht[146] also discusses retroperitoneal fibrosis with the use of methysergide in migraine therapy. He describes exploratory laparotomy in six patients whose urologic and vascular complaints led to the diagnosis of retroperitoneal fibrosis. All six patients had been on prolonged methysergide therapy. When the drug was discontinued, the pyelorenal dilation normalized in two patients. Four other patients required surgical ureterolysis and intraperitoneal transposition of ureters. Approximately 21 months after the diagnosis was made, kidney function and the status of the urogenital system were normal again in all six patients.

Farrel and co-workers[147] also found retroperitoneal fibrosis. They present a case of a 62-year-old female patient with a 2-month history of painless swelling of the left leg. She had been taking methysergide maleate tablets (2 mg two to three times daily) for 3½ years. There were no urinary tract complaints. A pelvic venogram showed complete obstruction of the left common iliac vein and an intravenous urogram showed partial obstruction of the left ureter. When a long midline laparotomy was performed, bilateral retroperitoneal fibrosis was noted. In addition to the obstructed left common iliac vein, marked stenosis of the left common iliac artery was present. There was no evidence of intravascular thrombosis. They further state that retroperitoneal fibrosis occurs in a small percentage of patients treated with methysergide—about 1%. Such patients commonly show symptoms of urinary tract obstruction that is often bilateral.

In a large series of patients with severe headache in whom methysergide was used, Graham[148] found that about 20% of patients gave up taking methysergide because of undesirable side effects. This percentage is influenced by the fact that about a third of these patients who suffered side effects during this experimental period were taking doses that exceeded the recommended 8 mg/day.

The most serious side effects are those involving the vascular system, whether arterial or venous. Methysergide should be used, if at all, only with the greatest caution in situations in which vascular disorders are known, suspected, or threatened. Pregnancy, sepsis, edematous states, and severe liver and renal impairment present further contraindications. The successful treatment of patients by drug withdrawal only had previously been reported, but only in cases in which no vascular obstruction was present. If obstruction occurs, surgery may be required.

RESULTS

There are probably more glowing reports on the use of methysergide in the prophylaxis of migraine than on any other oral form of medication.

Friedman and Elkind[131] used methysergide in 421 patients who previously had been treated unsuccessfully for recurrent headaches over periods as long as 55 years. The drug was given in amounts ranging from 6 to 16 mg/day in divided doses. The treatment, essentially prophylactic, was continued for periods up to 29 months. Side effects were frequent and adjustment of dosage was necessary. They concluded that methysergide maleate has no value in treating the acute attack but that it is effective in the prophylactic treatment of all forms of migraine headache.

Pedersen and Moller[149] used a dose of 6 mg of methysergide in adult patients daily, 3 mg in children. The sixty patients who completed the trial satisfactorily had classic or common type of migraine; patients with cardiovascular disease and pregnant women were excluded. Analysis showed that frequency of attacks was significantly reduced with the drug. In comparison with the preexperimental period, the frequency of attacks was reduced at least 50% in 57% of patients with methysergide (27% no attacks, 30% improved). The corresponding figure for placebo was 27% (7% no attacks, 20% improved).

Southwell and associates[150] did a double-blind trial of methysergide in fifty-three patients experiencing frequent severe attacks of classic migraine that had not responded to other treatment. The incidence of attacks was lower when methysergide was being taken. The difference between the groups was most significant ($p = 0.01$) when methysergide was taken in the second half of the trial period, suggesting that the effect of the drug was carried over after it had been stopped. Side effects occurred in one third of patients; this appeared to be related to dosage. It was concluded that methysergide exerted some beneficial prophylactic effect and was worthy of trial in cases of severe migraine refractory to other treatment.

Harris[151] made a similar study in which methysergide was used in the prophylactic treatment of forty-five patients with migraine and five with histaminic cephalalgia. Initial dosage was one 2-mg tablet every 4 hours, but since several patients experienced nausea and vomiting, the dose was reduced to 2 mg three times daily after meals. Six patients with migraine continued to have side effects in spite of reduced dosage and so discontinued the drug. Of the thirty-nine migraine patients completing the study, thirty had excellent results. Five continued to have headaches, but these were sporadic and did not last long. Four had no relief.

Lance and co-workers[152] studied the effectiveness of different serotonin antagonists in the prevention of migraine in a clinical trial involving 290 patients followed for periods up to 3 years. Considering only the initial treatment given to the patient on first attending the clinic, methysergide was more effective than BC-105 or placebo.

Lovshin[153] observed the use of methysergide in the treatment of extracranial vascular headache. Prophylactic treatment with methysergide was administered to 159 patients with histaminic cephalalgia. Some improvement was noted in 123 cases (77%). Marked improvement (good or excellent result) was noted in 110 patients (69%). Eighty-seven patients with chronic, severe migraine were also treated. Some improvement was noted in seventy patients (80%).

Marked improvement (good or excellent result) was noted in fifty-nine patients (68%).

In an early study, Abbott[154] concluded that methysergide represents a promising agent for prophylactic treatment, especially for chronic recurring migraine headaches, histaminic cephalalgia, cluster headache, and other vascular headaches. It reduces the frequency and severity of attacks. While the mechanism of action is not completely understood, there is some evidence that methysergide neutralizes some properties of serotonin which may play a role in the production and continuance of the migraine syndrome, histaminic cephalalgia, and other vascular headaches. Its mechanism of action may be a central modulating effect on the vasomotor centers.

Methysergide was used as a regular medication to prevent migraine in a series of eighty-seven patients with frequently recurring severe attacks of three types: common, classic, and cluster. The results were classified as excellent, good, fair, and nil. The total of patients reporting excellent and good results was 50.6%. In a few patients the drug appeared to lose effectiveness in long-term treatment.[140]

Graham[148] found methysergide to be effective in its ability to reduce the frequency or severity of headache attacks over a prolonged period of time in approximately 70% of the patients he followed.

From all these reports, its seems that methysergide is a useful drug in the prophylaxis of migraine and perhaps histaminic cephalalgia. It is of little or no value in mixed headaches or muscle contraction (tension) headache, the various neuralgias, or other types of head pain. This drug is quite expensive and quite potent. It should therefore be used only in patients who are severely enough handicapped by their headaches to warrant it. Methysergide is used only as a prophylactic agent, and only in extremely rare cases is it useful symptomatically.

Because of the severe side effects that can result from the use of this drug, the physician who uses methysergide should be thoroughly acquainted with its pharmacologic properties and with the total medical picture of the patient. Careful and close supervision of the patient is essential. However, if the drug is successful in relieving the patient from migraine attacks, such close management is worthwhile.

In summation, this drug can be helpful to the migraine patient, but it may also be harmful if used incorrectly.

Histamine

Histamine may be used either intravenously or subcutaneously in the prophylactic treatment of migraine. Nicotinic acid, given orally, may be helpful between injections, as may psychotherapy. In addition, if tension is present, diazepam (Valium), 2 mg three times a day, may be given; if depression is part of the picture, amitriptyline (Elavil), 10 mg three times a day and at bedtime, is administered.

We frequently employ intravenous histamine in the prophylactic treatment of migraine. The standard intravenous solution is 2.75 mg of histamine acid phosphate in 250 ml of isotonic solution of sodium chloride. This results in a solution containing approximately 0.0011% histamine acid phosphate, and each milliliter of the solution actually contains approximately 0.004 mg of histamine base. On occasion a more dilute solution is used composed of 0.00055% histamine acid phosphate; each milliliter then contains approximately 0.002 mg of histamine base. When histamine is used intravenously, the injection should begin at a very slow rate of speed. This slow rate should gradually be increased during the first treatment and in treatments to follow. This has to be done slowly so as not to cause any discomfort to the patient. The maximal vasodilation should be obtained. We usually limit the time of these intravenous treatments to 30 or 45 minutes. This prevents the patient from becoming fatigued or weak from the ordeal. It is important that the patient receiving the intravenous histamine have food in his stomach at the time of the administration, so that the excess gastric acid may be absorbed.

This form of treatment should start with the patient receiving 6 or 10 drops of the histamine each minute. If he tolerates this during the first treatment, the rate should be increased to 15 or 20 drops and gradually increased further. Some patients may tolerate 30 drops per minute. However, some patients can tolerate only 6 drops per minute and if the speed of first treatment is over 10 drops per minute, they will have a flushing reaction or even slight headache. If this occurs, the speed should be gradually reduced until a speed is obtained that will not cause the flushing or any throbbing of the head. This intravenous administration of histamine should be given for 30 to 45 minutes daily until the attacks have subsided, after which the interval between treatments may be increased.

In using histamine subcutaneously, the standard solution we use is 0.275 mg of histamine acid phosphate per cubic milliliter. The first dose should be 0.05 ml. Each succeeding injection is increased by 0.05 ml until 1 ml is reached. We have never given a migraine patient more than 1 ml of histamine subcutaneously. If a reaction occurs before reaching a level of 1 ml, the dosage level is reduced to that of the previous day, which did not produce any reaction. For example, if at 0.45 ml a typical headache attack occurs within 1 hour of the injection, the dosage is reduced to 0.4 ml and kept at that level throughout. In other words, adequate dosage is determined by each individual patient's response. If no flushing, throbbing, or headache is produced and if the symptoms seem to be decreasing in severity or frequency, the procedure may be considered adequate. However, if the symptoms seem to be aggravated or precipitated by the injections, the treatment is not being given correctly. In such a case, the reduction in amount should take place. There is no harm in continuing the maintenance doses for life, if that is necessary.

It is common for the patient, after a long period of freedom from the symptoms, to be lulled into a false sense of security. He then may discontinue his injections of the maintenance dose. If he does this, he will soon have a recurrence of his headache attacks. If this occurs, it is common to find that the maintenance dose level has changed. This may be due to the fact that his sensitivity to histamine is greater than it was during the previous episode. Each individual case differs. The maintenance dosage level cannot be determined by the patient's size, sex, age, occupation, or personality; it is individualized for each patient.

Histamine dilates the arterioles, venules, and capillaries. The intravenous use of histamine will produce cutaneous vasodilation that will appear first over the face and the neck. This vasodilation varies with the rate of administration. If the rate is too rapid, the cutaneous vasodilation will gradually extend down over the upper extremities, thorax, and lower extremities. The cutaneous vasodilation is often more marked in the lighter complexioned individual. Histamine will cause a definite increase in the skin temperature and the heart rate, but only a very slight decrease in the diastolic blood pressure. It has also been noted that flow in the extremities gradually increases in proportion to the dosage used. The changes in the skin temperature, heart rate, blood pressure, and blood flow gradually subside and the values return to normal shortly after the intravenous treatment is stopped.

The use of nicotinic acid in the preventive phase of the treatment of migraine was mentioned previously. We use this in the oral form, 100 to 200 mg before each meal. Nicotinamide should not be used, since it is not as good a vasodilator as is nicotinic acid. Nicotonic acid is used between the injections of histamine as a help in obtaining the desired results of preventing the migraine attacks. It is not as strong a cerebral dilator as is histamine, but it is a stronger dilator of the superficial skin vessels than is histamine. Because of this, the nicotinic acid will produce a much stronger flushing reaction in the skin. This flushing lasts only 15 to 30 minutes and is in no way harmful, but the patient should be warned that it might occur. If the patient is not forewarned he may become quite alarmed. Some physicians advocate the use of nicotinic acid alone in the preventive phase of the treatment of migraine, but we do not believe that the results obtained with nicotinic acid are as satisfactory as the results obtained with histamine.

BC-105 (Sandomigran, Pizotifen)

Another preparation that has stimulated considerable interest in the field of prophylactic treatment of migraine is BC-105. This drug is known in America merely as BC-105 because it is in the experimental stage of investigation and it has not been cleared for migraine therapy by the FDA. In various parts of the world BC-105 is marketed as Sandomigran and in other areas it is known as Pizotifen. Regardless of the name, BC-105, Sandomigran, and Pizotifen are one and the same preparation.

BC-105 structurally is a member of a tricyclic series, the derivatives of which exhibit specific antiaminic properties. Chemically, it is related to cyproheptadine but has a thiophene nucleus substituted for one of the benzene rings.

In pharmacologic tests, BC-105 demonstrated an antiserotonin effect equal to or greater than methysergide and an antihistamine effect equal to or greater than such potent antihistamines as chlorpheniramine or thenalidine. This compound also showed a marked inhibitory effect against tryptamine and a somewhat less pronounced antagonism against acetylcholine. In contrast, its adrenolytic properties are insignificant. Although BC-105 demonstrates marked central sedative properties, it is weaker in this respect than chlorpromazine. In animal tests, its antidepressant activity is clearly greater than that of imipramine and amitriptyline, which strongly suggests that

this preparation also possesses activating properties. In the dog, BC-105 has practically no hypotensive effect.

The activity profile of BC-105 is characterized by pronounced and prolonged antagonistic effects against biogenic amines, particularly serotonin. BC-105 is a derivative of benzocycloheptathiophene, a tricyclic system of a new type, having as the basic side chain a 1-methyl-4-piperidylidene-(4)-group similar to cyproheptadine. Its chemical designation is 4-(1-methyl-4-piperidylidene)-9, 10-dihydro-4H-benzo (4,5) cyclohepta (1,2-b) thiophene malate. The empirical formula of BC-105 is $C_{19}H_{21}NS \cdot C_4H_6O_5$. Its molecular weight is 429.54.

BC-105 is a white, fine crystalline powder with a bitter taste. As the hydrogen malate, BC-105 is soluble in water and organic solvents. In aqueous solution, the preparation is soluble.

On the basis of its pharmacological properties, which show it to be an extremely potent antiaminic agent capable of inhibiting the effects of serotonin, histamine, acetylcholine, and, to some extent, the plasma kinins, BC-105 should be evaluated for the interval treatment (prophylaxis) of vascular headache. The drug has little significant anticholinergic activity and in animals, at least, has no demonstrable sedative properties, while some activating effects are in evidence. However, this lack of sedation may not apply in humans.

In therapeutic doses, there are no toxic side effects. Moreover, on the basis of tolerance experiments in the conscious monkey, one would not expect any adverse effects on respiration and heart rate. However, experiments in the anesthetized dog show a minor transient increase in heart rate and decrease in blood pressure at dose levels of 1 to 10 mg/kg intravenously. BC-105 should not be administered in the presence of glaucoma, diabetes, impaired renal function, or predisposition to urinary retention. BC-105 should be used with caution in persons with hypertension, thyrotoxicosis, or cardiac disorders. Sensitive persons receiving BC-105 should be cautioned against driving, operating machinery, or performing other tasks requiring alertness.

Although anticholinergic activity seems to be of very low order, BC-105 should be used with caution in persons with prostatic hypertrophy, stenosing peptic ulcer, and pyloroduodenal or bladder neck obstruction. Possible side effects include drowsiness, hypotension, weight gain, increased appetite, dry mouth, and nervousness.

BC-105 was developed by Sandoz Pharmaceuticals in their search for headache remedies among the antihistamine, antiserotonin agents, hopefully one without frightening side effects of methysergide (Sansert).[155] The initial pharmaceutical and clinical studies were carried out in Florence by Sicuteri and associates,[156] who reported in 1967 that BC-105 was only slightly less potent than methysergide as an antiserotonin agent but with antihistamine effects greater than chlorpheniramine (Chlor-Trimeton). It also has potential antidepressant effects similar to the tricyclic compounds imipramine and amitriptyline.

BC-105 structurally resembles cyproheptadine (Periactin). Pharmacologically, the principal characteristics of BC-105 are due to its antiserotonin properties; in most in vitro and in vivo tests these effects were equivalent to or even superior to those of methysergide. BC-105 also has a powerful antagonistic action against histamine and tryptamine, and also against acetylcholine, although this is less pronounced. Thus BC-105 is characterized by its powerful and long-lasting antagonistic effects against the endogenous amines.

Declerck[157] says that BC-105 exerts an antiserotonin and antihistamine effect, it is a tryptamine inhibitor, and it acts as a central sedative and antidepressant.

Nelson[158] suggests that possibly BC-105 may work by blocking receptor sites for serotonin. There is a drop in serotonin prior to the onset of headaches, and this may be allayed by methysergide or BC-105. This may possibly maintain vasoconstriction in the face of lowered serotonin blood levels. However a central effect may also be present, because of the symptoms of weight gain, polyphagia, and drowsiness, which suggests some hypothalamic mediation.

Studies have been made on the carbohydrate metabolism in patients using BC-105. Fraipont-Guyot and associates[159] say that BC-105 was found to stimulate appetite, which resulted in an increase in weight. An attempt to confirm this effect was made in eleven patients free from endocrine disturbances. The serum glucose, nonesterified fatty acids (NEFA), and plasma insulin levels were measured. Intravenous injection of BC-105 was shown to cause a slight hypoglycemia after 3 hours but no alteration in the NEFA or plasma insulin levels. BC-105 was also tried after the intravenous injection of glucose in patients receiving 250 gm of carbohydrate per day. No effect was observed in the weight, blood pressure, glucose assimilation coefficient, or plasma insulin levels of any patient. There were no changes observed after the administrations of BC-105 during oral glucose tolerance tests. It is suggested that the hypoglycemic effect may be the result of inhibition of glycogenolysis by the liver.

Stary and co-workers[160] studied the vasomotor reactions in the areas of the superficial temporal and supraorbital arteries of the skin of the index fingers during auditory and optic stimulation and during the solution of a mental problem, both at the beginning and end of each period. A significant change was shown during BC-105 therapy in all types of vascular reaction in the superficial temporal and supraorbital arteries to all stimuli used; vasodilation, vasoconstriction, and nonreactive states were all affected. The amplitude of the vasodilator reaction in the region of the supraorbital artery was three times greater in these subjects during the administration of a placebo than in control subjects. After treatment with BC-105, the vasodilator reaction returned to normal. Similar changes were seen in all types of vascular reaction in the subcutaneous vessels of the index fingers after BC-105, with significant changes in the vasoconstrictor reactions to nonreactive states. A state of vasomotor inactivity was found to be present more often after the use of BC-105 than before it. This suggests a sedative action on the increased lability of the cranial vasomotor centers and the factor of hypersensitivity to vasoconstrictive stimuli.

Aellig[161] made some interesting clinical pharmacologic experiments with BC-105 on the superficial hand veins in humans. In his works he conducted experiments to investigate the effects of BC-105 on superficial hand veins in situ and also to study its interaction with 5-hydroxytryptamine. Local infusion of BC-105 produced a marked venoconstrictor effect, comparable to that seen after local infusion of dihydroergotamine (DHE-45). To test the antiserotoninergic effect of BC-105, local infusions of 5-hydroxytryptamine were administered to five patients before and after local infusion of BC-105. Aellig found that the venoconstrictor effect of a submaximal dose of 5-hydroxytryptamine was consistently reduced after the administration of BC-105. The venoconstrictor effect of ergotamine was examined in five patients, once without pretreatment and once after the local administration of BC-105. The results show that the venoconstrictor effect of ergotamine on superficial hand veins in humans was markedly reduced after the local administration of BC-105. Aellig concludes that venoconstrictor effect of ergotamine on

these veins was at least partly due to a stimulation of 5-HT receptors.

The chief side effect of BC-105 is drowsiness.[162] In a large study on BC-105 in migraine cases a common side effect was weight gain. This did not appear to be a fluid retention type but actual weight gain. Most of the patients who gained weight gained an average of 5 to 8 pounds in the 4-week period on BC-105. It required roughly 3 to 4 weeks for them to lose this weight following cessation of the use of the drug, but they all finally went back to their normal weight. Other side effects experienced with BC-105 consisted of dry mouth, nausea, cramps, increased appetite, and vertigo. However, these side effects were of a very minor nature. It is also interesting to note that many side effects were reported with the use of the placebo, such as drowsiness, nausea, vertigo, nervousness, and a dry mouth.

Schaer,[163] reporting on the use of BC-105 in 140 patients, found side effects in seventy-three patients, over 50%. None of these side effects was very serious. The main side effect was drowsiness (thirty-nine patients). In most cases, particularly in patients who were given a low dosage, this was mild and it disappeared in the course of a few days or weeks. In six cases the drowsiness was severe enough to cause considerable disruption of normal activities (job, housework, etc.) and as a result of this, the drug had to be discontinued. Another side effect observed quite frequently was a marked increase of appetite; this occurred in twenty-one patients. Seventeen patients gained a considerable amount of weight. However, this weight gain was usually only in evidence during the first months of treatment. Generally, the weight gain was 1 to 2 kg per month, although one woman put on 10 kg in 3 months. In spite of the favorable effect that BC-105 had on their headache, three patients chose to stop the drug because of this weight gain.

Brugger,[164] in a study of eighty patients, found similar side effects. The chief of these was an increase in appetite and weight:

seventeen patients showed a weight gain up to 10 kg in 2 to 3 months (average: 3 kg). One patient gained 13 kg in 6 months. Most patients experienced an increased drowsiness during the first week of treatment; while it usually vanished after 3 to 4 weeks, five patients had to abandon treatment for this reason. Two also showed a marked depression which disappeared when BC-105 was withdrawn.

In discussing BC-105 Andersson[165] says the side effects are not as serious as those of methysergide. This certainly is true. He found the chief side effect of BC-105 to be the rather pronounced weight gain most of the patients undergo. Other drugs as well cause increase in weight, but not as great as BC-105. This unfortunate side effect will undoubtedly limit the use of this drug to some extent. When the treatment is discontinued the patient regains his initial weight within about 2 months.

Prusinski and Niewodniczy[166] state that BC-105 was well tolerated. Slight side effects were noted in four patients: drowsiness in two, slight edema and redness of the face in one on the first day of treatment, and transient numbness of the upper extremities in one patient. All patients reported a greatly increased appetite, and body weight increases occurred in eight patients. The numbness in the extremities is truly a rare side effect of BC-105, and one that we have never seen.

Cerdan and associates[167] ran glucose tolerance tests and insulin levels on migraine patients. In this study, each patient was placed on a diet containing at least 200 gm of carbohydrate for 3 days and then, after overnight fasting (10 to 12 hours), the patients were given an oral glucose load of 100 gm. Blood samples were collected at 30, 60, and 120 minutes after the glucose load and analyzed for glucose and insulin. Thirteen healthy headache-free subjects served as controls. No significant differences were found in the blood glucose or serum insulin concentrations between the migraine and the control patients. The mi-

graine sufferers were then given 0.5 mg of BC-105 and the dose was increased by 0.5 mg a day until a total dose of 3 mg a day in three divided doses had been reached. Each patient was then maintained on this dose for 1 month, and the glucose tolerance test was repeated. No significant change in glucose levels was found, compared with those obtained before BC-105 medication. However, the insulin levels were significantly higher. Fasting insulin levels remained unaltered. All patients claimed that their migraine had improved while taking BC-105. Twelve patients gained weight (0.6 to 6 kg) while taking BC-105. It is concluded that the altered insulin secretion following administration of the drug is caused by enhanced pancreatic secretion due to BC-105.

An interesting observation on BC-105 in migraine patients was made by Biehl and Seydel.[168] BC-105 was tested in sixteen male students to evaluate its possible effects on the ability to drive a car. A control group of sixteen students received a placebo. The trial was conducted as a double-blind experiment. In no case was there any significant impairment of physical or mental fitness. Fatigue and headaches were reported far more often by members of the group taking the test drug than by the group receiving placebo. Side effects shown by those taking the active drug included vertigo, irritability, intellectual dulling, and intolerance to alcohol.

There are many other reports in the medical literature listing increased appetite, weight gain, and drowsiness as the chief side effects of BC-105.[169-172] This seems to be generally agreed on by all headache experts.

There have been many glowing reports on the successful results of using BC-105 in the prophylactic treatment of migraine. However, as is the case with clonidine all of these reports are from countries other than the United States. Schaer[163] concluded that BC-105 is effective in roughly the same percentage of cases of migraine as methysergide, and in some cases it exerts a prophylactic effect even after its administration has been discontinued.

At the Scandinavian Migraine Symposium in 1969, Stensrud and Sjaastad[173] used BC-105 as a prophylactic agent against migraine. It was compared with a placebo in twenty patients in a double-blind study. BC-105 and a placebo were given in a dose of 1 mg four times a day for 8 weeks each and the sequence of the substances was randomized. A significantly better effect of BC-105 than the placebo was apparent after eleven patients had finished the study. The average reduction in terms of headache days on BC-105 therapy was 43%, and as a rule the attacks were of shorter duration and lesser severity with BC-105. In three of twenty patients, there was no reduction in headache days. They concluded that BC-105 with the dosage used seems as favorable as methysergide in the prevention of migraine. While the results obtained were good, this is indeed a small number of patients.

Another study on BC-105, but again on a small number of patients, was made by Carroll and Maclay.[174] He conducted a double-blind randomized crossover, comparing BC-105 against a placebo. Prior to this trial, each patient had received BC-105 for 1 month in order to assess the effective dosage. The total duration of the trial was 5 months and 2 weeks. Each patient was given BC-105 for 1 month followed by a 2-month period on both a placebo and BC-105, with a 2-week washout between periods. BC-105 (0.5 mg) and the placebo were supplied in identical tablet forms. Laboratory investigations were carried out at the start of the trial, after 3 months and again at the end of the trial. Headaches were graded as severe, moderate, or mild, and their frequency was also recorded. Fifteen patients were given the Beck self-rating scale for depression. A total of twenty-seven patients was included in the trial, all having either classic or common migraine. None had hepatic and renal disorders or any diseases that might have interfered with the absorption or metabolism of BC-105. Fourteen patients completed the trial. Four out of the six patients receiving drug-placebo-drug improved, and two showed no change. Five out of the eight patients receiving drug-drug-placebo improved, two became worse, and one patient showed no change. Carroll concluded that BC-105 is a useful compound in the treatment of certain cases of migraine because it reduces the frequency and severity of the attacks of headache. The main drawback to its use is the weight gain experienced by some women in the 20- to 40-year age group. The drug does not appear definitely to alter the mood of the patient.

Barolin[175] found that BC-105 proved more suitable in cases of migraine with overtones of depression. He says the present indication for BC-105 appears to be the failure of other types of therapy. BC-105 had been found to be superior to methysergide. He also found a few cases of atypical facial pain that have responded well to BC-105.

Andersson[165] concluded that BC-105 is an effective drug in the treatment of migraine, as effective as methysergide, but its usefulness is restricted by its main side effect, increase in weight.

Dalsgaard-Nielsen[176] reported on thirty-eight cases successfully treated with BC-105. Each patient received 2 mg/day orally for 13 to 80 months (average: 28.8 months). Half (seven men, thirty-one women, aged 21 to 76 years) were subjected to an extensive tolerance investigation as well. All the patients reported a diminution in the frequency of attacks. Clinical neurologic examination was normal as regards motor and sensory function and tendon jerks. Ophthalmoscopy showed normal refractive parameters and fundi. Blood values were all within normal limits, as were the aspartate-aminotransferase and serum lactate dehydrogenase activities. Examination of the serum creatinine, urinalysis, and clinical examination revealed no signs of retroperitoneal fibrosis, which has been reported in patients receiving long-term treatment with methysergide. Electroradiography was normal and the blood pressure lay within the normal range. In twenty of the thirty-eight patients examined, an average gain in weight of 4.6 kg occurred (ranging from 2 to 15 kg), and this is assumed to have been due to a central appetite-stimulating effect. He concluded that BC-105 in a dose of 2 mg/day is an effective and well-tolerated prophylactic treatment of migraine.

In a study of thirty cases in wihch BC-105 was used in migraine, Pasquazzi and Anselmi[177] found that the therapeutic effects were good in seventeen cases (68% of the cases evaluable), with the beneficial effects occurring after the first week of treatment and giving rise to progressively fewer episodes of hemicrania, and finally to their elimination. In eight patients the treatment had no effect. This represents only a little better than 50% success and is not a striking percentage.

Anselmi[178] found BC-105 to be useful in treating migraine and also to be helpful in relieving the depression associated with the condition. He conducted a study including sixty patients in two parallel groups suffering from classic migraine, atypical migraine, or chronic cephalalgia who were treated under double-blind conditions with either BC-105 or fonazine for 4 weeks following a 4-week pretreatment placebo period. The therapeutic effect both on migraine and on the depressed mood was then evaluated. BC-105 was shown to be superior in the migraine field. Improvement in the depression associated with this condition was also demonstrated.

In still another report on fifty-two patients Arthur and Hornabrook[179] found excellent or good results—that is, at least 50% reduction in headache was achieved in twenty-one cases (40%) with BC-105 and in six cases (12%) with the placebo. This difference is statistically significant. There appeared to be no difference in response between the various forms of migraine. During the pretreatment period a total of

423 headaches were reported, of which 127 were severe. With placebo, the number rose to 457, with ninety-one severe headaches, and on BC-105, the figure dropped to 330, with fifty-three headaches graded as severe. This difference is also significant. BC-105 appeared not only to reduce the incidence but also the severity of the headaches.

Speight and Avery[180] say that BC-105 is indicated in the prophylaxis of severe and recurrent vascular headaches but is of no value in the treatment of acute attacks. Controlled studies have shown BC-105 to be significantly more effective than a placebo, but they found it to be less effective than methysergide. Exceptionally, patients with migraine respond to it after they have failed to respond to methysergide. They also point out that BC-105 is of little value in other forms of headache (tension or muscular contraction headache, posttraumatic headache, inflammatory headache, or trigeminal neuralgia).

Selby[181] in only forty cases gave BC-105 in a dose of 1.5 mg/day for 2 to 12 months. The results showed a definite improvement in about 40% of patients, with enhancement of the action of ergotamine. The chief side effect was a gain in weight. Drowsiness was not observed, possibly because of the use of lower initial doses. It is concluded that BC-105 is a useful drug in cases of classic migraine.

Wasilewski[182] conducted a study of twenty migraine patients treated with BC-105. The patients received up to six tablets per day for 3 to 8 months, while twenty control patients received a placebo. During the trial no other drugs were administered for headache. In twenty patients receiving the drug the attacks ceased completely during the course of treatment (fourteen in the first month of treatment, five in the second, and one in the fourth). In seven patients the frequency of the attacks decreased by at least 75%, in ten by 50% to 75%, and in seven by 25% to 50%. No improvement was seen in five patients. Of those receiving a placebo, the attacks ceased completely in one case, decreased in frequency by 50% or more in three cases, decreased by 25% in one case, were unchanged in fourteen cases, and increased in one case.

In Nelson's study[158] of thirteen patients with classic migraine, six showed an excellent reduction (75% to 100%) in the frequency of attacks, four a good reduction (50% to 70%), and three failed to benefit. Only fourteen of the thirty-five common migraine patients studied showed more than a 50% reduction in the frequency of attacks.

Most of the studies mentioned were on a very small number of patients. To say that a drug is either good or bad, more cases than reported in most of these reports would seem to be needed.

Not all reports in the literature show BC-105 to be successful. One of the first reports was by Lance and Anthony[183] in Australia. They said that a new preparation, BC-105, related chemically to cyproheptadine, proved less effective than cyproheptadine in the prevention of frequent migraine headaches. Indeed, it did not give significantly superior results to placebo medication in a short-term controlled trial.

Heyck,[184] in speaking of BC-105 and its use in migraine at the Scandinavian Migraine Symposium in 1969, found that six patients registered a reduction in attacks of more than 60%, six others a reduction in attacks of 40% to 60%, and in three cases a reduction in attacks of 20% to 30%. In eleven cases there was no effect. The side effects were for the most part fatigue (eleven cases). He concluded that the value of this polyvalent mixture of biogenic amines does not yet appear to be certain.

Ryan[162] made a study on BC-105 compared with methysergide and placebo in a double-blind study. In this trial the results obtained were good enough to require a second, more extensive trial. The results reported showed the number of headaches to be less with BC-105 (4.7) than when methysergide was used (6.2). Methysergide (6.2) actually was not much less than when the placebo was used (8.9). These figures were very interesting when one realizes that the same patients all received these three drugs (BC-105, methysergide, and placebo) for the same length of time. These results clearly showed the use of BC-105 to be superior to the use of methysergide in the prophylactic phase of migraine therapy. The headache index also favored the use of BC-105, which had a headache index of 8.9. On the other hand, methysergide had a headache index of 11.3, and the placebo headache index was 17.0.

In a second study on BC-105 compared with placebo there were much poorer results.[185] This was a double-blind clinical evaluation of the efficacy of BC-105, as compared with a placebo, in the interval treatment of migraine headaches. There were few statistically significant differences between treatments on measures of safety. While certain laboratory variables did show significant mean changes during the study, all were essentially within the normal range of laboratory values. The evaluation of efficacy was complicated by the fact that pretreatment mean differences were statistically significant on certain critical variables. There was no evidence to indicate that BC-105 was statistically significantly more efficacious than placebo in the interval treatment of migraine headaches in this study. Absolute mean values tended to make BC-105 appear less efficacious than placebo on most indices of efficacy. The evaluation of efficacy was complicated in this study by the fact that the treatment groups differed significantly before treatment with respect to several variables—frequency of migraine attacks, severity of migraine attacks, and migraine index. The differences in each case were weighted against BC-105.

This study indicated a progressive decrease in the incidence of side effects from week 8 to week 16 despite the gradual increasing dose schedule. There was an apparent development of tolerance with regard to side effects. The increase in body weight over control values resulting from BC-105 treatment appeared to be a true drug effect and is in agreement with similar findings from earlier studies. The mechanism responsible for the increased appetite and weight gain still remains to be elucidated. The stimulation of appetite is of special interest on both theoretical and practical grounds. It has been suggested that improved appetite is related to a diminution of nausea and vomiting in patients whose migraine headaches have been relieved. However, in this study analysis of the results showed no positive correlation between amount of weight gain and degree of migraine relief.

The results obtained in this double-blind study were not too encouraging as far as the ability of BC-105 to prevent migraine attacks from occurring is concerned. However, the fact that the group of patients receiving BC-105 apparently had more difficulty before the study began than did the group of patients receiving placebo should be borne in mind. The fact that this occurred is unfortunate and was not known until the study was completed. Perhaps if the scale had been more balanced in regard to this factor, the results obtained would have been more favorable for BC-105. This type of error is unavoidable in any double-blind study, so perhaps further investigation of this drug may still prove it to be a useful product in the prophylactic phase of the treatment of migraine.

It is evident from what has been presented here that there is at least some doubt as to the use of BC-105 in migraine prophylactic therapy.

Clonidine

In discussing the drugs advocated for the prophylactic form of treatment of migraine, clonidine must be included. A great deal of investigative work has been done on this drug within the past several years. To say that the results presented in the medical literature are contradictory would be put-

ting it mildly. Clonidine is known on the drug market as Dixarit. It has been approved as an antihypertensive type of drug in the United States but not as an antimigraine type of drug.

At the present time there are several reports in the medical literature on the use of clonidine. However, all of these reports came from England or the European continent. All headache patients desire to receive from the physician something which will prevent him from having headaches in the future (prophylactic treatment). These European and British reports deal with this type of treatment.

Reports from England dealing with clonidine for migraine therapy began as early as 1969; however, nothing appeared in the American literature concerning this drug until 1975.

Wilkinson found clonidine to be a useful drug in the prophylactic treatment of migraine in some 30% of the patients she observed.[186] She further stated that the success rate may be significantly improved by prior selection with tyramine. In her study she found drowsiness and depression to be the most common side effects, and she points out that these are the result of the central action of clonidine.

In previous studies of clonidine there are many cases of migraine which become more severe when this drug is used. This is a difficult factor to explain but it may be a dose-dependent effect.

Clonidine hydrochloride, a unique antihypertensive agent, was synthesized in the laboratories of Beohringer Ingelheim G.m.b.H., Republic of West Germany. Minute oral doses of clonidine (fraction of a milligram) were found to lower the blood pressure in humans. While its mode of action has not been completely defined, clonidine is distinctive from other antihypertensive agents in that it apparently acts centrally to inhibit or diminish the discharge of sympathetic impulses to the periphery. The most frequently observed side effects have been sedation, dry mouth, and constipation, which sometimes lessen or disappear with continued treatment.

Clonidine is an imidazoline with the chemical name 2-(2.6-dichlorophenyl-amino)-2-imidazoline hydrochloride. Its empirical formula is $CH_9Cl_2N_3$ and its molecular weight is 266.57. It is odorless, bitter-tasting, white crystalline powder with good solubility in water (1:7) and alcohol (1:10), and practically insoluble in chloroform or ether. A 10% aqueous solution has a pH of 4.5 to 5.5.

Clonidine is an imidazoline derivative chemically related to tologaline and phentolamine. Grabner and Wolf[187] found it to reduce blood pressure and to cause sedation, dry mouth, and bradycardia. Extensive pharmacologic investigations have shown that its actions differ from other antihypertensive drugs. It has no direct vasodilator action, it does not deplete catecholamine stores, and there is no block of ganglionic, postganglionic, or alpha- or beta-adrenergic transmission. It has vasoconstrictor and central depressant effects.

Zaimis and Hannington[188] found that in concentrations of 1 to 2 mg/kg body weight, clonidine decreases the responsiveness of peripheral blood vessels to circulating vasoactive amines and the blood vessels neither constrict nor dilate as much as normal. It was this that lead to the belief that possibly clonidine might be of some use in the treatment of migraine. The use of this drug in migraine in clinical trials in England gave encouraging results.[189,190] More recently in Europe, a statistically significant superiority of clonidine over placebo has been shown in a double-blind clinical trial.[191] In all of these studies the effective dose level in the prophylactic treatment of

migraine cases was considerably lower than these used to lower the blood pressure. Therefore, there were no hypotensive effects.

More recently clonidine was investigated in England in a study using a double-blind crossover comparison with placebo in the prophylactic aspect of migraine therapy.[192] In this study 59% of the patients with migraine benefited from the prophylactic administration of clonidine, whereas only 17% benefited from placebo. These patients with clonidine maintained their improvement for a period up to 1 year with continued administration of the drug. The dose range in this study was 1 to 2 mg/kg/day.

Clonidine is remarkably free from serious side effects and is therefore a relatively safe drug to use. No contraindications have been identified as yet for clonidine; however, it should not be used in pregnant women, regardless of the fact that reproductive studies in animals have revealed no teratogenicity with its oral use.

Studies have continued to show that sedation and dry mouth are the primary side effects of clonidine, being variously reported in 30% to 70% of patients. In most but not all instances, these symptoms abated with prolonged therapy. Constipation and orthostatic complaints were less frequently reported. Mild bradycardia often accompanied clonidine therapy, and electrocardiographic changes have been consistent with this finding. Impotence was noted infrequently. Interestingly, one patient with impotence and another with gynecomastia associated with a previous antihypertensive regimen improved when clonidine was substituted.[193] Depression or anxiety was reported in a few patients.[194,195] In most cases there was a previous history of these symptoms, so that a causal role of the drug was not apparent.

Adverse reactions associated with clonidine have been, for the most part, mild and often transient. Sedation and dry mouth predominated and were usually dose-related. In most instances they subsided during treatment, but occasionally they were poorly tolerated and dose-limiting. Constipation was reported less frequently but tended to be associated more often with long-term therapy. Bradycardia has consistently been observed in single-dose studies with clonidine and was often present to a mild degree during continuous therapy. However, extreme slowing of the pulse has been rare. Although the standing blood pressure is usually somewhat lower than the supine pressure during clonidine treatment, orthostatic complaints such as dizziness and headache are not often encountered and rarely are severe. Facial pallor is rarely seen during oral administration of clonidine, but it may be seen more often when the drug is given intravenously, as may be chills and piloerection. Weight gain responsive to an oral diuretic has been reported occasionally, but congestive heart failure and edema have rarely resulted.

Associated with clonidine have been rare instances of burning of the tongue; itching, dryness, or burning of the eyes; dryness of nasal mucosa; nasal stuffiness; urinary retention; muscle aching; thinning of the hair; and gynecomastia. Paralytic ileus and periorbital swelling with itching have occurred in one patient each.

Isolated (transient) elevations in creatine phosphokinase, alkaline phosphatase, serum bilirubin, serum transaminase, BUN, BSP retention, and uric acid have been observed. No adverse effect on the hemogram has been evident.

The circulatory effects of clonidine were studied in hypertensive patients at rest and when exercising. The results showed a lowering of the blood pressure was achieved by a variable reduction of cardiac output and systemic vascular resistance. The circulatory responses to blood in the supine and the erect position were unimpaired.

We[196] pointed out that in previous studies of clonidine some migraine patients noted that their headache attacks became more severe when this drug was used. This is a difficult factor to explain but it may be a dose-dependant effect. However, this is merely hypothetical.

In a study on the use of clonidine in migraine patients Kangasniemi and Rime[197] found that side effects with clonidine seldom occurred and were usually mild. Four patients, however, had rather severe giddiness, two showing orthostatic hypotension as well. In addition some patients experienced dry mouth or paresthesias, and surprisingly seven patients underwent a weight gain of 2 kg and two as high as 5 kg.

Wilkinson[186] found side effects in 22% of the patients studied in the use of clonidine for the prophylactic treatment of migraine. The most common side effects were drowsiness and depression, which are a result of the central actions of clonidine. The most difficult phenomenon to explain is that 12% were made worse by clonidine.

Shafar and associates[198] also report few or no side effects of clonidine in the prophylactic treatment of migraine.

Barrie and co-workers[192] report on the use of clonidine in migraine and found that the only side effect encountered was dry mouth (which is a recognized pharmacologic effect of clonidine) and minor gastrointestinal disturbances. The incidence of these unwanted effects was the same at all centers and in both responders and nonresponders to clonidine.

In general, it must be concluded that clonidine is a relatively safe drug to use if the proper doses are employed.

In 1971, Wilkinson[186] reported on a study dealing with clonidine in which she observed the success rate of the drug in patients who were tyramine-positive and in patients who were tyramine-negative. This study showed that in the tyramine-positive patients improvement of 73.5% was obtained. In the migraine patients who were tyramine-negative the improvement rate was 43.5%. In a third group, composed of unselected migraine patients, the improvement rate was found to be 46%. These results indicated that clonidine was far more effective in the prophylactic treatment of migraine when it is used by tyramine-positive patients.

Barrie and associates[192] state that the results obtained in a multicenter study indicate that 31% of patients with migraine benefited from the prophylactic administration of clonidine. Their impression was that at least 50% of patients who responded to clonidine have maintained improvement over periods of up to 1 year's continued administration of the drug.

Shafar, Tallett, and Knowlson,[198] in evaluating clonidine in the prophylaxis of migraine, found that both placebo and clonidine treatment gave lower rates as well as weighted scores, compared with the pretreatment phase. In the clonidine group, a statistically significant reduction in the number of severe attacks was found. In the severe group, the rate remained unaltered but the score was reduced in five cases by clonidine and in three by placebo. In neither group was the number of severe attacks affected by the placebo. They found that three of the severe group also showed marked improvement, which had not been seen in the shorter trial, perhaps indicating that the full benefit of clonidine may take several months to develop.

Carroll[199] made another report on clonidine and its use in the prophylactic treatment of migraine. His study consisted of a series of patients with migraine who were incorporated into a double-blind controlled clinical trial on an outpatient basis to test the efficiency of clonidine as a prophylactic agent. The severity and frequency of headaches were recorded at regular visits over a set period of time, and any side effects that occurred during treatment were noted. The results of the trial were evaluated and they indicated that clonidine can be an effective drug in the management of migraine.

A careful follow-up study was carried out on those patients in the trial who had responded to treatment with the drug. A significant proportion maintained their improvement while on the drug and some continued to do well after stopping treatment.

Kangasnieme and Rime[197] found nine (31%) out of twenty-nine patients who took clondine after placebo found improvement. Six showed fair (25% to 50%) and three excellent (50% to 75%) reduction of headache. Twelve (41%) patients found no difference compared to the placebo period and in eight (28%) cases headache got worse. Sixteen out of thirty-two (50%) on BC-105 reported that their headache improved. In ten cases pain was reduced by 25% to 50% and in six cases 5% to 75%. Nine (28%) patients found no difference compared to the placebo period and in seven cases (22%) the headache got worse.

These reports all were on the positive side and found clonidine to be helpful in preventing migraine attacks. All of them were from England or Europe.

Now let us look at the reports of clonidine in migraine which came from the United States. The first American report of clonidine and its use in prophylaxis of migraine was made by Ryan and Ryan.[196,200] They report that seventy-five patients were selected who gave a history of having three or more migraine attacks per month. These patients either had common or classic migraine. Both males (fifteen patients) and females (sixty patients) between the ages of 21 and 60 were included in the study. Their weights varied from 90 pounds to 229 pounds. None of the female patients was pregnant. None of the patients had liver disease, kidney disease, cardiovascular disease, or depressive illness. No other prophylactic medication was administered to these patients, but they were all instructed to use various medications for the symptomatic treatment of their headache attacks when they did occur. The name of the drug and the dosage used for each attack were all recorded in a medical diary which the patient used daily. The amount of the trial medication taken each day was also recorded in this diary.

The object of this study was to evaluate

the efficacy and safety of clonidine in the prophylactic treatment of migraine headache in comparison with placebo treatment. It was a double-blind, crossover type of study. Each patient received clonidine for a period of 8 weeks and then was crossed over to the placebo, or from the placebo to clonidine. Any patient who received poor results after a period of 6 weeks and did not seem to respond to the treatment was crossed over at that time. The order of treatment was randomized. At the time of the crossover, each patient was instructed not to take any of the test medication for a period of 2 days. After 2 days without medication had elapsed the patients returned for their second medication.

On the initial visit a brief history of the patient was recorded with certain leading questions being asked such as relation of headache attacks to emotional stress, menses, foods, seasons of the year, etc. Also recorded was the history of the patient with regard to other medication being used by the patient. Each patient received an examination, which included blood pressure, pulse, and electrocardiogram. Also certain laboratory tests were done; both the blood and urine were examined. All of these tests were rechecked at the crossover period and at the end of the procedure.

Patients were seen every 2 weeks. The vital signs were recorded on each patient then and also 48 hours after the patient had completed each course of drug treatment. At each visit the patient's diary was examined and a global evaluation was made concerning the frequency, duration, and severity of the headache attacks during the 2-week period. Side effects were also recorded.

At the beginning of the trial, each patient was instructed to take one tablet (25 mg) twice a day, one in the morning and one in the evening. After a period of 2 weeks, if there was no remission of the symptoms, the dosage was increased to two tablets in the morning and two tablets in the evening. This was the dosage level for another 2 weeks. If the desired degree of response was not achieved the dosage was increased to three tablets twice a day. This was the maximum dosage used. These patients who failed to receive the desired results with the six tablets per day dosage schedule were then crossed over to the second drug. In these cases, therefore, the crossover took place in 6 weeks. In the cases in which satisfactory results were obtained, the crossover took place 8 weeks after the investigation began.

Between the trial with drug 1 and that with drug 2, there was a 48-hour period in which no prophylactic medication was taken. After the 48 hours the patient returned for a recheck of the vital signs and evaluation.

This preliminary report includes the statistical analysis of the first half of the total study; in other words, up to the crossover point of the study. The final report of the entire study will be given at a later date. One of the outstanding features of the preliminary report is the lack of side effects reported. In this report, of the seventy-five patients, seventeen were found to be tyramine-positive and fifty-eight were tyramine-negative or non–tyramine-sensitive.[38]

A headache index was computed for each patient. This index was calculated by multiplying the number of severe, moderate, and mild headaches by 3, 2, and 1 respectively and summing to yield the index value. No statistically significant difference was found between the overall means for those patients receiving clonidine and those patients receiving a placebo for the tyramine-positive group or the tyramine-negative group. Another factor worth consideration is the headache frequency. Here it was found that there also was no statistically significant difference between the overall mean for those patients receiving clonidine and those patients receiving a placebo for both the tyramine-positive group of patients and the tyramine-negative group. In fact, the headache frequency tended to rise in both the groups of patients. This was true in the tyramine-positive, the tyramine-negative, and the tyramine-positive and placebo-positive groups of patients.

From the results obtained in this study it must be concluded that clonidine did not seem to produce any better result than did the placebo. This is true regardless of whether the patient was tyramine-positive or tyramine-negative.

In another study that failed to find clonidine useful in the prophylactic form of treatment of migraine, Ryan, Diamond, and Ryan[201] reported on a multiclinic study. This study was carried out at headache centers in Chicago and St. Louis. The studies, though done simultaneously, were independent, but the protocol used was identical. The objective was to evaluate the efficacy and safety of clonidine in the prophylactic treatment of migraine and compare this to placebo treatment in the same patients. There were similar results though evaluations were completely independent. Clonidine was not superior to placebo in preventing migraine attacks.

Still another report finding clonidine unsuccessful in the treatment (prophylactic) of migraine was made by Stensrud and Sjaastad[202] from Norway. They did a double-blind crossover study with clonidine and placebo in twenty-nine patients with migraine who had received clonidine in a 4- to 32-month pretest period and seemingly had responded beneficially to the treatment initially. Placebo and clonidine were each given for 7 weeks, and headache days and headache indices during the last 5 weeks in each period were used for the statistical evaluation. There did not seem to be any appreciable difference between the initial phase of clonidine treatment and the immediate pretest period as regards frequency and severity of attacks. In nine of the patients, however, the evaluation of the patient charts was difficult due to the various events of possible significance for the creation of attacks in one or both periods. For example, one patient lost a job in one period, whereas another patient prepared for final university examinations. If these

nine patients are excluded, there is no statistically significant difference between placebo and clonidine.

From the results presented here it is difficult to say that clonidine is successful in preventing migraine attacks. Because of this the FDA does not, at the present time, permit it to be sold in the United States for this purpose. However, it is used in Europe for this purpose.

Beta-blocking drugs

During the past few years there has been a considerable amount of interest in the experimental use of beta-blocking agents in the prophylactic treatment of migraine. Several of these drugs are experimental and have been investigated only in Europe. The only drug of this type which has been studied with migraine patients in the United States is propranolol (Inderal).

PROPRANOLOL (INDERAL)

Inderal is a beta-adrenergic receptor blocking drug, possessing no other autonomic nervous system activity. It specifically competes with beta-adrenergic receptor stimulating agents for available beta receptor sites. When access to beta receptor sites is blocked by Inderal, the chronotropic, inotropic, and vasodilator responses to beta-adrenergic stimulation are decreased proportionately.

Propranolol is almost completely absorbed from the gastrointestinal tract, but a portion is immediately bound by the liver. Peak effect occurs in one to one and one-half hours. The biologic half-life is approximately two to three hours. Propranolol is not significantly dialyzable. There is no simple correlation between dose or plasma level and therapeutic effect, and the dose-sensitivity range as observed in clinical practice is wide. The principal reason for this is that sympathetic tone varies widely between individuals. Since there is no reliable test to estimate sympathetic tone or to determine whether total beta blockade has been achieved, proper dosage requires titration.

The proper objective of beta blockage therapy is to decrease adverse sympathetic stimulation but not to the degree that may impair necessary sympathetic support.*

The observation that patients with vascular headaches who happened to be receiv-

---

*From Physicians' desk reference, ed. 32, Oradell, N.J., 1978, Medical Economics Co.

ing propranolol for angina pectoris were relieved of their headaches prompted the investigation of propranolol in the treatment of vascular headaches. Propranolol is on the drug market with FDA approval for use in cases of angina pectoris due to coronary atherosclerosis.

Because of the potential for adverse results, treatment should be carefully monitored. The patient should also be reevaluated periodically since the dosage requirement and the need to continue Inderal may be altered by clinical exacerbations or remissions.
Propranolol is contraindicated in 1) bronchial asthma; 2) allergic rhinitis during the pollen season; 3) sinus bradycardia and greater than first degree block; 4) cardiogenic shock; 5) right ventricular failure secondary to pulmonary hypertension; 6) congestive heart failure unless the failure is secondary to a tachyarrhythmia treatable with Inderal; 7) in patients on adrenergic-augmenting psychotropic drugs (including MAO inhibitors), and during the two week withdrawal period from such drugs.*

It is also contraindicated in pregnancy.

If propranolol is used it should not be abruptly discontinued. The dosage should be gradually reduced and finally discontinued. The patient should be warned of this because if he should decide to discontinue the drug on his own, he should be told to do it in a gradual, not abrupt, manner.

There have been numerous side effects of various degrees reported in the literature with the use of this drug. These were, of course, noted in conditions other than migraine for its use in migraine is still in the investigative phase. These side effects will merely be mentioned here and not elaborated on.

Cardiovascular: bradycardia; congestive heart failure; intensification of AV block; hypotension; paresthesia of hands; arterial insufficiency, usually of the Raynaud type; thrombocytopenic purpura.
Central nervous system: lightheadedness; mental depression, manifested by insomnia, lassitude, weakness, fatigue; reversible mental depression progressing to catatonia; visual disturbances; hallucinations; an acute reversible syndrome characterized by disorientation for time and place, short term memory loss, emotional lability, slightly clouded sensorium, and decreased performance on neuropsychometrics.

Gastrointestinal: nausea, vomiting, epigastric distress, abdominal cramping, diarrhea, constipation.
Allergic: pharyngitis and agranulocytosis, erythematous rash, fever combined with aching and sore throat, laryngospasm and respiratory distress.
Respiratory: bronchospasm.
Hematologic: agranulocytosis, nonthrombocytopenic purpura, thrombocytopenic purpura.
Miscellaneous: reversible alopecia. Oculomucocutaneous reactions involving the skin, serous membranes and conjunctivae reported for a beta blocker (practolol) have not been conclusively associated with propranolol.
Clinical laboratory test findings: Elevated blood urea levels in patients with severe heart disease, elevated serum transaminase, alkaline phosphatase, lactate dehydrogenase.*

When these vast possible side effects are compared with the use of histamine (which we have never found to produce a side effect), it makes one wonder if its investigation in the field of headache is worthwhile.

It has been pointed out by Blank and Rieder[203] that it is very hazardous to use propranolol in combination with the ergot preparations because of the possibility of severe peripheral vasoconstriction. This may be due to propranolol blocking a natural pathway for vasodilation and thus permitting ergot to produce marked vasoconstriction. The actual mechanism of the action of propranolol in migraine is as yet unknown. However, its main action may well be the blocking of vasodilator receptors in adrenergically innervated blood vessels.

Lechin and van der Dijs[204] advocate the use of propranolol in conjunction with d-amphetamine. They postulate that headache and depression are due to a predominance of the serotonergic over the noradrenergic system. Activation of the serotonergic system could be triggered by beta-adrenergic effects of the noradrenergic system. Then they suggest that serotonin acts like a weak alpha-adrenergic agonist and competes with norepinephrine for alpha receptors on cell membranes. Therefore,

---

*From Physicians' desk reference, ed. 32, Oradell, N.J., 1978, Medical Economics Co.

---

*From Physicians' desk reference, ed. 32, Oradell, N.J., 1978, Medical Economics Co.

low doses of *d*-amphetamine, by stimulating the noradrenergic system only, and propranolol, by interfering with serotonin synthesis in neurons, reestablish normal physiologic conditions.

Malvea, Gwon, and Graham[205] state that the rationale for using propranolol in the prophylaxis of vascular headache of the migraine type is based on its capacity to block the function of the beta-adrenergic system. Since the pain of migraine is alleviated by agents which produce cranial vasoconstriction, the ability of this "beta blocker" to prevent vasodilation may also be expected in an inverse fashion to be of potential benefit to migraine headache patients. They point out that although the effectiveness of propranolol in the prophylaxis of migraine as compared with a placebo is not dramatic, the study nevertheless strongly suggests that in some patients it is very effective and, in general, may have a useful role in the prophylaxis of migraine.

Diamond and Medina[206] tested propranolol against a placebo in sixty-two patients and found those preferring propranolol had a greater reduction in severity and frequency of headache and less consumption of ergotamine and analgesics than did those preferring the placebo. They found the side effects to be of a minor nature and suggest that propranolol is a safe drug to use in cases of this type.

Forssman and associates[207] observed the preventive effect of propranolol on migraine attacks compared to placebo in a double-blind crossover trial. Thirty-two patients with serious and prolonged migraine participated in the 12-week study. The effect of propranolol was significantly better than that of placebo. The number of migraine attacks during the propranolol period was reduced and the intensity of headache was significantly reduced during the propranolol period.

Borgesen and co-workers[208] did a double-blind, single crossover study to compare the effect of propranolol with that of a placebo in the prophylactic treatment of migraine in thirty patients, twenty-five women and five men. They found the patients receiving propranolol had a decrease in the frequency of attacks as compared to those receiving the placebo. Mild side effects such as drowsiness, fatigue, and diarrhea were noted. They concluded that propranolol is useful in these cases of migraine but point out that the mode of action is yet to be explained but may be due to some beta receptor antagonism.

Ludvigsson[209] tested propranolol in migraine in children and found it to be an excellent drug to use for this type of headache. The optimal dosage was 1 mg/kg three times a day. The only side effect he noted in this study was drowsiness.

Weber and Reinmuth[210] treated nineteen patients with refractory migraine with prophylactic propranolol (80 mg/day) and placebo in a 6-month double-blind trial. They concluded that propranolol is a safe and effective drug in the prophylaxis of migraine, provided that the patients are carefully selected. It should not be given to patients with a tendency to heart failure, asthma, or hypoglycemia, in which its beta-blocking effect could lead to complications. They point out that the precise mechanism of action of propranolol in migraine is unknown; they believe that it seems likely that its main effect is a blockade of vasodilator receptors in adrenergically innervated blood vessels.

Stensrud and Sjaastad[211] compared the effect of propranolol in racemic form (40 mg four times daily), *d*-propranolol (40 mg four times daily), and placebo in a randomized double-blind crossover study of 4 weeks duration each. They state that propranolol penetrates the blood-brain barrier, but only the racemic form, Inderal, has beta-blocking properties. Such a study might indicate the relative importance of the beta-blocking properties and the "central" action in migraine prophylaxis. They concluded that both the beta-blocking properties and other properties, such as the central action, may be of importance in migraine prophylaxis with propranolol because Inderal and *d*-propranolol produced similar results.

Blomberg[212] tested propranolol in seven patients with severe migraine who were using large daily doses of different preparations containing ergotamine. All were hospitalized and all analgesics were withdrawn. Propranolol in doses of 40 to 80 mg three times a day was given. Five of the patients were able to completely abandon analgesics and were free from migraine while regularly taking propranolol medication.

The oral administration of *d*-amphetamine with propranolol led to an immediate improvement of 161 out of 163 treated headache patients. Total disappearance of headache and other associated symptoms occurred after a few days. The addition of propranolol appears necessary to counteract undesirable side effects of amphetamines. Low doses of *d*-amphetamine are necessary for therapeutic success.[204]

Propranolol is the only drug of the beta-blocker type on the drug market in the United States. Other experimental investigative work has taken place in Europe. These results are also reported.

ALPRENOLOL

Ekbom[213] investigated the efficacy in migraine of alprenolol, a beta-receptor blocker with a weak beta-stimulating action. Alprenolol in a dosage of 400 mg daily was compared with placebo in a double-blind trial by means of the single crossover technique. A series of twenty-eight patients was studied. Eleven of these patients preferred alprenolol, twelve favored placebo, and five had no preference. Thus, this trial suggests alprenolol to be of little value in the prophylaxis of migraine. Side effects consisted of vertigo, dry mouth, drowsiness, and retrosternal burning on swallowing.

OPIPRAMOL

Jacobs[214] conducted a double-blind study comparing opipramol (Insidon) and a pla-

cebo. He found this drug to be of benefit in controlling mild attacks of migraine but no better than placebo in severe attacks. His results on the whole seem questionable as far as the overall relief of migraine attacks is concerned.

LB-46

LB-46 (*d*,1-4-[2-hydroxy-3-isopropylaminopropoxy], indol), an experimental drug, was tested in the prophylactic treatment of migraine by Ekbom and Lundberg[215] and by Sjaastad and Stensrud.[216] They were separate trials, one being conducted in Sweden (Ekbom) and the other in Norway (Sjaastad). However, both investigations proved this drug to be of no practical value in the prophylaxis of migraine.

PINDOLOL

Pindolol was observed by Reiger and associates.[217] This drug was administered intravenously (0.4 mg) after an electroencephalogram had been taken. Following the injection another electroencephalogram was taken during hyperventilation. It was concluded that there was no evidence of a central action of pindolol. This compared with the fact that there was also lack of relief from the headache attacks in these patients.

• • •

Of all of the various types of beta blocking drugs tested in the prophylaxis of migraine, the only one which may be of value at this date is propranolol, and its usefulness is indeed questionable. Much more investigation is needed.

Hormones
PROGESTERONE

There is some suggestion and evidence that a hormonal imbalance may be part of the etiology of migraine. This assumption has been made because very frequently attacks of migraine are found to occur either before, during, or immediately following menstruation, or at ovulation; or these patients' attacks are aggravated by estrogen-progesterone therapy (oral contraceptive pills); or they are free of their attacks during pregnancy. Another factor worth observing is that the initial attack in many cases of migraine occurs with certain endocrine changes occurring at the time of puberty. During all of these periods there are changes in the sex hormone levels, and it is only natural to suspect that this may have an influence on migraine attacks. From this it seems possible that migraine attacks might be abolished by suppressing the normal fluctuations in female sex hormone levels. This could possibly be accomplished by the administration of progesterone.

Somerville[218] studied the influence of hormone change on migraine and found that when plasma progesterone levels fell, migraine occurred in several patients. However, when these patients were given progesterone intramuscularly, prevention of the migraine attacks did not occur. Somerville concluded from this that perhaps a fall in the estrogen level is more important than the progesterone.

Epstein and associates,[10] studying sex hormones in migraine throughout the menstrual cycle, found that mean plasma progesterone and estrogen levels were higher in migraine patients than in normal patients, especially in the late luteal phase of the cycle. They concluded that there is no specific hormonal change occurring during an attack of migraine.

Somerville[219] in another study found a 41% improvement in migraine cases when given continuous progesterone treatment. He stated, however, that side effects frequently occurred in the form of polymenorrhea, breakthrough bleeding, and amenorrhea.

Somerville[220] believes that menstrual migraine is caused by the withdrawal of estrogen which affects a susceptible part of the vascular tree, and that progesterone withdrawal actually plays little or no part in the etiology of migraine.

Larsson-Cohn and Lundberg[28] found improvement in migraine attacks when female patients were given a low dose of progesterone sequential oral contraceptive. There was a decrease in the symptoms of migraine but no change in other types of headache. In an earlier study Lundberg[221] found progesterone therapy to give complete freedom from migraine in fifty-five of eighty-four patients. He found side effects to consist of menstrual irregularities, irregular bleeding, and weight gain.

The thinking behind the use of progesterone in the prophylaxis of migraine is that progesterone has a direct influence on the vascular tree, perhaps on the musculature of the walls of the artery in the affected region of the head. This has never been proved, but it does produce this effect on the myometrium. Progesterone also has an effect on muscular tone of the uterus. So it is apparent that the use of progesterone in the prophylaxis of migraine is quite controversial. We rarely find it to be effective.

ESTROGEN

A decrease in the estrogen level and the onset of migraine coincide.

Somerville[18] found that the injection of estrogen at an appropriate time to prevent the decrease of estrogen would often delay the migraine attack in patients with menstrual migraine.

Chaudhuri and Chaudhuri[222] report on two cases in which migraine was controlled with daily oral doses of 1.25 mg of estrogen for 21 days followed by 7 days without estrogen. Reduced dosages did not produce these results.

Somerville[11] found that a patient needed to be exposed to high doses of estrogen for several days before the estrogen withdrawal produced migraine. He also observed that the oral premenstrual administration of estrogen was of no value in the prophylaxis of migraine. Somerville[223] also used estrogen intramuscularly for this purpose but concluded that it did not offer a solution because of the menstrual irregularities which resulted.

It seems that the use of estrogen in the prophylaxis of migraine actually has little value. When this preparation is used for any great length of time it probably affects the blood vessels, making them more susceptible to the other facets which are implicated in migraine. Estrogen definitely alters vasomotor stability, but its effect on the cranial blood vessels, whether direct or indirect, is still uncertain.

Lisuride

Lisuride, a new preparation which is claimed to be beneficial in the prophylaxis of migraine, has been investigated both in Europe and in Australia. It has been tested against placebo and against methysergide. Lisuride chemically is known as lisuride hydrogen maleate. It is a derivative of isolysergic acid. Its formula is N-(d-6-methyl-8-isoergolenyl-)-N′-N′-diethyl urea hydrogen maleate.

Animal pharmacology studies have been conducted to assess the effect of lisuride on the biogenic amines. The results demonstrate marked peripheral serotonin-antagonistic as well as alpha-adrenolytic and histamine-antagonistic actions. Dopamine-antagonistic and serotonin-antagonistic effects on the central nervous system are very probable. Constrictor effects on the smooth muscles of blood vessels and the uterus are either absent or minimal.

In humans, the central action of lisuride is demonstrated by quantitative pharmaco-electroencephalographic analysis involving migraine patients and healthy volunteers. The results of these studies demonstrate a central action of lisuride 1 to 6 hours after a single oral administration. When lisuride is administered in a single dose of 25 to 75 μg the effects shown in the electroencephalogram can best be compared with that of psychostimulants of the dextroamphetamine type. The EEG effect typical for lisuride is a decrease of the delta and theta frequencies.

Lisuride shows a bimodal effect. Dosages lower than 10 μg have a centrally inhibiting effect, while higher dosages (between 10 and 100 μg) have predominantly centrally stimulating effects that can be seen in EEG recordings.

The maximum blood levels are found between 30 and 60 minutes after drug administration. The effects on the EEG are more pronounced 3 hours after administration than they are 1 hour after administration. This might suggest that the stimulatory action on the central nervous system follows the plasma level after a certain delay. One hour after drug intake, central inhibitory action is more predominant. It is possible that the blood plasma level runs parallel to these inhibitory effects.

According to the electrophysiologic data, a dosage regimen of three doses of 25 μg of lisuride per day provides a continuous action.

In in vitro and in vivo studies of experimental animals, lisuride hydrogen maleate as a serotonin antagonist is as potent as LSD but not quite as effective as methysergide. In contrast to other ergot derivatives, which have a hypertensive effect by virtue of their vasoconstrictor action, lisuride hydrogen maleate has a slight hypotensive effect in various species and particularly in narcosis. Human pharmacologic studies have shown that lisuride hydrogen maleate gives rise to considerably fewer central and vegetative effects than methysergide. In contrast to LSD-25 there are no hallucinations, states of intoxication or oneirism, tactile disturbances, or feelings of anxiety or uncertainty.

Herrmann and associates[224] did a study on this drug and compared it with methysergide. The therapy was initiated with a gradually increasing dose; the patient received only one capsule on the first 2 days of treatment, two capsules on the next 2 days, and three capsules of the preparation daily from the fifth day. The patients were advised to take the capsules at mealtimes.

The general case history and the history of attacks were recorded before the start of the trial. The following laboratory and measured values were determined before the start of therapy and at monthly intervals during it: hemoglobin, erythrocyte count, leukocytes, thrombocytes, differential hemogram, ESR, SGOT, SGPT, alkaline phosphatase, creatinine, BUN, blood pressure, and patient's weight. The patients were given patient's rating forms on which they were to enter the occurrence and a description of attacks, as well as the use of attack preparations.

A total of 130 patients were treated with lisuride and 123 with methysergide. The majority of patients had more than seven attacks per month, most of which occurred on one side only, lasted several hours to a whole day, and were of violent intensity.

With lisuride therapy, reduction of the frequency of attacks to two per month was demonstrated in twenty-eight patients (23%) after 1 month, thirty-six (35%) after 2 months, and thirty-six (41%) after 3 months, while the corresponding figures for the methysergide group are thirty-three (34%), thirty-two (41%), and thirty (49%). The observed differences are not statistically significant. If a reduction of the frequency of attacks by at least 50% is used as the criterion for the efficacy, then 53% of the patients in the lisuride hydrogen maleate group and 51% under methysergide are improved after 3 months of therapy.

There is also no significant difference between the two compounds as regards the improvement in the intensity and duration of attacks. With lisuride therapy the percentage of severe attacks was reduced from 78% before treatment to 23% after 3 months of treatment. The corresponding values for methysergide are 69% before and 25% after 3 months of treatment.

All these results show that, regardless of the evaluation criteria employed, after 3

months therapy with methysergide or lisuride between 50% and 60% of the patients reported a distinct improvement, while no statistical difference at all could be established between the two preparations. As regards the laboratory values, the use of covariance analysis failed to establish any statistical differences between the two treatment groups during the 3 months.

The therapy with lisuride was terminated prematurely by 17% of the patients because of side effects, while the corresponding proportion in the methysergide group was 39%. This difference is statistically significant. This means that side effects regarded by the trial user or patient as being so serious as to lead to termination of the therapy occurred significantly less frequently with lisuride.

A detailed analysis shows that 20% of the patients taking methysergide and 2% of the patients using lisuride terminated the respective therapy because of side effects as early as the first month. The reasons for dropout were categorized as "lack of effect," "side effects," and "other (nonmedical)." In the methysergide group the following symptoms are reported particularly frequently as the reason for dropping out (in most cases several symptoms per patient): nausea, twenty-one patients, usually accompanied by vomiting, eighteen patients; dizziness, sixteen patients; gastrointestinal complaints, ten patients; myalgia and neuralgia, six patients; drowsiness, five patients; paresthesia, five patients; hypotension or collapse, five patients; tachycardia, four patients. Anginous complaints, ophthalmalgia, and fatigue were each reported by three patients. In the lisuride group the following symptoms appeared as the main reason for terminating the therapy: nausea, seven patients; gastrointestinal complaints, six patients; drowsiness, four patients; dizziness, three patients; vomiting, two patients.

Dizziness was frequently given as a reason for dropout. But obviously many patients tolerated this symptom. About 15%

more patients complained about this symptom with methysergide therapy than with lisuride therapy. There were also relatively less cold feeling in the extremities (8%) and weakness in the muscles (8%) with lisuride therapy. Therefore, we conclude that in comparison to methysergide, lisuride has less vasoconstrictor effect. These findings have even more weight if it is taken into account that before treatment the two symptoms were more frequent in the lisuride group. Lisuride shows a blood pressure–lowering effect during resting and working (ergometry) conditions, together with the lower rate in the symptoms "cold extremities" and "muscle weakness." This may lead one to conclude that there are peripheral vasodilatory effects with lisuride rather than vasoconstrictory ones and that these effects are more like Hydergin than like methysergide.

The results of this study speak for the therapeutic value of lisuride in the prophylaxis of migraine. Lisuride is as effective as methysergide when given in a dose eighty times lower, and is much better tolerated. This finding is lent more weight by the fact that there are so very few alternatives to treatment with methysergide for migraine. Herrmann and associates point out that BC-105 is also better tolerated than methysergide, but the majority of clinical studies with this preparation seem to indicate that it is somewhat inferior to methysergide in efficacy. These researchers also state that clonidine is also well tolerated, but its efficacy is still in question. They conclude that if the efficacy and good tolerance of lisuride can be confirmed in further studies, this preparation could mean a significant advance in the therapy of migraine.

Another study by Somerville and Herrmann[225] compared lisuride to placebo. One hundred and fifty patients were in this study over a 3-month period. At the end of that time, patients with no significant improvement were allowed to leave the trial, and those who remained were asked to take the medication for a second 3-month period.

Patients in both groups showed a fairly high rate of dropout, primarily at the end of the first 3 months.

The dropout rate due to side effects for the lisuride-treated group significantly exceeds that of the placebo-treated group. At the end of the first 3 months, the figures are 4.4% and 1.5%, respectively.

Two patients experienced severe muscle aches and pains in the lisuride group (against none in the placebo group), and four patients experienced chest pains while taking lisuride compared to one in the placebo group. These chest pains were sharp in character and brief in duration and did not resemble clinically the pain of ischemic heart disease. One patient developed visual hallucinations while taking lisuride. All of these side effects subsided promptly on withdrawal of the medication.

Side effects of a less severe nature, not requiring the discontinuing of medication, were encountered frequently in both groups. Muscle aches and pains, dizziness, cold feelings in the extremities, and palpitations all occurred with more frequency in patients taking lisuride.

No significant deviation from normal was observed in any of the laboratory parameters or in blood pressure, body weight, or urinalysis in the lisuride-treated group compared to the group receiving placebo.

Somerville and Herrmann concluded that it is difficult to claim the efficacy of lisuride in the face of such a high rate of placebo response and a high dropout rate. The two findings from this trial which suggest that lisuride may have some value as a migraine prophylactic are:

1. The greater efficacy of treatment with lisuride compared to placebo. They suggest that the drug may exert its beneficial action only after a latent period of several weeks.
2. The fact that approximately twice as many patients taking placebo had dropped out by the end of the trial because of lack of efficacy compared to the lisuride-treated group.

Lisuride is another of the many preparations used in Europe for the prophylaxis of migraine that have not been cleared for investigational purposes by the FDA in the United States. Lisuride is perhaps the newest of all of these preparations, but from these two reports it does seem to be quite promising as far as prophylaxis of migraine is concerned. It seems to be as effective as methysergide, and certainly seems to have far fewer and far less serious side effects than methysergide.

Other prophylactic measures

A considerable amount of research has been done in the field of prophylaxis of migraine in the past 20 years. As in the field of symptomatic treatment of this condition, many articles appear announcing excellent results with a new or an old preparation. Many of these are soon discarded because they prove to be ineffectual, but some show promise and continue to be used in further research investigations. This is not unusual, for if it were not for research in this fashion, progress in this field would cease.

An attempt will be made in this text to present the various preparations that have been advocated in this field most recently. Some are still being investigated and some have already been discarded because of lack of effect on further investigation.

INDORAMINE

Carroll[226] at a headache symposium in Florence in 1976 reported on a new drug, indoramine. He administered indoramine in migraine patients in a double-blind study, comparing two dose schedules with a placebo. His preliminary results show that indoramine has some value therapeutically in reducing the frequency and the severity of migraine attacks. Further investigations with this drug are being made.

Indoramine is an alpha adrenoceptor blocker.

ERGO-LONARID

Ergo-Lonarid, a preparation containing 0.5 mg of dihydroergotamine tartrate, 400

mg of 4-acetylaminophenol, 10 mg of codeine phosphate, 30 mg of amobarbital, and 100 mg of caffeine has been used experimentally in Europe in cases of migraine.

Heide[227] reports on only four cases of migraine in which this preparation was used. He found good results in three cases and poor results in one case. The only side effect he encountered was a heavy feeling in the stomach in one patient.

Neumann-Mangoldt[228] tested the drug in thirteen cases and obtained nine satisfactory results, two moderate results, and two poor results. The side effects he found were four cases of drowsiness and four cases of local rectal irritation (from suppository administration).

Because of FDA regulations, this drug has not been investigated in the United States.

AMITRIPTYLINE

Amitriptyline has also been tested as a prophylactic agent for migraine.

Glaser[229] says that amitriptyline is effective in the prophylaxis of migraine. He suggests that the dosage requirement varies in relation to the patient's body weight.

Andersson[230] also reports good results with amitriptyline. His study consisted of twenty-six patients (twenty-two women, average age: 36.5 years; four men, average age: 46.8 years) with classic or common migraine. At the end of the treatment there was reduction in the frequency of attacks in 43% of the patients and average reduction in the migrainous severity in 51%. In five patients there was no reduction in either frequency or severity, and three showed a reduction in either frequency or severity. Side effect in the form of increase in weight was recorded in sixteen cases. Eight patients complained of tiredness, five of dryness of the mouth, five of marked constipation, and in five treatment had to be discontinued because of the side effects.

RESERPINE

Conflicting reports on the use of reserpine in the prophylaxis of migraine appear in the medical literature. Andersson[231] reports it to be ineffective in either reducing the frequency or the severity of migraine attacks. On the other hand, Nattero[232] states that it is quite successful when used for this purpose.

SULPIRIDE

Sulpiride has been tested in the prophylaxis of migraine in Europe but, because of FDA regulations, has not been used experimentally in the United States.

Sulpiride is a thymoanaleptic neuroleptic drug of the genzoamide group. It is described chemically as N-[(ethyl-i-pyrrolidnyl-2) methyl] methoxy-2 sulfonyl-5 benzamide, It has a powerful antiemetic action probably via medullary centers.

The mechanism of action of sulpiride in migraine is not understood: it may act as an antihistaminic or an antikinin agent.

Roge and De Roissard[233] used twenty-seven patients with migraine in a study of this drug. The results were excellent in twenty cases (74%), fair in four cases (15%), and negative in three (8%). In two cases there were side effects: in one, delayed menstruation with galactorrhea, and in the other, nervous crises with tachycardia and feelings of oppression.

Mosora and Boeriu[234] investigated the effect of sulpiride in migraine in twenty-six patients. The results were rated as very good (attacks allayed and made less frequent) in eleven cases, good (attacks only partly affected) in fourteen, and uncertain in one case. The only side effect observed was painful congestion of the breasts and galactorrhea in one patient on the sixth day of daily administration of two 100-mg vials of sulpiride; the untoward effect ceased 4 days after cessation of treatment. This adverse reaction may be due to the increase in the secretion of luteotropin by the pituitary gland following the diminution of hypothalamic inhibition, but it also connected with an individual neurohormonal factor.

Barre[235] tested sulpiride in thirty-one cases of migraine. The average oral dose was 100 to 200 mg daily and 200 mg intramuscularly daily for three patients. Tolerance was good with only one case of sleepiness and one of excitation. Excellent results were observed in thirteen patients, definite improvement in another thirteen, partial improvement in three, and poor improvement in two.

Pluvinage[236] found sulpiride to increase the tolerance to ergotamine tartrate.

Sulpiride was tested in thirty cases of migraine by Hakkarainen and Viukari.[237] They found that the number of migraine attacks during treatment with sulpiride was forty-eight, compared with sixty-four on the placebo, and the mean duration of the attacks was reduced from 3.3 hours to 2.4 hours. Sulpiride also significantly reduced the prodromal symptoms and the autonomic symptoms but had no significant effect on the psychiatric symptoms preceding the attacks. Gastrointestinal symptoms, especially nausea, were significantly reduced by sulpiride. Patients taking sulpiride required less analgesic than those taking the placebo and visual, mental or aphasic symptoms were less frequent. The only important side effect of sulpiride was congestion of the breast, which occurred in four patients. However, five patients had to interrupt the treatment.

VITAMIN B

Dalsgaard-Nielsen[238] used vitamin B in the prophylaxis of migraine but found it to be of no value.

MIGRALEVE

Migraleve has been tested in England, but it has not been found to be too successful in the prophylaxis of migraine.[239,240] It is available for investigation in the United States.

OPIPRAMAL

Opipramal was reported in 1972 by Jacobs[241] as being effective in migraine therapy, but nothing has been said about this drug since then.

DIMETHOTHIAZINE

Dimethothiazine was found to be more effective than methysergide and to have fewer side effects when used in the prophylaxis of migraine.[242]

SPASMALGAN

Spasmalgan, a compound with spasmolytic and analgesic properties was used in migraine prophylaxis in fifty-two patients.[243] In this study sixteen patients, experienced no benefit, and sixteen had satisfactory results, and twenty had excellent results. Infrequent side effects—erythema, gastric discomfort, giddiness, and drowsiness—did not necessitate discontinuation of medication in any patient. Side reaction to intravenous injections of Spasmalgan disappeared within 10 minutes.

BELLERGAL

Von Witzleben[244] believes that Bellergal, along with psychotherapy, is useful in the treatment of migraine. Bellergal acts as an inhibitor of the sympathetic and parasympathetic impulses of the autonomic nervous system, and it also quiets the central nervous system. Bellergal contains 0.3 mg of ergotamine tartrate, 0.1 mg of Bellafoline, and 20 mg of pentobarbital.

Hilsinger[245] states that Bellergal is the drug of choice in the prophylactic therapy of migraine cases.

We have tried Bellergal in a vast number of migraine cases and have found it to be of very little value. In over a hundred cases, we found only two patients who were helped. This certainly would not permit this preparation to be called a drug of choice.

Bellergal is an autonomic inhibitor.

CYPROHEPTADINE

Cyproheptadine, which is marketed as Periactin, has been used in the prophylaxis of migraine. This drug is a 5-HT antagonist and an antihistaminic. Early studies on this drug seemed promising, but since then its value seems to be quite doubtful. It has been described to be only of one slightly greater in value in this respect than placebo by Lance and associates.[152] These same results are described by Friedman.[142]

SALT

Brainard[246] advocates the restriction of salt from snack foods eaten on an empty stomach as a method of decreasing migraine attacks. He states that a sudden sodium chloride load may be a trigger mechanism. He found that migraine patients who avoided this trigger mechanism were improved in most cases in that their number of attacks were reduced.

Summary

In a vast number of cases of migraine there is an element of tension in the background which may often act as a trigger mechanism in producing the actual attack. If this is the case, it will naturally be necessary to offer the patient something to counteract this. This may be done by a bit of psychotherapy on the part of the physician. This does not mean that a psychiatrist should be ushered into the case for this purpose. In most cases this is not necessary. All that is usually required is a little time and effort on the part of the physician handling the case. The physician must show the patient what is causing the tension in the case and instruct the patient how to avoid this tension and its effects. Patients need reassurance that they can be helped, for they have usually tried many physicians and many preparations previously, usually to no avail.

If this psychotherapy is not enough, some mild form of tranquilizer may be employed for this purpose. We usually employ diazepam (Valium) in mild doses such as 2 mg three times a day. Another drug for this purpose is meprobamate (Equanil), 400 mg two or three times a day.

If there is an element of depression in the background of the case, some mild form of antidepressant may be employed. We usually use a drug such as amitriptyline

(Elavil) for this purpose. Mild doses such as 10 mg three times a day and at bedtime are usually sufficient for most cases of migraine accompanied by an element of depression.

Of course, all patients do not respond to the same drugs, so the choice of drugs are actually a matter of selectivity. If all patients responded to the same drug, only one drug for each purpose would be on the drug market. This certainly is never the case.

An attempt has been made to present the drugs whose names appear most prominently in the medical literature for the prophylaxis of migraine. Some of these seem to be of value and still others appear to be less effective. There are still others that seem to be not effective at all. However, because of conflicting reports on these drugs, all those that seem worth discussing are presented here. As mentioned previously, many of these drugs are not available in the United States due to FDA regulations, but many of these are being marketed elsewhere. If these drugs are actually ineffective it is better that the migraine patient not be subjected to them. If they are useful, the American patient is being deprived of receiving something that can prevent the painful headache attacks.

SYMPTOMATIC TREATMENT

In spite of the fact that migraine has been known to exist for over 200 years, the treatment is still in the experimental stage. This, of course, is partly due to the fact that the exact etiology is still theoretical. In 1869, Wilks[247] wrote about "sick headache." Fothergill[248] had previously described a condition under the name of "sick headache."

In migraine, therapeutic measures should be initiated as soon as the diagnosis has been completed. Migraine is helped by drugs which constrict the extracranial vessels. All migraine patients usually discover that black coffee constitutes the very best abortive headache medicine they can use.

Friedman[249] believes that about 15% of migraine patients are refractory to any form of symptomatic treatment and that at least 35% are refractory to preventive methods.

Migraine, like all types of headache, must be treated both symptomatically and prophylactically. Opiates should be avoided, not only because of the possibility of habit formation in this recurring difficulty but also because they are not very effective in relieving the pain of the migraine attack. Likewise, the analgesic group of drugs does not seem to be very effective in the symptomatic treatment of migraine.

If there is a tension element in the migraine case, this must also be taken into consideration. The tension must be combatted and removed, if possible. The patient must be shown his personality problems and must adjust his personality so as to free himself from this form of stimulus. Advice should be given to the patient concerning his change in habits or attitude and modification, acceptance, or avoidance of unhealthy environmental situations. This may not remove the obstacles, but will show the patient that they are present and that he must adjust himself to minimize their effects.

In treating migraine the physician must realize that both physical and emotional factors are present. Because of this, attainment of the objectives desired will depend not only on the physician and the drugs prescribed but also on the cooperation of the patient himself. The physician must remember that the successful management of any headache problem depends not only on the selection of the proper drug or drugs but also on the proper dosage of these drugs.

Many patients with migraine wait several years before they consult a physician. Their first medical consultation is often initiated by an increased frequency of attacks, which may be due to the use of oral contraceptives, weight-reducing diets, too much sleep, anemia, pain in the head or neck, or anxiety. Patients may also seek advice because of prolonged attacks, fear of intracranial disease, and depression.

These patients may often be referred to a

specialist if there is an increase of attacks, the development of some unusual symptoms, or a need for another opinion.

In the past, various preparations and procedures have been used to attempt to abort attacks of migraine. The breathing of pure oxygen for an hour or two was used in treating migraine in 1940.[250] Some have tried using pentobarbital (Nembutal) suppositories to abort the attacks,[251] but this also failed to produce the desired results.

The use of hormones has been attempted in treating migraine symptomatically. Among those tried have been chorionic gonadotropin (Follutein,[252] Antuitrin-S[253]), estrogen, and progesterone.[254] All of these attempts at treatment have been more or less discarded, as they do not seem to be the answer to the problem.

Pituitary extract was given migraine patients, but it too failed to abort most of the attacks experimented on.[255] Also tried in respect to hormone therapy, but again with negative results, was estrodiol (Progynon).[256] Another drug used in the past has been Emmenin. This is taken by mouth. Some have reported good results with it, but it has generally been discarded.[257]

Potassium thiocyanate was used by Hines and Eaton[258] in 1941, but it is now believed to be of little value in migraine therapy. Peptone was tried and thought to be of value but soon was disproved[259]; rarely, if ever, does it give good results.

Chondroitin sulfuric acid has been given to patients and scattered reports sound beneficial, but it too is generally believed to be of little value.[260] Other drugs which have been tried and have failed are carbachol,[261] neostigmine (Prostigmin),[262] vitamin B,[263] and calcium lactate.[264]

Different types of diet have been used unsuccessfully in the past. A ketogenic diet[265] and a high protein diet[266] were tried without success.

Nicotinic acid has been used in the past and is still found to be useful in many cases.[267] Other drugs listed under the failure heading in symptomatically treating

migraine are theophylline,[268] riboflavin,[269] diphenhydramine (Benadryl),[270] amphetamine sulfate (Benzedrine),[271] and thyroid extract.[272]

Vaisberg[273] reports satisfactory results in the symptomatic treatment of migraine by using 50 to 100 mg of dimenhydrinate (Dramamine), either intramuscularly or intravenously. We have not found this preparation to be very successful and cannot agree with his findings.

Certain surgical procedures have been attempted in the past, but it is now generally believed that surgery has no part in the treatment of migraine because usually the results were not very favorable. The use of procaine injections around the temporal arteries has been reported to be of some benefit.[274]

With all of the preparations just mentioned, an article would appear describing excellent results with a drug and then there would usually not be anything further on the subject. These preparations have no doubt been used by many, but, failing to produce the desired results, they are discarded and nothing is written or said about it. The literature is full of accounts of drugs said to cure certain percentages of migraine cases. However, in the actual application of these preparations with the migraine patient they do not seem to work so well as one would generally expect them to after reading the first enthusiastic literary reports. In many migraine cases, the physician is often desperate to produce relief for the patient. For this reason, both the physician and the patient are willing to try anything.

Let us now look at the drugs being used today in the treatment of migraine.

Ergotamine tartrate*

The first preparation to offer any real help in the symptomatic form of treatment for the migraine was ergotamine tartrate, which

---

*Other aspects of ergotamine tartrate are discussed further in Chapter 3.

is commonly known as Gynergen. Ergotamine is a very potent vasoconstrictor. This drug tends to restore the cerebrovascular system to its normal tone. This preparation given parenterally is highly effective, or it may be taken orally, which is less effective. The therapeutic effect of ergotamine tartrate depends on its ability to prolong vasoconstrictor action, thus interrupting the pain-producing mechanism. Ergotamine seems to act directly on the smooth muscles of the blood vessels and not as an antagonist to the sympathetics.

Gynergen acts best when it is administered as early as possible after the headache attack has started. Most investigators believe that it requires 30 to 45 minutes for the effects of Gynergen to become manifested. The best average dosage seems to be 0.5 mg injected either subcutaneously or intravenously. The oral form of Gynergen, the average dosage also being 5 mg, is not so effective as the injectable form, and it cannot be used in cases which have severe nausea or vomiting for two reasons. The first, of course, is that the vomiting will prevent the patient from keeping the preparation in his stomach, and the second, that the route of absorption through the stomach is much slower than normal during or following severe nausea, because of the inflammation which results in the stomach lining.

Gynergen is not indicated as a preventive measure in migraine, because it acts as a vasoconstrictor on the arteries which just before an attack have dilated and have allowed blood to go pounding through the brain.

The main side effects of Gynergen are nausea or vomiting. These occur in the majority of the cases after the injectable form has been used and are less common after the oral form has been used. Occasionally there is paresthesia, or cramps in the arms or legs can occur. Physicians are aware of the fact that Gynergen can produce gangrene, but actually this is ex-

tremely rare, and those cases that have been reported in the literature are cases in which Gynergen had been used in cases of severe jaundice and itching and not actually in cases of migraine at all.

Gynergen is not habit-forming. It is contraindicated in septic states, coronary diseases, any obliterative vascular diseases, or cardiac conditions.

If the oral preparation is used, it may prove to be more effective and less nauseating if the pills are crushed and taken sublingually. But even if taken this way it is not so efficient as the parenteral form. Neither form of the preparation should be used without the direct supervision of a physician. Gynergen has a very unpleasant taste and not many patients will care for the sublingual form of administration. If the oral treatment has to be extended beyond a period of 3 hours, the subcutaneous route of administration is preferred. No more than 0.25 mg of Gynergen should ever be given intravenously in any single dose. On the same basis, not more than 0.5 mg should be used when it is given subcutaneously. Not more than two subcutaneous injections should be given within a period of 24 hours. Daily doses of any amount are to be avoided, no matter what type of injection is used or which form of the preparation is used. If using the oral form, not more than 11 mg should be taken in 24 hours and not more than 33 mg a week.[275]

Friedman[276] points out that the beneficial effect of ergotamine probably is due to constrictive action on the smooth muscles of the blood vessels. The effectiveness of ergotamine tartrate has been improved by combining it with caffeine to potentiate its action and with other compounds to reduce side effects and control migraine symptoms. Rectal suppositories with ergotamine, caffeine, and an antispasmodic are used for ordinary and classic migraine. Parenteral or aerosol administration of ergotamine is also used. Because of its powerful vasoconstrictor action, ergotamine should not be given to patients with peripheral, cerebral, or coronary vascular disease of venous or arterial origin.

Ergotamine, an ergot alkaloid synthesized by a parasitic fungus of rye, *Claviceps purpurea,* has been used in the treatment of migraine for years. It is a nonpsychedelic polypeptide derivative of lysergic acid. Compared with ergot, the poisonous parent, it is relatively nontoxic when used in proper doses. Despite the great chemical and pharmacologic advances of the last few decades, ergotamine tartrate remains the best single agent for the control of individual attacks of migraine.

The beneficial action of ergotamine tartrate is probably related to its tonic action on smooth muscle, thus causing constriction of dilated, relaxed cranial arteries. Therefore, best results are obtained when the proper dose is used early in an attack. "Too little and too late" are the chief causes of unsatisfactory clinical results.

Whenever ergot preparations are used, caution must be employed, as side effects can occur. It can produce gangrene, but when it is used in migraine, the percentage of cases having this side effect is much lower than the percentage of gangrene produced by ergotamine when used in other conditions. Perhaps this is due to the fact that the liver function of migraine patients is usually good and permits rapid detoxification of the ergot preparations, preventing their accumulation and thus ergotism from developing.[277] The physician should instruct the patient to use the drug sparingly and not to abuse its use, because of the possibility of its toxic symptoms.

When ergotamine tartrate is used to terminate an attack of migraine, there is an increase in the tone in the dilated and strongly pulsating arteries, and there is also a return to normal of the pain threshold.

The disadvantages of parenteral administration of any drug are well known. For this reason, attention was centered on the development of an oral preparation of ergotamine tartrate which might be equally effective. One of the most efficient preparations of an oral type on the open drug market today, as far as aborting migraine attacks is concerned, is Cafergot. This preparation was introduced to the public as Cafergone and experimentally was known as EC-110. It is in tablet form, containing 100 mg of caffeine and 1 mg of ergotamine tartrate. The caffeine, when administered orally, acts as a vasoconstrictor. The addition of the caffeine seems to have improved the efficiency of ergotamine and also allows a smaller dosage of ergotamine to be given. It seems that the addition of the caffeine also cuts down the side effects and increases the rapidity of action. Caffeine is a cerebrovasoconstrictor. The first report on Cafergot was made in 1948.[278] Further reports made in 1949[279] and 1950[280] backed up the initial findings with the drug.

The side effects of Cafergot consist entirely of the gastrointestinal type. It produces nausea in about 15% of the cases in which it is used. It is very rare to find vomiting, but stomach cramps are experienced in 2% to 3% of the cases. Other than these, we have failed to observe any other type of toxic side effect produced by Cafergot. In our opinion, Cafergot is effective in about 80% to 85% of the cases in which it is used in attempting to abort an attack of migraine.

The best average dosage for Cafergot seems to be two tablets to be taken at the immediate onset of the headache attack. If Cafergot is taken after the headache is in full swing, it seldom produces the desired effects; therefore, taking this preparation at the immediate onset of the attack is of extreme importance. If, 30 minutes after taking of the two tablets of Cafergot, the headache still persists, but to a lesser degree, one additional tablet may be taken. If three tablets taken in this manner, at the immediate onset of the attack, fail to produce the desired results, taking of any additional tablets is not worthwhile.

Cafergot is contraindicated in organic heart disease, obliterative vascular disease, hypertension, pregnancy, and septic states associated with intervascular foci.

The chief cause of failure in using Cafergot, we have found, is the improper usage or dosage. In some cases Cafergot was given routinely so many times a day or every 6 hours, etc. This, of course, is useless, as Cafergot aborts migraine attacks and is not claimed to be, nor is it, a cure of migraine.

Friedman[281] lists six possible reasons for failure in using Cafergot:

1. Multiple etiology of headache, that is, vascular and nonvascular headaches
2. Incorrect diagnosis of type of headache, that is, migraine, tension headache, tumor
3. Medication not given early enough in the attack
4. Inadequate dosage
5. Residual muscle spasm, a source of pain in itself, that may follow a severe headache
6. Added emotional stress

The addition of caffeine to ergotamine tartrate does seem to produce results. Perhaps the fact that caffeine is a general circulatory stimulant is helpful, because usually patients having a migraine attack are going through a period of temporary circulatory depression.

In a study on the effect of caffeine on the internal absorption of ergotamine, Fanchamps[282] recorded the plasma level and urinary excretion of radioactivity. A detectable plasma level was present 1 hour after ergotamine tartrate alone was administered. However, after the combination of caffeine and ergotamine was administered the plasma level was detectable as soon as 30 minutes. Fanchamps concludes that there is a quicker and a greater internal absorption of ergotamine when used in combination with caffeine.

In a study of caffeine-ergot interaction Zoglio and Maulding[283] found that caffeine and other naturally occurring xanthines have been shown to exhibit an exceptional ability to form stable complexes with a wide variety of substances, and mixtures of ergot alkaloids themselves tend toward inter-molecular complexation. Study of the interaction of caffeine and ergotamine tartrate in aqueous solution has shown an increased solubility of the alkaloid in the presence of caffeine, an increased dissolution rate constant for the ergot alkaloid in the combination over pure ergotamine, and increased or decreased partitioning rates of the alkaloid in the presence of caffeine relative to ergotamine tartrate alone, depending on the pH studied. The attraction between ergotamine tartrate and caffeine appeared to be an extremely weak one. It was thought that the in vitro results might correlate with the clinical effectiveness of caffeine-ergotamine tablets and that caffeine acted by holding the ergotamine in solution in the intestine, providing increased drug activity through ease of absorption. They concluded that the ergot-alkaloid-xanthine inteaction is somewhat unusual, in that it represents an example of complexation in the gastrointestinal tract leading to enhanced rather than decreased absorption of a treatment drug.

All reports on these drugs for the symptomatic treatment were consistent in one thing: all drugs produced some side effects of a mild nature and a certain number of cases would not respond. The percentage of failures varies with each individual agent.

Many migraine patients experience so much nausea and vomiting with attacks that it is practically impossible for them to retain any type of medication taken orally. This plus the fact that absorption through the stomach is poor following nausea and vomiting has led to the idea of the rectal suppository form of administration. A previous report was made on four types of suppositories used in migraine which were found to be not too successful.[284]

As stated before[285] it is our opinion that a tension element causes these failures. If a true breakdown of most migraine cases were made. We believe that a majority of them would be found to consist of a combination of migraine and tension. The most logical solution to the problem is to remove the cause of the tension. However, this is often easier said than done, because in most of the cases the tension factor ties in with the patient's occupation, home life, age, or other factors which are not too easily changed in any complete form, although some minor adjustments can usually be made. Another method by which the tension factor can be combated is by giving a mild sedative. The ergotamine tartrate and caffeine combination has proved effective in relieving the headache phase of this problem. The addition of Bellafoline to Cafergot (ergotamine tartrate and caffeine) seems to cut down the gastric side effects in some cases.[284] Ergotamine tartrate is a sympathetic sedative and caffeine is a central stimulant. Bellafoline acts as a parasympathetic inhibitor, relieving smooth muscle spasm and controlling hypersecretion.[286] Bellafoline has been found to be less toxic than similar drugs used at the same dosage level.[287]

Therefore, in discussing the preparation for a new agent to be used in migraine, we suggested that in addition to the three drugs—ergotamine tartrate, caffeine, and Bellafoline—a sedative be added to try to combat the tension factor. A new agent was prepared that contained 2 mg ergotamine tartrate, 100 mg caffeine, 0.25 mg Bellafoline, and 60 mg pentobarbital sodium. This preparation was made in rectal suppository form and is known as Cafergot-PB.

In many cases it is rather confusing to the patient when he is told to take a preparation rectally for the purpose of relieving his headache attack. It should be explained to the patient that this suppository will in no way act as a laxative but is merely intended to help relieve the headache attack. One suppository seems to be the best average dosage. The suppository should be taken as soon as possible after the headache attack starts. However, it does not seem necessary that the suppository be taken exactly at the onset of the attack. In many cases the patient was unable to take the suppository

immediately, but it seemed to work about as well. This in itself is a great advantage of Cafergot-PB over the oral preparations.

The reason, of course, for the continued research in the field of headache is to find a preparation which will be successful in aborting the attacks but which will produce few or no side effects.

In a study on suppositories containing ergotamine tartrate El-Hamid Abdalla El-Shamy and associates[288] stated that ergotamine suppositories are often effective in refractory cases of migraine. However, they may undergo physical changes (discoloration) and chemical changes (oxidation and isomerization) on storage, which reduces their potency. They conclude that the following formula is recommended: ergotamine tartrate, 2 mg; tartaric acid, 4 mg; lactose, 40 mg; 1-hexadecanol, 100 mg; and Imhausen, 1 to 2 gm.

There are other oral preparations containing ergotamine tartrate available to the migraine patient. Migral is one of these. It contains ergotamine tartrate, 1 mg; caffeine, 50 mg; and cyclizine hydrochloride, 25 mg. The addition of cyclizine hydrochloride was made in an attempt to reduce the number and the severity of the gastric side effects that might be present with the migraine attack and also that might occur from the use of caffeine and ergotamine. Cyclizine hydrochloride has been proved to be effective in reducing nausea and vomiting in other conditions.[289,290] The first publication on Migral was by Ryan in 1959.[291] Two tablets of this preparation at the immediate onset of the headache attack seemed to be very beneficial in relieving both the headache attack and the nausea and vomiting associated with the headache.

Another widely used oral preparation containing ergotamine tartrate given for the symptomatic relief of the migraine attack is Wigraine.

Ergomar, a form of ergotamine tartrate used sublingually, is also available to the migraine patient. Each tablet containing 2 mg of ergotamine tartrate is placed under the tongue and allowed to dissolve and then the sputum is swallowed. This form of ergotamine tartrate absorption is based on buccal absorption.

Sutherland and co-workers[292] studied the buccal absorption of ergotamine. They point out that the oral route is the simplest method for self-administration of the drug, but it has the disadvantage of a possible loss of the dose due to vomiting. Absorption across the mucous membrane of the mouth might circumvent this problem. They measured the buccal absorption of ergotamine alone and also in the presence of caffeine, to access the potential effectiveness of the drug in migraine when given by this route. They found that over the range of concentration studied (limited by the solubility of ergotamine) there was no significant effect of concentration on ergotamine absorption. The data were consistent with ergotamine being absorbed passively across the buccal mucosa. The presence of caffeine did not significantly enhance ergotamine absorption.

Since the pH of saliva varies from 6 to 8, it is concluded that only about one sixth of an ergotamine dose in solution might absorb from saliva across the mucosa in 5 minutes. Because of the low solubility of ergotamine at the pH of saliva, it is unlikely that therapeutically useful amounts of the drug would have been absorbed during this period.

Ergotamine tartrate is also available to the migraine patient in the inhalation form. This is called Medihaler-Ergotamine. It was initially described by Ryan[293] in 1959. Further reports were made by Speed[294] and by Blumenthal.[295]

By the aerosol administration method the ergotamine tartrate is delivered per os to the respiratory tract epithelium and apparently is absorbed rapidly into the systemic circulation. The patient is instructed to:

1. Place the long end of the adapter deep inside the mouth and on the extended tongue, the vial being above the adapter. Close the lips around the mouthpiece.
2. After a slightly forced expiration and at the onset of a deep inspiration, press the vial against the adapter, releasing the metered dose.
3. Hold the breath in deep inspiration for as long as long as is comfortable, and then exhale slowly.

This method undoubtedly requires an intelligent patient or absorption will not be achieved. It is beneficial only if it is used correctly. Using it incorrectly is the main reason for therapy failure, and this occurs very easily.

Needless to say, for any of these preparations to be effective, the correct diagnosis must be made. If the correct diagnosis has not been established and the patient does not actually have migraine, none of these drugs will be effective. For example, a patient with a case of sinusitis would not respond to ergotamine any more than a case of migraine would respond to an antibiotic.

SUMMARY

The more successful preparations containing ergotamine tartrate which are on the market available for use by the physician in treating migraine patients have been presented. The drugs mentioned are the ones that seem to be the most useful at the present time. Research is constantly being undertaken to find even greater relief for the migraine patient, and it is our firm hope that some day we will find a most welcome "cureall" for these migraine patients. In all cases of migraine the symptomatic phase of the treatment program is a matter of selectivity. One patient may respond better to one preparation while the next patient may respond better to another. In this respect the symptomatic relief from the headache of a typical migraine attack is a matter of experimentation. It is safe to say that most patients obtain quicker and more complete relief from their migraine attacks by using ergotamine tartrate or one of its derivatives than any other drug obtainable on the open drug market today.

Ergonovine

Ergonovine has been used in cases of migraine for symptomatic relief, but it is less effective than ergotamine tartrate. It does produce less nausea and vomiting than ergotamine. This drug is a strong oxytoxic and is contraindicated in cases of pregnancy. Its dosage and routes of administration are the same as that of ergotamine tartrate. One writer[296] states that in some cases ergonovine is more effective than ergotamine tartrate when administered orally. This is the exception rather than the rule, in our opinion.

Dihydroergotamine tartrate (DHE-45)

The next important agent to appear on the drug horizon following ergotamine tartrate for the symptomatic form of therapy of migraine was DHE-45, called dihydroergotamine tartrate. This, as might be expected, is a powerful vasoconstrictor and is indicated if ergotamine tartrate is poorly tolerated and gives rise to undesirable side effects, such as nausea, vomiting, or muscular pain.

The first report on DHE-45 was made in 1945.[297] This preparation may be used intravenously or intramuscularly. More immediate relief is obtained if it is used intravenously. It is an extract of ergot in which the vasoconstrictor factor is present but the oxytoxic factor has been removed. For this reason, it is safe to use during the early stages of pregnancy. Its side effects are the same as those of Gynergen but occur less frequently. It also, on occasions, produces a little drowsiness or depression. In a nervous or excited patient this could prove beneficial. DHE-45 has no effect on the blood pressure but it may slow the pulse rate a little. It is generally considered that DHE-45 is one fourth as toxic as Gynergen. Many of the patients who do claim side effects from using DHE-45 are sensitive and extremely emotional types. This could account for some side effects in any preparation used.

DHE-45 is contraindicated in advanced cardiovascular disease, including angina pectoris, and toxemias.

The average dosage of DHE-45 is 1 ml (1 mg), either intramuscularly or intravenously. We have found in using DHE-45 intravenously that the more severe the headache actually is, the quicker the DHE-45 takes effect and starts bringing the patient much-desired relief.

DHE-45 has been used in the prophylactic phase of migraine therapy.

Girard[298] administered 20 drops of DHE-45 regularly three times a day to treat eighty patients with migraine. Improvement was recorded in fifty-eight (72.5%), of whom forty-four were women. Migraine disappeared in thirty-two patients and was greatly or partially reduced in the remaining twenty-six. Medication with DHE-45, which is much more manageable than methysergide maleate, must be continuous or nearly so. No significant side effects were encountered in Girard's study; one patient reported vertigo and another nausea.

Mercier-Carli[299] also used DHE-45 in the same fashion. He claims that to prevent attacks, dihydroergotamine is preferable to ergotamine tartrate for women or in patients in whom orthostatic arterial hypotension is present. In certain conditions, including hypertension, renal insufficiency, and pregnancy, the use of ergot derivatives should be avoided.

We personally have never found DHE-45 to be useful as a prophylactic agent in cases of migraine. However, we would say that it is probably the best symptomatic drug for migraine when used intravenously (1 ml).

Heyck[300] claims that of the hydrogenated ergot preparations, dihydroergotamine is recommended when hypotension or disturbed circulatory conditions are present, especially in adolescence.

Zenglein[301] believes that DHE-45, if it is combined with 40% glucose, has an even stronger effect. We have had no experience with this procedure.

Since DHE-45, several other preparations have been introduced for aborting the pain of migraine.

Isometheptene (Octin)

Isometheptene has been used hypodermically and orally. Peters and Zeller[302] reported on this preparation in 1949 but were not impressed by their finding. MacNeal[303] reported isometheptene to be useful in the injectable form but not orally. He states, however, that its side effects and its contraindications are so few that it is a very safe drug to use. He further states that the percentage of patients obtaining relief from this agent when taken orally is very low.

Isometheptene is a sympathicomimetic, vasoconstricting, smooth-muscle relaxing agent. It may safely be used during pregnancy and does not produce dysmenorrhea, even if taken just before the beginning of a menstrual period. It does not produce nausea or vomiting. It may produce a transient hypertension and therefore should not be used in any case of hypertension.

The average dosage of isometheptene given intramuscularly is 100 mg. The average oral dose is one tablet, which is 130 mg (2 gr). We have not had as much success with Octin as with some of the other preparations, such as Cafergot, Gynergen, and DHE-45.

Seltzer[304] states that the average case of migraine requires about 1 ml of isometheptene intramuscularly for relief from an attack.

Diamond and Medina[305] observed the effect of isometheptene on thirty-six patients in a double-blind, two-way crossover study of isometheptene and placebo. Seventeen had a better response on isometheptene than on placebo. Placebo was superior to isometheptene in eight cases. Of seventy-two courses of treatment with each drug, isometheptene produced good or complete relief of pain in 42%, while placebo produced a similar response in 29%. When the severity of pain and the degree of relief were considered, the superiority of isometheptene did not reach statistically significance at the 5% level. They found side effects due to isometheptene were few and of mild or moderate severity. They concluded that isometheptene may be an alternative treatment when ergotamine is contraindicated.

Midrin

Midrin is a drug indicated for relief of migraine headache. The usual dose is two capsules at once, followed by one every hour until relief is obtained, up to a total of five capsules within a 12-hour period. Each capsule of Midrin contains: isometheptene mucate, 65 mg; dichloralphenazone, 100 mg; and acetaminophen, 325 mg. This combination of drugs is intended to relieve both vascular headaches such as migraine and headaches of the tension type. The basic pharmacology of each of this product's components is briefly reviewed here.

Isometheptene, available as the mucate, is an unsaturated aliphatic amine with sympathomimetic properties. Animal experimentation conducted in the years immediately following its synthesis indicated that this drug acts at both alpha and beta postganglionic adrenergic neuroeffectors. Thus the drug can both cause the contraction and the relaxation of visceral and vascular smooth muscle.

This agent was originally employed clinically for its antispasmodic action on the smooth muscle of the intestinal and genitourinary tracts. It was effective for this purpose and occasionally for relaxing bronchial smooth muscle, because these inhibitory effects are elicited at lower doses than are required for bringing about cardiovascular system stimulation.

It was later learned that although large parenteral doses are required to produce generalized vasoconstriction, the vessels of certain vascular beds are constricted at dose levels far below those that affect the systemic blood pressure. The mechanism by which isometheptene is believed to exert its desired effect in relieving vascular headache is through constriction of cranial and cerebral blood vessels.

Dichloralphenazone is a molecular complex of chloral hydrate and phenazone. In the dose contained in this product, it is the sedative effect of the chloral hydrate rather than the analgesic action of the phenazone component that predominates. The calming effect of this drug is considered desirable for reducing the patient's emotional reaction to the pain of both vascular and tension headaches. Sedation may also help to exert a prophylactic effect in patients who are susceptible to such headaches. That is, it may prevent the onset of a headache by reducing the patient's reaction to emotionally stressful experiences.

In the recommended doses, it is believed that dichloralphenazone's actions are largely limited to those subcortical areas of the brain that subserve emotional reactivity and that its mild but definite depressant effects at these central sites are of a kind that produce sedation and tranquilization without causing drowsiness. However, higher doses can presumably depress the brainstem reticular formation neurons that activate the cerebral cortex, and such depression can lead to hypnotic effect.

Acetaminophen, a natural metabolite of both acetanilid and phenacetin, is, like these drugs, a true analgesic. That is, it acts centrally to raise the threshold of the thalamic neurons which receive impulses generated by painful stimuli and relay them on to higher cortical centers. Thus, the drug's main mode of action is through the reduction of the patient's perception of the pain impulses that originate in dilated cerebral vessels or in the tense muscles of the neck and scalp. In addition to this subcortical effect, this drug appears to possess a peripheral antiinflammatory or antiprein-flammatory effect that may help to lessen the number of painful stimuli set off by locally releasing chemicals in certain types of vasodilator headaches.

Briefly, the sites and modes of action of Midrin's components are as follows:

1. Isometheptene acts by constricting dilated cranial and cerebral arterioles, thus reducing the stimuli that lead to vascular headaches.

2. Dichloralphenazone tends to reduce the patient's emotional reaction to the perception of headache pain, and by reducing emotional reactions to stressful environmental situation it may even prevent tension and vascular headaches.

3. Acetaminophen raises the threshold of certain subcortical centers to painful stimuli, thus exerting an analgesic effect against all types of headaches. The phenazone component of dichloralphenazone is thought to have an additive analgesic effect.

Midrin acts directly on dilated cerebral arteries to reduce throbbing and intracranial pressure. Midrin relieves pain by reducing the perception of pain impulses originating in dilated cerebral vessel, controls the reactive component of the pain experience, and prevents the development of pain by constricting the cranial blood vessels which exert pressure on adjacent nerve tissue. Midrin controls emotional stress that causes both cerebral vasodilation and muscular contraction in the nuchal and scalp region.

Midrin is contraindicated in severe renal, hepatic, organic heart, and peripheral vascular diseases, severe hypertension, or glaucoma. It is also contraindicated in those patients who are taking monoamine-oxidase inhibitors and those who have had recent cardiovascular attacks.

Adverse reactions to this drug consist of a transient dizziness and skin rash. Usually these, if they do occur, will be eliminated by either a reduction of the dosage or the, complete discontinuation of the drug.

This preparation produces no peripheral or coronary vasoconstriction. Its use is desirable in patients who are predisposed to nausea, vomiting, and dysmenorrhea. It does not aggravate or increase the frequency of headache nor does it produce withdrawal symptoms with resultant recurrent headaches, as is so often seen with ergotamine tartrate.

In a study on the use of Midrin in vascular headache Johnson[306] reported that drowsiness and lightheadedness occurred in only a few patients. However, no patients experienced any gastrointestinal side effects or withdrawal symptoms, numbness or tingling of the extremities, or increases in frequency or aggravation of the headache.

Ryan made an experimental study to compare the effects of Midrin with those of isometheptene mucate alone and of a placebo.[307] It involved three treatments, each with one replication, in a randomized block design. Fourteen male and forty-six female patients of age range 22 to 77 years (mean 45) with classic or common migraine were involved. Each patient was provided with a total of six treatment units (each consisting of a vial containing five capsules): two units of Midrin, two of isometheptene mucate, and two of a placebo. The period of study was six attacks of migraine. The patient received each of the three treatments during his first three attacks and again each of the treatments for his last three attacks. Diary cards were issued on which the patient had to record the severity of the headache, the degree of relief afforded by the drug, and the number of capsules taken. In addition, a medical assessment was made of the patient's global response to each drug. The efficacy of each drug was determined by quantifying the degree of relief (complete, 3; good, 2; fair, 1; and none, 0), the reduction in the number of the capsules taken, and the medical assessment (excellent, 3; poor, 0). Statistical analysis of the results showed that Midrin and isometheptene mucate were more effective than the placebo but the efficacy of Midrin did not differ significantly from that of isometheptene mucate. Neither drug produced significantly more side effects than the placebo. The results of this study demonstrate that Midrin and isometheptene mucate are efficacious in the treatment of migraine and produce no side effects when taken in the dose advised.

Midrin is beneficial in the symptomatic treatment of migraine headache in selected cases. In general it has fewer toxic side effects than does ergotamine tartrate, but on the whole it is usually not as effective.

Midrin can be used in many cases where ergotamine tartrate is contraindicated and for this reason alone it is a very useful drug for the symptomatic phase of the treatment program in cases of migraine.

Yuill and associates[308] did a double-blind study with Midrin and ergotamine tartrate in thirty-eight patients who had a total of 122 episodes of migraine. The duration of headache was the same, irrespective of whether ergotamine or Midrin was used. The duration and frequency of the nausea were significantly less in the attacks treated with Midrin. Palpitations and drowsiness were seen in a few cases treated with it. It was concluded that in this trial Midrin is superior to ergotamine combined with caffeine.

As a broad general statement we would say that if ergotamine tartrate fails to relieve the symptoms of the migraine attacks, one should try Midrin next. Also if ergotamine tartrate produces undesirable side effects or is contraindicated in the case, Midrin should be tried. This is because in the average case of migraine we have observed few or no side effects with the use of Midrin. This cannot be said of ergotamine tartrate.

Other therapeutic measures

There are constant investigations in the field of migraine therapy. We still see articles in the medical literature claiming this or that about a new or an old preparation which is successful in aborting migraine attacks. Many of these investigations have not been found to be of much value. Still others seem to have some promise and are still in the experimental stage of investigation. An attempt will now be made to present a brief description of the more recent investigations in this field.

LEVODOPA

Levodopa was tried in 1970 in a case of migraine by Antunes and co-workers.[309] The patient had Parkinson's disease and levodopa was used for the purpose of alleviating this condition. During the first week on levodopa therapy she had a typical migraine attack. After this no further attacks were observed for the 7 months she remained on levodopa therapy. However, when the levodopa was replaced with a placebo, without the knowledge of the patient, the attacks recurred.

These researchers suggest that further inquiry into the role of levodopa in migraine is in order. However, in our experience this drug has not proved to be successful in migraine therapy.

FOLIC ACID

The use of folic acid was suggested by Kopjast[310] to be successful in relieving migraine attacks. Folic acid is a vasodilator. Kopjast tested the drug in only thirty-one patients. The average age of the patients was 39.

The patients were divided into a younger group of ten patients, aged 23 to 35 years, with a history of migraine of less than 3 year's duration, and an older group of twenty-one patients with a history of migraine of over 5 years. Each patient was given 15 mg folic acid (as sodium folate) by slow intravenous injection: no other treatment was given. If the headache persisted, the injection was repeated on the following day. It was found that 60% responded favorably to the first injection, the headache subsiding within 1 hour. The best response occurred in the younger patients. In all but three of the older patients, the headache was abolished by the second injection. As far as side effects are concerned, five patients experienced nausea and vomiting at the end of an attack. Kopjast concluded that folic acid reduces the edema of migraine and the low toxicity of the substance recommends it as

a therapeutic agent. We have never found this preparation to be of any value in the field of migraine therapy.

DIAZEPAM (VALIUM)

We used diazepam when it was still in the experimental stage and found it useful in tension headache but not in pure migraine.

Bleger[311] found in four patients with true migraine that two showed response to diazepam; both had previously responded to 5-allyl-5-(2-hydroxypropyl) barbituric acid. The two failures with diazepam had not improved under previous treatment with 5-allyl-5-(2-hydroxypropyl) barbituric acid, dimethothiazine mesylate, dihydroergotamine, or Transoddi. Further tests showed better results when diazepam was combined with 5-allyl-5-(2-hydroxypropyl) barbituric acid, dimethothiazine mesylate, or dihydroergotamine.

ANALGESICS

The use of the analgesic type of drug in the symptomatic phase of migraine therapy is nothing new; in fact, the analgesics are probably the oldest form of treatment for this purpose. In some cases they are still the best. Many patients can control their migraine attacks quite adequately by the use of the analgesics. It would be poor advice on the part of the physician to take these patients off of the analgesics if they are used successfully and to have them use the ergotamine preparations. In the first place the analgesic preparations are by far less expensive than the ergotamine preparations. The main reason for not switching, of course, is the possible toxicity which can be produced by the ergotamine type of drug.

Analgesics, like the ergotamine preparations, should be taken at the immediate onset of the attack if they are to be successfully used. If not used in this fashion even large doses will not be successful.

Edmeads[312] suggests that the action of the salicylates may be more than a simple peripheral analgesic effect. They may inhibit the synthesis and release of prostaglandins which may be involved in the genesis of migraine.

Volans[313] studied the absorption of effervescent aspirin during migraine attacks. He reported that poor absorption was found more often with an increasing severity of headache and also with nausea. Since the subjects who were poor absorbers during a migrainous attack showed normal absorption when free from headache, and since aspirin is mostly absorbed through the small intestine, it seems likely that delayed gastric emptying causes reduced absorption of the drug during the attack. He concluded, therefore, that preparations which either bypass the gastrointestinal tract or are rapidly absorbed will produce the best effects in relieving the pain of migraine attacks.

Effervescent aspirin is more commonly used for the symptomatic relief in migraine in Great Britain than it is in America. It is certainly a safer drug to use than is ergotamine, but probably not quite as successful.

Lance and associates[314] report on fifteen cases in which the carotid body was removed in patients with frequent intractable headache. They report relief of headache on the operated side in five patients and partial relief in four. They conclude that the proportion of patients receiving benefit from the procedure was not considered high enough to warrant an extended trial of carotid glomectomy for the treatment of migraine.

MAGNESIUM GLUTAMATE

Vosgerau[315] used magnesium glutamate in only 10 cases of migraine. He reports it to be successful but admits that it is difficult to explain the therapeutic effect of magnesium in genuine attacks of migraine. Perhaps magnesium produces vasodilation in the first phase of the attack, when there is still a vasoconstriction present. In the second phase, the hypotensive effect of magnesium may prevent major hypertension and, consequently, relieve headache. We have never used this preparation for migraine relief.

INDOMETHACIN (INDOCIN)

Indomethacin is another drug which on occasions has been tried in the symptomatic form of therapy in cases of migraine. This is the type of drug which is used as a "last resort."

Indomethacin is a potent, nonsteroidal drug with antiinflammatory, antipyretic, and analgesic properties. It therefore has capabilities of relieving pain and reducing fever and tenderness. The exact mode of action of this drug is unknown.

This drug is helpful in relieving the pain of rheumatoid arthritis and degenerative joint disease. It is also effective in rheumatoid spondylitis. However, it has never been used to any extent in any controlled migraine study.

This drug is contraindicated in children, during pregnancy, in patients with gastrointestinal lesions, or in patients who are allergic to aspirin or the drug itself.

Because of the possibility of side effects, the drug should be used at low dosage level (under 150 mg/day). The possibility of side effects being produced by indomethacin increases in direct proportion to the age of the patient.

This is not the type of drug that can be used as simply as one would an aspirin. It should not be used, therefore, without strict supervision of the physician because of the possibility of adverse reactions which might occur.

We do not recommend this drug in the symptomatic phase of migraine treatment. It is merely being mentioned because it has been tried on rare occasions. We have never found it to be effective in cases of migraine. But again, we have only used it when everything else has also failed.

PSYCHOTHERAPY

Bosburg[316] believes that the treatment of migraine may require psychotherapy in order to improve the patient's response to psychologic stimuli and drugs to modify the cerebrovascular reaction.

The average case of migraine certainly does not require psychotherapy. If it does, it is the type the average family physician could provide, if he or she takes the necessary time.

PHYSICAL THERAPY

Hornbacher[317] used physical therapy in seventy-four cases in which headache was the main complaint. Of these 50% showed good improvement and 46% some improvement. In cases of migraine, physical therapy seems to produce very little effect. In fact, if overdone it may make the pain more severe. Simple massage may help relieve symptoms if applied in a gentle fashion, but if to vigorous it may increase the patient's discomfort.

HYPNOSIS

Hypnosis has been reported to be useful in the field of migraine therapy.[318,319] Simple relaxation techniques which prevent increase in anxiety and tension, which in turn produces headache, are claimed to be the most beneficial in these cases. Actually, this form of therapy for migraine seems to have very little value.

Wilkinson[320] says a small dose of some form of tranquilizer such as diazepam (Valium), 5 mg, or sodium amytal, 60 mg, may help migraine patients to relax and to be able to lie down and get some sleep. When they awaken, they frequently are free from their migraine attack. She states that perhaps in place of a tranquilizer, this effect can be obtained with some form of sedative. She states that the treatment of an acute attack of migraine should be directed toward the headache and the nausea that usually accompanies it. She concludes that in the majority of the cases frequently the only treatment required is an analgesic and an antiemetic. The most frequent analgesic she employs is aspirin.

Summary

The most useful drugs in the field of the symptomatic treatment of migraine have been presented. Other drugs presented are still in the investigational phase of their development. Some drugs which do not seem to be of value have been presented. This is done so that the physician may determine their use with migraine patients. These patients experience real, severe, and dreadful pain. It is the hope of all investigators in the headache field that someday the ideal drug will be found which will alleviate the pain of the attack and that will also be free from side effects. This the wish of the physician and the migraine patient most of all, for after all, he is the one who has to put up with this condition.

CASE HISTORY

The following is an example of a typical case of migraine.

M. S. was a single, white, 38 year-old female. Her headache was usually associated with nausea and sometimes with vomiting. Photophobia was often present along with scotomas. She had a periodic type of headache with a duration of many hours or even a few days. There was a family history in her case, and her attacks were more severe during, or just preceding, her menstrual periods. She was a conscientious person with a responsible position. When she had had a hard, tense day at the office she usually had some form of headache attack that evening or during her early sleeping hours.

A typical account of her use of Cafergot-PB follows. She awakened at 6:00 A.M. with pain in the eyes, across the forehead, and in the top of the head. The pain subsided slightly after she had breakfast, but it did not leave entirely. By 9:00 A.M. the pain was much more intense, at which time she took two Cafergot tablets. At 10:00 A.M. she took another two more tablets. She worked hard and continuously all day and, while the pain lessened, it did not entirely leave. By 4:00 P.M. the pain became much more severe and was mainly on the left side of the face and head. At 6:00 P.M. she had dinner. By 7:00 P.M. the pain was extremely severe, with a nervous reaction. Her stomach was upset and she was nauseated but was unable to vomit. At 10:00 P.M. she took one Cafergot-PB suppository. In about 20 minutes she was slightly drowsy and went to bed. By approximately 10:30 P.M. she had fallen asleep. She slept for about 3 hours and awakened completely relaxed; the upset stomach and pain in the head, neck, and face had vanished completely. She stayed awake for about a half hour, then went back to sleep. She slept until 7:30 A.M., at which time she had no pain and felt fine throughout the day.

This patient also received histamine injections according to the method advocated in this chapter, and the frequency and severity of her attacks were lessened. In this case in which Cafergot failed, Cafergot-PB definitely was successful in relieving the typical migraine headache attack.

SUMMARY

Symptoms and signs

1. More frequently seen in women
2. Nausea
3. Scotomas
4. Frequently associated with menstruation
5. Often associated with tension element
6. Patient always states that the headache is a "sick headache"
7. Family history
8. Vomiting
9. Photophobia
10. Anorexia

Pain is

1. Throbbing
2. Hemicranial
3. Periodic
4. Present for several hours or days

Negative

1. X-ray of skull
2. General physical examination
3. Neurologic examination
4. Electroencephalogram
5. Eye grounds

Treatment

Prophylactic
1. Histamine
2. BC-105
3. Lisuride
4. Tranquilizers
5. Reassurance
6. Methysergide
7. Clonidine
8. Nicotinic acid
9. Antidepressants
10. Personality adjustment

Symptomatic
1. Cafergot tablets or suppositories
2. Cafergot-PB tablets or suppositories
3. DHE-45
4. Octin
5. Migral
6. Medihaler-Ergotamine
7. Midrin
8. Gynergen
9. Ergomar
10. Analgesics

REFERENCES

1. Ostfeld, A. M., Reis, D. J., Goodell, H., and Wolff, H. G.: Headache and hydration, Arch. Intern. Med. **96**:142, 1955.
2. Schumacher, G. A., and Wolff, H. G.: Experimental studies on migraine, Arch. Neurol. Psychiatry **45**:199, 1941.
3. Simons, D. J., Day, E., Goodell, H., and Wolff, H. G.: Experimental studies on headache: muscles of the scalp and neck as sources of pain: a research, Nerv. Ment. Dis. Proc. **23**:228, 1943.
4. King, G. S.: Every man his own headache, Med. World, p. 207, May 1943.
5. Peters, G. A.: Migraine: diagnosis and treatment, Proc. Staff Meet. Mayo Clin. **28**:673, 1953.
6. Dalsgaard-Nielsen, T., Engberg-Pedersen, H., and Holm, H. E.: Clinical investigations of the epidemiology of migraine, Dan. Med. Bull. **17**:138-148, 1970.
7. Greene, R., and Dalton, K.: The premenstrual syndrome, Br. Med. J. **1**:1007-1014, 1953.
8. Greene, R., and Dalton, K.: Discussion on the premenstrual syndrome, Proc. R. Soc. Med. **48**(5):337-347, 1955.
9. Kessel, N., and Coppen, A.: The prevalence of common menstrual symptoms, Lancet **2**:61-64, 1963.
10. Epstein, M. T., Hockaday, J. M., and Hockaday, T. D. R.: Migraine and reproductive hormones throughout the menstrual cycle, Lancet **1**(7906):543-548, 1975.
11. Somerville, B. W.: Estrogen-withdrawal migraine: I. Duration of exposure required and attempted prophylaxis by premenstrual estrogen administration, Neurology **25**(3):239-255, 1975.
12. Kashiwagi, T., McClure, J. M., Jr., and Wetzel, R.: The menstrual cycle and headache type, Headache **12**:103-104, 1972.
13. Dalton, K.: The premenstrual syndrome, Springfield, Ill., 1964, Charles C Thomas, Publisher, p. 9.
14. Grant, E. C. G.: Venous effects of oral contraceptives, Br. Med. J. **4**:73-77, 1969.
15. Grant, E. C. G., and Pryse-Davies, J.: Effect of oral contraceptives on depressive mood changes and on endometrial monoamine oxidase and phosphatases, Br. Med. J. **3**:777-780, 1968.
16. Coppen, A., Eccleston, E. G., and Peet, M.: Total and free tryptophan concentration in the plasma of depressive patients, Lancet **2**:60-63, 1973.
17. Grant, E. C. G.: Relation of arterioles in the endometrium to headache from oral contraceptives, Lancet **1**:1143-1144, 1965.
18. Somerville, B.: The role of estradiol withdrawal in the etiology of menstrual migraine, Neurology **22**(4):355-365, 1972.
19. Kudrow, L.: The relationship of headache frequency to hormone use in migraine, Headache **15**(1):36-40, 1975.
20. Carroll, J. D.: Migraine and oral contraception, Proceedings of the International Headache Symposium, Elsinore, Denmark, May 16-18, 1971.

21. Carroll, J. D.: Migraine and oral contraception, Hemicrania 1(4):4-6, 1970.
22. Diddle, S. W., Gardner, W. H., and Williamson, P. J.: Oral contraceptive medications and headache, Am. J. Obstet. Gynecol. 105(4):507-511, 1969.
23. Desrosiers, J. J.: Headaches related to contraceptive therapy and their control, Headache 13: 117-124, 1973.
24. Dalton, K.: Migraine and oral contraceptives, Headache 15:247-251, 1976.
25. Cohn-Larsson, U., and Lundberg, P. O.: Headache and treatment with oral contraceptives, Scandanavian Migraine Society Symposium, 1969.
26. Carroll, J. D., and Grant, C. G.: The effect of oral contraceptives on blood-vessels and migraine, Klin. Monatsbl. Augenheilkd. 163(3):212-215, 1970.
27. Pluvinage, R.: Migraine, headache and oral contraceptives, Concours Med. 92(9):1946-1955, 1970.
28. Cohn-Larsson, U., and Lundberg, P. O.: Headache and treatment with oral contraceptives, Acta Neurol. Scand. 46(3):267-278, 1970.
29. Gardner, J. H., Hornstein, S., and ven den Noort, S.: The clinical characteristics of headache during impending cerebral infarction in women taking oral contraceptives, Headache 8:108-110, 1968.
30. Pendl, G., Jellinger, K., and Kietter, G.: Clinical and morphological aspects of acute cerebrovascular episodes during oral contraception, Verh. Deutsch, Ges. Pathol. 56:413-417, 1972.
30a. Ryan, R. E.: A controlled study of the effects of the oral contraceptives on migraine, Headache 17(6):250, 1978.
31. Vaughan, W.: Practice of allergy, St. Louis, 1939, The C. V. Mosby Co.
32. Rowe: Allergic migraine, J.A.M.A. 99:912, 1932.
33. Wolff, H. G.: Headaches and other head pain, New York, 1948, Oxford University Press, p. 359.
34. Hannington, E., and Harper, A. M.: The role of tyramine in the etiology of migraine, and related studies on the cerebral and extracerebral circulations, Headache 8:84-97, 1968.
35. Sandler, M., Youdin, M. B. H., Southgate, J., and Hannington, E.: The role of tyramine in migraine: biochemical mechanics, Background to Migraine 3:103-112.
36. Blackwell, B., and Mabbitt, L. A.: Tyramine in cheese related to hypertensive crisis after monoamine oxidase inhibition, Lancet 1:938, 1965.
37. Smith, I., and others: A clinical and biochemical correlation between tyramine and migraine headache, Headache 10:43-51, 1970.
38. Ryan, R. E., Jr.: A clinical study of tyramine as an etiologic factor in migraine, Headache 14: 43-48, 1974.
39. Forsythe, W. I., and Redman, A.: Two control trials of tyramine in children with migraine, J. Dev. Med. Child. Neurol. 16:794-799, 1974.
40. Mofett, A. M., and others: Effect of chocolate in migraine: a double-blind study, J. Neurol. Neurosurg. Psychiatry 37:445-448, 1974.
41. Osvald-Cernes, I.: Tyramine and migraine, a clinical study, presented at Headache Symposium, Florence, Italy, June, 1976.
42. Shaw, S. W. J., and others: RO tyramine and dietary migraine sufferers, unpublished report.
43. Hannington, E.: Food for thought, Ranson 2: 1148, 1974.
44. Sandler, M., and others: Phenylethylamine oxidizing defect in migraine, Nature 250:335-337, 1974.
45. McCulloch, J., and others: Phenylethylamine and cerebral circulation, presented at the International Migraine Symposium, London, England, September 16, 1976.
46. Hilton, B. P., and Cumings, J. N.: An assessment of platelet aggregation induced by 5-hydroxytryptamine, J. Clin. Pathol. 24:250-258, 1971.
47. Sicuteri, F., Anselmi, B., and DelBianco, P. L.: 5-Hydroxytryptamine supersensitivity as a new theory of headache and central approach with P-chlorophenylalanine, Psychopharmacologia 29: 347-356, 1973.
48. Grammeltvedt, A., Hovig, T., and Sjaastad, O.: Electronmicroscopy of blood platelets in migraine and cluster headache, Headache 14(4): 226-230, 1974.
49. Carroll, J. D., and Hilton, B. P.: The effects of reserpine injection on methysergide treated control and migrainous subjects, Headache 14:149-156, 1974.
50. Shore, P. A., Silver, S. L., and Brodies, B. B.: Interaction of reserpine, serotonin, lysergic acid diethylamide in brain, Science 122:284-285, 1955.
51. Sicuteri, F.: Headache as a possible expression of deficiency of brain 5-hydroxytryptamine (central denervation supersensitivity), Headache 12: 69-72, 1972.
52. Sjaastad, O.: The significance of blood serotonin levels in migraine: a critical review, Acta Neurol. Scand. 51:200-210, 1975.
53. Hilton, B. P.: Effects of reserpine and chlorpromazine on 5-hydroxytryptamine uptake of platelets from migrainous and control subjects, J. Neurol. Neurosurg. Psychiatry 37:711-714, 1974.
54. Hale, K.: Are 5-HT neurons of importance for central control of pain sensitivity? Bergen Migraine Symposium, Bergen, Norway, June 1975.
55. Fanchamps, A.: The role of humoral mediators in

migraine headache, J. Can. Neurol. Sci. **1:**189-195, 1974.

56. Berde, B., and Fanchamps, A.: Importance of humoral mediators for the pathogenesis and treatment of migraine, Kopfschmerz Headache, Innsbrook, Austria, pp. 55-74, 1975.

57. Fanchamps, A.: Humoral factors in the pathogenesis of migraine, Praxis **64:**226-230, 1975.

58. Deshmukh, V. D., and Harper, A. M.: The effect of serotonin on cerebral and extracerebral blood flow with possible implications in migraine, Acta Neurol. Scand. **49:**649-658, 1973.

59. Tretyakova, K. A., and Fets, A. N.: Total blood serotonin concentration in patients with migraine during and between attacks, Zh. Nevropatol. Psikhiatr. **69:**831-835, 1969.

60. Hilton, B. P., and Cumings, J. N.: 5-Hydroxy-tryptamine levels and platelet aggregation responses in subjects with acute migraine headache, J. Neurol. Neurosurg. Psychiatry **35**(4):505-509, 1972.

61. Rydzewski, W.: Serotonin (5-HT) in migraine: levels in whole blood in and between attacks, Headache **16:**16-19, 1976.

62. Hardebo, J. E., and Evinsson, L.: Mechanical action of serotonin and the effect of related inhibitors in intracranial and extracranial vessels, Headache **76:**11-13, 1976.

63. Somerville, B. W.: The fall in platelet serotonin during migraine is not accompanied by a rise in the free plasma level of serotonin, Bergen Migraine Symposium, Bergen, Norway, June 1975, pp. 77-78.

64. Thonnard-Neumann, E., and Taylor, W. L.: The basophilic leukocyte and migraine, Headache **8:**98-107, 1968.

65. Thonnard-Neumann, E.: Some interrelationships of vasoactive substances and basophilic leukocytes in migraine headache, Headache **9:**130-140, 1969.

66. Sicuteri, F.: Mast cells and their active substances: their role in the pathogenesis of migraine, Headache **3:**86, 1963.

67. Thonnard-Neumann, E.: Studies of basophils: basophilic leukocytes and gonadal activity in the rabbit, Acta Haematol. **32:**358, 1964.

68. Graham, H. T., Lowry, O. H., Wheelwright, F., Lenz, A. M., and Parrish, H. H., Jr.: Distribution of histamine between leukocytes and platelets, Blood **10:**467, 1955.

69. Braunsteiner, H.: Mast cells and basophilic leukocytes. In Braunsteiner, H., and Zucker-Franklin, editors: The physiology and pathology of leukocytes, New York, 1962, Grune and Stratton, Inc., p. 46.

70. Archer, G. T.: Release of heparin from the mast cells of the rat, Nature **191:**90, 1961.

71. Riley, J. D.: Histamine and heparin in mast-cells: why both? Lancet **2:**40-41, 1962.

72. Sicuteri, F., Michelazzi, S., Lonbardi, V., and Franchi, G.: Coagulation changes during migraine, Angiology **14:**580, 1963.

73. Kimball, R. W., Friedman, A. P., and Vallejo, P.: Effect of serotonin in migraine patients, Neurology **10:**107, 1960.

74. Lance, J. W., Anthony, M., and Hinterberger, H.: The control of cranial arteries by humoral mechanisms and its relation to the migraine syndrome, Headache **7:**93, 1967.

75. Appenzeller, O., and Scott, D.: Migraine vasomotor function and the basophilic leukocyte, Proceedings of the International Headache Symposium, Elsinore, Denmark, May 1971, pp. 1-8.

76. Barolin, G. S., and Sperlich, D.: Migraine families—a contribution to the genetic aspect of migraine, Fortschr. Neurol. Psychiatr. **37**(10):521-544, 1969.

77. Young, G. R., Leon-Barth, C. A., and Green, J.: Familial hemiplegic migraine, retinal degeneration, deafness, and nystagmus, Arch. Neurol. **23**(3):201-209, 1970.

78. Grant, E. C. G., Pryse-Davies, J., Goodwin, P. M., and Carroll, J. D.: The influence of hormones on headaches in women and the associated endometrial patterns, Headache Symposium, Innsbruck, Austria, May 1974.

79. Espin Herrero, J., and Barcia Marino, C.: Etiological aspects of migraine, Med. Esp. **71**(419):115-124, 1974.

80. Ziegler, D. K., Hassanein, R. S., and Harris, D.: Headache in a non-twin population, Headache **14:**213-217, 1975.

81. Barraquer-Bordas, L., Peres-Serra, J., Grau-Veciana, J. M., and Sagimon-Rabassa, E.: Familial prosoplegic migraine, Acta Neurol. Belg. **70**(3):301-308, 1970.

82. Wolff, H. G., Goodell, H., and Lewontin, R.: Familial occurrence of migraine headaches: a study of heredity, Arch. Neurol. Psychiatr. **72:**325, 1954.

83. Wolff, H. G.: Migraine. In Barr, D. P.: Modern medical therapy in general practice, Baltimore, 1940, The Williams & Wilkins Co., p. 2068.

84. Friedman, A. P., von Storch, T. I. C., and Merritt, H. H.: Migraine and tension headaches: a clinical study of 2,000 cases, Neurology **4:**773, 1954.

85. Hirsch, S.: Clinical observations on migraine and its treatment, N. Y. J. Med. **54:**663, 1954.

86. Lippman, C. W.: Ever had migraine? Coronet, p. 162, March 1955.

87. Dalsgaard-Nielsen, T.: Migraine—a reaction pattern, Manedsskr. Prakt. Laegegern **48**(12):541-558, 1970.

88. Horrobin, D. F.: The role of prostaglandins in migraine, presented at the meeting of the American Association for the Study of Headache, June 18, 1976, San Francisco, California.

89. Carlson, L. A.: Metabolic and cardiovascular effects in vivo of prostaglandins. In Bergstrom, S., and Samuelsson, B.: Prostaglandins, Nobel Symposium II, New York, 1967, Inter Science, pp. 123-132.

90. Carlson, L. A., and others: Clinical and metabolic effects of different doses of prostaglandin F in man, Acta Med. Scand. **183:**423-430, 1968.

91. Karim, S. M. M., and Somers, K.: Cardiovascular and renal actions of the prostaglandins. In Karim, S. M. M.: The prostaglandins: progress and research, Lancaster, 1972, MTP, pp. 165-203.

92. Ferreira, S. H., and Vane, J. R.: Prostaglandins: their disappearance, their release into the circulation, Nature **216:**868-873, 1967.

93. Alabaster, B. A., and Bakhle, Y. S.: The release of biologically active substances from isolated lungs by 5-hydroxytryptamine and tryptamine, Br. J. Pharmacol. **40:**582-583, 1970.

94. Yamamoto, Y. L., and others: Experimental vasoconstriction of cerebral arteries by prostaglandins, J. Neurosurg. **37:**385-397, 1972.

95. Welch, K. M. A., and others: Observations on the vascular effects of serotonin and prostaglandins in a model for the experimental study of migraine mechanisms. In Diamond, S., editor: Vasoactive substances relevant to migraine, Springfield, Ill., 1975, Charles C Thomas, Publisher.

96. Pickard, J. D., and others: Serotonin and prostaglandins: intercranial and extracranial effects with reference to migraine, presented at the British Migraine Symposium, September, 1976, London, England.

97. Olesen, J., and others: Regional cerebral blood flow in man determined by the initial slope of the clearance of intra-arterially injected xenon, Stroke **2:**519-540, 1971.

98. Pennink, M., and others: The role of prostaglandin F2 alpha in the genesis of experimental cerebral vasospasm: angiographic study in dogs, J. Neurosurg. **37:**398-405, 1972.

99. Anthony, M.: Plasma free fatty acids and prostaglandin El in migraine and stress, Headache **16:**58-63, 1976.

100. Sicuteri, F.: 5-Hydroxytryptophan in the prophylaxis of migraine, Pharmacol. Res. Commun. **4:**213-216, 1972.

101. Fanciullacci, M., and others: Free and total plasma tryptophan in spontaneous and pharmacologically induced headaches, presented at the British Migraine Symposium, September, 1976, London, England.

102. Sicuteri, F., Buffoni, F., Anselmi, B., and Del Bianco, P. L.: Monoamine oxidase activity in migraine and arterial hypertension. In Dalessio, D. J., Dalsgaard-Nielsen, T., and Diamond, S., editors: Proceedings of the International Headache Symposium, Elsinore, Denmark, 1971, American Association for Study of Headache and Danish Migraine Society, pp. 195-200.

103. Dalessio, D. J.: Headache mechanisms. In Vinken, P. J., and Bruyn, G. W., editors: Headaches and cranial neuralgias, Amsterdam, 1968, North-Holland Publishing Co., pp. 15-16.

104. Sulman, F. G.: Serotonin-migraine in climactic heat stress, its prophylaxis and treatment. In Dalessio, D. J., Dalsgaard-Nielsen, T., and Diamond, S., editors: Proceedings of the International Headache Symposium, Elsinore, Denmark, 1971, American Association for Study of Headache and Danish Migraine Society, pp. 205-210.

105. Bróca, P.: Anatomie comparée des circumvolutions cérébrales: le grand lobe limbique et la scissure limbique dans la serie des mammiferes, Rev. Anthrop. **1:**385-498, 1878.

106. Papez, J. W.: A proposed mechanism of emotion, Arch. Neurol. Psychiatr. **38:**725-743, 1937.

107. Raffaelli, E., Jr., and Menon, A. D.: Migraine and the limbic system, Headache **15:**69-78, 1975.

108. Sicuteri, F.: Migraine, a central biochemical dysnociception, Headache **16:**145-159, 1976.

109. Sicuteri, F.: Headache: disruption of pain modulating. In Bonica, J. J., and Abbe-Fessard, D., editors: Advances in pain research and therapy. vol. 1, New York, 1976, Raven Press.

110. Sicuteri, F., and Fonda, C.: Sulla natura centrale o periferica del dolore nelle cafalee essenziali, Minerva Med. **67:**1826-1833, 1976.

111. Schrire, L.: Permanent scotoma in migraine, S. Afr. Med. J. **43**(7):170-172, 1969.

112. Olsen, C. W.: The hemodynamics of preheadache scotoma in migraine, Bull. Los Angeles Neurol. Soc. **39**(1):14-16, 1974.

113. Aring, C. D.: The migrainous scintillating scotoma, J.A.M.A. **220**(4):519-522, 1972.

114. Alvarez, W. C.: Migrainous scotoma, Am. J. Ophthalmol. **49:**489-504, 1960.

115. Nick, J.: The borders of migraine: the place of migraine among headaches of vascular origin, Nouv. Presse Med. **3**(17):1087-1093, 1974.

116. Alvarez, W. C.: Migrainous personality and constitution; essential features of disease; study of 500 cases, Am. J. Med. Sci. **213:**1, 1947.

117. Shea, J. J.: Therapy of headache, J. Omaha Mid-West Clin. Soc. **11:**71, 1950.

118. Williams, H. L.: Headache from the standpoint of the otolaryngologist, J. Iowa Med. Soc. **37:**34, 1947.

119. Briggs, J. F., and Bellomo, J.: Precordial migraine, Dis. Chest **21:**635, 1952.

120. Ask-Upmark, F.: Inverted nipples and migraine, Acta Med. Scand. **147:**191, 1953.

121. Blan, J. N., and Pyke, D. A.: Effect of diabetes on migraine, Lancet **2:**241-243, 1970.

122. Barolin, S. G.: Migraine and trauma, Wien Z. Nervenheilkd. **27**(1):45-76, 1969.

123. Whiteley, J. S.: Migraine: a psychosomatic investigation, Clin. Med. **73**:33-34, 1966.

123a. Scollo-Lavizzari, G.: Electroencephalography in the diagnosis of migraine, Praxis **64**(8):234-237, 1975.

123b. Jacobi, G., Emrich, R., Ritz, A., and Herranz-Fernandez, J.: Headaches in childhood: headache and migraine: comparison of clinical and EEG findings, Fortschr. Med. **90**(6):199-204, 1972.

123c. Gschwend, J.: EEG findings and their interpretation in simple migraine, Z. Neurol. **201**(3):279-292, 1972.

123d. Hughes, J. R.: EEG in headache, Headache **11**(4):162-170, 1972.

124. Barolin, G. S.: The significance of the EEG in the differential diagnosis of headache, Ost. Arzteztg. **24**(8):945-946, 963-970, 1969.

124a. Smyth, V., and Winter, A.: EEG in migraine, Electroencephalogr. Clin. Neurophysiol. **16**:194-202, 1964.

124b. Weil, A. A.: EEG findings in dysrhythmic migraine, J. Nerv. Ment. Dis. **134**:277-281, 1962.

124c. Barolin, G. S.: Headache symposium, Innsbruck, Austria, May, 1974, pp. 142-149.

124d. Towle P. A.: The electroencephalographic hyperventilation response in migraine, Electroencephalogr. Clin. Neurophysiol. **19**:390-393, 1965.

125. Dalsgaard-Nielsen, T.: Migraine and epilepsy, Ugeskr. Laeger. **126**:185, 1964.

125a. Ninck, B.: Migraine and epilepsy, Europ. Neurol. **3**(3):168-178, 1970.

125b. Greene, C. A., Sudhakar, R. V., Maragos, G. D., and Mitchell, J. R.: On the relationship of migraine . . . epilepsy, Neb. State Med. J. **56**(4):136-139, 1971.

125c. Lance, J. W., and Anthony, M.: Some clinical aspects of migraine, Arch. Neurol. **15**:356-361, 1966.

125d. Panzani, R.: Migraine: Similarity to asthma, Allerg. Asthmaforsch. **8**(1):1-15, 1962.

126. Basser, L. S.: The relation of migraine and epilepsy, Brain **92**(2):285-300, 1969.

126a. Lees, F., and Watkins, S. M.: Loss of consciousness in migraine, Lancet **2**:647-650, 1963.

126b. Savoldi, F., Tartara, A., Nappi, G., and Bono, G.: EEG findings in migraine. In Headache—new vistas, Florence, Italy, 1977, Biomedical Press, pp. 34-35.

126c. Rios Mozo, M.: Migraine and abdominal epilepsy: correlations with biliary disease and rheumatic fever, Rev. Clin. Esp. **132**(2):115-124, 1974.

126d. Serratrice, G., Acquaviva, P., Gastaut, J. L., and Gastaut, J. A.: Migraine and epilepsy, J. Med. Montpellier **8**(2):76-80, 1973.

127. Sicuteri, F.: Prophylactic and therapeutic properties of 1-methyl lysergic acid butanolamide in migraine, Int. Arch. Allergy **15**:300, 1959.

127a. Friedman, A. P.: Clinical observations with 1-methyl lysergic acid butanolamide (UML-491) in vascular headaches, Angiology **11**:364, 1960.

127b. Graham, J. R.: Use of a new compound, UML-491, in prevention of various types of headache, N. Engl. J. Med. **263**:1273, 1960.

127c. Friedman, A. P., and Losin, S.: Evaluation of UML-491 in treatment of vascular headache, Arch. Neurol. **4**:241, 1961.

128. Dalessio, D. J., and others: Studies on headache: responses of bulbar conjunctival blood vessels during induced oliguria and diuresis, and their modification by UML-491, Arch. Neurol. **5**:590, 1961.

129. Karlsberg, P., Adams, J. E., and Elliot, H. W.; Inhibition and reversal of serotonin-induced cerebral vasospasm, Surg. Forum **13**:425-427, 1962.

130. Sicuteri, F., Franchi, G., and Fanciullacci, M.: Serotonin potentiation of methysergide, LSD-25 and ergotamine in man: an informal approach to migraine pharmacology, Symposium on Headache, Innsbruck, Austria, May 1974, pp. 101-104.

131. Friedman, A. P., and Elkind, A. H.: Appraisal of methysergide treatment of vascular headaches of migraine type, J.A.M.A. **184**:125-128, 1963.

132. Rooke, E. D., Rushton, J. G., and Peters, G. A.: Vasodilating headache: suggested classification and results of prophylactic treatment with UML-491 (methysergide), Proc. Staff Meet. Mayo Clin. **37**:433-443, 1962.

133. Dalessio, D. J.: On migraine headache: serotonin and serotonin antagonism, J.A.M.A. **181**:318-321, 1962.

134. Saxena, P. R.: On the mechanism of action of methysergide in vascular headaches of migraine type, Headache Symposium, Innsbruck, Austria, May 1974.

135. Saxena, P. R.: The effects of antimigraine drugs on the vascular responses by 5-hydroxytryptamine and related biogenic substances on the external carotid bed of dogs: possible pharmacological implications to their antimigraine action, Headache **12**:44-54, 1972.

136. Saxena, P. R.: Selective vasoconstriction in carotid vascular bed by methysergide: possible relevance to its antimigraine effect, Eur. J. Pharmacol. **27**:99-105, 1974.

137. Owen, D. A. A., Herd, J. K., Kalberer, F., Pacha, W., and Salzmann, R.: The influence of ergotamine and methysergide on the storage of biogenic amines, Proceedings of the International Headache Symposium, Elsinore, Denmark, May 1971, pp. 153-156.

138. Hilton, B. P., and Zilkha, K. J.: Effects of ergotamine and methysergide of blood platelet aggregation responses of migrainous subjects, J. Neurol. Neurosurg. Psychiatry **37**:593, 1974.

139. Persyko, I.: Psychiatric adverse reactions to

methysergide, J. Nerv. Ment. Dis. **154:**299, 1972.

140. Lloyd-Smith, D. L., and McNaughton, F. L.: Methysergide (Sansert) in prevention of migraine, Can. Med. Assoc. J. **89:**1221, 1963.

141. Lindeneg, O., and Kok-Jensen, A.: Pleurisy and pleural fibrosis developing during treatment with methysergide, Nord. Med. **79:**681, 1968.

142. Friedman, A. P.: Prophylaxis of migraine, Headache **13:**104, 1973.

143. Pedersen, E., and Moller, C. E.: Prophylaxis of migraine with methysergide, Nord. Med. **74:**1282, 1965.

144. Daniell, H. W.: Vasospastic reaction to methysergide maleate simulating Leriche's syndrome: ineffective treatment with adrenergic blockade, Ann. Intern. Med. **60:**881, 1964.

145. Utz, D. C., Rooke, E. D., Spittell, J. A., and Bartholomew, L. G.: Retroperitoneal fibrosis in patients taking methysergide, J.A.M.A. **191:**983, 1965.

146. Wagenknecht, L. V.: Retroperitoneal fibrosis after methysergide therapy, Munch. Med. Wochenschr. **114:**585, 1972.

147. Farrel, W. J., Nolan, J. J., and Tessitore, A.: Unilateral eg edema, migraine and methysergide: a clinical presentation of retroperitoneal fibrosis, J.A.M.A. **207:**1909, 1969.

148. Graham, J. R.: Methysergide for prevention of headache: experience in five hundred patients over three years, N. Engl. J. Med. **270:**67, 1964.

149. Pedersen, E., and Moller, C. E.: Clinical trial of methysergide in migraine prophylaxis, Clin. Pharmacol. Ther. **7:**520, 1966.

150. Southwell, N., Williams, J. D., and Mackenzie, I.: Methysergide in the prophylaxis of migraine, Lancet **1:**523, 1964.

151. Harris, M. C.: Migraine headache and histamine cephalalgia: treatment with antiserotonin agent, Ann. Allergy **19:**500, 1961.

152. Lance, J. W., Anthony, M., and Somerville, B.: Comparative trial of serotonin antagonists in management of migraine, Br. Med. **2:**327-329, 1970.

153. Lovshin, L. L.: Use of methysergide in the treatment of extracranial vascular headache, Headache **3:**107-11, 1963.

154. Abbott, K. H.: Clinical studies on the treatment of vascular headaches, a progress report on methysergide (Sansert), Headache **4:**261-271, 1965.

155. Graham, J. R., Suby, H. I., Lecompte, P. R., and Sadowsky, N. L.: Fibrotic disorders associated with methysergide therapy for headache, N. Engl. J. Med. **274:**359-368, 1966.

156. Sicuteri, F., Franchi, G., and DelBianco, P. L.: An autonomic drug in the prophylaxis of migraine, Int. Arch. Allergy **31:**78-93, 1967.

157. Declerck, A.: A comparative study of two methods of treatment of vascular headaches with mi-

grainous components, Tijdschr. Diergeneeskd. **25:**931-939, 1969.

158. Nelson, R. F.: BC-105—a new prophylactic agent for migraine—four years experience in seventy-five patients, Headache **13:**96-103, 1973.

159. Fraipont-Guyot, C., Luyekx, A., and Lefebvre, P.: Study of the effects of serotonin antagonist (BC-105 Sandoz) on carbohydrate metabolism, Rev. Med. Liege **25:**414-421, 1970.

160. Stary, O., Jansky, M., Figar, S., and Stein, J.: Clinico-physiological studies of the action of BC-105 (Sandoz, Basle) in the interval treatment of migraine, Eur. Neurol. **11:**353-362, 1974.

161. Aellig, W. H.: Clinical-pharmacological experiments with Pizotifen (Sandomigran) on superficial hand veins in man, International Headache Symposium, London, England, September 1976.

162. Ryan, R. E.: Double blind cross over comparison of BC-105, methysergide and placebo in the prophylaxis of migraine headache, Headache **8:**118-126, 1968.

163. Schaer, J.: BC-105: A new serotonin antagonist in the treatment of migraine, Headache **10:**67-73, 1970.

164. Brugger, A.: Differential diagnosis of headache, and experience of BC-105 in the treatment of migraine, Praxis **59:**1360-1365, 1970.

165. Andersson, P. G.: BC-105 and Deseril in migraine prophylaxis, Headache **13:**68-73, 1973.

166. Prusinski, A., and Niewodniczy, A.: Use of Pizotifen (Sandomigran; BC-105) in cervical migraine, Wiad. Lek. **27:**297-300, 1974.

167. Cerdan, A., Acosta, M., and Jolin, T.: Long-term administration of Pizotifen to migraine patients: effects on oral glucose tolerance tests and on insulin levels, Headache **15:**126-128, 1975.

168. Biehl, B., and Seydel, U.: Experimental studies on the influence of the new anti-migraine preparation BC-105 on the ability to drive an automobile, Zentrabl. Verkehrs-Med. **17:**67-72, 1971.

169. Forssman, B., Henriksson, K. G., and Kihlstrand, S.: A comparison between BC-105 and methysergide in the prophylaxis of migraine, Acta Neurol. Scand. **48:**204-212, 1972.

170. Hernandez-Cossio, O.: A new drug, BC-105, in the treatment of migraine, Rev. Cuba Med. **11:**607-610, 1972.

171. Pichler, E., and Suchanek-Frohlich, H.: Interval treatment of migraine with BC-105, a new serotonin antagonist, Wien. Klin. Wochenschr. **82:**208-211, 1970.

172. Tedeschi, G., Lettieri, M., and Turra, M. V.: The treatment of vasomotor headache with a new drug, BC-105: preliminary report, Acta Neurol. (Napoli) **26:**61-65, 1971.

173. Stensrud, P., and Sjaastad, O.: Appraisal of BC-105 in migraine prophylaxis, Scandinavian Migraine Symposium, 1969.

174. Carroll, J. D., and Maclay, W. P.: Pizotifen (BC-

105) in migraine prophylaxis, Curr. Med. Res. Opin. **3**:68-71, 1975.

175. Barolin, G. S.: Long-term treatment of intractable migraine with BC-105, Z. Allgemeinmed. **46**:1130-1133, 1970.

176. Dalsgaard-Nielsen, T., and Ulrich, J.: Long-term effect and tolerance during prophylactic treatment of migraine with a benzo-cycloheptathiophene derivative, Pizotifen, Headache **13**:12-18, 1973.

177. Pasquazzi, M., and Anselmi, E.: Results with Pizotifen (BC-105: Sandomigran) in the treatment of migraine (30 cases), Roma Rif. Med. **88**:267-274, 1974.

178. Anselmi, B.: Sandomigran as treatment of choice in anxious, emaciated and anorectic migraine-sufferers, Schweiz Med. Wochenschr. **102**:487-492, 1972.

179. Arthur, G. P. and Hornabrook, R. W.: The treatment of migraine with BC-105 (Pizotifen): a double-blind trial, N.Z. Med. J. **73**:5-9, 1971.

180. Speight, T. M., and Avery, G. S.: Pizotifen (BC-105): a review of its pharmacological properties and its therapeutic efficacy in vascular headaches, Aust. Drug Inform. Serv. **3**:159-203, 1972.

181. Selby, G.: A clinical trial of an antiserotonin drug, BC-105, in the prophylaxis of migraine, Proc. Austr. Assoc. Neurol. **7**:37-43, 1971.

182. Wasilewski, R.: The value of Pizotifen (Sandomigran) in the treatment of migrainous syndromes, Pol. Tyg. Lek. **28**:1320-1321, 1973.

183. Lance, J. W., and Anthony, M.: Clinical trial of a new serotonin antagonist, BC-105, in prevention of migraine, Med. J. Aust. **1**:54-55, 1968.

184. Heyck, H.: Prophylactic treatment of migraine, Scandinavian Migraine Symposium, 1968.

185. Ryan, R. E.: BC-105: A new preparation for the interval treatment of migraine—a double blind evaluation compared with a placebo, Headache **11**:6-12, 1971.

186. Wilkinson, M., and others: Clonidine in the treatment of migraine at the city migraine clinic in patients selected with tyramine, Proceedings of the International Headache Symposium, Elsinore, Denmark, May 16-18, 1971, pp. 219-221.

187. Grabner, W., and Wolf, M.: Kritische Behachlanger zum wirkungsmechanism des 2(2-6 Dichlorphenylamine)2-imidazolin hydrochloride, Arzeim. Forsch. **16**:1055, 1966.

188. Zaimis, E., and Hannington, E.: A possible pharmacological approach to migraine, Lancet **2**:298-300, 1969.

189. Wilkinson, M.: Clonidine for migraine, Lancet **2**:430, 1969.

190. Wilkinson, M.: Clonidine for migraine, Proceedings of the International Migraine Headache Symposium, Florence, Italy, May 26-28, 1970, pp. 117-118.

191. Sjaastad, O., and Stensrud, P.: 2-(2-6 dichlorophenylamine-2 imidazoline hydrochloride ST 155 or Calopresan) as a prophylactic remedy against migraine, Acta Neurol. Scand. **47**:120-122, 1971.

192. Barrie, M. A., and others: The use of clonidine (ST-155) in migraine and the problems encountered in a multicenter trial, Proceedings of the International Headache Symposium, Elsinore, Denmark, May 16-18, 1971, pp. 23-26.

193. Horwitz, D., and others: Presented at the Second Catapres Symposium, September 18-19, 1968.

194. Fairbairn, J. F., II, and others: Presented at the Second Catapres Symposium, September 18-19, 1968.

195. Gifford, R. W., Jr.: Presented at the Second Catapres Symposium, September 18-19, 1968.

196. Ryan, R. E., and Ryan, R. E., Jr.: Clonidine—its use in migraine therapy, Headache **14**:190-192, 1975.

197. Kangasniemi, P., and Rime, V. K.: Clonidine and pizatiphene in the internal treatment of migraine patients. In Headache—new vistas, Florence, 1977, Biomedical Press, pp. 15-16.

198. Shafar, J., Tallett, E. R., and Knowlson, P. A.: Evaluation of clonidine in prophylaxis of migraine, Lancet **1**(7747):403-407, 1972.

199. Carroll, J. D.: Clonidine (Dixarit) in the prophylaxis of migraine, Berlin International Migraine Symposium, June 1975, p. 22.

200. Ryan, R. E., and Ryan, R. E., Jr.: The effects of clonidine in the prophylactic treatment of migraine, Headache **14**:200-212, 1975.

201. Ryan, R. E., Sr., Diamond, S., and Ryan, R. E., Jr.: Double blind study of clonidine and placebo for the prophylactic treatment of migraine, Headache **15**:202-205, 1975.

202. Stensrud, P., and Sjaastad, O.: Catapresan (clonidine)—double blind study in patients after long term treatment with the drug, Bergen International Migraine Symposium, Bergen, Norway, June 1975, p. 82.

203. Blank, N. K., and Rieder, M. J.: Paradoxical response to propranolol in migraine, Lancet **2**:1336, 1973.

204. Lechin, F., and van der Dijs, B.: A new treatment for headache: pathophysiologic considerations, Headache **16**:318, 1977.

205. Malvea, B. P., Gwon, N., and Graham, J. R.: Propranolol prophylaxis of migraine, Headache **12**:163, 1973.

206. Diamond, S., and Medina, J. L.: Double blind study of propranolol for migraine prophylaxis, Headache **16**:24, 1976.

207. Diamond, S., and Medina, L.: Double blind study of propranolol for migraine prophylaxis, Headache **16**:24, 1976.

208. Børgesen, S.-E., Nielsen, J. L., and Møller, C. E.: Prophylactic treatment of migraine with propranolol: a clinical trial, Acta Neurol. Scand. **50**:651, 1974.

209. Ludvigsson, J.: Propanolol used in prophylaxis of migraine in children, Acta Neurol. Scand. **50**:109, 1974.

210. Weber, R. B., and Reinmuth, O. M.: Treatment of migraine with propranolol, Neurology **22**:366, 1972.

211. Stensrud, P., and Sjaastad, O.: Short term clinical trial of propranolol in racemic form ("Inderal"), D-propranolol, and placebo in migraine, Bergen Migraine Symposium, Bergen, Norway, June 1975, p. 81.

212. Blomberg, L.-H.: Propranolol as an antidote in ergotamine addiction, Bergen Migraine Symposium, Bergen, Norway, June 1975, p. 19.

213. Ekbom, K.: Alprenolol for migraine prophylaxis, Headache **15**:129, 1975.

214. Jacobs, H.: A trial of opipramol in the treatment of migraine, J. Neurol. Neurosurg. Psychiatry **35**:500, 1972.

215. Ekbom, K., and Lundberg, P. O.: Clinical trial of LB-46 (d,1-4-[2-hydroxy-3-isopropylaminopropoxy] indol), an adrenergic beta-receptor blocking agent in migraine prophylaxis, Headache **12**:15, 1972.

216. Sjaastad, O., and Stensrud, P.: Clinical trial of a beta-receptor blocking agent (LB 46) in migraine prophylaxis, Acta Neurol. Scand. **48**:124, 1972.

217. Rieger, H., Regli, F., Enkelmann, R., and vom Brocke, I.: Effects of a beta-adrenoceptor-blocker on the EEG in vascular headaches of migraine type, Mk. Arztl. Fortb. **25**:306, 1975.

218. Somerville, B. W.: The influence of hormonal changes upon migraine in women, Proc. Austr. Assoc. Neurol. **8**:47, 1971.

219. Somerville, B. W., and Carey, H. M.: The use of continuous progestogen contraception in the treatment of migraine, Med. J. Aust. **57**:1043, 1970.

220. Somerville, B. W.: The influence of progesterone and estradiol upon migraine, Headache **12**:93, 1972.

221. Lundberg, P. O.: Migraine prophylaxis with progesterone, Acta Endocrinol. **40**(Suppl. 68):1-22, 1962.

222. Chaudhuri, T. K., and Chaudhuri, S. T.: Estrogen therapy for migraine, Headache **15**:139, 1975.

223. Somerville, B. W.: Estrogen-withdrawal migraine: II. Attempted prophylaxis by continuous estradiol administration, Neurology **25**:245, 1975.

224. Herrmann, W. M., Horowski, R., Danmehl, K., Kramer, U., and Luiat, K.: Clinical effectiveness of lisuride hydrogen maleate, a new migraine prophylactic: results of a double blind trial v. methysergide, Headache **17**:54-60, 1977.

225. Somerville, B. W., and Herrmann, W. M.: Migraine prophylaxis with lisuride hydrogen maleate—a double blind study of lisuride vs. placebo, Headache **18**:75-79, 1978.

226. Carroll, J. D.: Indoramine in the prophylaxis of

migraine. In Headache—new vistas, Florence, 1977, Biomedical Press.

227. Heide, M.: Treatment of headache with Ergo-Lonarid, Ther. Gwg. **110**:371-378, 1971.

228. Neumann-Mangoldt, P.: Treatment of vasomotor headaches and migraine, Z. Ther. **8**:156-159, 1970.

229. Glaser, A.: Migraine—vasomotor headaches and their therapeutic approach, Med. Welt. **25**:1435-1438, 1974.

230. Andersson, P. G.: Treatment of migraine patients with amitriptyline, Nord. Psykiat. **28**:227-230, 1974.

231. Andersson, P. G.: Migraine patients treated with reserpine tablets—an open study. In Headache—new vistas, Florence, 1977, Biomedical Press.

232. Nattero, G.: Reserpine in the prophylaxis of migraine, Bergen Migraine Symposium, June 1975, p. 61.

233. Roge, J., and De Roissard, F.: Migraine and sulpiride, Cah. Med. **12**:295-303, 1971.

234. Mosora, N., and Boeriu, I. N.: Sulpiride in the treatment of migraine, Clujul Med. **47**:245-249, 1974.

235. Barre, Y.: Sulpiride in treatment of migraine, Sem. Hop. Paris **46**:80-86, 1970.

236. Pluvinage, M. R.: Treatment of migraine and vasomotor headache with a tranquillizer, J. Med. Chir. Prat. **141**:291-296, 1970.

237. Hakkarainen, H., and Viukari, M.: Sulpiride in the treatment of migraine, tension headache and psychosomatic symptoms, Duodecim **89**:1504-1509, 1973.

238. Dalsgaard-Nielsen, T., and Trautmann, J.: Prophylactic treatment of migraine with vitamin B, Ugeskr. Laeger. **132**:339-341, 1970.

239. Scopa, J., Jorgensen, P. B., and Foster, J. B., Migraleve in the prophylaxis of migraine, Curr. Ther. Res. **16**:1270-1275, 1974.

240. Jorgensen, P. B., Weightman, D., and Foster, J. B.: Comparison of migraleve and buclizine in prophylaxis of migraine, Curr. Ther. Res. **16**:1276-1280, 1974.

241. Jacobs, H.: A trial of opipramol in the treatment of migraine, J. Neurol. Neurosurg. Psychiatry **35**:500-504, 1972.

242. Foldes, E. G.: Comparative treatment study of migraine headache, Int. J. Clin. Pharmacol. **6**:60-66, 1972.

243. Beier, R., and Vehreschild, T.: Clinical and electroencephalographic findings during treatment of migraine and similar headache with spasmalgan, Dtsch. Gesundh. Wes. **28**:1814-1817, 1973.

244. Von Witzleben, H. D.: Adjunctive therapy in migraine, J. Mo. Med. Assoc. **49**:486, 1952.

245. Hilsinger, R. L.: Vascular headache and related conditions, Laryngoscope **64**:403, 1954.

246. Brainard, J. B.: Salt load as a trigger for migraine, Minn. Med. **59**:232-233, 1976.

247. Wilks, S. M.: Diseases of the nervous system, Med. Times, Jan. 2, 1869.
248. Fothergill, J.: Remarks of that complaint commonly known under the name of the sick headache, Med. Observ. **6:**103, 1784.
249. Friedman, A. P.: Treatment of migraine, N. Engl. J. Med. **250:**600, 1954.
250. Alvarez, W. C., and Mason, A. Y.: Results obtained in the treatment of headache with the inhalation of pure oxygen, Proc. Staff Meet. Mayo Clin. **15:**616, 1940.
251. Alvarez, W. C.: What to do in a rebellious case of migraine, Gastroenterology **9:**754, 1947.
252. Moffat, W. M.: Treatment of menstrual migraine with small doses of gonadotropic extract of pregnancy urine, J.A.M.A. **108:**612, 1937.
253. Leyton, N.: A new approach to the treatment of migraine, Med. Press **211:**302, 1944.
254. Riley, H. A., Brickner, R. M., and Kurzrol, R.: The abnormal excretion of theelin and prolan in patients suffering from migraine; a preliminary report, Bull. Neurol. Inst. N. Y. **3:**53, 1943.
255. Eggleston, C., and Wiss, S.: The treatment of migraine with extract of the anterior lobe of the pituitary, Am. J. Med. Sci. **183:**283, 1932.
256. Dunn, C. W.: Male migraine treated with female sex hormone, Delaware Med. J. **13:**89, 1941.
257. Glass, S. J.: Migraine and ovarian deficiency, Endocrinology **20:**333, 1936.
258. Hines, E. A., Jr., and Eaton, L. M.: Potassium thiocyanate in the treatment of migraine; a preliminary report, Proc. Staff Meet. Mayo Clin. **17:**254, 1942.
259. Brown, T. R.: The treatment of migraine and hypertrophic arthritis based on metabolic studies, Trans. Assoc. Am. Physicians **44:**215, 1929.
260. Crandall, L. A., Jr., and Roberts, G. M.: The treatment of periodic headache with chondroitin sulphuric acid, Ill. Med. J. **63:**513, 1933.
261. James, A. K.: Prevention of migraine by oral administration of carbachol; an analysis of 12 cases, Br. Med. J. **1:**663, 1945.
262. Pelner, L.: The treatment of periodic occipital headache with "desensitizing" doses of prostigmin, Dis. Nerv. Syst. **4:**177, 1943.
263. Palmer, H. D.: Treatment of migraine with vitamin B_1: resume of one year's experience, Arch. Neurol. Psychiat. **45:**368, 1941.
264. Riggs, C. E.: Calcium lactate as a preventive in migraine, Minn. Med. **9:**87, 1926.
265. Barborka, C. J.: The ketoginic diet and its uses, Med. Clin. North Am. **12:**1639, 1929.
266. Goldzieher, J. W., and Popkin, G. L.: Treatment of headache with intravenous sodium nicotinate, J.A.M.A. **131:**103, 1946.
267. Atkinson, M.: Meniere's syndrome and migraine: observations on a common causal relationship, Ann. Intern. Med. **18:**797, 1943.
268. Marin, R. B.: Theophylline in the treatment of migraine; a preliminary report, J. Med. Soc. N. J. **43:**274, 1946.
269. Smith, C. B.: The role of riboflavin in migraine, Can. Med. Assoc. J. **54:**589, 1946.
270. Friedman, A. P., and Brenner, C.: Principles in the treatment of chronic headache, N. Y. J. Med. **45:**1969, 1945.
271. Gottlieb, J. S.: The effect of benzedrine sulfate on migraine: a preliminary report, Am. J. Med. Sci. **204:**553, 1942.
272. Moehlig, R. C.: Migraine, a study based on one hundred cases, Endocrinology **15:**11, 1931.
273. Vaisberg, M.: Relief of migraine, Ann. Allergy **12:**180, 1954.
274. Nadler, S. B.: Paroxysmal temporal headache, J.A.M.A. **129:**334, 1945.
275. Ayash, J. J.: Headache and headache pain, Lancet **69:**389, 1949.
276. Friedman, A. P.: Pharmacotherapy for headache, Neurology **13:**27-33, 1963.
277. Peters, G. A., and Horton, B. T.: Headache: with special reference to the excessive use of ergotamine preparations and withdrawal effects, Proc. Staff Meet. Mayo Clin. **26:**9, 1951.
278. Horton, B. T., Ryan, R. E., and Reynolds, J.: Clinical observations on the use of E. C.-110, a new agent for the treatment of headache, Proc. Staff Meet. Mayo Clin. **23-**105, 1948.
279. Ryan, R. E.: Cafergone for relief of headache, Postgrad. Med. **5:**330, 1949.
280. Ryan, R. E.: Cafergot for relief of headache—a further study, J. Mo. Med. Assoc. **47:**107, 1950.
281. Friedman, A. P.: Method of Arnold P. Friedman. In Conn, H. F.: Current therapy 1950, Philadelphia, 1950, W. B. Saunders Co., p. 563.
282. Fanchamps, A.: The effect of caffeine on the internal absorption of ergotamine. In Saxena, P. R., editor: Migraine and related headaches, Rotterdam, 1975, Erasmus University, pp. 131-138.
283. Zoglio, M. A., and Maulding, H. V.: Complexes of ergot alkaloids and derivatives: II. Interaction of dihydroergotoxine with certain xanthines, J. Pharmacol. Sci. **59**(2):215-219, 1970.
284. Ryan, R. E.: ECB-210, a new agent for the treatment of headache, a comparison with Cafergot, J. Mo. Med. Assoc. **47:**178, 1950.
285. Ryan, R. E.: Treatment of headache, J. Mo. Med. Assoc. **48:**106, 1951.
286. Kramer, P., and Ingelfinger, F. J.: Use of antispasmodics and spasmodics in the treatment of gastrointestinal disorders, Med. Clin. North Am. **32:**1227, 1948.
287. Cushney, A. R.: Atropine and the hyoscyamines—a study of the action of optical isomers, J. Physiol. **30:**176, 1904.
288. El-Hamid Abdalla El-Shamy, A., El- Anwar, F. M., and Kassema, A. A.: Formulation and sta-

bility of ergotamine tartrate in suppositories, J. Drug Res. **5:**159-168, 1973.

289. Moore, D. C., and others: Control of postoperative vomiting with Marezine: a double blind study, Anesthesiology **17:**690, 1956.

290. Dent, S. J., and others: Postoperative vomiting: incidence, analysis, and therapeutic measures in 3000 patients, Anesthesiology **16:**564, 1955.

291. Ryan, R. E.: A new agent for the symptomatic relief of migraine attacks, Clin. Med. **6**(11):2111-2116, 1959.

292. Sutherland, J. M., Hooper, W. D., Eadie, M. J., and Tyrer, J. H.: Buccal absorption of ergotamine, J. Neurol. Neurosurg. Psychiatry **37** (10):1116, 1974.

293. Ryan, R. E.: A new agent approach to the symptomatic treatment of migraine, Arch. Otol. **72:**325-328, 1960.

294. Speed, W. G., III: Ergotamine for vascular headache, Am. J. Med. Sci. **240:**327, 1960.

295. Blumenthal, L. S., and Fuchs, M.: Vascular headaches: transpulmonary absorption of ergotamine, Med. Ann. D. C. **30:**10-12, 1961.

296. Lenox, W. G.: Ergonovine versus ergotamine as a terminator of migraine headache, Am. J. Med. Sci. **195:**458, 1938.

297. Horton, B. T., Peters, G. A., and Blumenthal, L. S.: A new product, Proc. Staff Meet. Mayo Clin. **20:**241, 1945.

298. Girard, M.: The action of dihydroergotamine alone in the prevention of migraine: a study of 80 cases, J. Med. Lyon **50:**371, 1969.

299. Mercier-Carli, R.: Treatment and prevention of the attack of migraine, Angiologia **25:**179, 1973.

300. Heyck, H.: Treatment of migraine, Paediatr. Prax. **8:**419, 1969.

301. Zenglein, R.: Treatment of migraine, Dtsch. Med. Wochenschr. **100:**557, 1975.

302. Peters, B. A., and Zeller, W. W.: Evaluation of a new agent in the treatment of vasodilatory headaches, Proc. Staff Meet. Mayo Clin. **24:**565, 1949.

303. MacNeal, P. S.: Headache as an emergency complaint, Med. Clin. North Am. **33:**1581, 1949.

304. Seltzer, A.: The use of octin in migraine and related headaches, Med. Ann. D. C. **17:**3945, 1948.

305. Diamond, S., and Medina, J. L.: Isometheptene—a non-ergot drug in the treatment of migraine, Headache **15:**211-213, 1975.

306. Johnson, D. E.: Alternative to ergotamine in the treatment of vascular headaches, Clin. Med. **77:**33-36, 1970.

307. Ryan, R. E.: A study of Midrin in the symptomatic relief of migraine headache, Headache **14:**33-42, 1974.

308. Yuill, B. M., Swinburn, W. R., and Liversedge, L. A.: A double-blind crossover trial of isometheptene mucate compound and ergotamine in migraine, Br. J. Clin. Pract. **16:**76-79, 1972.

309. Antunes, J. L., Macedo, C. and Damasio, A. R.: Levodopa and migraine, Lancet **2:**928, 1970.

310. Kopjast, T. L.: The use of folic acid in vascular headache of the migraine type, Headache **8:**167-170, 1969.

311. Bleger, G.: Therapeutic trials of diazepam (Valium) in cases of headaches and migraine, J. Med. Nordest **11:**114-119, 1974.

312. Edmeads, J.: Management of the acute attack of migraine, Headache **13:**91-95, 1973.

313. Volans, G. N.: Absorption of effervescent aspirin during migraine, Br. Med. J. **4:**266-268, 1974.

314. Lance, J. W., Anthony, M., and Gonski, A.: Serotonin, the carotid body, and cranial vessels in migraine, Arch. Neurol. **16:**553-558, 1967.

315. Vosgerau, H.: Treatment of migraine with magnesium glutamate, Ther. Gwg. **112:**640-648, 1973.

316. Bosburg, R.: Conjoint therapy of migraine: a case report, Psychosomatics **13:**61-63, 1972.

317. Hornbacher, W.: Physical therapy for sleep disturbances, depression and migraine, Z. Phys. Med. **2:**499-503, 1971.

318. Blummenthal, L. S.: Hypnotherapy of migraine and other types of chronic headache, Am. J. Clin. Hypn. **3:**174-178, 1961.

319. Rubottom, R. L.: Hypnosis made practical for the general practitioner: migraine headaches and obstetrics, J. Am. Inst. Hypno. **14:**184-193, 1973.

320. Wilkinson, M.: The treatment of acute migraine attacks, Headache **15:**291-292, 1976.

SUGGESTED READING

Friedman, A. P.: The (infinite) variety of migraine. In Cochrane, A. L., editor: Background to migraine, Third Migraine Symposium, London, 1962, p. 172.

CHAPTER 5

Vascular headaches: atypical forms of migraine

HEMIPLEGIC MIGRAINE

Hemiplegic migraine is an uncommon variant of migraine with a familiar background in which there are striking signs of a unilateral neurologic deficiency superimposed on the usual classic symptoms. These symptoms consist of nausea, vomiting, photophobia, and scotoma, usually begin in childhood, and are found more frequently in females and in those having a family history.

The neurologic symptoms present in hemiplegic migraine are usually transient and often vary in individual patients. These symptoms may vary in severity, being mild with one attack and severe in another. The hemiplegia may consist of brief sensory symptoms, varying through moderate numbness and weakness or pronounced to the point of unconsciousness.

Headache and paresthesia occur in practically every case. Visual disturbances are present in about 90% of the cases. Weakness is present in half the patients, as are speech disturbances. Unconsciousness is not as commonly seen as these other symptoms.

The paresthesia accompanying hemiplegic migraine is usually described as a tingling or numbness, often resulting in poorly coordinated movements. The hand is usually the most commonly involved location. Other areas involved (but to a much lesser extent) are the face and the leg.

The neurologic symptoms reach their peak in only a short time, usually within 10 minutes or so. The duration of the symptoms varies from 1 to 24 hours in most cases. However, in some cases they may persist for as long as a week, but this is not very common. Usually attacks which have the greater duration are associated with a marked weakness and tend to occur less frequently.

The visual disturbances associated with hemiplegic migraine consist of teichopsia, homonymous hemianopia, diplopia, blindness, or central scotoma. Speech disturbances associated with this condition are usually dysphasia, but occasionally a slurring dysarthria may be present.

Hemiplegic migraine is usually not fatal, but if brain damage should result, death can occur.

In hemiplegic migraine a diminution of consciousness is not uncommon. This usually occurs at the height of the actual headache. This tends to come on rather slowly and may be present for up to an hour or less. Full unconsciousness may occur, but it is very infrequent. If it does occur in patients with hemiplegic migraine, it may be preceded by blurred vision, slight vertigo, and/or sweating.

According to Heyck,[1] hemiplegic migraine should not be considered as a disease heterogenic from classic or common migraine. Its classificatory separation is justified only from a clinical point of view. It is not true that hemiplegic migraine mostly runs in families with hemiplegic migraine. It runs in families with ordinary migraine as often as common or classic migraine does.

As mentioned, hemiplegic migraine has a family history in its symptomatology. Young and associates[2] traced it in four successive generations of a family. In this family four individuals had hemiplegic migraine and at least seven others had common migraine. The two adults with hemiplegic migraine had in addition Usher's syndrome (retinitis pigmentosa and sensorineural deafness) and nystagmus; one also had mild ataxia. The two children with hemiplegic migraine had nystagmus but not ataxia or Usher's syndrome. The time of onset of the ataxia, retinitis pigmentosa, and deafness was such that they could not have been caused by recurrent migraine attacks. Gilbert and co-workers[3] describe a case of nonfamilial hemiplegic migraine associated with progressive multifocal retinal and macular degeneration of the "complicated migraine" variety. It is believed that this case was due to a migrainous vasospasm. The general consensus of opinion is that the pathology involved in the transient neurologic symptoms of hemiplegic migraine might be a vasospasm of the cerebral cortex. This, however, is only theoretical.

Glista, Mellinger, and Rooke[4] report a family of twenty-six, ten of whom had hemiplegic migraine. Familial hemiplegic migraine with a high incidence in the members is rare; there are few reports in the literature. They suggest that the neurologic deficit is due to focal edema which develops secondary to the vasospasm. They further point out that the ideal treatment for hemiplegic migraine should be twofold—the prevention of neurologic symptoms and the prevention of headache. Ergotamine tartrate as well as other vasoconstrictors are contraindicated. There is evidence to suggest that propranolol is an effective prophylactic in hemiplegic migraine.

Gastaut and associates[5] believe that each attack of hemiplegic migraine is accompanied by electroencephalographic anomalies. The anomalies vary considerably and concern delta activity, but a pattern emerges with a 2- to 5-second interval. The electroencephalogram shows the anomaly over the hemisphere opposite the hemiplegia, being most marked in the anterior half. Only occasionally is it found over the posterior half of the hemisphere. It is almost certain that it occurs during the actual attack, and it may last from 5 to 36 hours. Regression of the attack is signaled by depression of the alpha rhythm in the relevant hemisphere. Between attacks the electroencephalogram is completely normal.

Hemiplegic migraine is a rare type of migraine in which the headache many times may be of only a moderate severity. The neurologic symptoms accompanying this condition may actually persist long after the headache has subsided.

It is believed that ischemic episodes in cerebrovascular disease may resemble those of so-called hemiplegic migraine. Thus, when symptoms of migraine occur in patients with known atheromatous lesions or in an age group where atheroma is likely, the possibility of a migrainous mechanism operating against a background of cerebrovascular disease should be considered.

The treatment of this condition is symptomatic. The antiserotonin compounds are often found to be effective. As these patients become older (assuming that they have their onset in childhood) the attack may become less severe and frequent, and a more characteristic picture of regular migraine may result.

BASILAR ARTERY MIGRAINE

Basilar artery migraine is another migraine variant. This condition occurs primarily in females under 35 years of age. A family history is present in 75% of these cases.

Basilar artery migraine was initially described by Bickerstaff[6] in 1961.

The attacks of this condition begin with a bilateral loss or partial loss of vision which is of short duration. This is followed by vertigo, tinnitus, ataxia, dysarthria, and occasional bilateral tingling or numbness in the toes and fingers. These symptoms persist for usually less than an hour and after their disappearance, the headache begins.

The headache of basilar artery migraine is usually quite severe, throbbing, and located in the occipital area. It is not a generalized type of headache, nor is it hemicranial. Vomiting usually occurs with the headache.

Between attacks, these patients are symptom-free. Sharf and Bental[7] present four cases of basilar artery migraine, three in women in their forties and one in a woman aged 37 years. The main symptoms were frequent attacks of severe pain at the back of the head and neck, vertigo with tinnitus, nausea and vomiting, visual disturbances such as photophobia, scintillating scotomas, nystagmus, hemianopias of various patterns, and sometimes total transient blindness. In all four cases, no neurologic residua were found after the attacks, nor any disturbances emanating from the inner ear (audiometric or vestibular).

According to Bickerstaff[6] the symptoms depend on transient ischemia in the region of the basilar artery, contrary to typical migraine attacks, in which the carotid artery is affected.

The visual disturbances, amounting at times to total transient blindness, depend on an impaired blood supply in the posterior cerebral arteries. In every case of sudden appearance of basilar symptoms, migraine should be suspected as the cause.

Classic migraine is due to disorders of carotid blood flow, but basilar artery migraine arises from disturbed circulation in the basilar artery.

Kramer[8] believes that the transient neurologic deficits are attributed to impaired circulation in the posterior fossa due to congenital dysplasia of the basilar artery. Most of the observed symptoms and signs can be accounted for by transitory hypoxia of the distal part of the dorsal thalamus.

Golden[9] reported eight children with recurrent attacks of neurologic dysfunction referable to the brainstem and cerebellum. The episodes occurred suddenly, cleared completely, and left the patient without residue. The most frequent signs were ataxia, alternating hemipareses, and vertigo. The majority of patients were girls and most had the onset of the condition prior to the age of 4 years. Headache was definitely present in three children and possibly present in four. A history of migraine was obtained in seven families, accounting for sixteen affected relatives. Fifteen of these were female and fourteen were related on the maternal side.

CAROTODYNIA

Carotodynia was initially described in 1927. It is associated with the presence of tenderness over the carotid arteries in the neck. It is related to overdistention, relaxation, and an increase in pulsation in the carotid artery.

This condition is actually a syndrome of vascular neck pain which has no age range. Most cases, however, are seen in persons between the ages of 40 to 50. It is more commonly seen in females, and many of the patients give a history of having vascular headaches prior to the appearance of carotodynia.

The pain is usually unilateral and centered around the carotid bulb, radiating up along the course of the carotid artery, behind the mandible to the postauricular area. The pain may go to the opposite side of the neck.

While the pain is not severe, it is of a chronic nature and may be continuous for a matter of several days or weeks. The etiology of this condition is unknown. Some believe it to be a migraine variant.

Treatment consists of using such drugs as the ergotamine tartrate preparations orally. Propranolol may be useful. The use of the steroids may be beneficial.

Patients with carotodynia sometimes need reassurance that the disease is not serious. This plus the analgesic type of medication may be enough to bring about a satisfactory result.

ABDOMINAL MIGRAINE

To the average patient there is more to the symptomatology of migraine than just headache. Most migraine patients usually suffer from abdominal symptoms (gastrointestinal symptoms) and also ophthalmic symptoms. Nausea is usually present. Other symptoms of abdominal origin may consist of vomiting (the second most frequently found gastrointestinal symptom), bloating, abdominal pain, and even occasionally diarrhea. In some patients the abdominal symptoms may often be more troublesome than the actual headache itself.

Some researchers like to distinguish different forms of migraine. If the abdominal symptoms are more pronounced than anything else, they call it abdominal migraine. In the same way, when the ophthalmic symptoms are the most prominent part of the picture, it is called ophthalmic migraine. Regardless, they all represent migraine, call it what you may.

The episodes of abdominal pain may be one of the chief symptoms of the case, and it may be a headache equivalent.[10,11]

It is not unusual to see some authors refer to this type of migraine attack as a form of abdominal epilepsy. Attempts have been made to differentiate between abdominal migraine and abdominal epilepsy.[12,13] Abdominal epilepsy is an uncommon cause of recurrent abdominal pain and/or other epigastric symptoms occurring uniquely in children or young adolescents.[14] There is often quite a bit of confusion in the medical literature between abdominal migraine and abdominal epilepsy.

Abdominal migraine is a subject which seems to be rather sadly neglected in the medical literature when it is compared with the abundance of articles found on migraine and even ophthalmic migraine.

Symptomatology

In the abdominal form of migraine, there may be violent pain in the upper abdomen, in the hepatic area. This may, at times, simulate biliary colic. The vomiting and retching in these cases are incessant. In some severe instances, there have been reports of latent jaundice[15] in which the scleras assume an icteric tint and the bilirubin, when checked by the van den Bergh method, is found to be elevated, as is the icteric index, but not enough to overstep the renal threshold. The urobilinogen in the urine may become markedly increased in some of these cases.

Usually, constipation is the rule rather than the exception in most cases of abdominal migraine. The spasticity of the bowel in abdominal migraine is invariably intensified during an attack. This condition can often be mistaken for some form of gallbladder pathology, and because of this, no doubt, there have been many innocent gallbladders removed in surgery following the mistaken diagnosis. If such is the case, it would certainly fall under the heading of unsuccessful cholecystectomies, because the biliary symptoms will reappear after the gallbladder has been removed. This mistaken diagnosis can be prevented if the physician takes the time to take a good history. In the history the physician will find that the attacks will usually begin with headache and constipation and that, in contradistinction to biliary colic, the abdominal pain develops subsequently and follows in the wake of the of the cranial symptoms. In abdominal migraine, the cranial pain experienced does not radiate to the back and to the shoulder, as is often the case in the pain associated with gallbladder disease.

In a typical case of abdominal migraine, we might expect to find severe vomiting. This is seen more often in younger individuals, in adolescents, or even in children. It is so severe at times that it often may have hysterical manifestations. As might be expected, there is frequently a family history in these cases of abdominal migraine.

These attacks seem to have a more or less sudden onset and terminate in like manner. The attacks usually will persist for 24 hours or even as long as 3 to 4 days. There are epigastric tenderness and severe abdominal pain.

In abdominal migraine a striking feature is the fact that the disorder is not limited to the head, but if may manifest itself in a widespread disorganization of bodily functions.[16] There may be polyuria and even diarrhea present, and also chilliness, edema, vertigo, and abdominal distention. There may also be tremor and pain in the extremities in these patients. Frequently they have the usual migraine personality make-up. Some of these cases do not present much of a headache problem or the frequently found prodromal symptoms.

The gastrointestinal tract, not the cranium, is the chief target in these cases. However, the diagnosis will indicate that the mechanism of abdominal migraine is similar to that of the classic migraine attack. Abdominal migraine is generally seen in a younger age group than is classic migraine. It is more commonly seen in children, adolescents, and young adults. The head pain in abdominal migraine, when it is present, is of the same type as in classic migraine but of a less severe nature. The pain is throbbing, periodic, and hemicranial. As in classic migraine, with the abdominal migraine patient we usually find a negative x-ray of the skull and sinuses, negative electroencephalogram, negative general physical examination, and negative eye grounds and neurologic examination.

Carroll[17] made some interesting observations on the electroencephalogram in abdominal migraine. He found that while there is no specific EEG pattern diagnostic of abdominal migraine, a large proportion of children suffering from this condition may exhibit one or more of the following features in the electroencephalogram:

1. Posterior temporal or temporal slow wave activity in excess of that normally seen in the age range
2. Generalized slow wave activity, which can be paroxysmal, in excess of that seen in the age range
3. Spike/wave complexes which may be generalized or confined to the temporal regions, expecially the posterior temporal areas
4. Positive photosensitivity

Lundberg[18] observed that recurrent attacks of abdominal pain occur in migraine sufferers but not in patients with tension headaches. This supports the suggestion that both migraine and abdominal pain may have a common etiology in these patients. Abdominal pain is a frequent complaint. The clinical features, the duration, the interval between attacks, the occurrence of headaches and abdominal pain together, and the results of treatment will indicate whether the attacks of abdominal pain are migraine equivalents.

Bille[19] found that of seventy-three school children with migraine, aged 9 to 15 years, forty-eight had digestive symptoms and fifteen had paroxysmal attacks of abdominal pain. He regarded this as a manifestation of autonomic dysfunction, but stated that this may also be found in other "psychosomatic diseases." It appears that recurrent attacks of abdominal pain are more common in childhood migraine but this occurs also in adults.

To establish the diagnosis of abdominal migraine certain factors seem to be necessary. Usually there is the family history and the patient presents a history of either classic or common migraine. In abdominal migraine the patient has recurrent attacks of abdominal pain which are identical in character, and between the attacks there is no symptomatology referable to the abdomen whatsoever. The abdominal pain usually persists for several hours and for at least 1 to 2 hours. These abdominal pain attacks usually begin before the age of 40 and are predominately seen in the female patient, just as is ordinary migraine. The pain in the abdomen is primarily experienced in the upper portion of the abdomen.

Farquhar[20] points out that abdominal migraine may be referred to in the literature as various other conditions. He states that considerable interest has been shown in the condition variously known as cyclic vomiting, abdominal migraine, abdominal epilepsy, or the periodic syndrome. By whatever name it may be called the clinical manifestations are of a remarkable constancy, consisting of recurrent attacks of abdominal pain, vomiting, and headache, occurring alone, consecutively, or in combination. Laboratory investigations and radiologic examination seldom help in the diagnosis, which remains in doubt unless this syndrome is recognized.

Recurrent abdominal pain can be a manifestation of migraine in children. Nonspecific abnormalities of the electroencephalogram may be present. All patients with migraine have tenderness on palpation in the right upper abdominal quadrant, but no explanation for the pain mechanism is at hand.

Treatment

In treating abdominal migraine the same formula as prescribed for classic migraine should be followed. There should be the usual practical psychotherapy, which should consist of some good sound advice by the physician to the patient. The patient's activities should be reorganized so that the stimulus which may be causing his troubles can be avoided or its effects be minimized if it cannot be completely avoided. This emotional guidance is very important.

If any abnormalities are noted in the general physical examination, they should be corrected. The improvement of general health is vital in all cases of migraine, whether it be classic, abdominal, or ophthalmic migraine.

The symptomatic treatment of the attacks is the same as for classic migraine. The oral preparations, however, are rather useless because of the severe gastric disturbances, namely, the nausea and severe vomiting. The rectal suppository, Cafergot-PB, can be used if diarrhea is not present. The injectable preparation, DHE-45, is more useful than Gynergen because it produces fewer gastric side effects. With all of the gastric symptoms present in abdominal migraine, the addition of any gastric side effects in the treatment program would merely be adding insult to injury.

The use of sedatives helps in these cases, as do antispasmodics of the gastrointestinal tract. Such preparations are best given rectally or by injection.

In treating abdominal migraine, Suckling[21] describes patients with this syndrome who were treated in a variety of ways including the use of chlorpromazine, glucose, and miscellaneous dietetic restrictions, such as use of citrus fruits, pork, and chocolate, but with no particular success.

After diagnosis the patients were maintained on a low oxalate diet. All foods containing more than 10 mg oxalate per 100 gm (such as oranges, chocolate, cocoa, tea, and rhubarb) were forbidden; foods containing less than 10 mg oxalate per 100 gm (such as bananas, pears, cabbage, and lettuce) were permitted in small quantities; and oxalate-free foods such as meat, fish, eggs, milk (less than 500 ml per day), lemons, and bread were unrestricted.

Within 3 weeks all patients showed an improvement and migraine attacks were abolished, to recur only when a forbidden item of food had been taken. After 6 weeks the dietary items in the second category (less than 10 mg oxalate per 100 gm) were restored, and thereafter items in the first category (more than 10 mg oxalate per 100 gm) were restored individually (except chocolate and oranges). After 3 months it was usually possible to restore the diet to normal without any ill effects.

Although the administration of oxalate (10 to 2,000 mg per day) to nonmigrainous subjects does not cause ketosis, it is suggested that in migraine sufferers a genetic defect altering succinic dehydrogenase could result in relatively low doses of oxalate precipitating ketosis. This would explain the vomiting. The headache may result from an undue sensitivity to oxalate in the brain.

The occurrence of headache simultaneously with abdominal pain strengthens but is not necessary for the diagnosis of abdominal migraine. A surgical cause for abdominal pain should be excluded before the patient is treated with antimigraine medication which is usually successful in abolishing the recurrent attacks of abdominal pain.

SUMMARY

Symptoms and signs	Treatment
1. Family history	1. Histamine
2. Sudden onset	2. DHE-45
3. Sudden termination	3. Sedatives
4. Duration–1 to 4 days	4. Cafergot-PB suppositories
5. No fever	5. Antispasmodics
6. Severe nausea and vomiting	
7. Epigastric tenderness	
8. Pain of a cutting type	
9. Constipation	
10. Vertigo	
11. Chilliness	
12. Severe abdominal pain	
13. Other symptoms of migraine	
14. Polyuria	
15. Abdominal distention	

OPHTHALMOPLEGIC MIGRAINE

J. D. CARROLL

Ophthalmoplegic migraine is an uncommon condition which can occur in all age groups. It may develop in a patient who has had common or classic migraine for many years, or it can be the first manifestation of this disorder. It is the term applied to recurrent attacks of unilateral headache associated with partial or complete paralysis

of the oculomotor nerve. Less commonly, the abducens or trochlear nerve is involved, and rarely all three nerves are involved giving rise to a total external ophthalmoplegia. When the oculomotor nerve is only partially involved, there may well be only some difference in the size of the pupils, defects in divergence and convergence, and loss of accommodation.

The ocular palsy is transient or short-lived at first, but with later attacks the paralysis may persist for days or months and rarely may become permanent. The headache always precedes the extraocular paralysis by some hours or indeed it may not develop until the headache subsides. Symonds[22] concluded that the paralysis tended to occur at the stage of dilation of the artery. Partial or complete paralysis of the ocular nerves only occurs if the headache lasts longer then 24 hours. Rarely there can be a period of some days between the onset of a prolonged headache and the development of the palsy.

The headache is invariably situated behind or above one or other eye and is gnawing or boring in type. It is never a paroxysmal throbbing pain. The ocular palsy develops on the side of the headache but is sometimes bilateral. If the headache is very severe there are often associated symptoms of nausea, vomiting, and vertigo. The usual visual disturbances associated with migraine may precede the headache. The attacks occur at intervals of months or years but with repeated attacks there is a tendency for the intervals between attacks to become shorter.

It has been observed that an elevated protein level and an abnormal number of lymphocytes may be found in the cerebrospinal fluid of some patients after an attack of ophthalmoplegic migraine. However, the constituents of the fluid are found to be normal if the lumbar puncture is repeated a few days later. The cause of these abnormal findings in the fluid is not known.

It can be extremely difficult to differentiate between ophthalmoplegic migraine and an aneurysm on the bifurcation of the internal carotid artery or the posterior cerebral artery when the former condition presents for the first time, even in a patient who has a previous history of classic or common migraine. It is common practice in such cases to perform a carotid angiogram to exclude with absolute certainty the presence of an intracranial aneurysm. Meadows,[23] however, clarified the position somewhat when he stated that multiplicity of attacks, a frequent onset in childhood, and the complete recovery of the ocular palsy, at least in the earlier attacks, were all unusual features in intracranial aneurysm. There is also the relevant clinical observation that with an aneurysm, the pupil on the affected side is always fixed and dilated, whereas in only a small proportion of patients with ophthalmoplegic migraine with a third nerve palsy is the pupil similarly affected.

The relationship of ophthalmoplegic migraine to common or classic migraine was always considered in the past to be dubious, for it was believed that the paralysis was due to the effects of an aneurysm which compresses the ocular nerves. However, angiography has always failed to show such a lesion on the vascular tree.

Alpers and Yaskin[24] described two patients with this condition in whom a carotid angiogram failed to show an aneurysm. One of these patients subsequently died and an autopsy showed that the vascular tree was normal and, in particular, there was no aneurysm present. Ostfied and Wolff[25] suggested that ophthalmoplegic migraine was the result of pressure exerted on the ocular nerves by greatly dilated, thickened, and edematous arterial walls, together with persistent edema associated with such headaches. Bickerstaff[26] made an interesting point when he drew attention to the angiogram in which a localized constriction on the internal carotid artery within the cavernous sinus on the affected side is seen in some patients during an attack and not when the attack abates. He believes that the condition is due to localized arterial spasm.

Table 5-1. Analysis of permanent cranial nerve palsies

Patient	Sex	Nerve	Number of attacks prior to onset of permanent palsy
1 (A. B.)	F	Third	16
2 (C. K.)	F	Third	11
3 (S. H.)	M	Third	12
4 (M. K.)	F	Fixed pupil	9
5 (J. S.)	M	Fixed pupil	13

It is, however, relevant to record that Walsh and O'Doherty[27] had suggested that the appearances in the angiogram of such patients was due to edema which develops in the arterial wall, rather than spasm with consequent narrowing of the lumen.

There have been alternative suggestions for the ophthalmoplegia by other workers over the years. These have consisted of constriction of the small vessels to the ocular nerves in relation to the attacks, or actual edema of the orbital contents. There has also been unlikely suggestion that there is edema of the brain itself causing shift of the uncus which as a result impinges on the oculomotor nerve in relation to the attacks.

I have had a very great interest in this form of migraine and so analyzed in detail a personal series of twenty cases of this condition which were fully investigated from 1966 to 1973.

Third nerve	10
Third, fourth, and sixth nerves (complete external ophthalmoplegia)	2
Third and sixth nerves	1
Fourth nerve	2
Sixth nerve	1
Fixed pupil	4

General review of these cases shows that the oculomotor nerve was the most common ocular nerve affected by the paralysis. The clinical courses of the various cranial nerve palsies were studied and they show that 25% of the cases were left with a permanent palsy.

Table 5-2. Lumbar puncture: cerebrospinal fluid findings (normal, 18; abnormal, 2)

Patient	Sex	Day	Cerebrospinal fluid			
			Pressure	Protein (mg/100 ml)	Polymorphonuclear leukocytes	Lymphocytes
1 (D. K.)	M	2	Normal	120	0	18
		6	Normal	35	0	2
2 (C. P.)	F	2	Normal	95	0	20
		5	Normal	30	0	3

Transient palsies	15
Permanent palsies	5
Third nerve	3
Fixed pupil	2

Detailed analysis of these palsies showed that each patient had to experience quite a number of attacks before being left with a permanent lesion (Table 5-1). It is clearly advisable to investigate patients with ophthalmoplegic migraine. These investigations should include hematology, radiographs of skull and chest, electroencephalography, brain scan, and lumbar puncture. A carotid angiogram should be included if the patient has not had this investigation before and especially after the first attack to exclude, with absolute certainty, an intracranial aneurysm. The rise of protein and the cellular response in the cerebrospinal fluid, which can occur in the early stages following an attack in a small proportion of cases, should also be taken into account in the diagnosis of the condition (Table 5-2).

This variant of migraine is just one more manifestation of a condition which in recent years has produced a resurgence of interest both from the clinical and research angles.

RETINAL MIGRAINE

Another so-called migraine variant is the retinal migraine. This was described by Carroll[28] in 1970.

Retinal migraine is defined as an uncommon condition usually presenting in a young adult with recurrent episodes of unilateral or bilateral impairment or loss of vision, lasting for a matter of seconds or up to 10 minutes as a maximum. The episodes may be triggered by a bright light. Headache and preceding fortification spectra are absent. Typical migraine may or may not coexist. There is a relatively high incidence of permanent complications, including permanent field defect or total blindness, and optic atrophy.

The differential diagnosis includes internal carotid artery insufficiency, retinal vessel emboli, giant cell arteritis, and other diseases of arteries including syphilis, diabetes, and collagen disorders.

The patient is usually a young adult and is subject to recurrent attacks of complete loss or dimness of vision either unilaterally or bilaterally without prior fortification specta. Although visual distrubance may affect both eyes, one eye is always involved predominantly. Such episodes can often be brought on by a bright light and can vary in frequency and severity. The visual disturbance usually lasts no longer than 10 minutes but in rare instances it can persist for an hour or more. The unusual feature is the invariable absence of headache, making the diagnosis of a possible migrainous basis for the visual symptoms very difficult. However, the patient may complain of typical attacks of migraine at other times, although the visual manifestations without headache may predominate, whereas in other patients the visual disturbances may be the sole manifestation of a possible migrainous predisposition to migraine.

The visual field disturbances of retinal migraine are almost always reversible, but nevertheless permanent complications are more common in this form of migraine because of the intraocular pressure. The probable cause of the permananent disability is considered to be due to retinal ischemia following constriction of ophthalmic rather then retinal vessels, producing a fall in intraocular blood pressure.

Retinal migraine is indeed a rare condition.

CERVICAL MIGRAINE
Etiology

The bony deformities of degenerative cervical arthritis may cause distortion and compression of the vertebral arteries which results in an impairment of vertebral blood flow. Therefore, in certain patients cervical arthritis plays an important role in producing the various clinical manifestations of vertebral artery insufficiency, including severe, intermittent headache. This was initially suggested by J. Barre[29] in 1924. He believed that cervical arthritic deformities might produce vascular compression resulting in ischemia of the medulla with resultant motor dysfunction.

Cervical spondylosis is an important cause of vertebral artery compression leading to the clinical syndrome of vertebrobasilar insufficiency.

The distribution of the vertebral arteries and the sympathetic plexus is such that in certain postures an osteophyte may readily compress the artery. Irritation of the sympathetic plexus per se may cause a reduction in blood flow. Congenital absence or malformation of the vertebral arteries (which is not uncommon) can be a further predisposing factor.

Disorders of the cervical spine are thought by Blumenthal[30] to be a not uncommon cause of headache. He believes that if history and physical examination provide no explanation for chronic headache, a careful search should be made for disorders of the cervical spine. Stretching or tearing of the supporting ligaments or tendons at the fibroosseous junction may have occurred, followed by malalignment of the articular facets, muscular spasm and

atrophy, and reflex vasomotor and autonomic interference. The resulting cycle may cause headache and associated symptoms for many years.

Symptomatology

In 1926, M. Barre described a "syndrome sympathetique cervical posterieur" which consisted of occipital headache, vertigo associated with head and neck movements, and visual and auditory symptoms.[31] He claimed that the primary disturbance was irritation of the vertebral sympathetic nerve plexus by cervical arthritic deformities, with secondary alteration of blood flow through the intracranial vessels supplied by the plexus.

It was not until 1948 that Bartschi-Rochaix[32] established the name "migraine cervicale" to designate the syndrome of headache, auditory symptoms, paroxysmal vertigo, scotomas, and pain and sensory changes in the arms occurring as late sequelae of cervical trauma.

Many patients with migrainous headaches are seen whose complaints are referable to disorders of the cervical spine. Mechanical lesions of the cervical nerve roots and disturbances of the vertebral arteries are thought to be chiefly responsible. Triggering causes include postural anomalies such as prolonged typing and working with compressed air tools. The pain is often associated with circulatory disorders of the arms and hands.

Treatment

A surprising number of intractable chronic headaches respond to a complete regimen of treatment to alleviate muscle spasm, to relax and break up scar tissue and adhesions, and to realign the facets.

Jackson[33] states that it can be said with certainty that many headaches are the result of disorders of the cervical portion of the spine and that treatment directed to the cervical spine will, in most instances, give relief of the pain in the head as well as the neck and its related structures.

Sheldon[34] found in a study of so-called migraine headaches that cervical nerve root compression is very important as an etiologic factor. He points out that the chiropractors, osteopaths, masseurs, and neuropaths have been treating headache and its associated variegated symptoms with therapy directed toward the cervical spine area for years. Medical doctors may be either reluctant to or possibly afraid to admit the truth of the sometime success of these fringe therapeutic groups. To a great degree their success lies in the medical profession's neglect of the patient with headache caused by cervical spine pathology.

In dealing with this condition Dutton and Riley[35] state that although treatment with cervical traction has been successful in the past (and may be of diagnostic value), surgery is recommended after full radiologic and angiographic investigation. The surgery could be cervical fusion, excision of the offending osteophyte, or both.

Rahn[36] reports good results in treating this condition with the preparation Venopyronum, which contains extract of horse chestnut, rutin, and cardiac glycosides. The vasotonic properties of horse chestnut extract and its favorable effects on vascular permeability have been demonstrated empirically.

Braaf and Rosner[37] believe that trauma produces a mechanical derangement of the structures of the cervical spine which may involve the cervical nerve roots, the cervicocranial autonomic system, and/or the vertebral vessels. Compression of these structures, even on an intermittent basis, may result in headache and a wide range of other symptoms.

They say that cervical traction is specific for headaches of cervical origin, and is the simplest and most effective method. If all other conservative methods of treatment have failed to give the patient adequate relief of headache, myelography of the cervical spine may be advisable, followed by cervical laminectomy, if indicated.

Cervical migraine is a relatively rare condition. Despite this there seems to be a wide variance of opinion as to the effective form of treatment program to be employed. Most headache authorities believe that cervical spine abnormalities play only a minor role in the production of headache.

HARRIS' MIGRAINE

In a report on migraine Bickerstaff described what he called the periodic migrainous neuralgia of Wilfred Harris. This was initially described by Harris in 1926. Ten years later Harris termed this condition "ciliary neuralgia."

Actually, this form of headache is a variant of migraine and is an involvement primarily, if not entirely, of branches of the external carotid artery. These patients all seem to have personality patterns comparable to patients having classic migraine. Most patients seem to have their attacks on the right side. Many patients believe that muscular activity drains off whatever is causing their pain.

This condition is also referred to as migrainous neuralgia in the medical literature. Some researchers believe that this condition is actually the same thing as histaminic cephalalgia (cluster headache); however, it is similar but not the same entity.

Symptomatology

The syndrome is characteristic in its symptomatology and signs but nevertheless it frequently is initially unrecognized when seen.

The condition is seen more frequently in males than it is in females, and it usually begins between the ages of 30 and 50.

The pain is very severe but the duration is relatively short, usually a few minutes to up to 1 hour. The pain is the constant boring type, usually located lateral to one eye. The pain, however, may spread and eventually involve the remainder of the cheek, forehead, temporal scalp, and occasionally even the neck.

The pain is unilateral and it is usually on the same side.

In cases of Harris' migraine the patient cannot recline. This is in contrast to the average case of a typical migraine attack. In these cases, there definitely seems to be a relationship between the pain and the muscular activity that it occasions.

On the side involved there is usually congestion of the conjunctiva. In some cases, on the side involved there is stuffiness of the nostril.

Few patients experience any vomiting. In some cases there is a flushing of the forehead and cheek on the side involved.

Many cases of this type have typical trigger mechanisms as are found in trigeminal neuralgia. Some of these are the act of chewing, washing of the face, or brushing the teeth.

These attacks tend to occur at approximately the same time of the day or night. The patient usually has an attack every day or night for several weeks and then is free from attacks until another series of attacks occurs. Between attacks, the patient is perfectly well.

Many patients have previously had a more classic form of migraine in their history.

Treatment

Harris' migraine is relieved symptomatically by using ergotamine tartrate, usually 0.25 mg injected intramuscularly three times a day for 5 days. Occasionally a slightly larger dose (0.5 mg) may be required. These injections are discontinued, gradually because on occasion sudden withdrawal of the drug will produce a generalized type of headache.

This condition seems to actually be a variant of histaminic cephalalgia in which there is little or no periodicity (cluster). It is rather uncommon and actually would be less than 10% of the total cases of histaminic cephalalgia.

Harris' migraine may often be found to be difficult to diagnose differentially from such conditions as trigeminal neuralgia, temporomandibular joint syndrome, acute glaucoma, retrobulbar neuritis, cranial arteritis, or diseases of the paranasal sinuses or the teeth. However, if the symptomatology is known, these conditions can clearly be ruled out.

Usually this condition may be treated both symptomatically and prophylactically just as a case of ordinary migraine. The ergotamine preparations are drugs of choice. They may be given by injection, by mouth, by rectum, by inhalation, or sublingually.

In cases where medical prophylactic treatment fails, surgical procedures may be attempted, but they also are not very effective. Such procedures as section of a greater superficial petrosal nerve along with neurolysis of the trigeminal sensory root has been used. Another surgical procedure used in this condition which is not entirely satisfactory is resection of the greater superficial petrosal nerve or division of the intermediate nerve.

None of these surgical procedures seems to be satisfactory; they are only used as a last resort.

MISCELLANEOUS VARIANTS

Articles appear in the medical literature in which a new type of migraine is described. These usually represent a small group of patients who vary from the usual case of migraine. The authors of these articles group these cases and call them a migraine variant.

Examples of this are as follows.

Familial prosoplegic migraine

Familial prosoplegic migraine is extremely rare. It consists of migraine associated with paresis of the facial nerve. There is recurrent facial paralysis often alternating from one side to the other. It is sometimes accompanied by paralysis of other cranial nerves or brainstem lesions.

The paralysis is usually over the lower part of the face. This could indicate central origin of the pathology. The pathology involved is probably a segmental arterial constriction. Compression of the cranial nerves by edema of the artery walls (internal auditory artery) and compression of the facial nerve in the facial nerve canal also occur.

Cardiac migraine[38]

Cardiac migraine consists of actual migraine accompanied by chest pain. The chest pain in this small segment of migraine is believed to be due to the same type of arterial spasm which produces migraine. The fact that both migraine and angina may be treated with the beta-blocking agents is interesting in these cases. The term "cardiac migraine" has been used in cases in which there is the combination of angina with a negative coronary arteriogram, positive exercise test, and migrainous headaches. The arterial vasoconstriction is believed to be due to sympathetic overactivity, but the exact details of this remain unknown.

Biliary migraine

Many patients complaining of biliary disorders also complain of headache. Serious liver diseases, however, seldom are accompanied by headache. Headache, often of the migrainous type, is seen in cases of viral hepatitis and in cases of gallstones. However, these conditions are very unlikely to be the causative etiology of migraine.

Complicated migraine

Complicated migraine is defined as migraine having prolonged episodes of focal cerebral deficit associated with or occurring independently of the headache.

There are no established regimes of treatment for a prolonged attack of complicated migraine, but ergotamine tartrate may be helpful.

The prognosis of complicated migraine occurring in infancy is less favorable than the prognosis of the usual childhood migraine case. This is due to the fact that retardation, seizures, or other disorders may be involved.

Classic migraine is seen when transient focal cerebral dysfunction is present. These dysfunctions may become prolonged. The exact cause of this condition remains unknown.

Recurrent headache problems which do not fit into any obvious classification often present a problem both diagnostically and therapeutically. Many cases of this type may actually be an atypical case of migraine or a migraine variant.

Because of the difficulty in diagnosing cases of this type, the patient afflicted with this type of headache often becomes depressed and despondent. These cases present a difficult problem; the physician must apply more effort and diligence to give the patient the desired relief.

Weil's dysrhythmic hemicrania

Weil's dysrhythmic hemicrania has similar characteristics of common migraine but also there are associated paroxysmal variations in the electroencephalogram. These variations consist of type 1 tracings, with groups of 50 to 500 mv delta and theta waves; type 2 tracings, which have a 6 to 8 cps spindle of 100 to 150 mv occasionally mixed with slower components; and a type 3 tracing, which has a marked response to hyperventilation.

Isolated visual migraine

Isolated visual migraine is the term Rydzewski and Pozniak-Patewicz[39] give to the condition characterized by visual symptoms of a positive and a negative character. They claim the positive character manifests itself mainly by scintillating zigzag lines that spread outward from the paracentral area of the field of vision toward its periphery. The negative character consists of a bilateral central or paracentral scotoma. On occasion blurred vision may persist for a short period of time, and on rare occasions a permanent bilateral hemianopia or even blindness may occur.

Rydzewski and Pozniak-Patewicz claim this condition is encountered in young adults, either occurring spontaneously without cause or being brought on by bright lights. In most of these cases these eye complaints are the only complaints, but in about 40% they alternate with typical attacks of migraine. The prognosis of this condition is usually good but in some cases permanent visual field deficits may develop or optic atrophy may even occur. The etiology of this condition is probably a periodic transient ischemia.

Occlusive migraine

Occlusive migraine is a rare form of migraine. Actually this may be considered to be more of a complication of migraine rather than a migraine variant.

This condition occurs when there is an occlusion of one of the cerebral arteries, which may be any vessel from the ophthalmic artery to the posterior cerebral artery.

Symptoms besides headache may be scotomas, blurred vision, temporary loss of vision which may become permanent, and homonymous hemianopia.

In these cases, the vasoconstriction and reduced cerebral blood flow are the etiologic factors responsible for the neuro-ophthalmologic prodromes. However, it is impossible to predict which patients will develop a permanent visual loss or neurologic dysfunction.

If a patient with migraine has a marked visual loss or pronounced neurologic deficits prior to the actual headache attack, it is wise not to prolong the vasoconstriction phase of the attack. In other words, the use of vasoconstrictive drugs such as ergotamine tartrate and methysergide should be avoided.

Fortunately, this is a rare condition or complication of migraine, because little, if anything, can be done about the visual loss.

Focal migraine[40]

Occasionally in the medical literature there are articles referring to focal migraine. This condition is not commonly seen; in fact, it is extremely rare.

This condition is usually seen initially in children or in adolescents.

Focal migraine usually has a prolonged history of recurrent headaches accompanied by a family history and transient cerebral symptoms. These cerebral symptoms may consist of a unilateral paresthesia, motor or mixed aphasia, and hemiparesis.

Along with the general nervous disorders these cases often have major electroencephalographic abnormalities present. The electroencephalographic changes may be recorded as slight to moderate generalized involvement with focal signs which show up in the form of a delta focus. These electroencephalographic abnormalities are often suggestive of some severe lesion which may simulate a severe vascular deficit or even a neoplastic tumor.

Neurologic defects may actually be seen rather infrequently. However, if they are present they may be persistent for several weeks. If they are present arteriographic studies should be done to aid in the diagnosis. The diagnosis in these cases may often cause some difficulties because the first attack is usually seen in childhood.

REFERENCES

1. Heyck, H.: Varieties of hemiplegic migraine, Headache **12:**135-142, 1973.
2. Young, G. F., Leon-Barth, C. A., and Green, J.: Familial hemiplegic migraine, retinal degeneration, deafness, and nystagmus, Arch. Neurol. **23:** 201-209, 1970.
3. Gilbert, G. J., Rappaport, A., and Trump, P.: Retinal degeneration in hemiplegic migraine, Headache **14**(2):77-80, 1974.
4. Glista, G. G., Mellinger, J. F., and Rooke, E. D.: Familial hemiplegic migraine, Mayo Clin. Proc. **50**(6):307-311, 1975.
5. Gastaut, J. L., Giraud, J., and Saint-Jean, M.: Electroencephalographic manifestations of hemiplegic migraine, Rev. Electroencephalogr. Neurophysiol. Clin. **5**(1):23-28, 1975.
6. Bickerstaff, E. R.: Basilar artery migraine, Lancet **1:**15-17, 1961.
7. Sharf, B., and Bental, E.: Basilar artery migraine, Harefuah **86**(7):361-362, 1974.
8. Kramer, W.: Basilar artery migraine, Ned. Tijdschr. Geneeskd. **114**(25):1037-1042, 1970.
9. Golden, G. S., and French, J. H.: Basilar artery

migraine in young children, Pediatrics **56**(5):722-726, 1975.

10. Blumenthal, L. S., and Fuch, M.: Abdominal migraine, Am. J. Proctol. **8**:370-379, 1957.

11. Catino, D.: Ten migraine equivalents, Headache **5**:1-11, 1965.

12. Hagberg, B.: Abdominal migraine in children, Acta Paediatr. **46**:645-646, 1957.

13. Prichard, J. S.: Abdominal pain of cerebral origin in children, Can. Med. Assoc. J. **78**:665-667, 1958.

14. Babb, R. R., and Eckmas, P. B.: Abdominal epilepsy, J.A.M.A. **222**(1):65-66, 1972.

15. Diamond, J. S.: Migraine—pathogenesis and treatment, Med. Rec. **139**:634, 1934.

16. Friedman, A. P.: The migraine problem, N. Y. State J. Med. **49**:1831, 1949.

17. Carroll, J. D.: The EEG in abdominal migraine, International Migraine Symposium, Bergen, Norway, June 1975.

18. Lundberg, P. O.: Abdominal migraine—diagnosis and treatment, Headache **15**:122-125, 1975.

19. Bille, B.: Migraine in school children, Acta Paediatr. **51** (Suppl.): 136, 1962.

20. Farquhar, H. G.: Abdominal migraine in children, Br. Med. J. **1**:1082-1085, 1956.

21. Suckling, P. V.: The management with a low oxalate diet of abdominal migraine in children: with a note on oxalate metabolism, S. Afr. Med. J. **48**(3): 89-92, 1974.

22. Symonds, C.: Migrainous variants, Trans. Med. Soc. Lond. **67**:237, 1951.

23. Meadows, S. P.: Intracranial aneurysms, Mod. Trends Neurol., p. 391, 1951.

24. Alpers, B. J., and Yaskin, H. E.: Pathogenesis of ophthalmoplegic migraine, Arch. Ophthalmol. **45**:555, 1951.

25. Ostfield, A. M., and Wolff, H. G.: Studies on headache; participation of ocular structures in migraine syndrome, Mod. Probl. Ophthalmol. **1**:634, 1957.

26. Bickerstaff, E. R.: Ophthalmoplegic migraine, Rev. Neurol. **110**:582, 1964.

27. Walsh, J. G., and O'Doherty, D. S.: A possible explanation of the mechanism of ophthalmoplegic migraine, Neurology **10**:1079, 1960.

28. Carroll, D.: Retinal migraine, Headache **10**(1): 9-13, 1970.

29. Barre, J. A.: Troubles pyramidaux et arthrite vertebrale chronique, Medecine **5**:358, 1924.

30. Blumenthal, L. S.: Injury to the cervical spine as a cause of headache, Postgrad. Med. **56**(3):147-152, 1974.

31. Barre, M.: Sur un syndrome sympathetique cervical posterieur et sa cause frequente: arthrite cervicale, Rev. Neurol. **45**:1246, 1926.

32. Bartschi-Rochaix, W.: Le diagnostic de l'encephalopathic posttraumatic de l'origine cervicale (migraine cervicale), Praxis **37**:673, 1948.

33. Jackson, M. D.: Headaches associated with disorders of the cervical spine, Headache **6**:175-179, 1967.

34. Sheldon, K. W.: Headache patterns and cervical nerve root compression—a 15 year study of hospitalization for headache, Headache **7**:180-188, 1967.

35. Dutton, C. B., and Riley, L. H., Jr.: The cervical migraine, not merely a pain in the neck, Am. J. Med. **47**(1):141-148, 1969.

36. Rahn, E.: Treatment of cervical migraine with venopyronum, Munch. Med. Wochenschr. **114**:992-994, 1972.

37. Braaf, M. M., and Rosner, S.: Trauma of cervical spine as cause of chronic headache, J. Trauma **15**(5):441-446, 1975.

38. Leon-Sotomagor, L. A.: Cardiac migraine, Angiology **25**(3):161-171, 1974.

39. Rydzewski, W., and Pozniak-Patewicz, E.: The syndrome of isolated visual migraine, Neurol. Neurochir. Pol. **24**:181, 1974.

40. Beck, U., and Manz, F.: Focal migraine in childhood and adolescence, Arch. Psychiatr. Nervenkr. **215**:407-416, 1972.

CHAPTER 6

Other types of vascular headache

MUSCLE CONTRACTION (TENSION) HEADACHE

In the past, the term "tension headache" represented many different clinical entities to various physicians. However, most of these individuals will agree that tension headache results from sustained contraction of the skeletal muscles of the head and of the neck.

In 1962 tension headache was classified as muscle contraction headache by a committee on classification of headache.[1] This committee defined muscle contraction headache as an ache or sensation of tightness, pressure, or constriction widely varied in intensity, frequency, and duration. They stated that the ambiguous and unsatisfactory terms "tension," "psychogenic," and "nervous" headache refer largely to this group. They further stated that it is associated with sustained contractions of the skeletal muscles in the absence of permanent structural change, usually as part of the individual's reaction during life stress.

The muscle contraction headache is one of the most common of all headache syndromes. Many so-called tension headaches have a combined muscle contraction element and a vascular element. The term is used to include a majority of the types of chronic recurring headaches, regardless of the cause.

Years ago Ogden[2] stated that tension is a factor in all headaches, and that the classification of a headache type as being a "tension headache" is too all-embracing to be definitive.

Throughout the past few years the problem of tension headache has been prominently exploited to the American public. This has been done primarily through the advertising employed by various companies in the pharmaceutical industry. These companies are using the media of television, radio, and the newspapers daily to show how their product is the finest preparation on the drug market for the symptomatic relief of tension headache. If the American public were to believe everything they see, hear, and read about the effects of these various preparations, they should be quite confused because each preparation is claimed to be the best of its kind. Many new preparations have been introduced to the tension headache patient for the relief of his pain.

Muscle tension headache may be a primary condition, or it may be secondary to other forms of headache. Patients who experience a sustained head pain may produce a chronic state of tension in the musculature of the head and neck which can be a secondary source of pain in the areas involved. This was shown by Simons and co-workers.[3] Tension and spasm of the muscles along the back of the neck is a cause of pain in these patients. Such muscle contraction is, in some cases, the primary factor causing the headache in some of these cases. However, in other patients the headache may be secondary to a sustained vascular headache; if so, the pain will tend to develop somewhat toward the end of the attack and will cause a further prolongation of the headache discomfort.

Wolff and Wolf[4] in various experiments on this form of headache concluded that sustained muscle contraction would produce the headache. However, if there is in addition vasoconstriction of the arteries, the severity and the duration of the skeletal muscle contraction necessary for the production of the headache are far less, and at the same time the severity of the headache from the muscle contraction is much greater.

Headache sufferers frequently experience stiffening of the muscle at the back of the neck as an accompaniment of sustained headache. Such muscle tension pain is not limited to the tension headache patient but develops during the course of sustained headaches of other types as well. This residual muscular pain may persist even after the initial headache has been terminated by specific treatment.

Etiology

Muscle contraction headache may often be due to an axiety-tension state. When this condition exists the muscles are in a state of hypertonicity for a prolonged period of time. Some muscle tension headaches may actually be of a psychogenic origin. Other muscle tension headaches may be occupational in origin.

Possibly the cause of this type of headache is a reduced blood supply which is brought on by a vascular reflex constriction. This constriction results in the production of ischemia with the end result being the headache.

A general increase in muscle tone often accompanies anxiety, emotional distress, and apprehension. This mechanism can be a cause of muscle tension headache.

It has been shown that the pain in tension headache is caused by prolonged, excessive contraction of the muscles of the head and neck. These vigorous contractions have been demonstrated by recording of the action potentials (electric measurements) from these muscles. When a muscle remains long in contraction it develops areas of local spasm and tenderness. Neck muscle (nuchal) contractions pull taut the fascia (galea) underlying the scalp and produce tension on its anterior supraorbital attachment. Thus occipitonuchal and/or frontal localization of pain is most common.[5]

Headache may be a complaint in practically any mental or nervous disorder. If the pain is caused by unconscious sustained contraction of the voluntary muscles of the scalp and neck, it is known as tension headache. The emotional component of muscle contraction headache usually is uncovered readily. The syndrome is caricatured by the anxious, fearful, overworked, and underpleasured housewife, unhappy in a drab existence that appears to have no resolution.[6]

Lance and Curran[7] state that many cases of persistent and chronic tension headache may actually be caused by hidden depressions or mixed anxiety and depressive states, with the depression being paramount.

In describing tension headache Blumenthal and Fuchs[8] point out that some of the leading factors which may be responsible for this emotional disturbance are occupational, financial, sexual, domestic, social, physical, allergic, or endocrine.

Patewicz[9] studied the electromyographic examinations of neck and temporal muscles with various types of headache. She states that "cephalgic" muscular spasm appears to be a consequence rather than the cause of headache. Perhaps it is an expression of a psychosomatic defensive reaction which protects the patient against provocation or exacerbation of headache by excessive movements of the head.

The results of this investigation do not support the assumption that there is a specific type of headache of muscular origin. Spasm of the head and neck muscles occurs in all types of headaches both during the attacks and in the headache-free interval. This spasm as judged by the amplitude of action potentials in temporal and neck muscles is even less intense in so-called tension headaches.

Martin[10] believes that emotional conflicts are often manifested by way of increased contraction of skeletal muscles in the head and neck to produce muscle contraction headache. The vast majority of headaches are vascular headaches (migraine type), muscle contraction headaches, or a combination of these two types. Emotional factors appear to be of significance in most of them. The particular nature of the psychologic difficulties may be highly variable.

Williams[11] believes that a much more frequent cause of headache arising from muscles of the head and neck is the "continued muscle tension which is secondary to an anxiety state, which is usually termed as anxiety tension state." When a person is in this anxiety-tension state, the shoulder and neck muscles are maintained in a state of hypertonicity. After the muscles are in this hypertonic state for a prolonged period of time, an occipital headache will occur. This type of headache in the occipital area often will radiate toward the vertex of the head.

Some of these muscle tension headaches may actually be of a psychogenic nature.

Williams[12] states that a chronic state of tension in the postural muscles of the head and neck will produce a deep referred type of pain.

Muscle tension headache may be associated with an infectious disease, such as scarlet fever or typhoid fever. It is common for some diseases such as these to produce pain in the musculature of the neck and of the head.

It is common to see a spasmodic condition of the musculature of the neck in cases of arthritis of the cervical spine.[13] This is frequently seen as a protective mechanism. In such cases the pain will originate in the neck and will migrate to the occipital area of the head. Any excessive movement of the head will tend to increase the pain in such a condition.

Cervical neuralgias may also give rise to a state of muscle spasm or muscle tension. In many cases of cervical neuralgia, muscular contraction and tenderness of the musculature of the involved area are quite frequently seen.

Some researchers[14] have pointed out that they believe the cause of this type of headache is primarily a reduced blood supply, which is the result of a vascular reflex constriction. This in turn results in the production of ischemia and the end result is the headache.

The daily work of some individuals tends to force them to hold the head in a particular position for long intervals of time. Muscles are not designed for continuous tonic contraction. The average individual frequently changes the position of the head and transfers the strain of holding the head erect from one muscle group to another and prevents the accumulation of substances capable of irritating the nerve endings subserving pain. This is an automatic process for most people as they go about their daily chores.

In fatigue headache there is a tendency for the head to be maintained in one position. This type of headache frequently occurs among truck drivers, typists, operators of business machines, and the like who may hold the head in a more or less rigid position throughout the day's work. This headache frequently can be relieved by an explanation of its cause, pauses at intervals for muscular relaxation, and local application of heat and massage. Muscle spasm can be the primary cause of head pain in telephone operators or in a salesman driving for miles with the window open and getting a stiff neck. More often muscle spasm is secondary to some other condition, such as acute cervical strain, cervical arthritis, diskogenic disease of the cervical spine, or occipital neuralgia or is part of a migraine or tension headache attack.[15]

Irritation and spasm of the muscular elements at the back of the head and neck can produce muscle tension headache. The same tissues can go into spasm from any heightened emotional condition such as anxiety, apprehension, fatigue, fear, guilt, resentment, or frustration.

An increase in innervation of the skeletal muscles accompanies anxiety, so that in anxious patients attempting to relax, not only will muscle tension be greater than in a healthy person, but those patients with most clinical evidence of anxiety and tension will have the most muscle tension, and the physiologic mechanism underlying the common symptoms of anxiety is increased muscle tension. This was brought forth in a study by Sainsbury and Gibson[16] of the relations between the symptoms complained of by anxious patients and the activity of skeletal muscles.

Severe jarring or jolting of the head may frequently result in a tenderness and in a stiffness of the musculature of the head and of the neck, and in turn this may produce a muscle contraction type of headache.

It is common to find that alcoholic beverages may precipitate an attack of muscle contraction headache.

Marmion[17] believes that reflex spasms of the musculature in the neck and head may occur as a result of painful lesions in these areas and that the spasm may, in itself, give rise to further pain. Muscle contraction headache resulting from spasm may be confused with the muscular soreness frequently seen in the terminal stages of a migraine attack.

A general increase in muscular tone often accompanies anxiety, emotional tension, and apprehension, and this mechanism can be a common cause of headache.

Muscle contraction headache may also be a secondary headache in such conditions as nasal sinusitis, dental pathology such as diseased teeth, acute ear infections, or certain forms of ophthalmologic pathology. Occasionally it is seen in the so-called temporomandibular joint syndrome.

Nervous tension is one of the most important and one of the least understood components of the headache syndrome. Nervous tension and periods of anxiety give rise to a state of vessel hypertonicity. That the muscle contraction type of headache belongs to the vascular group of headaches is generally agreed. Horton and associates apply the term "tension headache" to a commonly occurring type of head pain that is caused by heightened nervous tension and occurs immediately following such an episode.[18] Liddell and associates[19] believe that some tension states are in fact epilepsy, possibly latent at the time of examination. They also point out that the epileptic prodrome is likewise a tension state, lasting a day or so and being relieved by the epileptic discharge. These patients have a lower hormonic response to photic stimulation. This type of headache belongs in the vascular group because the headache is not caused by the nervous tension per se, which gives rise to a state of hypertonicity (vasoconstriction), but by the hypotonicity (vasodilation) which follows.

The muscle contraction headache patient will usually show a definite relation between the headache and a stress situation. Another factor that may play an important part in the development of this type of head pain is physical fatigue. Because of this, muscle contraction headache is frequently found among members of the medical profession. It is not uncommon for the physician to do excessive work while fatigued and under severe nervous and emotional strain. The headache in such a case usually occurs in the letdown phase which follows the stress situation, without any associated psychogenic disturbances.

These headache patients will usually give

no specific hereditary factor in their histories. These patients usually will state that the pain develops without any prodromal symptoms. There are no prominent ocular symptoms preceding the actual headache phase, such as are found in the migraine type of head pain. However, there are underlying emotional disturbances present, and, because of them, the patient must learn to make adjustments to those situations or to minimize their effects.

From all of the facts presented we can see that the etiology of muscle contraction headache is quite varied and can actually be of multiple causes.

Symptomatology

As a rule, the symptoms of the muscle contraction headache will depend on the emotional state of the patient. Because so many conditions can produce muscle contraction headache, the general picture can be widely varied.

The muscle contraction headache is usually of a continuous type, not intermittent. It may occasionally be seen in the temporal muscles and in the frontal muscles to a small degree, but primarily it affects the musculature of the neck and of the occipital area. Naturally these muscle tension headaches can be either bilateral or unilateral, depending on the musculature involved in each case. However, the majority of muscle contraction headache problems are found to be bilateral.

The character of muscle contraction headache is usually a dull, steady ache; it is not the throbbing type of pain. The pain is usually described by the patient as being deep. The duration of the headache can vary from a matter of a few hours to several days. The variation, again, is due to the many different types of conditions which can produce this type of headache.

Frequently there will be associated tenderness at the points where the involved muscles are inserted. This may result in painful and tender nodular formation, with an accompanying sensation of stiffness.

Some of these cases have a psychogenic basis. If this is the situation, the symptomatology may be bizarre. The description of the headache may be extremely variable in such cases.

In many cases of muscle contraction headache the symptoms may be increased in severity by the movement of the musculature which is involved.

This type of headache usually comes on gradually, not suddenly, and as a rule the attacks tend to terminate in a like manner.

The patient with a muscle contraction type of headache will usually have normal physical findings and will generally reveal no organic basis for the headaches.

If nervous tension is present in these cases, a typical history shows that the headache will come on at the end of an excessively hard working period. Quite often the pain will come on several hours after the patient has finished his work, when he has left his work problems behind him, and is relaxing at home or even asleep. This may be very confusing to the patient, but this again shows that the actual headache attack is due to the secondary state of hypotonicity which results from the vascular fatigue, and not to the state of hypertonicity which usually prevails during the period of nervous tension. The hypotonicity leads to vasodilation of the cranial vessels, with the result that the adjacent pain-sensitive areas are stimulated.

As for the general characteristics of the typical muscle contraction headache pain, it is usually found to spread over the entire head and quite frequently is most severe in the occipital area. The patient will frequently describe his pain as a tight band around the head, which seems to become increasingly tighter. The pain is nonthrobbing and of a dull character. The severity of the attack is often seen to vary, and the attacks may be rather periodic and recurrent in nature. There are usually no gastrointestinal upsets associated with these headache attacks, which in itself is a great difference from the classic migraine type of headache, in which there is almost always nausea and, very frequently, vomiting. There are usually no nasal or ocular symptoms present.

It is common to find an element of tension in migraine headache cases. However, the symptomatology of the muscle contraction headache per se and that of the migraine headache are entirely different.

The age incidence of this headache group has a very wide range and is definitely not an important factor.

Blumenthal and Fuchs[20] describe three distinct types of head pain. One type of pain feels as if the head were in a vise, causing a constricting pain in the forehead. The second type of pain, according to Blumenthal, is located in the vertex of the head and feels as though the top of the head had been blown off. The last type of pain is located in the occipital area of the head and is often accompanied by muscular stiffness in the neck.

Both the history-taking and the observation of the patient should help the physician to evaluate the patient's nervous tension. The presence of nervous tension serves to illustrate the importance of treating the patient, not merely the headache. If they are not both attacked at the same time, there will be no success in the therapy administered.

No drug will be entirely effective until the etiologic significance of nervous tension has been fully determined by the physician and thoroughly explained to the patient. The physician must help the patient to recognize the situations and activities in his daily routine which result in nervous tension. This undertaking must be done very skillfully and tactfully. The patient will resent or be especially sensitive to any implication that the reaction is "all in the head."[21]

If an anxiety state exists, these patients may also exhibit the symptom of dizziness. This may result from hyperventilation, which is frequently found to be a conditioned reaction to the state of anxiety. If persistent hyperventilation should exist,

tachycardia and palpitation may occur which may be associated with faintness and a sensation of tightness in the chest.

Anorexia is commonly found in cases of muscle contraction headache. This is especially true if there is an excessive emotional tension factor involved in the case.

The patient with muscle contraction headache is very often found to be of the perfectionist personality type and one who is unable to adapt to situations encountered in his average home life or working environment. He is often a rather nervous person who is very conscientious in his work and his daily pattern of life. The basic factor in the etiology of the muscle contraction headache problem is that the patient does not know how to relax and rest. Because of this, nervous tension will develop, and this in turn will bring about the physiologic reaction which produces the headache attack.

Nervous tension may result when a person who has an inadequate personality attempts to respond to any extraordinary demands. The physician has a duty to help the patient to recognize the limitations of his nervous system and how he might live within these limitations. Perhaps the patient will be unable to understand the situation which is the stimulus of his headache attacks. On the other hand, the patient may be unable to meet the demands of the situation if he does recognize it. It is important that both the physician and the patient realize the role which tension plays in the production of headache in each individual case.

Because of the physiologic mechanism behind the tension type of headache, these patients may often be awakened at night by the headache attacks. They will usually not find it necessary to get out of bed immediately because of the pain; they are more likely to be restless in bed. If they do get up, it is not until several minutes have passed. This is a marked distinction between the muscle contraction type of headache and the pain of histaminic cephalalgia, in which the patient is forced to get out of bed almost immediately because of the severity of the pain.

In the average case of headache, the etiologic significance of nervous tension is all too frequently overlooked. This may be chiefly due to a poor history of the case or too much significance being placed on the results of the physical examination and the laboratory tests which are ordered.

In speaking of the emotional aspects of chronic tension headache Weiner[22] points out that one may think of chronic tension headache as the end result of a psychoneurotic response to anxiety created by various stresses. It is important to note that headache appears to be but one of many symptoms in a multisystem complex and not simply a psychophysiologic disorder. The patients with tension headache have a higher frequency of family history of headache, history of head trauma, somatic complaints (neuromuscular, gastrointestinal, cardiorespiratory, gynecologic, and general review of systems), problems of everyday living (particularly marital and financial difficulties), and work problems.

Headache of conversion reaction is thought to be clinically indistinguishable from classic muscle contraction headache. The conversion reaction usually meets the immediate needs of the patient and is associated with obvious secondary gain.[23]

Bakol and Kaganov[24] believe that many patients have trouble describing precisely the location of the head pain. Although functional headache is usually discussed in terms of muscle contraction or migraine, clinical observation suggests that many patients show symptoms associated with both classes of headache.

There is also variability in the site of head and neck pain symptoms among patients with muscle contraction and migraine headaches. Thus, a muscle contraction headache sufferer might experience pain predominantly in the forehead, one or both sides of the neck, the back of the head, behind the eye, or any combination of these and other locations.

In describing muscle contraction headache Friedman[25] believes that it usually causes no problem in diagnosis and is clearly differentiated from migraine. However, many patients with migraine will also have muscle contraction headaches between their attacks of migraine.

MacNeal[26] states that any headache occurring "all day, every day" for a period of 1 year without demonstrating objective changes to the examiner is almost certainly a tension headache. This headache practically never awakens a patient from a sound sleep. He may awaken for some other purpose and find that the head hurts, however. The psychodynamics of tension headaches of sufficient severity or frequency to represent disability is most likely to be repressed hostility. This hostility is always directed against persons who should be "loved." These individuals are usually parents, siblings, spouse, child, God, employer, or self. This hostility creates such strong guilt feelings that it must be repressed and, by the time this recurring headache has driven a patient to consult a physician, the source and object of the feelings have been "forgotten." Such patients are likely to suffer also from varying degrees of depression.

Patients usually present a normal blood pressure. The urinalysis and routine blood tests are also usually negative. Skull x-rays and nasal sinus x-rays are negative, as are the electrocardiogram and electroencephalogram. Therefore, the taking of a complete, thorough case history is important in these cases.

Treatment

In treating muscle contraction headache the causative agent should be removed. If there is any focus of infection causing the disturbance, it should be removed. If there is any psychogenic element present, psychotherapy should be employed. The patient should be shown that there is an emotional factor involved and should be reassured that there is no form of organic pathology present and that he will be able to master the condition by readjusting his own handling of his daily problems.

If the condition is due to a patient's occupation, which requires the holding of his head in one particular position, as in the case of a stenographer or a machine worker, the only logical solution of course, is for the individual to change jobs. However, this is not always an easy thing for a person to do satisfactorily, and if the patient cannot make this readjustment, he must be instructed how he may shift the strain on the musculature of the head from one group of muscles to another.

If the condition is primarily one that is basically due to the presence of an anxiety tension state, it can often be overcome by reassurance and readjustment. The placing of the patient in an occupation which will distract him from his state of anxiety will also be helpful.

The treatment of this syndrome requires very careful judgment. The physician must weigh the risks against the possible benefits of therapy, depending largely on the severity and frequency of the symptoms. An occasional tension headache may be safely relieved by any simple analgesic and sedative combination. Attempts to prevent more frequent episodes should be made with gentle tranquilizers or mixtures of these with antidepressant medications. Appropriate warnings in referene to automobile driving and other dangerous occupations should always be issued when these medications are prescribed.[26]

Probably the basic approach to treatment of chronic tension headache involves the concept that it is an overt manifestation of a psychoneurotic state. Use of analgesics and proper psychopharmacologic agents such as antidepressants when depression is present is important, but the physician's support in the patient's attempt to overcome environmental stresses and to make personality adjustments is invaluable.[22]

During the various states of fatigue, exhaustion, and nervousness, physicians commonly prescribe rest and relaxation without instructing the patient in a technique by which such relaxation may be obtained. Physical therapy, especially hydrotherapy and light generalized massage, will often give marked relaxation. Patients frequently volunteer the information that marked relief has been obtained from a facial massage.

Bernik[27] states that tension headache arises in states of continuing emotional crisis. It is generally bilateral and accompanied by various symptoms. It varies in frequency and duration. The cause of tension headache, as of migraine, is unknown, but it usually arises from psychologic pressure due to economic, social, physical, or intellectual problems. The aim of treatment is to lessen the emotional tension. This is often within the scope of the general practitioner, but some patients require formal psychiatric treatment. The actual symptoms may be treated with analgesics and sedatives.

Chronic headache is a serious problem and requires careful and adequate management. Both physiologic and psychologic aspects must be considered; both are necessary for recovery.

Most muscle contraction headaches are linked with either muscular contraction or changes in the caliber of the cranial blood vessels. Treatment must take into consideration the selection of the proper medication, the mode of administration, and the dosage and tolerance.

Practically speaking, once the diagnosis of muscle contraction headache has been established, the physician should immediately decide on the type of therapy which would be most effective for the patient. Of course, this will vary with each individual patient depending on the etiology involved with the case. There are three different forms of treatment programs which may be used: psychotherapy, drug therapy, and physiotherapy. One of these or any combination of the three may be used.

In the average case, the help of a trained psychiatrist is not needed for psychotherapy. Any physician can usually accomplish this by taking the time and the effort. Martin[50] states that psychotherapy may vary from supportive or gentle reassurance to more formal intensive psychotherapy by a psychiatrist. If the patient is well motivated and insightful and if such care is available, the more intensive approach may be most curative. It seems that all such patients can benefit from psychotherapy; however, the nature of such therapy will vary greatly.

Among the important psychologic considerations are the patient's personality, the physician-patient relationship, environmental factors, and the symbolism of medication to the patient.

In using drug therapy for the treatment of muscle contraction headache, the analgesics (such as Fiorinal, Empirin Compound, Phrenilin, and aspirin) and/or muscle relaxants are useful. The use of tranquilizers may also prove to be of benefit, depending on the etiology of the case. Drugs are used to counteract the muscle spasm in the case involved and its painful vascular consequences. Addictive drugs should not be used for muscle contraction headaches.

In speaking of drug therapy for muscle contraction headache, Martin[10] says that drug therapy may be helpful but is rarely of permanent benefit. Mild tranquilizers, especially those with muscle-relaxing qualities, often are used as an effective adjunct. If depression is significant, a trial of antidepressant therapy may be helpful. Mild analgesics may be used for the symptomatic treatment of an ache in the head or the neck. Analgesics and sedatives are of greater help when they are used in combination. Narcotics should never be used for the treatment of muscle contraction headaches.

A new analgesic, ibuprofen (Motrin), is reported to be effective for the relief of muscle contraction. It appears that as far as the relief of muscle contraction headache is concerned, there is very little difference between ibuprofen and aspirin. One drug seemed to produce as good a result as the other. The same can be said for side effects. Both drugs seemed to produce very little in the way of side effects, and those produced were mild. The placebo seemed to produce as severe and as many side effects as either of the active drugs, but it was not as effective as the two active drugs as far as relief of pain was concerned. In conclusion, this investigation merely proved that ibuprofen was as effective as aspirin in relieving muscle contraction headache. Neither drug produced much in the way of side effects, and none which was either severe or incapacitating.[28]

Such muscle relaxers as orphenadrine citrate (Norflex) are often helpful in obtaining relief from the pain of muscle contraction headache. Orphenadrine has proved to be a useful adjunct in the treatment of any type of head or neck pain in which skeletal muscle spasm is a factor. The drug acts on the higher levels of the central nervous system, interfering with reflex pathways for pain and skeletal muscle contraction. Thus, orphenadrine relaxes skeletal muscle spasm but does not reduce the general tonus of skeletal muscles.[15] Orphenadrine gave good to excellent results in 73% of twenty-six patients with tension headaches.[29] Use of an analgesic was required in addition in some cases. Use of opiates is contraindicated except in emergencies because of the addictive potential.[29]

There have been numerous reports in the medical literature which claim that meprobamate (Equanil) is useful in cases of tension headache. Meprobamate is said to act to alleviate both the underlying anxiety and the tension of the head and neck muscles associated with tension headache. Some report that this drug is also useful in the prophylactic phase of tension headache therapy. However, we have found this drug and others of a similar nature to have an extremely limited value in this type of case. Many of the authors who report good results in treating the symptoms of tension headache with meprobamate also report almost as satisfactory results with the use of a placebo.

Amitriptyline has also been reported in the medical literature as being effective in the treatment of muscle contraction headache. Diamond and Baltes[30] did a double-blind randomized clinical evaluation of the comparative efficacy of 10 mg and 25 mg of amitriptyline against placebo in the treatment of depressed and/or anxious patients with chronic tension headaches. Eight target symptoms, one of them being headache, plus a global evaluation were measured. The 10 mg of amitriptyline showed statistically significantly larger reductions in symptom scores than placebo for all eight of the target symptoms, including a reduction in headache during the first period. The patients' overall response based on three weekly evaluations compared with a pretreatment evaluation during the 4-week course of therapy was statistically significantly better with 10 mg of amitriptyline than with either 25 mg of amitriptyline or placebo.

Lance and Curran[7] reported that amitriptyline (Tryptanol, Tryptizol, Laroxyl) is effective in treatment of chronic tension headache. Best results are in illness of long duration and in older people. Success of the drug is unrelated to its antidepressant effect but may result from vasodilation in overcontracting scalp muscles. Patients characteristically are unable to relax muscles of face, scalp, and neck. They frown, look worried, are apt to clench jaws, and cannot permit a raised arm to fall limply. Vasoconstriction occurs in the conjunctiva with frontal tension and persists as long as the headache. Overcontraction of the muscle is not limited to time of emotional crisis.

In studying the effects of an analgesic and a tranquilizer, Martins and associates[31] concluded that in patients with tension headache the administration of methyl-melubrin (methampyrone) with medazepam reduces the incidence of crises to a tolerable minimum, that it reduces their duration, and that it causes the patient to recover more rapidly. The only appreciable side effects were slight dizziness and dryness of the mouth. These effects were attributed to medazepam.

The effects of sulpiride, a thymoanaleptic neuroleptic drug of the benzoamide group, in the prevention of migraine and tension headache were studied. In cases of tension headache, the total number of days with a headache was 236 while taking the placebo but only 161 while taking sulpiride ($P < 0.001$). The frequency of days with a headache was also reduced by sulpiride ($P < 0.05$) and the duration of the headaches was significantly reduced from 7.9 to 5.4 hours ($P < 0.01$). Although the difference in the intensity of the headache was not significant, the mean number of analgesics taken during the course of sulpiride (1.5) was significantly less ($P < 0.001$) than during the placebo period (2.5). Sulpiride also significantly reduced nausea ($P < 0.01$) but not vomiting or diarrhea, autonomic symptoms, vertigo ($P < 0.05$), or psychic symptoms ($P < 0.01$). Of the thirty tension headache patients, twenty preferred sulpiride, three preferred the placebo, and seven found no difference. In the total series, sulpiride was more effective in thirty-three patients, placebo was more effective in twelve, and no clear-cut difference was found in ten patients. It is concluded that sulpiride is significantly ($P < 0.001$) more effective than a placebo.[32]

If a state of ischemia of the muscles is suspected, the use of a vasodilator such as nicotinic acid or nicotinyl alcohol (Roniacol) is indicated. It is important that nicotinic acid be used in such cases, and not nicotinamide, because the amide of nicotinic acid is not an efficient enough vasodilator to be of much value. We believe that in this type of headache problem the use of nicotinic acid is better than the use of histamine. Histamine is a better cerebral vasodilator, but nicotinic acid is a stronger vasodilator than histamine in the skin and musculature structures. In these cases we recommend giving 100 mg of nicotinic acid intramuscularly daily until the pain recurs. Then the patient can switch to the oral route of administration, taking 200 to 300 mg daily.

If the musculature is in a spasmodic state, physical therapy may help. This form of therapy is often overlooked in the treatment of muscle contraction headaches. Physiatrists can offer much relief by using muscle-relaxing techniques. Heat and massage may relax taut muscles and help relieve the ache of a chronically tense, therapeutically frustrated patient. Once temporary relief is obtained, subsequent drug or psychotherapy becomes much easier.[10] At home the patient can employ wet heat in the form of wet, hot towels. We believe that the application of wet heat is more useful than dry heat in these muscle tension headache cases. However, sometimes deep penetrating heat may be required, and in such cases diathermy is often helpful.

The muscle contraction can also be relieved temporarily by a hot bath, an ounce or two of brandy or whiskey, posterior neck and scalp massage, or 0.2 to 0.5 gm of amobarbital (Amytal) given intravenously. Isotonic neck exercises are also useful. With his hands placed on his forehead, the patient resists strong flexion of the neck for a minute or so, then resistance to neck extension is practiced with his hands folded over the back of his head, and finally inclination of the head to one side and then to the other is resisted.[16]

This form of headache is accompanied by contracture of craniocervical muscles. Electric stimulation of the muscles served by the motor roots of the cranial nerves and the first, second, and third cervical nerves is palliative. Current of low amperage with an impulse frequency less than sixty per minute is employed.[33]

Attempts to stretch the involved muscles increase, rather than relieve, the fatigue spasm, since fatigued muscles do not stretch. Conditioned relaxation and light myopulse exercise restore energy and flexibility to the muscles.

In some of cases the use of a mild sedative is helpful. In severe cases, the local injection of procaine (1% Novocain) into the tender areas may be required in order to obtain muscular relaxation. The effect of this procedure may persist for several days or even as long as 2 or 3 weeks.

Rest of the musculature involved is helpful in most muscle tension headaches.

Reducing the number of the attacks is a difficult problem and one which depends on the discovery of the ultimate causes of the patient's emotional upsets. To do this, the entire life situation of each individual patient must be taken into consideration. Each patient will differ, as there is no distinct pattern. The patient's personality must be analyzed, as should his ability to handle these conditions.

When this type of headache problem is discussed with the patient, it must be done tactfully, because this type of person can be extremely sensitive when the physician suggests that his headaches are primarily due to nervous tension. Some of these patients bluntly resent such an explanation. They often base their assumptions on the fact that their attacks awaken them from their sleep and that they certainly could not be tense while they are asleep. If this is the case, it is certainly the wise thing to explain, step by step, the physiologic mechanism of their headache attacks. A patient of average intelligence will understand this if he is honestly seeking a solution to his headache problem. The patient should be told that it is not the nervous tension per se which is causing the headache, but that this tension does result in a constriction of the blood vessels. Then it should be explained to him that while he is relaxing, as in his sleep, there is an overrelaxation of the cranial blood vessels and that it is this overdistention of the vessels that actually causes the head pain.

The psychosomatic implication in most of these patients is great, and they must be approached along the lines designed to clarify their emotional and personality conflicts.

Recently a great deal has appeared in the medical literature concerning the use of biofeedback in muscle contraction tension headache.* Actually, headache experts are divided on the effectiveness of biofeedback and the relief it affords this or any type of headache patient. Biofeedback systems measure a particular physiologic function in an individual and then feed the information back to him as visual or auditory signals. Spontaneous changes in the physiologic variable in a desired direction will thus be recognized and reinforced by the subject. This procedure will lead to some degree of voluntary control over the physiologic function itself. There are three basic areas of biofeedback research—electromyographic feedback, electroencephalographic feedback, and feedback from autonomic functions.

Volunteer patients with a history of tension headache participated in a controlled experiment for the purpose of evaluating the effect of electromyographic feedback training on the frequency and severity of tension headaches.[34] Eighteen patients were randomly allocated to one of three groups. Group A patients received electromyographic feedback training. Group B patients received "pseudofeedback"; the feedback signal produced and heard by group A patients was recorded and played back to group B patients. Group C patients received no training.

The levels of frontalis electromyograms in all groups of patients were on average double those of young healthy subjects. The mean electromyographic level for group A patients showed a sustained and consistent decrease following the baseline sessions. The mean electromyographic level for group B showed a decrease after the baseline sessions but the decrease was not as great or as consistent as for group A patients. The average headache score for both groups A and B declined over the experimental period, but only the group A difference was statistically significant. During the training period there was a high correlation between headache activity and frontalis electromyographic levels for group A patients while group B patients showed no such correlation.

Sustained contraction of the scalp and neck muscles appears to be associated with tension headache. Electromyographic feedback seems useful in the induction of muscular relaxation.[35] Budzynski and associates[36] described an electromyographic instrument and feedback training procedure which appeared to reduce both the intensity and frequency of tension headache.

In a study on the electromyographic feedback on the tension type of headache Wickramasekira[37] states that the clinical impression and the more dramatic decline in frontalis electromyogram associated with the feedback training procedure appears to suggest that the addition of response-contingent electromyographic feedback training results in a more specific and powerful procedure for the clinical management of tension headache.

Studies on patients with tension headache unrelated to neurologic or any other organic disorders have been carried out with electromyographic feedback training in which the activity of the frontalis muscle is translated into audible signals. The patients, who were trained to relax this muscle during sixteen training sessions over a period of 8 weeks, found that their condition showed significant improvement with reductions in headache and in drug requirements. This improvement appeared to be permanent.[38]

In a trial study to evaluate a simple and rapid method of relaxation training in the management of the patients with chronic headache, Warner and Lance[39] found improvement after relaxation therapy. The patient's response to a course of relaxation therapy was assessed three months after its

---

*See also Chapter 3.

conclusion. Six months after completion of the trial each patient filled in a detailed questionnaire regarding the frequency, duration, and severity of their headaches. The technique of relaxation therapy combined muscular relaxation (emphasized in the earlier training sessions) with mental relaxation. A classic conditioning technique was used, involving the use of the word "relax" as the conditioning stimulus.

Nineteen of the twenty-five patients showed substantial improvement after relaxation therapy. Seventeen either reduced or dispensed with their medication, only four reported no change, and none reported a deterioration.

CASE HISTORY

Mrs. K. A., a 39-year-old housewife, came to the office complaining of severe frontal headaches. These had been present for several months and were occurring daily. The attacks usually occurred at night, and the pain was of a throbbing nature. If she ingested alcoholic beverages, she could precipitate an attack. She also had noticed that the headaches were associated with nervous tension. On some occasions, she could obtain temporary relief with Empirin Compound and codeine (¾ grain). She had a phobia about a brain tumor causing her trouble, and this it itself helped to increase the nervous tension element. On some occasions, the headache attacks incapacitated her, and she was unable to perform her usual duties.

Her routine examinations, otolaryngologic examinations, and blood pressure were within the normal limits for a person of her age. She admitted that she was conscientious and rather tense, regardless of whether she was working or engaged in some form of recreational activity. She had never learned how to relax properly and was always "high strung." She was literally unable to live within the limits of her nervous system. Her housework at times was difficult because of several young children who would often "get on her nerves." She never had an actual vacation and was constantly going through the same daily routines. She complained of never being able to obtain sufficient rest or sleep.

Psychotherapy was administered in that the patient was reassured that there was no brain tumor present. The fact that she was not relaxing in any form of her daily routine was explained to her, and she was instructed how to relax and how to live and enjoy her life. She recognized these facts and made a quick and excellent personality adjustment, and the headache attacks soon became a thing of the past.

Symptomatically she responded to the analgesics with the addition of a muscle relaxant.

SUMMARY

Symptoms and signs

May be varied

Pain is
1. Continuous
2. Bilateral or unilateral
3. Neck area
4. Occipital, frontal, or temporal area
5. Dull
6. Deep
7. Nonthrobbing
8. Few hours to several days
9. Possibly tender to touch
10. Gradual onset
11. Gradual termination
12. Chronic periodic

Patient is
1. Conscientious
2. Nervous personality
3. Does not know how to rest or relax
4. Any age
5. Anorexic

Negative

1. Physical examination
2. Gastrointestinal symptoms
3. Nasal symptoms
4. Family history
5. Laboratory findings

Treatment

1. Removal of causative agent
2. Analgesics
3. Lessening of emotional tension
4. Muscle relaxants
5. Tranquilizers
6. Sedative, mild
7. Vasodilators
8. Biofeedback
9. Physical therapy
10. Psychotherapy
11. *Never* narcotics

MIXED TYPE OF HEADACHE

The headache problem referred to as a "mixed type of headache" probably presents more difficulties to the practicing physician than any other type. The mixed type of headache problem is characterized by having two definite forms of headache, in any combination, occurring in the same patient. For example, the patient may have a migrainous type of headache at certain times and at other times attacks of sinusitis headache. Or he may have a myalgia type of head pain and a tension headache. In other words, the patient has two or more forms of headache which may occur at the same time but more frequently occur separately.

Some call a headache problem a mixed headache (combined headache) only when it is a combination of a vascular headache (such as migraine) and a muscle contraction headache. We think that this classification is too restrictive and prefer to include any combination of headaches.

The only way in which the physician can discover the two or more separate problems is by carefully taking the case history. In doing this, the physician will note that the patient will mention that he experiences another type of headache which seems to him to be altogether of a different nature and in an entirely different location of the head. Since the patient himself may or may not be aware that he has two distinct types of head pain, the physician cannot expect too much help from the patient in this regard and usually has to determine this factor personally.

However, most patients with a mixed type of headache are aware of the fact and will tell the physician that they have two problems. When this occurs the physician actually has two case histories to obtain.

We have seen many patients with headache problems of a mixed type, who have received treatment over various periods of time, but the treatment was directed toward only one of the patient's headache patterns. Many times these patients experienced relief from this one phase of their headache problem but continued to experience pain from the second, untreated type of headache. For example, if a patient had an obvious sinusitis headache and also a myalgia problem and received treatment and relief for the sinusitis only, the pain of the myalgia would naturally continue to occur, and the patient would still be in distress. If this is not then corrected by the physician, the patient will naturally seek the advice of another physician, primarily through despair.

The symptomatology of a mixed headache will naturally depend on what two forms of headache the patient has.

The treatment program instituted after the correct diagnosis has been made also depends on the diagnosis of the two forms of headache of which the patient complains.

The patient, if he is unaware of the fact, should be given a clear explanation that two different forms of headache are present in his case. This will be a form of reassurance to the patient and perhaps explain to him why he has not had successful treatment for his problem in the past, because only one type of headache was being treated.

The best way to demonstrate the mixed type headache problem is to present a few case histories.

It is common in some vascular headache problems to find an element of hypertension in the background which acts as an independent entity and has no general bearing on the migraine problem at all. A typical case of a situation such as this is the following:

P. K., a 43-year-old white male, had experienced periodic attacks of headache since about the age of 17. His headache attacks were associated with severe gastrointestinal disturbances, always nausea and quite frequently attacks of vomiting. His head pain was of a throbbing nature and occurred on the average about once every 2 weeks and with a duration of 2 or 3 days. There was a family history of headache attacks in this case, as his mother had headaches which had many years ago been diagnosed as migraine. He located his headaches in the left temporal area and around and behind the left eye. At times, he would experience head pain which would radiate back to the occipital area, and there was always a residual soreness of the musculature of the occipital area following these attacks. Many attacks were so severe that the patient was often confined to bed for a few days.

On further questioning, he stated that the pain in the temporal area seemed to differ in many respects from the pain in the occipital area. There was no gastrointestinal upset associated with the headache in the occipital area, but the headache was quite often associated with excitement. However, the headache which was in the temporal area was always associated with nausea, occasionally with vomiting, and frequently with tension or fatigue, but not with excitement. The pain in the occipital area usually was gone on awakening in the morning, but the head pain in the temporal area persisted for 2 or 3 days and was much more severe. With the head pain in the temporal area, he noticed scotomas and was quite sensitive to light during these attacks (photophobia). However, with the occipital form of his headache problem there were no ophthalmologic manifestations.

This patient's otolaryngologic examination was negative. His general examination was essentially negative except for an elevated blood pressure of 182 systolic and 108 diastolic. This, of course, represented a condition of hypertension.

The history in this case gave a clear-cut description of two distinct types of head pain. The type of pain which this patient had been experiencing in the temporal area was a typical case of migraine. This conclusion was based on the history. The head pain experienced in the occipital area was due to the hypertension. This diagnosis was based on the history plus the physical examination, which revealed the elevated blood pressure, with everything else being normal.

This patient had to be treated for his migraine and also for his hypertension, which was handled by the referring physician. As soon as the blood pressure was lowered and brought under control, the hypertension headache also was controlled. The migraine also responded to vasodilatory treatment and to ergotamine tartrate, so both of his headache problems had been solved and the result was a happy and comfortable patient.

The big point in this case was that the patient had been treated for hypertension, and hypertension alone, as that was thought to be the sole cause of the patient's headache problem. This mistake was probably due to two prime factors. The first was that an incomplete history must have been taken because the migraine factor was very obvious in this case. The second factor, which no doubt led to the conclusion that the headaches were entirely of a hypertensive origin, was the elevated blood pressure. It was so obvious that it was too easy to accept as being the cause of the problem. The fact that this patient had had headaches since the approximate age of 17 should have

led one to search for another cause for the headaches.

Patients too frequently do not recognize that they may have a headache problem in which more than one type of headache is occurring. However, if they are aware of this fact they will help the physician tremendously because they are then able to give a rather clear-cut description of their attacks and their symptoms. By doing this, they give the physician an extreme advantage in trying to establish an accurate and correct diagnosis of the headache problem.

Many of these patients who have a mixed type of headache problem can tell the physician merely that they have severe head pain. It is only by carefully questioning the patient about this pain that the two or more separate forms of headache can be distinguished. However, with many headache patients, the only important symptom seems to them to be the severe head pain which they find hard to endure. This complicates any headache problem, especially if it is a mixed type of headache problem.

Mrs. K., a 40-year-old white housewife, had had headache attacks since about the age of 30. Her attacks were always associated with any form of temperature change. She was very susceptible to drafts, air conditioning, and cold, damp weather. Her headaches would come on gradually and increase until they reached their peak and then would gradually subside. The pain would migrate from one area of the head to the other, and she stated that the areas of the head which were involved were excessively tender during an attack. Her headache attacks were not associated with any nasal, ocular, or gastrointestinal disturbances. They were in no way associated with her menstrual periods. The pain was usually in the right temporal area, migrating to the right occipital area and down the right side of the neck to the right shoulder.

This patient had been in an automobile accident 6 weeks before the examination. Following this accident, she had become severely nervous and emotionally upset, and she was noticing that she would awaken from her sleep at night with a severe headache of a more or less generalized nature. This pain seemed to differ from that she had been having for many years. The "night headache," as she called it, was extremely severe and throbbing, whereas the pattern of the headaches before the accident had been of a general, dull, aching type. At night the pain would not migrate and was not associated with any element of tenderness. She still would have her headaches during the day, but they seemed to her to be of an entirely different nature. She was aware that there was something different about her headache attacks since the accident occurred, but she was not fully aware that she was experiencing two distinct types of attacks.

The headache attacks which she had experienced for over 10 years had all the classic symptoms and signs of myalgia of the head. For this she was given nicotinic acid by mouth, 100 mg three times a day. This, along with heat and massage, symptomatically gave her relief from the myalgia phase of her headache problem.

The physical examination, routine laboratory examinations, and otolaryngologic examinations of this patient were essentially negative. She had previously had a complete neurologic examination, and this was also negative. The headache which this patient called her "night headache," which had been occurring only since the automobile accident, was diagnosed as a tension type of headache. She was reassured that the accident had not produced any pathologic condition within her head and that emotional upset was the basis for her new type of headache. Personality adjustment was essential in this case, and she was given a mild tranquilizer (diazepam, 2 mg three times daily) to combat her emotional upset.

This patient responded very well to both phases of her headache problem. After 3 weeks the mild sedative was discontinued. She continued to take the nicotinic acid for several months, and it seemed to keep the attacks of myalgia of the head in check.

If this case had been managed only as a case of tension headache or only as a case of myalgia of the head, the results would not have been satisfactory for the patient because head pain still would have been present. However, by attacking both elements of the problem the patient was freed of her headache attacks and once again was able to enjoy a pleasant life.

A 50-year-old white male had had irregularly occurring headaches for "over 20 years," as he put it. These attacks would occur two or three times a year. The attacks would last usually less than an hour and sometimes only a few minutes. When he had one attack, he could usually expect to have one attack a day for a week or 10 days. Then there would be a period of remission for perhaps several months. His attacks would usually occur at night and would awaken him from a sound sleep. They would be so severe that they would force him to get out of bed. The pain was primarily located over the left temporal area and was always of a throbbing nature. During the attack, he would notice a nasal stuffiness on the left side and also some lacrimation from the left eye. There were no gastrointestinal symptoms associated with the headache attacks. These attacks were postural, however, and if he was in a horizontal position, the pain was much more severe.

Between these severe attacks of headache, this patient had noticed that he would experience some severe head pain in the right antral area, during and following some acute upper respiratory infections. These head pains were associated with right nasal obstruction and congestion for several days and also a purulent nasal and postnasal discharge for about a week from the right nasal passage. The right antral area was usually tender during these attacks. No ophthalmologic or gastrointestinal symptoms were associated with these attacks. The pain was relieved on a temporary basis with Empirin Compound.

This patient realized that he had two different types of headache. Of course, the two types of headache were of such an extreme difference that it would be hardly possible for either the physician or the patient to miss the diagnosis of a mixed type of headache in this case.

The severe form of headache in this mixed headache problem was easy to diagnose as histaminic cephalalgia (cluster headache). He responded excellently to vasodilatory therapy with histamine. He also received ergotamine tartrate and reassurance that something could be done for this type of severe head pain problem.

The head pains this patient associated with his acute upper respiratory infections were diagnosed as right maxillary sinusitis. In his particular case, surgical care was needed to bring about the desired results. A right nasoantral window operation was performed, and the attacks of right maxillary sinusitis were thus held in check.

From these few case histories, one can gather that any two or more types of headache can be found in an individual, and this merely tends to make the headache problem more complicated in most cases. The pitfalls of a mixed type of headache problem can be avoided if the physician takes the time to make a sufficient examination and, most of all, to get a complete case history from the patient.

A cardinal rule in the mixed type of headache problem should be that if more than one type of headache is encountered in an individual, all types should be treated independently and simultaneously.

From the few case histories just outlined, it is quite apparent why we prefer to call the combination of any two forms of headache in the same patient a mixed headache. Mixed headaches should not be limited merely to the combination of a muscle contraction headache and a vascular headache.

HISTAMINIC CEPHALALGIA (CLUSTER HEADACHE, HORTON'S SYNDROME)

On March 30, 1936, at a general staff meeting of the Mayo Clinic, Bayard T. Horton[40] first described what is now called histaminic cephalalgia. He stated that this was a new type of headache which had not been described adequately in the literature. This headache was a distinct entity in itself, classic in its symptomatology, and unique in its response to histamine. This type of headache seemed to respond to histamine treatment but not to the usual methods of treatment. Most patients with this type of headache were willing to submit to anything in order to obtain relief. Horton further stated that they had been diagnosed as suffering from everything from psychoneurosis to organic lesions, and most of them had pain of such severity that they had to be constantly watched for fear of suicide.

Histaminic cephalalgia is probably the most severe type of head pain we know. It is not nearly so frequent a headache as migraine or some other types of vascular head pain. Riggs,[41] when speaking of histaminic headache, stated that it is one of the most common types. We totally disagree with this statement. Typical histaminic cephalalgia is not a common type of headache, but it does appear frequently in the field of headache.

Horton found the majority of his patients in his first report were from 40 to 50 years of age. Today we claim that the average histamine headache patient is a middle-aged male.

Etiology

The etiology of histaminic cephalalgia is still not known. There are many pertinent facts which have appeared in the literature, but the etiology of this condition is mainly theoretical. The factors which seem to be best received by headache authorities will all be mentioned.

Horton[40] states that the attacks of pain of histaminic cephalalgia are associated with the phenomena of vasodilation. The pathogenesis of the pain lies in the phenomenon of abnormal vasodilation. As proof of this, he offers the fact that spontaneous attacks can be induced by subcutaneously injecting 0.3 ml of histamine diphosphate (2.75 mg per milliliter). If this injection is given to a patient with histaminic cephalalgia, a typical headache attack will be precipitated.

Williams[42] states that histaminic cephalalgia is based on the mechanism of a local capillary constriction and dilation in the adventitia of the wall of the affected artery. He further states that histaminic cephalalgia is associated with signs of autonomic overactivity of the homolateral side, such as nasal mucosa congestion, vasomotor rhinitis, and lacrimation.

Horton[21] states that when histamine is used as a provocative agent, the immediate reaction is a generalized histamine headache; this is a physiologic response. This will occur generally 5 to 50 minutes following the injection and is useful as a diagnostic procedure.

In studying the cerebral and ocular circulation in cluster headache, Broch and associates[43] found that electromagnetic flowmetry showed no changes in mean or pulsatile blood flow on either side during the headache attacks. They also found that dynamic tonometry showed an increase in intraocular pressure during attacks and an increased corneal indentation pulse. They suggest that a vasodilation is present in the pulsatile intraocular vascular bed during the headache attack, being more pronounced on the headache side.

In studying the cutaneous blood flow in patients with histaminic cephalalgia, Sjaastad and co-workers[44] recorded in six patients the cutaneous blood flow in the frontotemporal region of the forehead and the pulse synchronous variation in intraocular pressure during and between attacks, and he compared these results with those from twenty-two control patients. The lowest mean flow was found on the side involved during an attack. Although the mean flow was reduced during an attack, in two of the cluster headache patients flow was increased during an attack. Pulse synchronous variations in intraocular pressure were shown to increase during attacks and were associated with both increased and decreased blood flow through the skin of the forehead.

Bruyn and others[45] present the thought that dysfunction in the medulla oblongata is the etiologic factor in this type of headache. This, they claim, is brought on by an increased central alpha-adrenergic activity.

Carotid angiography was done in eighteen patients with histaminic cephalalgia by Ekbom and Greitz.[46] They found that there was a localized narrowing of the extradural part of the internal carotid artery during an attack, in the final stage of which the narrowing had spread to the upper part of the carotid canal. They concluded that these changes were possibly due to constriction and edema of the arterial wall.

Many believe that an attack of histaminic cephalalgia may be due to the sudden discharge of histamine from the body stores. If this be the case, this condition would be similar to an allergic or hypersensitivity reaction and the corticosteroids would be of value in the treatment program or the use of the antihistamines. Occasionally steroids are of benefit, but not antihistamines.

It has been observed that cluster headaches may be caused by the dilation of extracranial blood vessels, possibly due to vasodilator agents. The possible roles of histamine and serotonin have therefore been investigated by measurement of their blood levels before, during, and after attacks.

In this respect, Anthony and Lance[47,48] believe that attacks of this type of headache are associated with histamine release, but serotonin release may only be a compensatory response. Anthony, Lance, and Lord[49] further point out that in spite of the marked elevation of blood histamine during an attack of cluster headache, H_1 or H_2 blocking agents are only partly effective in preventing these headache attacks. This would mean that histamine may not play a major role in the production of this type of headache, or the blocking agents used were not of sufficiently high dosage, or these agents are not effective at all.

Sadjadpour[50] suggests that cigarette smoking may be an etiologic factor in this type of headache. We do not find this in the average case of histaminic cephalalgia. However, in less than 5% of these people we have seen some correlation between tobacco and the onset of an attack. On the other hand, alcohol is seen as a causative agent in almost 100% of these cases.

Electron microscopy studies of the blood platelets have been performed in patients with cluster headache.[51] These studies produced evidence that release of serotonin from the platelets during a headache attack cannot be demonstrated.

Sometimes in the literature histaminic cephalalgia (cluster headache) is referred to as a migraine variant. Because of the extreme difference in the symptomatology of migraine and histaminic cephalalgia, we do not accept this classification. We believe that these two forms of headache problems are two distinct clinical entities. Ekbom[52,53] also shares this opinion, as do many others. There are patients who have both histaminic cephalalgia and migraine. However, in general, the incidence of migraine in histamine headache patients is probably no different from that of migraine in the general population.

Histaminic cephalalgia and histamine headache should not be regarded as synonymous terms.[54] When histamine is used as a provocative test agent, the immediate reaction is a generalized histamine headache. This will occur in a normal person as well as in one having histaminic cephalalgia. However, in the patient with histaminic cephalalgia, reproduction of the syndrome will occur approximately 15 to 50 minutes following the histamine headache. This delayed response occurs as a pathologic response only in cases of histaminic cephalalgia.

Boies[55] states that histaminic cephalalgia is produced by a localized capillary constriction with the result being the release of histamine. He lists histaminic cephalalgia under the type of headache which results from the stretching of the pain-sensitive structures along the blood vessel's course.

The absence of trigger areas in cases of histaminic cephalalgia and the fact that the distribution is vascular and not confined to the branches of the trifacial nerve will help to distinguish the pain of these histamine headaches from the pain of tic douloureux.[56] This point is worth mentioning because we have stated that the pain of the histaminic cephalalgia attack is very severe, and we know that the pain of an attack of tic douloureux is also very severe.

There is some suggestion that in headache cases of this type there is a change of vegetative balance in a vagotonic direction during the headache phase.[57]

Gilbert[58] points out that vasodilation of a recurrent, focal, paroxysmal nature is known to underlie cluster headaches, and a similar mechanism may precipitate episodes of vertigo or tinnitus in certain young or middle-aged adults presenting the symptom constellation of recurrent paroxysmal Meniere's syndrome.

Horven, Nornes, and Sjaastad,[59,60] when studying dynamic tonometry and the corneal indentation pulse, found the corneal indentation pulse to increase in attacks of histamine headache, especially on the side of the head involved with the headache. These changes were not observed in cases of migraine. In fact, the pulse was lower in migraine patients than it was in normal control patients. This shows a pathophysiologic difference between the two types of headache.

In another study showing that these two types of headache are different and distinct entities, Sjaastad and Sjaastad[61] proved that with most migraine patients there is an excessive amount of histamine excreted in the urine during the headache-free period. However, in areas of cluster headache the urinary excretion of histamine was similar to that of normal, healthy control patients in most cases, and an increase in histamine excretion was found in only a few cases. In a similar study[61] these same authors found that the urinary excretion of histamine was increased on one or more occasions in seven of twenty-two patients with cluster headache. In six of these patients the increase appeared only on the days of the attacks. In migraine, increased excretion was found in five of thirty-one patients on days of the headache; however, on the headache-free days this occurred in seven of the twenty-four patients. Three patients showed increased histamine excretion during the attacks as well as between attacks.[62]

Symptomatology

The pain experienced by a patient suffering with histaminic cephalalgia is constant but of a very short duration. The pain begins and ends suddenly. The attacks actually persist for only a matter of a few minutes up to an hour or so, as an average, but the pain is so excruciating during these few minutes that the patient is often exhausted and fatigued following an attack.

The pain is of a burning, boring nature and as a rule always unilateral. The same patient may have an attack on one side of the head and later experience the pain of another attack on the opposite side of the head. However, the pain does not occur on both sides at the same time.

With histaminic cephalalgia there are no vasospastic phenomena or auras, and usually there are no pulsations to the pain.

The time of onset of this type of headache is of more significance than that of most other forms of headache. This may provide the clue to the classification of the headache. The typical attack of histaminic cephalalgia will occur at night, mainly during sleep. The patient is suddenly awakened from his sleep by the pain of the attack, and the pain is of such severity that he is forced to get out of bed immediately. He will then usually pace the floor in a vain attempt to obtain relief from the pain. In some cases of histaminic cephalalgia the pain is so severe that the patient rams his head against the floor or the wall. In general, it might be said of histaminic cephalalgia that the pain is far more severe and of a shorter duration than any other type of nocturnal headache.

The histamine headache patient usually cannot relate the onset of the headache to any definite cause. The attacks are more frequent when the patient is lying down, and the habit of sleeping flat without a pillow will encourage the headache to start. A few patients will obtain relief to small degrees by sitting up, but most patients must arise and walk about. Most patients normally sleep with their heads propped up with two or three pillows because they know that any position of the body which will cause engorgement of the vessels of the head will cause marked exacerbations.

There are no familial characteristics connected with histaminic cephalalgia, which in itself is quite different from the ordinary case of migraine, which has about a 50% element of family history background. This was pointed out by Ekbom,[32] Farias De Silva,[63] and many others.

The majority of the cases will not show any periodic characteristics. Most of the attacks occur at irregular intervals, with no definite pattern.

Usually these patients experience the pain in the area of the temple and the eye, and occasionally the face or neck. The signs and symptoms are limited to the distribution of the carotid arteries.

Ekbom[52] describes two different types of cluster headache, which he names the upper syndrome and the lower syndrome. The upper syndrome presents pain from the eye to the forehead, the top of the head and the temporal area, and back to the nape of the neck. The lower syndrome presents pain in the infraorbital area. The upper syndrome has an earlier onset than the lower syndrome, and in the upper syndrome there is a swelling of the superficial temporal artery whereas in the lower syndrome there is not. Ekbom bases his findings on the fact that different segments of the carotid artery are involved; in the upper syndrome the external carotid artery is involved, and the internal carotid artery is involved in the lower syndrome. He believes that both types are probably due to a stimulation of the pain-sensitive fibers either by vasodilation or vascular edema.

In most cases of histaminic cephalalgia, coincident with the onset of the pain, the patient invariably describes the onset of the phenomena of vasodilation on the same side of the head as the pain. These phenomena consist of engorgement of the temporal vessels, conjunctival inflammation, plugging of the nasal passage causing nasal obstruction, profuse watering of the eye (lacrimation), rhinorrhea, flushing of the side of the face, and an increase in the surface temperature over the eyebrow and in the frontal area.

Horner's syndrome is not uncommonly seen in patients with histaminic cephalalgia. This may remain permanently, or it may disappear after a series of attacks has ceased.[64]

Graham[65] believes that patients with cluster headache tend to have rugged leonine features and a muscular mesomorphic build. The incidence is much higher in men, and women suffering from such headaches tend to have a rather masculine appearance. The leonine facies is also a feature of patients with the carcinoid syndrome. He believes that it is possible that the constant outpouring of serotonin or bradykinin during cluster headaches is responsible for the leonine facial appearance.

Kudrow[66] did a study on the physical and personality characteristics found in patients with histaminic cephalalgia. He found the patient with this type of headache to be 2.7 to 3.2 inches taller than the control groups, to have hazel-colored eyes, and to have a higher hemoglobin concentration (16.2 gm per 100 ml blood, compared with 15.5 gm per 100 ml of blood for control persons).

Kudrow states that patients with this type of headache were all heavy drinkers and heavy smokers. Graham[65] also believes these patients to be heavy drinkers. We find that it is truly rare to see a patient with histaminic cephalalgia who will drink at all. These patients know that alcohol will precipitate a headache attack, and they actually have a fear of alcohol. They usually have not had a drink for some length of time because of this. In most of these cases, we find that alcoholic beverages will have a relationship to exacerbations of pain; however, the mere staying away from the alcohol will not prevent future attacks from occurring. Abstaining from alcohol will, however, cut down on the frequency of the attacks. Tobacco does not seem to have as strong an effect on these patients but, as a prophylactic measure, it is better for them to refrain from smoking.

Since ingestion of alcohol may precipitate an attack of histaminic cephalalgia, this is often a helpful diagnostic aid. Williams[64] believes that in addition to alcohol, the exposure to severe cold will precipitate an attack. We have failed to find much evidence of this in our cases. We believe that temperature or weather has little or nothing to do with bringing about an attack of histaminic cephalalgia.

In a study on the personality profiles in patients with cluster headache, Rogado and associates[67] found high scores on low back pain and low scores on social introversion, psychasthenia, and hypochondriasis.

Lovshin[68] claims this type of headache is more commonly seen in black males than in white males. We have not found this to be true.

A high incidence of gastroduodenal ulcer is claimed to be associated with patients with histaminic cephalalgia.[68-71] This may be due to a hypersensitivity to histamine. This relationship is obscure, but both conditions have a known tendency to periodic occurrence frequently in the spring and the fall.

Ekbom and Lindahl[57] report a case of histaminic cephalalgia in a patient with angina pectoris in which there was a marked remission of angina attacks during the headache periods. They suggest that this may mean that the periods of cluster headache are associated with a changed vegetative tone.

Jacobsen[72] presented a case of cluster headache associated with a marked sinus bradycardia during the actual headache attacks. This is indeed a rare thing to find with headache cases of this type. He believes it to be due to a parasympathetic discharge emerging from the brainstem over the third, seventh, and tenth cranial nerves.

There is absolutely no correlation in the female patient between attacks of histaminic cephalalgia and menstrual periods. However, the majority of the females afflicted with this type of headache will have a remission of their headaches during pregnancy. They also experience an exacerbation immediately following the delivery of the child. Similar symptoms in this regard are found in migraine. However, a large percent of female patients afflicted with migraine associate their headache attacks with their menstrual periods.

In a study with male cluster headache patients, Ekbom[73] studied the heart rate and blood pressure during cluster attacks precipitated by nitroglycerin. He found the heart rate to be reduced and the blood pressure to be increased (both systolically and diastolically). These changes seemed to be directly related to the intensity of the pain of the attacks. In these patients the electrocardiograms showed changes in the P waves. This may be indicative of an increased vagal tone during attacks.

Gilbert[74] claims that cluster headache and cluster vertigo may be found in the same patient, which suggests that they are a part of the same pathophysiologic process, which could be a recurrent paroxysmal focal vasodilation.

These patients do not complain of having a "sick headache" and as a rule have no gastrointestinal symptoms. Neither are scotomas and photophobia listed among their symptoms.

In many cases, compression of the common carotid artery on the side involved will give relief of a temporary nature, but when the pressure is released the pain will recur. Strong pressure over the eye and the temporal vessels will give slight relief to some patients.

Diagnosis

The diagnosis of the histaminic cephalalgia type of headache depends a lot on the taking of a good history. However, this problem is somewhat simplified if use is made of provocative tests. The failure of treatment is often due to the fact that the physician has not seen the patient in the actual attack of the head pain. The reproduction of the headache and its subsequent abortion are of great value to the physician, but this is not always possible. Both the reproduction and the abortion are of medical and psychologic significance.

In doing a provocative test, it is of utmost importance that the physician not let the patient know that he is trying to reproduce the pain. If this is the case, the results will be far more reliable because it will rule out any element of nervous tension and any degree of suggestibility to which the patient might be subject. Both the suggestibility and the nervous tension factors are unmeasurable quantities, and this may interfere with the evaluation of the particular drug which is used to reproduce the head pain. When this headache is actually reproduced it helps to establish a situation in each individual case where the physician and the patient have a common understanding of the headache. When such a reproduced attack is aborted, there is a certain element of confidence established in the patient's relationship with the physician. This confidence will give the patient some freedom from the fear and tension that developed when his attacks of pain became incapacitating and all his attempts to obtain relief were unsuccessful.

Reproducing the head pain and subsequently aborting the attack will also give the physician confidence that he or she will be able to cope with the condition and give the patient the desired relief. This will create a successful relationship between the physician and the patient in every respect.

Ekbom[75-77] advocates the use of nitroglycerin as a provocative agent in these cases. He uses 1 mg sublingually for this purpose. He claims that this will provoke an attack in 30 to 50 minutes. We generally find that histamine will work within 5 to 10 minutes.

Differential diagnosis of histaminic cephalalgia and sphenopalatine neuralgia should not be too difficult a task. If the sphenopalatine ganglion is cocainized, relief of the pain occurs while it does not in histaminic cephalalgia. On the other hand, an intravenous injection of 1 ml of DHE-45 will relieve a patient of the pain of an attack of histaminic cephalalgia in 5 minutes or so. On the contrary, it will do nothing for the pain of sphenopalatine ganglion neuralgia.

The differential diagnosis of this type of headache includes the pain of intracranial aneurysm, acute glaucoma, temporal arteritis, and sinus headache. An important point to remember is that cluster headache is the only functional headache which commonly arouses a patient from sleep. Thus, if other features typical of cluster headache are lacking, then intracranial aneurysm must be seriously considered. A tense tender bulb and funduscopic changes should distinguish glaucoma.

The history alone should differentiate histaminic cephalalgia from migraine. The same is true for histaminic cephalalgia and acute nasal sinusitis.[78] Migraine and histaminic cephalalgia can also be differentiated by electron microscopy of the blood platelets. Grammelvedt and co-workers[79] point out that during attacks of migraine the blood serotonin level has a marked drop at the onset of the attack, whereas in cluster headache no such drop occurs.

Treatment

In treating histaminic cephalalgia, as with any other type of headache, the program should be of both a prophylactic and a symptomatic nature. By that we mean that the prevention of future attacks should be one aim and the abortion of any attacks which do occur another.

PROPHYLACTIC TREATMENT

There is much discrepancy concerning the prophylactic treatment of histaminic cephalalgia. The methods presented in the medical literature include surgery, methysergide, histamine, amobarbital, psychotherapy, BC-105, and various other preparations.

Methysergide (Sansert).* Methysergide is a lysergic acid derivative, and many successful reports are found in medical literature on its use in the prophylactic treatment of histaminic cephalalgia. The usual daily dosage is 2 mg three times a day. If this dosage is successful in preventing attacks, it may be used for 8 weeks or so, and then gradually tapered. Many patients tend to become refractory to this drug after various lengths of time. However, the chief obstacle with the use of this drug is the possibility of the development of serious side effects. The most dangerous side effects encountered are retroperitoneal fibrosis or cardiac valve damage. Because of these side effects, this drug should be one of the last drugs tried in the prophylactic treatment of this or any other type of headache. The side effects which might be produced are sometimes more dangerous than the headache problem itself. This drug is often effective prophylactically but never symptomatically.

BC-105 (Sandomigran, Pizotifen).* BC-105 has been used in cases of histaminic cephalalgia, primarily in Europe.

Prusinski and Klimek[80] tried BC-105 in a series of only eight cases. They found that in six cases complete cessation of attacks

---

*See also Chapter 4.

was obtained, improvement usually taking place at the end of the first week of treatment. Side effects of general weakness and somnolence occurred in only one patient during the short time of treatment. The improvement achieved by treatment with BC-105 was usually maintained for 2 months up to 1 year. The patients were treated for from 4 to 6 weeks, starting with one tablet a day and increasing up to three a day.

Ekbom[81] found BC-105 to be a valuable alternative drug to use in twenty-eight patients in whom ergotamine drugs were contraindicated. Nelson[82] found this drug to be helpful in breaking up cluster headache. He points out that it is a much safer drug to use than is ergotamine or methysergide.

We have had considerable experience with the use of BC-105 in migraine but not in cluster headache. On the whole we found this drug to be no better than placebo in migraine, so we doubt that it works any better in this type of headache.

Histamine. The use of vasodilating drugs has been found to be effective in the prophylactic treatment of histaminic cephalalgia. The vasodilating drug we use in histaminic cephalalgia is histamine. This form of therapy is often referred to as histamine desensitization.

Histamine is a vasodilator and it will flush out the arterial loop of the localized capillary constriction which is present in these patients.

We administer histamine intravenously in a solution containing 2.75 mg of histamine acid phosphate in 250 ml of normal saline (isotonic sodium chloride). This solution is administered at a rate of 6 to 10 drops per minute on the first administration. The rate of flow actually depends on what rate of flow each individual patient can tolerate. This solution is given to the patients for 30 minutes while the patient sits up in a chair with a special arm rest. We find this position to be most satisfactory, for most of the attacks of histaminic cephalalgia occur when the patient is lying down or asleep. The patient receives this treatment daily until the cluster pattern has been broken and then the injections are gradually tapered off. If the patient tolerates the rate of 6 to 10 drops per minute, on the second visit the rate of flow is increased to 10 to 15 drops per minute. The rate is increased with each treatment until a flush or the start of a headache occurs. Then the rate is put back to the rate of the previous treatment and kept at that level. If the patient cannot tolerate 4 to 6 drops per minute and receives a headache from it, a half-strength solution is used (0.5 ml histamine acid phosphate in 250 ml saline) or even 0.25 ml histamine acid phosphate in 250 ml saline if the one-half strength solution is too strong.

It is always best if the patient's stomach is not empty when the intravenous histamine is administered, because it will cause an increase in the gastric secretion of hydrochloric acid. This route of administration is continued as long as improvement is indicated and until the patient has completely recovered.

Histamine dilates both the intracranial and the extracranial blood vessels. Histamine dilates the arterioles, venules, and capillaries. Nicotinic acid produces more vasodilation in the extracranial vessels than it does in the intracranial vessels. It is important that the physician have a thorough knowledge of the physiologic action of the drugs used in treating an organic condition.

Some researchers[83] suggest that the diet should be low in sodium in cases of histaminic cephalalgia and that the patient should abstain from any food or combination of foods that in the past may have produced the headache. We have not found the diet to be of any great significance in the cases of histaminic cephalalgia that we have seen and treated, and we believe that it is now generally agreed that both histaminic cephalalgia and migraine are not caused by an allergy.

It has also been suggested[56] that the fluid intake in these patients should be reduced. But once again we cannot see where this has any bearing on the physiologic basis of histaminic cephalalgia.

The avoidance of specific allergens by a strict elimination diet has been recommended[84] by starting on a practically starvation regimen. New foods are then added one at a time until symptoms of headache are reproduced. The foods which seem to bother the patient are then restricted from the diet. This program is continued until all of the allergenic foods are isolated. Here again histaminic cephalalgia does not have an allergic basis physiologically, and we cannot see the value of such a procedure in treating such a patient, either prophylactically or symptomatically.

If the intravenous type of treatment of these cases is not feasible, the drug may be used subcutaneously. However, this route of administration of histamine is not as successful in treating histaminic cephalalgia as is the intravenous type of administration. When using this drug subcutaneously, we employ histamine acid phosphate in a solution containing 0.275 mg per milliliter. This preparation, readily obtainable in 1-ml vials, is injected subcutaneously on a daily basis. The first dose consists of 0.1 ml. This dosage schedule may be increased in 0.05-ml increments to as high as 1 ml, but we have never exceeded this amount at any single injection. If at any time during this procedure the patient notices the typical symptoms of his routine headache attack or its prodromal symptoms within 60 minutes following the injection, the dosage is reduced to the dosage level of the day before, which did not produce these symptoms. This level is then taken as the patient's individual dosage tolerance level. For example, if the patient experiences a typical headache attack or its prodromal symptoms within 1 hour of receiving 0.45 ml, the dose the following day is cut to 0.4 ml and his injections are kept at that level in the future. If this does not occur, the injections are progressively increased until a level of 1 ml is reached. The dosage level is kept at this amount but never above it.

Horton[21] used a similar method, but he gave the patient two injections each day in place of one.

After the attacks have disappeared, it is often necessary to administer a maintenance dose for an indefinite period of time. We gradually increase the interval between the injections, cutting them from daily to three times a week, then twice a week, and gradually to once a week. Finally the injections are reduced to once every 2 weeks. If the patient at any time has an attack, the injections are given more frequently for a short period of time.

In treating these cases, along with the histamine injections, it is often helpful to give the patient nicotinic acid by mouth, 100 to 200 mg three times a day before each meal. It is important not to use nicotinamide, as it is not as effective as a vasodilator as is nicotinic acid. In fact, as far as the cerebral vessels are concerned, nicotinic acid is not as good a dilator as histamine.[83]

Hilsinger[85] believes that the prophylactic treatment of histaminic cephalalgia should consist of psychotherapy, Bellergal, and histamine desensitization. We have personally found Bellergal to be of no benefit in either the symptomatic or the prophylactic form of therapy of histaminic cephalalgia. We also find psychotherapy to be of no avail in cases of this type. The only employment of psychotherapy which we have found helpful in histaminic cephalalgia is to reassure the patient that his case is not hopeless and that he can find relief by the use of histamine desensitization intravenously.

These patients actually obtain good results with the use of histamine. They are not cured merely by the power of suggestion, because histaminic cephalalgia is an organic pain of a very severe nature and not on any psychogenic basis whatsoever.

Histamine is a very tricky drug to use in cases of this type. If too rapid a rate of administration or too strong a solution is used, it can produce a headache. This is similar to the provocative test which was described under diagnosis. If too slow a rate

of flow or too weak a solution is used, the desired results will not be obtained. We believe that this is the primary reason why some people think that histamine does not work in these cases; it is not used correctly.

Stern[86] also reported good results with the use of histamine in histaminic cephalalgia. He reported that desensitization by the subcutaneous method gave headache-free periods of 10 to 20 months and by the intravenous method periods of 11 to 22 months. Some signs of peptic ulceration were shown by a patient treated by the former method.

Harsh[87] reported excellent results in the prophylactic treatment of histaminic cephalalgia using histamine by iontophoresis.

Blumenthal[88] reported excellent results when employing histamine in histaminic cephalalgia. He points out that the proper dosage must be employed. He also found it to be of benefit in Meniere's syndrome, migraine, and urticaria.

Hanes[89] used histamine combined with hydrochloric acid orally and reported good results. This is the only report we know of in the medical literature where this combination of drugs is used in histaminic cephalalgia therapy.

Nattero and associates[90] also report a small number of cases of histaminic cephalalgia in which histamine desensitization was successful in the treatment program.

McGovern and Haywood[91] reported that many patients afflicted with histaminic cephalalgia have responded favorably to histamine hyposensitization.

Histamine is a powerful therapeutic agent and the physician must know how to use it properly to make it a useful drug. Its dosage schedule has to be "tailor-made" to fit each individual patient, so as not to provoke an attack and still be effective prophylactically. We have never seen a serious side effect from the use of histamine. This is more than can be said of any other drug commonly used in the prophylactic treatment of histaminic cephalalgia.

Amobarbital. The use of intravenous

amobarbital in cases of cluster headache is advocated by Coddon.[92] The amobarbital solution contains 50 mg per centimeter sterile water. The patient is hospitalized and receives the solution intravenously at the rate of 50 to 100 mg per minute. The patient is flat in bed without a pillow. Usually 250 to 300 mg is the average dosage used to produce relief of the pain. The total dosage is increased to 5000 mg, which produces narcosis. The patient then sleeps 1 to 6 hours. Coddon also says the amobarbital may be given intramuscularly or orally. He claims no side effects from this form of treatment.

Surgery. According to Horton,[54] who originally described this condition, histaminic cephalalgia is a medical, not a surgical, problem. In spite of this, nearly 50% of the patients we see with this condition have previously undergone various minor or major surgical procedures in a vain attempt to obtain relief of their pain. Many of these patients have had various types of intranasal surgery or even fifth nerve surgery, all to no avail.

Stowell[93] in these cases performed surgery when medical treatment was ineffective. He states that supraorbital nerve blocking or avulsion gave relief in sixteen out of twenty-one cases and petrosal nerve section gave relief in thirty-two out of thirty-six cases. Eight of this latter group had recurrences of pain after 1 year, three after 2 years, and four after 3 years, due to the regeneration of nerve fibers. Four underwent reoperation, in three cases with relief. Sectioning of the first division of the fifth nerve produced relief in all five cases in which it was carried out.

Cook[94] advocates the use of cryosurgery. This consists of applying extremely low temperatures to the sphenopalatine, superficial temporal, occipital, middle meningeal, or internal maxillary arteries, with the type of pain determining the site or sites of treatment. In cases of retroorbital and facial pain, the physician freezes the sphenopalatine or internal maxillary area; if the pain is in the temporal or frontal areas, the physician works on the superficial temporal artery.

Safer[95] reports a case of histaminic cephalalgia which did not respond to medical therapy and in which the common carotid artery was ligated. This produced dramatic relief of the headache attacks without causing any neurologic signs. We know of no other reports of such a procedure in the literature.

Psychotherapy. Like any other form of headache problem, the psychologic aspects of histaminic cephalalgia have to be considered. However, as stated before, anyone seeing one of these patients in an actual attack would never believe the condition to be psychogenic. It is wise to reassure patients that they can obtain relief from their attacks. They usually will have received a variety of treatments for the condition, perhaps even some forms of surgery, all to no avail. So perhaps this reassurance may be considered a form of psychotherapy.[96]

Supportive psychotherapy and manipulation of the environment may sometimes terminate a seemingly intractable episode of cluster headache. Proper treatment of anxiety or accompanying depression may also significantly influence the clinical course.

Diet. While diet may possibly be influential in producing migraine, this is not true in the case of histaminic cephalalgia. We do not believe that any form of restricted or elimination diet is beneficial in the treatment program of histaminic cephalalgia. We know many allergists who state that they never see cases of histaminic cephalalgia. This is because it does not have an allergy factor in its etiology.

Other drugs. There are reports in the medical literature dealing with the prophylactic treatment of histaminic cephalalgia in which various other drugs have been successfully employed. Reports are few and will only be mentioned here for reference. Such drugs as prednisone,[97] propranolol,[98] ergotamine tartrate,[139] diphenhydramine,[100] and lithium[101] have been used.

SYMPTOMATIC TREATMENT

Symptomatic relief is directly related to the mechanistic pattern of these headaches. The pain associated with vascular headaches is caused by the dilation of cerebral arteries.

It must be remembered that histaminic cephalalgia represents a distinct clinical entity and must not be confused with migraine, ophthalmic migraine, or any other type of headache found in humans.[102] It seems to represent a localized anaphylactic reaction. Sensitized cells and tissues in the region of the painful area liberate histamine, which in turn accounts for the localized vasodilation and edema. It is this against which the symptomatic form of treatment should be directed.

The first preparation to be of any significant value in the aborting of attacks of histaminic cephalalgia was DHE-45, dihydroergotamine.[103] This preparation gives fewer side effects than does ergotamine tartrate (Gynergen), which is effective in cases of migraine but not so effective in histaminic cephalalgia. DHE-45, when used in severe cases, should be administered intravenously. We have found in histaminic cephalalgia that the more severe the attack, the quicker DHE-45 seems to take effect. In such cases, we have found that the slow intravenous injection of 1 ml of DHE-45 is most satisfactory.

Side effects of DHE-45 are comparatively few, and most cases show no toxicity whatsoever. Some patients will complain of slight nausea or vomiting or a general malaise. Occasionally, some experience mild pains in the legs, but this is not too common. The blood pressure does not seem to be affected by the administration of DHE-45. Of course, the usual precautions should be observed in advanced cardiovascular disease. King[104] finds DHE-45 to have a mild depressive effect which may be beneficial in the nervous type of patient or in dealing with anxiety states.

In 1948 an oral preparation was intro-duced for the aborting of attacks of histaminic cephalalgia. This preparation was experimentally known as EC-110 and was first reported on by Horton, Ryan, and Reynolds.[18] This preparation was at first known as Cafergone but, since its introduction to the public, its name has been changed to Cafergot.* Cafergot contains 1 mg of ergotamine tartrate and 100 mg of caffeine; it is prepared in tablet form. The preparation, to be effective, has to be administered at the immediate onset of the headache attack. If it is not taken at an early stage in the attack, it will not abort the average attack of histaminic cephalalgia. One of the chief causes for the failures found in using Cafergot in the symptomatic treatment of histaminic cephalalgia is using it incorrectly.[105] We know of cases in which the patient had been told to take the preparation routinely, such as four times a day, every 4 hours, or after each meal. This, of course, is useless, for Cafergot will not cure any case of histaminic cephalalgia and is useful only in attempting to abort the attacks. To take the preparation when not having an attack will, therefore, produce no results whatsoever and will cause the patient to become disappointed, whereas the drug might have produced the desired effects if used correctly. A standard rule in regard to this preparation should be that Cafergot is used to abort the attack and not used as a cure for the headache.

We find that the proper dosage of Cafergot is two tablets taken at the immediate onset of the headache attack. If the attack is dulled but not aborted, we advise the patient then to take two more tablets 40 to 60 minutes after talking the first two. The company manufacturing Cafergot advises taking up to six tablets for one headache attack. We believe that if six tablets do not abort the attack, sixty-six will not either. Cafergot also comes in the suppository form, with each suppository containing 2

---

*For additional information see Chapter 4.

mg ergotamine tartrate and 100 mg caffeine.

The only toxic effects of Cafergot are gastrointestinal. Some patients experience nausea, and a few have some mild vomiting attacks. Other than these, we have found Cafergot to produce no toxic side effects. Cafergot has proved effective in relieving the headache phase of this problem. Another type of preparation to be used in the symptomatic form of treatment of histaminic cephalalgia has been Cafergot-PB.[106] This agent contains 2 mg ergotamine tartrate, 100 mg caffeine, 0.25 mg Bellafoline, and 60 mg pentobarbital sodium. This preparation was made in the rectal suppository form as well as the tablet form. The addition of Bellafoline seems to cut down the gastric side effects in some cases.[56] Ergotamine tartrate is a sympathetic sedative and caffeine is a central stimulant. Bellafoline acts as a parasympathetic inhibitor, relieving smooth muscle spasm and controlling hypersecretion,[107] and it has been found to be less toxic than similar drugs used at the same dosage level.[108]

The initial results reported were remarkable, especially in regard to the gastric side effects. Cafergot produced gastric side effects in about 11% of the cases reported. But, with Cafergot-PB, there was not a single case of gastric side effect reported. However, a large percentage of the patients who used Cafergot-PB did experience side effects. Sixty percent experienced a tired or sleepy sensation, to various degrees. Some of the patients felt only a little sleepy, while others felt the sedative effect much more and slept for 2 or 3 hours. The usual report was that the patient took the suppository and about 20 or 30 minutes later the headache began to be less severe but the patient felt sleepy. He would sleep usually from 1 to 3 hours and then would awaken entirely free from the headache. The sedative effects usually were no longer present when the patient awakened. It seemed that the degree of this sedative side effect was in direct proportion to the patient's size and body weight. The larger male adults experienced no sedative effects at all. This side effect was the only one produced by Cafergot-PB. The majority of histaminic cephalalgia patients were rather desirous of rest after one of their attacks, and most patients were not at all alarmed or disturbed by this sleepy sensation when it did occur. Since many real histaminic cephalalgia patients are near the exhaustion stage following an attack, perhaps this side effect helps in the "recovery" stage.

CASE HISTORY

T. T., a married, white, 39-year-old male, was a high-pressure businessman who had unilateral headaches of short duration. His attacks would commence and terminate rather suddenly, and frequently he would be awakened from his sleep by an attack a few hours after he had retired. Sitting up or standing often would ease his attacks but would not relieve them completely. With his attacks he had nasal congestion on the side involved (right), rhinorrhea, and stuffiness of the right nostril. On occasion, he also had congestion of the right eye and swelling of the right temporal vessels. Severe pain was the chief complaint, being constant and boring in character, involving the right frontal area just above the eye. His report of an attack in which he successfully used Cafergot-PB is as follows. The patient had had an exceptionally heavy day at the office and went home tired. He retired about 11:00 P.M., his usual hour. At about 2:45 A.M. he was awakened suddenly from his sleep, with a severe pain over the frontal area. The right temporal vessels were engorged. The right nostril was congested and the right eye was watery and congested and had a burning sensation. The pain was boring and severe. At 3:00 A.M. he took one suppository of Cafergot-PB and fell asleep in about 20 minutes. At about 5:00 A.M. he awakened and the pain was completely gone and the vessels in the right temporal area were no longer swollen and engorged. The right eye felt normal and the mouth and nose felt dry. He felt a little drowsy at that time, and this feeling continued until about lunch time but was not severe enough to interfere with his work. He had no signs of headache.

This case is of a typical severe attack of histaminic cephalalgia which was relieved completely by the taking of one suppository of Cafergot-PB. This patient received prophylactic histamine injections according to the method advocated in this chapter.

SUMMARY

Symptoms and signs
on side involved

1. Rhinorrhea
2. Nasal congestion
3. Eye congestion
4. Watering of eye
5. Swelling of temporal vessels
6. Increased surface temperature

Pain is

1. Constant
2. Excruciating
3. Burning
4. Boring
5. More severe when reclining
6. Unilateral
7. Of short duration (few minutes)
8. Of sudden onset
9. Terminated suddenly

Treatment

Prophylactic

1. Sansert
2. Histamine
3. BC-105
4. Surgery
5. Amobarbital
6. Psychotherapy
7. Prednisone
8. Propranolol
9. Nicotinic acid

Symptomatic

1. DHE-45
2. Cafergot-PB
3. Cafergot
4. Migral
5. Ergomar
6. Ergostat
7. Wygraine
8. Midrin

REFERENCES

Muscle contraction (tension) headache

1. Ad Hoc Committee on the Classification of Headache, J.A.M.A. **179**:717-718, 1962.
2. Ogdon, H. D.: Headache and tension, Ann. Allergy **11**:329-331, 1953.
3. Simons, D. J., Day, E., Goodell, H., and Wolff, H. G.: Experimental studies on headache; muscles of scalp and neck as sources of pain, A. Res. Nerv. Ment. Dis. Proc. **23**:228, 1943.
4. Wolff, H. G., and Wolf, S.: Pain, ed. 2, Springfield, Ill., 1958, Charles C Thomas, Publisher.
5. Finch, J. W.: Chronic headache, Clin. Med. **69**(1):117-121, 1962.
6. Aring, C. D.: Emotion-induced headache, Postgrad. Med. **56**(3):191-195, 1974.
7. Lance, J. W., and Curran, D. A.: Treatment of chronic tension headache, Lancet **1**:1236-1239, 1964.
8. Blumenthal, L. S., and Fuchs, M.: Chronic headache, Med. Am. D. C. **26**:589-594, 1957.
9. Patewicz, E. P.: Cephalgic spasm of head and neck muscles, Headache **15**:261-266, 1976.
10. Martin, M. J.: Tension headache, a psychiatric study, Headache **6**:47-54, 1966.
11. Williams, H. L.: Headache from the standpoint of otolaryngologist, J. Iowa Med. Soc. **37**:45, 1947.
12. Williams, H. L.: Treatment of certain common forms of headache confused with sinus headache, Ill. Med. J. **105**:53, 1954.
13. Bisgard, J. D.: Arthritis of the cervical spine; some neurological manifestations, J.A.M.A. **98**:1961, 1932.
14. Ayash, J. J.: Headache and head pain, Lancet **69**:389, 1949.
15. Blumenthal, L. S., and Fuchs, M.: Muscle relaxation in the treatment of headache, Headache **1**:8-20, 1961.
16. Sainsbury, P., and Gibson, J. G.: Symptoms of anxiety and tension and accompanying physiological changes in muscular system, J. Neurol. Neurosurg. Psychiatry **17**:216, 1954.
17. Marmion, D. E.: The role of muscles in the etiology of headache, J. R. Army Med. Corps **100**:99, 1954.
18. Horton, B. T., Ryan, R. E., and Reynolds, J.: Clinical observations on the use of a new agent for the treatment of headache, Proc. Staff Meet. Mayo Clin. **5**:105, 1948.
19. Liddell, D. W., Robin, A. A., and Darby, C. E.: Latent epilepsy as a factor in tension states, J. Nerv. Ment. Dis. **121**:215, 1955.
20. Blumenthal, L. S., and Fuchs, M.: What have you got for a headache? Am. Druggist, August, 1950.
21. Horton, B. T.: Headache; clinical varieties and therapeutic suggestions, Med. Clin. North Am. **33**:973, 1949.
22. Weiner, L. P.: Emotional aspects of chronic tension headache: a study of soldiers and their dependents, Headache **9**:162-171, 1969.
23. Friedman, A. P., de Sola Pool, N., and von Storch, T. J. C.: Tension headache, J.A.M.A. **151**:174, 1953.
24. Bakol, D. A., and Kaganov, J. A.: A simple method for self-observation of headache frequency, intensity, and location, Headache **16**:123-124, 1976.
25. Friedman, A. P.: Current concepts in the diag-

nosis of chronic recurring headache, Med. Clin. North Am. **56**(6):1257-1271, 1972.

26. MacNeal, P. S.: Useful therapeutic approaches to the patient with "problem headache," Headache **14**:186-189, 1975.

27. Bernik V.: Migraine and tension headache: clinical forms, diagnosis and treatment, Rev. Paul. Med. **80**(4):173-180, 1972.

28. Ryan, R. E.: Motrin—a new agent for the symptomatic treatment of muscle contraction tension headache, Headache **16**:280-283, 1977.

29. Harris, M. C.: Tension and migraine headaches: treatment, West. Med. **2**:234-237, 1961.

30. Diamond, S., and Baltes, B. J.: Chronic tension headache—treated with amitriptyline—a double-blind study, Headache **11**:110-116, 1971.

31. Martins, L. E., Viera de Douza, F., Antonini, R., and Bernik, V.: Tension headache and its treatment in 60 patients: a double blind comparison of the action of an analgesic with that of a tranquilizer, Rev. Assoc. Med. Bras. **17**(1):19-26, 1971.

32. Hakkarainen, H., and Viukari, M.: Sulpiride in the treatment of migraine, tension headache and psychosomatic symptoms, Duodecim **89**(22):1504-1509, 1973.

33. Dixon, H. L., and Dickel, H. A.: Tension headache, Northw. Med. **66**:817-820, 1967.

34. Budzynski, T. H., Stoyva, J. M., Adler, C. S., and Mullaney, D. J.: EMG biofeedback and tension headache: a controlled outcome study, Psychosom, Med. **35**(6):484-496, 1973.

35. Green, E. E., Walters, E. D., Green, A. M., and Murphy, G.: Feedback technique for deep relaxation, Psychophysiology **6**:372-377, 1969.

36. Budzynski, T. H., Stoyva, J. M., and Adler, C.: Feedback induced muscle application to tension headache, J. Beh. Ther. Exp. Psychiatr. **1**:205-211, 1970.

37. Wickramasekira, I.: The application of verbal instructions and EMG feedback training to the management of tension headache—preliminary observations, Headache **13**:74-76, 1973.

38. Hoffmann, E.: Biofeedback training: a new therapy in the treatment of migraine and tension headache? Dan. Med. Bull. **22**(3): 97-99, 1975.

39. Warner, G., and Lance, J. W.: Relaxation therapy in migraine and chronic tension headache, Med. J. Aust. **1**(10):298-301, 1975.

Histaminic cephalalgia (cluster headache, Horton's syndrome)

40. Horton, B. T., MacLean, A. R., and Craig, W. M.: A new syndrome of vascular headache: results of treatment with histamine: a preliminary report, Proc. Staff Meet. Mayo Clin. **14**:257, 1939.

41. Riggs, J. P.: Headache, Eye Ear Nose Throat Mon. **29**:311, 1950.

42. Williams, H. L.: Headache from the standpoint of the otolaryngologist, J. Iowa Med. Soc. **37**:45, 1947.

43. Broch, A., Horven, I., Nornes, H., Sjaastad, O., and Tonjum, A.: Studies on cerebral and ocular circulation in a patient with cluster headache, Headache **10**:1, 1970.

44. Sjaastad, O., Rootwelt, K., and Horven, I.: Cutaneous blood flow in cluster headache, Headache **13**:173, 1974.

45. Bruyn, G. W., Bootsma, B. K., and Klawans, H. L.: Cluster headache and bradycardia, Headache **16**:11, 1976.

46. Ekbom, K., and Greitz, T.: Angiography in cluster headache, Acta Radiol. Diag. **10**:1, 1970.

47. Anthony, M., and Lance, J. W.: Whole blood histamine and plasma serotonin in cluster headache, Aust. Assoc. Neurol. **8**:43, 1971.

48. Anthony, M., and Lance, J. W.: Histamine and serotonin in cluster headache, Arch. Neurol. **25**:225, 1971.

49. Anthony, M., Lance, J. W., and Lord, G.: Migrainous neuralgia—blood histamine levels and clinical response to H_1 and H_2 receptor blockade, International Migraine Symposium, London, September, 1976.

50. Sadjadpour, K.: Studies on cluster headaches—role of cigarette smoking and incidence of oculosympathetic palsy, Bergen Migraine Symposium, Bergen, Norway, June 1975, p. 66.

51. Grammeltvedt, A., Hovig, T., and Sjaastad, O.: Electronmicroscopy of blood platelets in migraine and cluster headache, Headache **14**:226-230, 1975.

52. Ekbom, K.: A clinical comparison of cluster headache and migraine, Acta Neurol. Scand. **46**:1, 1970.

53. Ekbom, K.: Migraine in patients with cluster headache, Headache **14**:69, 1974.

54. Horton, B. T.: Histaminic cephalalgia, J.A.M.A. **160**:468, 1956.

55. Boies, L. R.: Causes of head pain, Ann. Otol. Rhinol. Laryngol. **59**:507, 1950.

56. Shea, J. J.: The therapy of headache, J. Omaha Mid-West Clin. Soc. **11**:71, 1950.

57. Ekbom, K., and Lindahl, J.: Remission of angina pectoris during periods of cluster headache, Headache **11**:57-62, 1971.

58. Gilbert, G. J.: Meniere's syndrome and cluster headaches, J.A.M.A. **191**:691, 1965.

59. Horven, I., Nornes, H., and Sjaastad, O.: Different corneal indentation pulse pattern in cluster headache and migraine, Neurology **22**:92, 1972.

60. Horven, I., Nornes, H., and Sjaastad, O.: Dynamic tonometry in migraine and cluster headache, Proceedings of the International Headache Symposium, Elsinore, Denmark, May 16-18, 1971, pp. 103-110.

61. Sjaastad, O., and Sjaastad, O. V.: The histamin-

uria in vascular headache, Acta Neurol. Scand. **46:**331, 1970.

62. Sjaastad, O., and Sjaastad, O. V.: Histamine metabolism in Horton's headache (cluster headache) and migraine, Bergen Migraine Symposium, Bergen, Norway, June 1975, p. 74.

63. Farias De Silva, W.: A study of migraine and Horton's syndrome, Neurobiologia **37:**171, 1974.

64. Williams, H. L.: The treatment of certain common forms of headache confused with sinus headache, Ill. Med. J. **105:**53, 1954.

65. Graham, J. R.: Cluster headache, Headache **11:**175, 1972.

66. Kudrow, L.: Physical and personality characteristics in cluster headache, Headache **13:**197, 1974.

67. Rogado, A. Z., Harrison, R. H., and Graham, J. R.: Personality profiles in cluster headache, migraine and normal controls, Arch. Neurobiol. **38:**229, 1974.

68. Lovshin, L. L.: Clinical caprices of histaminic cephalalgia, Headache **2:**7, 1961.

69. Graham, J. R.: The physical and physiological characteristics of patients with cluster headache, Third International Symposium on Migraine, National Hospital, London, April 24-25, 1969.

70. Ekbom, K.: Patterns of cluster headache with a note on the relations to angina pectoris and peptic ulcer, Acta Neurol. Scand. **46:**225, 1970.

71. Horton, B. T.: Histamine cephalgia resulting in production of acute duodenal ulcer, J.A.M.A. **122:**59, 1943.

72. Jacobson, L. B.: Cluster headache: a rare cause of bradycardia, Headache **8:**159, 1969.

73. Ekbom, K.: Heart rate, blood pressure, and electrocardiographic changes during provoked attacks of cluster headache, Acta Neurol. Scand. **46:**215, 1970B.

74. Gilbert, G. J.: Cluster headache and cluster vertigo, Headache **9:**195, 1970.

75. Ekbom, K.: Clinical aspects of cluster headache, Headache **13:**176, 1974.

76. Ekbom, K., and Lindahl, J.: Effect of induced rise of blood pressure on pain in cluster headache, Acta Neurol. Scand. **46:**585, 1970.

77. Ekbom, K., and DeFine Olivarius, B.: Chronic migrainous neuralgia—diagnostic and therapeutic aspects, Headache **11:**97, 1971.

78. Ryan, R. E.: Histamine cephalalgia differentiated from acute nasal sinusitis, Eye Ear Nose Throat Mon. **49:**18, 1970.

79. Grammeltvedt, A., Hovig, T., and Sjaastad, O.: Electronmicroscopy of blood platelets in migraine and cluster headache, Headache **14:**226, 1974.

80. Prusinski, A., and Klimek, A.: Horton's type headaches and their treatment with Sandomigran (BC-105), Lodz Wiad. Lek. **26:**367, 1973.

81. Ekbom, K.: Prophylactic treatment of cluster headache with a new serotonin antagonist—BC-105, Acta Neurol. Scand. **45:**601, 1969.

82. Nelson, R. F.: Cluster migraine can be relieved but is seldom recognized, Mod. Med. **39:**115, 1971.

83. Dille, R. S., and Horton, B. T.: Effects of various agents on pulsations of human brain, Proc. Central Soc. Clin. Res. **19:**58, 1946.

84. MacNeal, P. S.: Headache as an emergency complaint, Med. Clin. North Am. **33:**1581, 1949.

85. Hilsinger, R. L.: "Vascular" headaches and related conditions, Laryngoscope **64:**403, 1954.

86. Stern, F. H.: Histamine cephalalgia—an often overlooked cause of headache, Psychosomatics **10:**53, 1969.

87. Harsh, G. F.: Histamine by iontophoresis; a long neglected modality in the prevention of migraine and other vascular headaches, Headache **6:**208, 1967.

88. Blumenthal, L. S.: Current histamine therapy, Mod. Med. **18:**51, 1950.

89. Hanes, W. J.: Histamine cephalalgia resembling tic douloureux: differential diagnosis and treatment, Headache **8:**162, 1969.

90. Nattero, G., Gastaldi, L., and Gai, V.: Clinical and therapeutical observations on so-called "migraine variants," Minerva Med. **61:**1613, 1970.

91. McGovern, J. P., and Haywood, T. J.: Histaminic cephalalgia, Headache **3:**39, 1963.

92. Coddon, D. R.: Results of intravenous amobarbital therapy in 14 patients with cluster headache over a five-year period, Proceedings of the International Headache Symposium, Elsinore, Denmark, May 16-18, 1971, p. 51.

93. Stowell, A.: Physiologic mechanisms and treatment of histaminic or petrosal neuralgia, Headache **9:**187, 1970.

94. Cook, N. C.: Latent word in headache relief is cryosurgery, Med. World News **12:**15, 1971.

95. Safer, L. A.: Cluster headache—case report of a variant type, Ohio State Med. J. **58:**917, 1962.

96. Ryan, R. E.: Modern concepts of the management of histaminic cephalalgia, South. Med. J. **56:**1384, 1963.

97. Jammes, J. L.: The treatment of cluster headaches with prednisone, Dis. Nerv. Syst. **36:**375, 1975.

98. Vallat, J. N., Tapie, P., DeMarti, D., Vallati, I., and LaBaume, A.: So-called "cluster headaches" (a note on the treatment of facial vascular pain with a beta-blocking agent), Rev. Med. Limoges **5:**41, 1974.

99. Wentges, R.: Cluster headache, Ned. Tijdschr. Geneeskd. **119:**348, 1975.

100. Tucker, W. I., and O'Neill, P. B.: Benadryl in histamine headache, Lahey Clin. Bull. **7:**218, 1952.

101. Kudrow, L.: Compared results of prednisone, methysergide, and lithium therapy in cluster headache, International Migraine Symposium, London, England, September 1976.

102. Horton, B. T.: Use of histamine in the treatment of specific types of headaches, J.A.M.A. **116:**377, 1941.

103. Horton, B. T., Peters, G. A., and Blumenthal, L. S.: New product in treatment of migraine; preliminary report, Proc. Staff Meet. Mayo Clin. **20:**241, 1945.

104. King, G. S.: Headaches and their treatments, N. Y. State J. Med. **51:**255, 1951.

105. Ryan, R. E.: Cafergone for relief of headache, a further study, J. Missouri Med. Assoc. **47:**107, 1950.

106. Ryan, R. E.: Migraine and histaminic cephalalgia, a new agent for their treatment, J. Missouri Med. Assoc. **48:**963, 1951.

107. Kramer, P., and Ingelfinger, F. J.: Use of antispasmodics and spasmodics in the treatment of gastrointestinal disorders, Med. Clin. North Am. **32:**1227, 1948.

108. Cushney, A. R.: Atropine and the hyoscyamines—a study of the action of optical isomers, J. Physiol. **30:**176, 1904.

CHAPTER 7

Cranial neuralgias

TRIGEMINAL NEURALGIA (TIC DOULOUREUX)

The term "tic douloureux" is descriptive, meaning unbearable pain associated with contortions and grimaces of the face. This disease is characterized as follows:

1. There is paroxysmal unilateral facial pain in the distribution of one or more branches of the trigeminal nerve.
2. The pain can be provoked by sensory stimuli such as touch or movement of the face in chewing, talking, or yawning.
3. There is no objective trigeminal loss or motor weakness.

These symptoms have been grouped together and called idiopathic trigeminal neuralgia, in contrast to symptomatic trigeminal neuralgia, in which other neurologic deficits have been implicated in the etiology of the trigeminal pain.

Tic douloureux is a unique disease in several aspects. Patients give a very consistent history and are often older in age. Their clinical picture may show seasonal exacerbations of pain, which may be relieved by drugs not commonly considered as analgesics. These patients commonly manifest trigger zones. Such zones are quite precise areas of skin and mucous membrane which, when excited by the most trivial stimuli, are capable of producing pain in one or another of the divisions of the trigeminal nerves. These patients very carefully avoid these zones and often develop different behavioral patterns in order to protect themselves from contacting these trigger zones.

Etiology

In the past it has been accepted that there were no specific pathologic findings in the trigeminal system to explain the clinical picture of idiopathic trigeminal neuralgia. There have been many conditions which have been indicated as causing trigeminal neuralgia, but it is doubtful whether they can be regarded as more than inciting or precipitating causes. Trigeminal neuralgia is found in intoxication, such as lead, alcohol, and arsenic, and in infections such as influenza, syphilis, herpes zoster, tuberculosis, malaria, and other diseases. It is found also in gout, rheumatic diseases, and diabetes, and there has also been an association seen in patients with multiple sclerosis.

Recently there has been a revival of interest as to a possible viral etiology of trigeminal neuralgia. It was suggested by Behrman and Knight that herpes simplex might play an etiologic role in trigeminal neuralgia based on the similarity of the periodicity and location of lesions in herpes simplex and trigeminal neuralgia. Herpes simplex was recovered from the trigeminal ganglion in six of seven patients studied by Baringer and Swoveland at autopsy of unselected cadavers. However, Rothman and Munson found no association between a history of frequent cold sores and trigeminal neuralgia in the 526 patients with trigeminal neuralgia that they studied. They stated that while this historical information may not be a sensitive index of the presence of the virus, it does not support the herpes simplex viral etiology.

So numerous are the cases for which there is no cause found that the term "idiopathic" has been used for them. Exhaustion, overwork, and nervous strain have frequently been observed as predisposing causes. The fact is that after the many exciting conditions and predisposing factors are mentioned, it is still impossible to state the cause.

Lindsay[1] discussed the possibility that trigeminal neuralgia may sometimes be an extreme manifestation of a disordered temporomandibular joint with the pain arising in the muscles of mastication. He postulated that the cause of trigeminal neuralgia may be a defect in the nervous mechanism of the temporomandibular joint. Experience with his series of cases suggested that correction of the occlusion, particularly establishment of the correct vertical dimension, should be the first treatment after the diagnosis of trigeminal neuralgia has been made.

Smolik and Hempstead[2] believed that a reconsideration of the entire trigeminal area and its relation to the masticatory apparatus was mandatory. They noted that trigeminal neuralgia occurred most often in an older age group, specifically those over 40 years of age, and especially in edentulous women, and the pain was initiated frequently by chewing, sneezing, or coughing—in other words by some movement of the mandibular mechanism. They remarked that little consideration is usually given to the examination of the occlusion of the natural teeth and less to the fit of the artificial dentures in cases of trigeminal neuralgia. They noted that malocclusion produces a shift of the condylar mechanism, and the condylar capsular components and the diseased tissue associated with this shifting may produce tension on the chorda tympani and on branches of the auriculotemporal nerve innervating the capsular area. This is a suitable clinical method.

Gonzalez-Revilla found a posterior fossa etiology for trigeminal neuralgia in 48.5% of his patients.[3] Gardner[4] has underlined this fact and insisted that trigeminal neuralgia is a symptom and not a disease. He states that a causative factor for the symptom may often be found. The common factor in all of these "extrinsic" etiologies for pain lies in the insidious compression with local myelin dysfunction of the fifth nerve roots, which fails to produce overt signs but may result in paroxysms of facial pain. He believed that it was reasonable to suggest that this occult compression of the fifth nerve might result in a disturbance of the motor root detectable by electromyography.

Abbott[5] studied a series of fifty-seven patients with trigeminal neuralgia. In his series five were found to have an underlying extrinsic lesion responsible for the facial pain. In three of these cases the clinical picture was indistinguishable from typical trigeminal neuralgia, with no historical or physical evidence indicative of the underlying pathology.

In case 1 a tumor was found arising from the undersurface of the tentorium and right petrous ridge; the brainstem was distorted and the ipsilateral fifth nerve completely obscured. In case 2 there was extensive vascular malformation in the left posterior fossa. In case 3 a firm mass was visualized arising from the trunk of the nerve. Case 4 had an aneurysm of the internal carotid artery in the area of the cavernous sinus. In case 5 a bony proturbance was arising from the apex of the petrous bone which was found to be obscuring the origin of the fifth nerve in the brainstem. Therefore in his series the total number of cases with trigeminal pain secondary to lesions was found to be 8.7% and 5.3% of the total. These patients had histories typical of trigeminal neuralgia and were normal on examination. An important feature in these secondary cases is the early age of onset of the facial pain, being 20 years below the overall average. A large variety of lesions may be responsible, but Abbott stresses that the absence of neurologic defects is essential to the diagnosis of trigeminal neuralgia.

Physiology

Kugelburg and Lindblom[6] have described the physiology of trigeminal neuralgia as being a "temporal summation of afferent impulses. That is, the disease can be reviewed as a problem of recurrent input, evoking eventually an increased neuronal firing to a threshold which thereafter triggers an antidromic paroxysmal discharge in the distribution of the trigeminal nucleus. These discharges represent the attack of pain the patient experiences." In 1969 Dalessio[7] used a tactile stimulator and showed by this method that if a great number of impulses per second were delivered, pain occurred rapidly; if a few impulses were given, pain was latent, if occurring at all. This confirmed Kugelburg and Lindblom's observation of temporal summation of afferent impulses and thus is a suitable clinical method.

Erokhina[8] studied electroencephalographic recordings in patients with bilateral or unilateral trigeminal neuralgia. During and immediately after an attack signs of irritation were noted in both hemispheres, together with desynchonization of cortical activity and in some cases bursts of bilateral waves, mainly of beta or alpha type. Diffuse beta waves sometimes dominated the electroencephalogram, and then bilateral bursts of high amplitude beta or beta waves were seen. Desynchonization is considered to be due to the constant inflow of impulses to the cortex along the nonspecific afferent system and the inflow of pain impulses to the parietal cortex along a specific afferent system, with subsequent descending parietal cortical influences on the activating system of the brainstem.

Erokhina stated that in trigeminal neuralgia, when the inflow of pain impulses along the nonspecific system is prolonged and the continuous, articular activation of the cortical rhythm is depressed, the electroencephalogram then shows not only desynchronization but also synchonization, manifested as bursts of bilateral waves of varied frequencies, thereby demonstrating the role of midline brain structures in the mechanism of pathogenesis of trigeminal neuralgia.

Symptoms

The history in typical trigeminal neuralgia is quite characteristic; pain cannot be mistaken readily for other types of pain. The onset is sudden and the details as a rule are lost in obscurity. Usually no precipitating causes are found by the patient, and no antecedent twinges of pain were experienced before the onset.

These patients experience a paroxysmal pain which is severe and lasts only seconds to minutes, with intervals between severe attacks being either pain-free or with only mild, dull, aching sensations. The pain is often described as beginning at the ala of the nose and radiating along the maxilla toward the temporomandibular joint. Not infrequently it spreads along the side of the nose and toward but not into the eye. It may begin along the corner of the mouth and spread along the lower jaw or start over the eye and radiate over the forehead.

Patients with trigeminal neuralgia have a reasonably consistent pain response from one day to the next during an exacerbation of their disease. Their pain may often be elicited by recurrent and precise stimulation of a minute area, when such stimulation is little more than a slight tug or pull on the skin. Stimulation of even a single hair has been reported to produce pain in the trigger zone of the susceptible individual.

The trigger zones of these patients are small, usually 2 to 4 mm in size, and cluster about the nares and mouth. Attacks of pain may be produced by some form of stimulation of the trigger zone, as when washing the face or brushing the teeth, or by simple movements of the mouth and jaw in talking or mastication. Different forms of stimuli affect the trigger zones in strange ways. Painful stimulation of the trigger zone may not be an effective stimulus. Thermal stimuli are usually not effective. The application of pressure on a trigger zone almost always evokes an attack in susceptible individuals, and vibratory stimulus is also effective in these patients.[7]

In most instances, the pain is paroxysmal, the paroxysms occurring at irregular intervals, sometimes often and other times infrequently. It may, however, give the appearance of constant pain when the paroxysms are repeated frequently. The pain may arouse the patient from his sleep. A history of previous bouts of pain with a pain-free interval between is obtainable in most cases. If the patient is seen during a period of paroxysms, there is often a history of failure to eat over a period of days for fear of precipitating attacks of pain.

Pain is usually limited to one side of the face in any one attack. Attacks are bilateral in fewer than 5% of persons with trigeminal neuralgia. Pain rarely occurs on both sides of the face at the same time. In these patients with trigeminal neuralgia, there is an absence of objective hypesthesia or hypalgesia on examination of the trigeminal distribution. Objective sensory loss suggests symptomatic trigeminal neuralgia.

The number of attacks varies from a few per day to pains every few minutes. In the usual case, the pain lasts 1 to 2 minutes, but in some typical cases the pain may last 30 to 60 minutes. Remissions from the pain are not uncommon and may last from a few weeks or months to years.

Kalyanaraman[9] reviewed a series of 331 cases of trigeminal neuralgia. He found the maximum incidence to be in the fifth decade of life. In 62% of the subjects, the pain was on the right side of the face and in 2% it was bilateral. While the most common duration of pain was less than 1 year, 30% of the men and 29% of the women had suffered from tic douloureux for 2 to 5 years. In 197 patients in whom the blood group was determined out of the 331 in the total group, a significantly greater incidence of group O was found. Trigeminal neuralgia begins after age 40 in more than 90% of the patients and has been reported to occur in families on rare occasions, but there is no definite hereditary tendency. A report from the Mayo Clinic reported an average incidence rate of 4 per 100,000 for a 25-year period in people living in Rochester, Minnesota.

Physical examination

Physical examination in these patients is very unrewarding. This examination usually reveals nothing in the majority of cases. There is often evidence of retinal arteriosclerosis, but apart from this little else. Sensation over the face is unaffected, and the corneal reflex is active. At the time of examination, the patient is extremely apprehensive and is often afraid to talk because of fear of precipitating his pain. Manipulation of the face is resented, and there is usually a warning to avoid the areas of the trigger zones.

Associated diseases
MULTIPLE SCLEROSIS

In any discussion of the clinical aspects of trigeminal neuralgia, the possible relationship to multiple sclerosis must be considered. According to Friedlander and Zeff,[10] facial pain experienced by patients with multiple sclerosis is sometimes erroneously attributed to dental disease. The disorder may be a result of an idiopathic type of neuralgia that originates in the trigeminal nerve and resembles tic douloureux. There have been reports in the literature which indicate that approximately 1% of patients with multiple sclerosis have trigeminal neuralgia. In some cases the trigeminal neuralgia is the first symptom of the multiple sclerosis. The trigeminal neuralgia seen in association with multiple sclerosis is similar to the idiopathic type. However, neuralgia associated with multiple sclerosis differs from trigeminal neuralgia in certain respects: The multiple sclerosis patients are usually 20 to 40 years of age rather than the 40 to 60 years seen in trigeminal neuralgia; the pain in the multiple sclerosis patient is usually bilateral, where in trigeminal neuralgia it is unilateral; and the trigger zones of the face are observed in patients with trigeminal neuralgia but not in patients with multiple sclerosis. In the case of the multiple sclerosis patient, the dentist should carry out a thorough oral and extraoral examination. If the origin of the pain proves to be not in the teeth, definite therapy depending on the general physical condition of the patient and the intensity of the pain should be undertaken.

The most consistent pathologic finding in this group of patients is a demyelinated plaque in the root entry zone of the fifth nerve in the pons on the side of the clinical symptoms. The involvement is in the primary afferent pathway. Although some patients also have secondary afferent pathways involved, it appears that the primary afferent lesion is the significant one.

Sectioning of the peripheral branches of the trigeminal nerve is a simple and safe procedure which is preferable to preganglionic sectioning of the root of the gasserian ganglion, nerve compression, or nerve decompression.

Successful medical treatment with carbamazepine or phenytoin has been reported. Carbamazepine is more effective in reducing pain, but adverse side effects may indicate the use of phenytoin which, although less effective in reducing pain, is usually accompanied by fewer side effects.

DIABETES MELLITUS

According to Finestone,[11] diabetic neuropathy is not uncommon and sensory symptoms including hyperalgesia frequently occur in patients with trigeminal neuralgia. He reviewed a series of ninety-two cases of trigeminal neuralgia to investigate whether there existed any etiologic relationship between trigeminal neuralgia and diabetes mellitus. These patients varied in age from 25 to 94 years, with the majority over the age of 45 years. Of the forty patients in the 65- to 85-year age group, almost 50% had confirmed or suspected diabetes. This was an unusually high figure as far as the incidence of diabetes was concerned. For this reason, he recommends performing a glucose tolerance test in all patients with trigeminal neuralgia in whom the diabetic status is not known.

Treatment
MEDICAL TREATMENT

Many medical therapies have been described for treatment of trigeminal neuralgia.

Vitamin B$_{12}$. In 1954 Surtees and Hughes[12] reported that the use of massive doses of vitamin B$_{12}$ held out new hope for patients with trigeminal neuralgia. They used this treatment in eighteen patients with trigeminal neuralgia. Patients were given 100 μg daily for 10 days followed by 1,000 μg twice weekly for five doses. Some patients received 1,000 μg twice each day for periods up to 3 weeks without any apparent harm. Considerable improvement or great relief was obtained in fourteen cases, moderate improvement in one case, and little or no immediate improvement in three cases. Though in some cases the neuralgia subsided only slowly during treatment, in most of those in whom improvement took place it was noted after the second or third injection. There was considerable variation in the total amount of vitamin B$_{12}$ necessary to give relief, but the minimum appeared to be about 5,000 μg. These authors concluded that vitamin B$_{12}$ in large doses can produce a remission that may be continued for a long time, but there is no evidence that this treatment will permanently cure trigeminal neuralgia.

Fields[13] also reported on thirteen patients treated with intramuscular injection of vitamin B_{12}. In his series the typical response consisted of relief of the sharp paroxysmal type of pain on about the third day of treatment. Residual paresthesias disappeared shortly thereafter. Of the thirteen patients in his group, the nine without previous treatment had complete and prompt remission; the other four, all of whom had had surgical or alcohol nerve block therapy, were more refractory, although ultimate results were equally good.

This method of therapy is not commonly used these days as further advancements in the line of medical treatment have been developed.

Stilbamidine. This drug has been known to produce anesthesia, hypesthesia, or hypalgesia and paresthesia by its effects on the trigeminal structures in the brainstem. The dose of stilbamidine is 150 mg intravenously each day to a total of 1 to 2 gm. In the original series, good relief of pain within 1 to 14 weeks with freedom from pain for 2 to 6 years was reported. With the recurrence of pain, the medication can be given orally for several days. Woodhall and Otem[14] began to use stilbamidine therapy for treatment of trigeminal neuralgia in 1953. They found that intravenously administered stilbamidine controlled the pain of trigeminal neuralgia in thirty-six of forty-one patients in this preliminary series for a period ranging between 9 months and 2 years. The relief of pain was associated with sensory changes over the trigeminal and upper cervical dermatomes, which suggested a true chemical neuropathy. In a small percentage of cases, unpredictable paresthesias occurring over the face tended to decrease the potential value of this therapeutic agent. Although this drug in its intravenous form might not be the definitive medical therapy for trigeminal neuralgia, the original authors believed that it represented a valuable adjunct to the care of this complex pain syndrome.

This drug falls in the same group as vitamin B_{12} in that it has been replaced by some of the newer anticonvulsive medications.

Histamine. In 1962, Hanes[15] reported that in a series of seventy-five cases of trigeminal neuralgia it was found that 91% of the patients had either achlorhydria or a decrease in free hydrochloric acid. It was thought that improper protein digestion resulting from this condition might lead to the release of histamine or histamine-like substances into the general circulation. The symptoms of neuralgia might be attributable to urticaria of the trigeminal nerve ganglion. Hanes believed that as a result of the antacidity, temporary or permanent, in a hypersensitive and allergic individual, histamine or histamine-like substances are possibly absorbed from the stomach into the general circulation and carried to the trigeminal nerve root. The exposure to the excess histamine results in a localized urticaria, which then gives rise to a secondary neuralgia. Thus, just as the swelling of the nerve root due to infection or trauma results in the pain of neuralgia, he thought the swelling of the nerve root of the gasserian ganglion in these cases of trigeminal neuralgia due to the localized urticaria in the hypersensitive allergic individual might easily result in the same sort of neuralgic pains down along the branch of the fifth nerve.

The patients in Hanes' series were treated by administration of supplementary hydrochloric acid, the use of an antihistamine, and histamine desensitization. This treatment produced relief of symptoms in 79% of the patients and in 70% of them the relief was permanent.

Dobaczewski[16] treated patients in a similar manner on the theory that trigeminal neuralgia was caused by a vascular spasm. Fifteen cases were submitted to systemic treatment by intravenous histamine drip. In his patients, improvement of variable duration occurred in 64% of the cases. In none of the cases was a permanent cure achieved, the longest period of freedom from pain being 6 months in two patients. However, in his series, most patients improved following histamine infusion initially whereas all other previous treatment had failed to alleviate their pain even temporarily.

The histamine theory as a cause of trigeminal neuralgia has fallen into disfavor, and this form of therapy is not often used in the treatment of trigeminal neuralgia at the present time.

Phenytoin. Phenytoin first received notoriety by several reports in the European literature regarding its use in the treatment of trigeminal neuralgia. The basis of its use was apparently on the assumption that an epileptiform mechanism was involved in the trigeminal neuralgia. Animal experience had shown that systemic phenytoin abolished the rebound spike of the peripheral nerve induced by a constant current stimulation. It was assumed that the pain of peripheral nerve origin was related to repetitive discharge in the afferent fiber or end organ. Various reports in the literature have reported inconsistent findings with the use of this drug in the treatment of trigeminal neuralgia. It is used orally in doses of 300 to 700 mg per day. Intravenous therapy offers no advantage over oral administration. The relief of pain is only transient in the majority of patients. Within months or years, control of pain requires combined treatment with carbamazepine or mephenesin. It appears that phenytoin itself has only a limited beneficial effect. It may have continuing usefulness in the medical management of this condition, but only in combination with other methods of treatment.

Anticonvulsants. Strychnine disinhibition may serve as a model for trigeminal neuralgia. The trigger zones of trigeminal neuralgia appear to represent a peripheral manifestation of a hyperactive and a hyperexcitable area of the nervous system, as though a portion of the sensory input through a small area of the trigeminal nerve were operating in a strychnine circuit, lacking inhibition. If this model was correct, drugs effective in trigeminal neuralgia should inhibit convulsions induced by strychnine.

One possibility of a pharmacologic mechanism in the management of trigeminal neuralgia is that the drugs depress synaptic transmission in either the spinal trigeminal nucleus, or the gasserian ganglion, or both. Another possible mechanism of drug action is that it affects the afferent projection system by reducing sensitivity, hence the therapeutic use of anticonvulsants such as phenytoin and carbamazepine. These anticonvulsants have met with moderate clinical success. Laboratory studies have shown that these anticonvulsants depress synaptic transmission in the trigeminal system, as evidenced by decrease in amplitude and increase in latency of the volt potentials.

Mephenesin. Mephenesin (Tolseram) is a carbamic acid ester used in patients with idiopathic trigeminal neuralgia. Attacks of pain occurring in clusters can be relieved by intravenous mephenesin in a dosage of 4 gm per 500 ml in 5% glucose every 6 to 12 hours.

Sixty percent of patients treated in this manner maintain sufficient comfort to make a surgical procedure unnecessary. In the 40% in whom the results are unsatisfactory, surgical procedure is necessitated because of complaints of lightheadedness, unsteady gait, and continuation of the pain.

Carbamazepine. Carbamazepine (Tegretol) is an iminostilbene derivative. Like other tricyclic drugs, it cannot be safely used concurrently with monoamine oxidase inhibitors. This drug was initially studied in Europe, and there have been several reports regarding its usefulness in the treatment of trigeminal neuralgia. In one report of thirty-three cases treated with the carbamazepine, 70% obtained a good result. The usual daily dose is 400 to 600 mg orally, although occasionally up to 1,200 mg per day has been used. It is suggested that the drug be started with meals at 100 mg twice a day on the first day. It should be gradually increased in 100-mg increments every 12 hours until freedom from pain is accomplished.

The most common side effects seen in these patients are occasional vomiting, nausea, vertigo, and drowsiness. These side effects are usually dose-dependent. There are more serious side effects seen in these patients occasionally, such as hypertension, transient or persistent leukopenia, and skin rash, which may necessitate discontinuation of the drug temporarily or permanently. Because of the toxicity of the drug and the tendency for drug resistance to develop with prolonged therapy, it is recommended that attempts be made to reduce dosage to a minimum or discontinue therapy every 3 weeks.

RECOMMENDED TREATMENT

The treatment of choice in trigeminal neuralgia requires the use of anticonvulsant drugs. Once the diagnosis of trigeminal neuralgia has been made, we generally begin therapy with the administration of carbamazepine orally. This is given at a dosage of 200 mg two or three times a day. If this is tolerated well and the pain is relieved, it may be continued for several weeks or months, depending on the course of the disease. The dosage of the drug is usually regulated depending on the severity of the patient's symptoms. After the patient has been free of pain for a period of several weeks, it is well to attempt to stop the medication altogether, hoping that by reducing the pain paroxysms and the irritability of the spinal trigeminal nucleus the patient has been put into a period of remission. We have found that a dosage of 800 mg per day of carbamazepine is the upper limit, since the commonly produced side effects are usually attained at dosages above this. In patients who are refractory to this form of therapy, we add phenytoin to the carbamazepine. When this is done, the dosage of the carbamazepine should be reduced to 200 mg two or three times a day while the phenytoin is given at a dosage of 100 mg two or three times a day. There are some patients in whom the pain still persists in spite of this combination of the two drugs. At that point, we add mephenesin to the regimen. This drug is given at a dosage of 400 mg two or three times a day in these patients with severe pain that is unresponsive to other medical therapy, and in these patients we receive some good results. It must be emphasized here that one must be very careful in using this combination of the three drugs for a prolonged period of time. It is unwise to do this as unwanted side effects may be produced in these patients.

Unfortunately, there are some patients who are refractory to all forms of medical therapy. In these patients, if the pain continues unabated, surgical therapeutic procedures should be considered.

SURGICAL TREATMENT

A review of the literature in regard to surgical therapy of trigeminal neuralgia reveals that there are numerous different surgical procedures that have been tried to relieve the pain. Since so many different types of procedures have been applied, it is obvious that the perfect operation for the relief of trigeminal neuralgia has yet to be devised. There is a need for sound surgical principles in the manipulative treatment of trigeminal neuralgia. "In these patients, the least serious operative procedure carrying the lowest mortality and morbidity rate producing the most minimal disability yet providing relief is the procedure of choice in the surgical therapy of trigeminal neuralgia. Each patient should be carefully evaluated and therapy designed to fit the individual problem."[17]

Peripheral injections and neurectomies. For several years it has been known that injections of destructive substances into the peripheral branches of the trigeminal nerves producing anesthesia in the trigger areas or in areas of distribution of the spontaneous pain, can be effective in relieving this syndrome, usually as long as the peripheral anesthesia persists. Ninety-five percent alcohol is the most common substance injected into the peripheral trunk, and this can at times produce pain relief for several years. Unfortunately, this is not the usual case. Most times the injection of alcohol is ineffective for significant periods of time while it carries with it the risk of damage to the neighboring tissues.

Peripheral neurectomy, according to Quinn,[18] is a conservative method of relieving the pain of trigeminal neuralgia. It acts by interrupting the flow of a significant number of afferent impulses to the central trigeminal apparatus. Not only does neurectomy remove the sensory receptors of the peripheral nerves, but the resulting trauma causes temporary degenerative changes in the ganglionic cells. Although the relief is temporary, the procedure can be repeated if the pain recurs. This form of treatment is indicated in patients in whom craniotomy, a more traumatic procedure which may cause complete anesthesia, is contraindicated because of age, debility, or significant systemic disease. Except for extremely old and debilitated patients, neurectomy is performed as an outpatient procedure under local anesthesia.

According to Ransohoff,[17] patients with second division pain harboring trigger areas in the nasolabial fold or in the upper gum usually at the level of the first incisor have been treated by avulsion of the infraorbital nerve through an incision carried out transorally in the upper gum. Patients suffering third division trigeminal pain in the lower jaw and harboring trigger areas in the lower gum along the lateral margin of the tongue have been subjected to section of the lingual and mental branches of the mandibular nerve, also by a transoral incision.

Injections into major divisions or into the gasserian ganglion. In patients not responding to drug therapy and whose pain is too widespread to consider for peripheral avulsion, consideration must be given to more proximal procedures. The injection of hot water into the ganglion via a foramen ovale approach as developed by Jaeger[19] was by all reports successful in a high percentage of cases but once again has fallen into disuse. Jefferson[20] reported on a series of his cases of trigeminal neuralgia in which, applying a radiographic method for control, phenol solution was injected into the gasserian ganglion. Phenol usually causes no more than a partial sensory loss and it may be regarded as causing a chemical gangliolysis. He believed that this method was relatively simple, safe, and remarkably free from complications.

Utilizing techniques of controlled radiofrequency, Sweet[21] developed a modification of the Jaeger procedure with considerable success in his own series of patients.

Rhoton[22] describes the technique of radiofrequency, stereotactic lysis of the gasserian ganglion, and sensory root lesions, techniques which overcome the need for general anesthesia, reducing the risk of injury to facial or extraocular nerves and lowering the risk of recurrent pain. By this manner the lesion is placed within the ganglion rather than in its peripheral branches. Using this method, the head of the patient is hyperextended and rotated to the opposite side from the pain and the foramen ovale is identified using the image tube. The needle is directed into the foramen ovale and its depth determined by x-ray. The depth the needle has passed through the foramen ovale varies according to the area of neuralgia. When the needle is in place, a stimulating current is passed and the needle readjusted until paresthesia occurs in the area of the trigeminal neuralgia. Barbital, 20 to 30 mg, is then administered intravenously in order to produce general anesthesia for 2 or 3 minutes. During this period the lesion is produced at 80° to 85° for 60 seconds. When the patient awakens, sensory testing is carried out in order to determine the extent of the analgesia. If not as extensive an area as desired is produced, the procedure is repeated until the desired result is achieved. The needle is then removed. Rhoton used this technique on eighteen patients, and all obtained relief of pain and none had any recurrence of pain after a 2-year period. This technique should produce a 1-year cure rate of approximately 80% and less than a 0.5% complication rate. Long-term relief seems to be about 50% at 5 years. This technique is particularly valuable in elderly or debilitated patients. The only undesirable side effect in these patients was extension of the numbness beyond the confines of the involved division in three patients.

Kirschner[23] introduced electrocoagulation of the gasserian ganglion as a treatment for trigeminal neuralgia, but later he abandoned this procedure because of the spread of heat and uncontrollable damage to neighboring structures. The technique was reintroduced in 1965 when stereotaxis and a highly effective radiofrequency generator made it possible to produce precise lesions causing only partial destruction of the trigeminal ganglion. A further technical advance was introduction by Tew of anesthetic techniques which allowed sensory testing of the patient during the operation.[24] Tew claimed successful results in 90% of 120 procedures. A submentovertex radiogram of the skull is used to demonstrate the bony landmarks, and the needle is placed in the foramen ovale and advanced until cerebrospinal fluid is obtained, indicating that the trigeminal cistern has been reached. The needle is maneuvered until low threshold electric stimulation produces paresthesia in the appropriate division without any contraction of the masseter muscle. The patient is then anesthetized by means of a short-acting technique. A thermistor is inserted into the hollow needle and the radiofrequency current is passed to produce a temperature of 65° at the needle tip for 60 seconds. About three lesions are required in each patient if dense hypalgesia is to be produced in the appropriate division. Tew treated sixty patients in this manner and follow-up ranged from 6 months to 4 years. Six of his patients had recurrences, three of which had no postoperative hypalgesia in the appropriate division. Diminished corneal sensation was present in 28% of his patients, troublesome numbness in 15%, corneal anesthesia in 10%, weakness of the masseter in 10%, keratitis in 4%, and cranial nerve palsies in 2%.

Intracranial operations directed toward the posterior root of the trigeminal nerve. Retrogasserian section of the posterior root of the trigeminal nerve by the subtemporal approach was the procedure of choice in the earlier days. In recent years, however, surgeons have shied away from this procedure, being somewhat hesitant to produce major areas of total anesthesia. The development of the procedure for decompression of the posterior root introduced a new era in the neurosurgical therapy of tic douloureux in which a large number of patients were afforded relief of pain without the production of major sensory loss. Disturbing incidences of recurrence, however, led to further refinement in this procedure in which the area of the ganglion and posterior root were selectively compressed. A small but significant number of recurrences have been reported in the series using the compression procedure.[25] Because of this, many surgeons have been hesitant to carry out this procedure, feeling that once a patient is subjected to the risks of an intracranial procedure he should be afforded the least likelihood possible of a recurrence requiring a second procedure of similar magnitude.

Transtentorial and posterior fossa procedures for the relief of trigeminal neuralgia. There are a number of advantages to this approach. Not only are the anatomical relationships more standard when approaching the posterior root via the intradural route, but in addition, unsuspected tumors and vascular malformations are more readily delineated and handled in this procedure. With the advent of the use of the operating microscope in surgical procedures, a significant refinement to the field of surgery has been added. With the use of this microscope Jannetta and Rand were able to confirm Dandy's original opinion that accessory fibers existed and might be concerned with the perception of light touch on the face.[26] These same authors have reported a number of successful procedures in which the major sensory root of the trigeminal nerve was sectioned and the accessory fibers preserved. In these patients complete relief of trigeminal pain has been afforded with preservation of light touch and corneal sensation in all instances.

Posterior root coagulation via the posterior fossa route. By this approach it has been possible to clearly visualize the entire nerve and coagulate the rostral two-thirds of the major sensory root and in some instances to a point of profound blanching and when desired to a point of tissue dissolution, depending on the voltage employed.

Ransohoff[17] used this method in twenty patients and there were no deaths by this means of treatment. The motor root was inadvertently sacrificed in two instances in this series and a partial lower facial weakness occurred in one patient. Pain relief was achieved in all patients in his series. Three patients had the interesting finding of pain relief with preservation of spotty sensation of touch throughout the face. In these three patients, who had originally suffered from pain in all divisions of the nerve, the rostral two-thirds of the root was coagulated to the point of dehiscence while the cephalad one-third was preserved with cauterization only to a point of tissue blanching. Ransohoff speculated that he inadvertently spared the accessory fibers of the posterior root or that a differential susceptibility to heat between the pain and touch fibers accounted for the fortuitously good result.

Trigeminal tractotomy. Incision of the descending trigeminal tract near the cervico-medullary junction will reliably cause the loss of pain and temperature sensation in the ipsilateral face and pharynx and usually will relieve the pain of trigeminal neuralgia. When gangliolysis or another surgical procedure has failed, tractotomy may succeed. It is especially helpful in a patient with pain perceived in both the glossopharyngeal or nervus intermedius and trigeminal distribution. It should not be the initial surgical procedure for trigeminal neuralgia.

GLOSSOPHARYNGEAL NEURALGIA

Glossopharyngeal neuralgia is a disorder characterized by paroxysms of severe lancinating pain in the tonsillar area, throat, and ear. Weisenberg[27] is credited with the original description of pain due to glossopharyngeal nerve irritation. However, Wilfred Harris[28] was the first to recognize glossopharyngeal neuralgia as a distinct pain syndrome.

Etiology

In addition to idiopathic glossopharyngeal neuralgia, etiologies which have been established include elongation of the styloid process, atheromatous plaques of the vertebral artery, tuberculous laryngitis, ossification of the stylohyoid ligament, and nasopharyngeal and intracranial tumors.

Symptoms

This type of neuralgia, often precipitated by chewing, swallowing, or yawning, is characterized by sudden paroxysms of pain of increasing intensity which seem to radiate from the throat to the deeper portions of the ipsilateral ear. The pain lasts 20 to 30 seconds and is often followed by an intense burning sensation lasting 2 or 3 minutes in these same areas. Glossopharyngeal neuralgia may be associated with cardiac arrest and syncope.[29] Males are affected more frequently than females.

Differential diagnosis

In establishing a diagnosis of glossopharyngeal neuralgia, one must exclude diseases of the throat and ear, such as tumors and inflammations. Actually the only disorder that strongly enters into the differential diagnosis is trigeminal neuralgia. Careful questioning will elicit the classic radiation of pain confined to the distribution of the ninth nerve in patients with glossopharyngeal neuralgia, whereas in patients with trigeminal neuralgia, the patient usually has a trigger zone which will precipitate the pain. This is in contrast to the different maneuvers which will precipitate the pain in glossopharyngeal neuralgia. An important step, which should be undertaken early in the treatment of this disease, is to rule out a local musculoskeletal lesion, neoplasm, or a bony or soft tissue abnormality as the cause of the pain and to make sure that it is not the usual kind of depressive pain affecting structures of the face and the neck.

Treatment

Once the physician is satisfied that glossopharyngeal neuralgia is present, conservative medical therapy should be attempted initially. This should consist of therapy with carbamazepine, using the lowest possible dosage. The dosage should begin at 200 mg a day and increase only as necessary. It should be kept to a minimum because there are definite toxic effects on the bone marrow, liver, and kidneys as well as less serious minor side effects, the chief one being lightheadedness. Baseline chemical studies, such as blood urea nitrogen, serum glutamic oxaloacetic transaminase, and complete blood count, should be taken, and these tests should be repeated every 4 to 6 weeks. Phenytoin is also used in the treatment of this condition. However, both phenytoin and carbamazepine are much less effective for treatment than they are for trigeminal neuralgia.

Before specific agents were available, vitamin B was the treatment of choice. This might be used if carbamazepine fails.

If carbamazepine is effective, the question of the duration of its use arises. The medication may be withdrawn at about the time a pain-free interval would normally be expected. Alternatively, it could be after 6 months. If pain recurs the carbamazepine treatment is started again and the hematologic, renal, and hepatic statuses are checked at regular intervals. Atropinization before an anticipated attack prevents cardiac and syncopal symptoms, but not throat and ear pain. After the effects of atropine have worn off, the carotid sinuses are massaged with the head in different positions. Manipulation will usually precipitate syncope or cardiac arrhythmia if the patient has hyperirritable carotid sinus disease. No symptoms will occur if the patient has true glossopharyngeal neuralgia with a vagal component, unless massaging the neck causes the patient to swallow and secretions flow over the triggered area. Anesthetizing the posterior wall of the pharynx may abort the attack, confirming the diagnosis. However, complete cocainization of the pharyngeal wall is difficult.

As mentioned earlier, medical therapy of this problem is not nearly as rewarding as in the treatment of trigeminal neuralgia. When medical therapy is unsuccessful, the physician has to resort to surgical therapy.[30] Anatomically, part of the ninth nerve may be included with the vagus nerve, where it emerges from the skull, and section of the ninth nerve alone will usually relieve pain in both groups. Extracranial block of the glossopharyngeal nerve is not recommended. Injection of alcohol in the region of the jugular foramen where these nerves exit would cause paralysis of the tenth, eleventh, and twelfth cranial nerves and also involve the sympathetic trunk. The nerve has been divided extracranially in the past, but this permits regeneration of the nerve with the recurrence of the pain.

The most satisfactory treatment consists of intracranial section of the ninth nerve. If both glossopharyngeal pain and ear pain are present, the auricular branches of the vagus nerve are probably also active in the process and the cephalic fibers of the vagus nerve should be cut. Following section of the ninth nerve, there is permanent unilateral anesthesia of the soft palate and pharyngeal wall from the eustachian tube to the epiglottis, including the posterior third of the tongue.

The upper two or three filaments of the ipsilateral vagus nerve should be cut only if the ninth nerve appears unusually thin, if the diagnosis cannot be made on clinical grounds, if there is a demonstrable trigger zone, if stimulation of the ninth nerve fails to reproduce the pain, or if the pain is incompletely reproduced. Section of the upper roots of the tenth nerve may be followed by intense irritation in the throat with prolonged, excessive, and troublesome coughing.

Postoperative sensory and reflex changes usually occur following section of the ninth nerve alone. The variability of the sensory changes probably results from the degree of sensory overlap of the field supplied by the ninth and tenth nerves in any particular instances. There are recurrences of minor or major degree despite the fact that the nerve is sectioned between a brainstem and its ganglia, which suggests that the positive mechanism of glossopharyngeal neuralgia probably lies within the brainstem.

We have seen a case where the patient was diagnosed as having a glossopharyngeal neuralgia of his left side and treated by intracranial section of his nerve. The patient responded very well to this form of therapy, but he returned 7 years later with similar symptoms on the opposite side. The patient was treated in like manner but had no benefit from the intracranial section of the nerve. After close follow-up, 1 year later it was observed that the patient had a small carcinomatous lesion in his piriform sinus, which was believed to be the precipitant of the symptoms on the second side.

Patients treated by the intracranial section of the nerve do remarkably well, with very low incidence of morbidity and mortality. They usually are awake the next morning and able to eat and perform acts which prior to surgery they had been completely afraid to attempt.

SPHENOPALATINE GANGLION NEURALGIA

An unusual type of neuralgia is attributed to involvement of the sphenopalatine ganglion, which lies just beneath the maxillary division of the trigeminal nerve and the lateral bony wall of the nose. The pain of sphenopalatine ganglion neuralgia is said to be due to nasal constriction of the vascular bed supplying the nasal mucous membrane, but there is doubt whether such nasal constriction is accompanied by pain. This ganglion gives nerve supply to the orbit, the sphenoidal and ethmoidal cells, the nose, the hard and soft palates, the tonsils, the

nasopharynx, and the gums. From this diffuse nerve supply it can be seen that the pain in this type of neuralgia is diffuse and widespread. It is believed by some that sphenopalatine ganglion neuralgia is, in fact, due to neuritis of the vidian nerve, caused in most instances by infection of the sphenoidal sinus. According to this concept, sphenopalatine ganglion neuralgia is a vidian neuralgia and is due to an irritation or inflammation of the vidian nerve.

The cause of this condition is not specifically known. Among the more commonly attributed causes are infection of the sphenoidal and ethmoidal sinuses, which was advocated by Sluder, who originally described this condition.[31] Also implicated are intumescence of the nasal membrane associated with intranasal deformities and such systemic disorders as toxemia and anemia. Pertinent intranasal deformities include deviation of the nasal septum, nasal spurs, prominent turbinates, adhesions, and osteomas. Many patients with sphenopalatine ganglion neuralgia have an intranasal deformity involving contact with the middle turbinate. The pain is said to be due to irritation of branches of the sphenopalatine ganglion supplying the middle turbinate. In other instances infection of the sphenoidal or ethmoidal sinuses appears to be responsible.

Symptoms

Sphenopalatine ganglion neuralgia is a disorder characterized by pain arising in or around the nose of the patient and spreading to the ipsilateral cheek, the upper teeth, the retroorbital and frontal temporal areas, and, posteriorly, the mastoid area on occasion. The pain is always unilateral, of high intensity, and continuous. It lasts from several hours to many weeks and, in severe cases, it lasts more than a year. It is usually described as a burning, aching sensation.

During the attacks, the nasal mucosal membrane in the involved side is swollen and the mucosa appears inflamed. Clear rhinorrhea and nasal obstruction are evident on the involved side. About half the patients in the series reviewed at the Mayo Clinic had a deviated nasal septum, but no case was causing pressure on the sphenopalatine ganglion as such.[30] These patients may also present with conjunctivitis or lacrimation, but this is not a strict criterion for the diagnosis of sphenopalatine ganglion neuralgia.

A majority of the patients had previously been treated for dental or sinus infection in the period immediately before the onset of their facial pain. These attacks occurred more commonly in women by a ratio of 2 to 1, and had the onset in the fourth to sixth decades of life in most instances.

Differential diagnosis

Among the conditions requiring differentiation are migraine, trigeminal neuralgia, cluster headache, dental abscesses and septal impaction, maxillary and ethmoidal sinus disease, brain tumors, intracranial aneurysms, and temporomandibular joint disease. Migraine is readily distinguished by the history of unilateral headache associated with nausea and vomiting, often with scotomas, hemianopias, or other transient phenomena, and relieved by ergotamine. Trigeminal neuralgia is characterized by sudden severe paroxysmal pain affecting one or more branches of the trigeminal nerve. Here the pain is not as diffuse as in sphenopalatine ganglion neuralgia. The pain, which is aching and burning, may occur spontaneously but is often initiated by a trigger mechanism that discharges pain into the involved area. These trigger mechanisms include such maneuvers as talking, eating, blowing the nose, scratching the face, and shaving. Cluster headache has been divided into two different types, lower-half cluster headache and upper-half cluster headache. This was described initially by Ekbom[32] and it was divided according to the varying distribution of the pain. In patients with lower-half cluster headache the pain is located in the orbital region where it radiates to the infraorbital area, over the cheek, and into the upper teeth. The pain is unilateral, sudden in onset, and severe. It lasts for only about 30 minutes to 2 hours. These attacks occur cyclically, lasting a few weeks to months, and then remitting only to recur. These attacks occur in a greater number of men than women by a ratio of 4 to 1. Individual attacks can be precipitated by alcohol consumption or tobacco smoking, and the attacks frequently occur after the patient reclines. Dental abscesses or impactions are easily diagnosed by inspection and roentgenograms. Brain tumor rarely gives a history of profuse pain such as is found in sphenopalatine ganglion neuralgia, and it is associated with bilateral headache, awareness of increased pressure, and signs of focal brain disease. Cerebral aneurysm may cause unilateral headache of the paroxysmal type, often behind the eye, but it is associated with cranial nerve palsies of varying sorts and often has signs of skull erosion as seen on a roentgenogram.

Treatment

The ideal form of treatment for sphenopalatine ganglion neuralgia would consist of prophylaxis. These patients often become addicted to narcotic preparations because of the chronicity of their pain.

Throughout the years, many different forms of therapy have been tried. Sluder suggested injecting the ganglion with a phenol solution.[31] Lillie[33] and Childrey reported relief from this type of a pain by cauterization of the ganglion with silver nitrate solution. If a severely deviated septum is involved in the pathogenesis of the symptoms, then a nasoseptal reconstruction should be performed. Other patients may be kept free of pain by the use of 0.5% cocaine nasal spray once or twice daily. Some patients are not relieved by this treatment or develop a tolerance to decongestants. Also, the repeated application of a nasal spray can cause severe irritation to the nasal mucosa. Sphenopalatine ganglionectomy has been resorted to in severe cases, with a fair degree of success reported, but side effects from this procedure, such as a dry eye, make this procedure a last resort.[34]

We recommend in a patient suspected of having sphenopalatine ganglion neuralgia that his nasal mucosa be treated with a local vasoconstricting agent to enable better visualization of the posterior aspect of the nose. A cocaine-treated applicator is then applied to the sphenopalatine ganglion, which is located immediately posterior to the medial end of the middle turbinate. If this procedure produces relief of the patient's symptoms, the diagnosis is confirmed after an unsuccessful attempt using a placebo and the condition is then treated. While the nasal mucosa is still reduced and visualization is good, the sphenopalatine ganglion is treated with a silver nitrate applicator or is cauterized by an electrocautery probe. This produces a traumatic injury to the ganglion and interferes with the transmission of pain impulses. In a series of twenty cases treated in this manner, each patient had a prolonged symptom-free interval, in each case achieving a longer symptom-free period than had been experienced before. The pain did recur in these individuals, but the procedure was then repeated with identical results.

VIDIAN NEURALGIA

Vidian neuralgia, according to Vail,[35] is a pain in the nose, face, eye, ear, head, neck, and shoulder occurring in severe attacks and essentially similar to that described by Sluder as sphenopalatine ganglion neuralgia. It is Vail's conclusion that the syndrome described as sphenopalatine ganglion[36] neuralgia is actually a vidian neuralgia and is due to an irritation or inflammation of the vidian nerve. For this reason, it seemed proper to Vail that the term "vidian neuralgia" be applied to this syndrome, rather than the term "sphenopalatine ganglion neuralgia."

Etiology

The vidian nerve is formed by the junction of the greater superficial petrosal nerve and a greater deep petrosal nerve at the beginning of the cranial opening of the vidian pterygoid canal of the sphenoid bone. The vidian nerve passes through the vidian canal to end in the sphenopalatine ganglion. The vidian nerve does not enter into the sphenomaxillary fossa, since the sphenopalatine ganglion sends a prolongation a short distance into the vidian canal. This fact is of prime importance, as it would be impossible by electric stimulation or alcohol or procaine injection in the sphenomaxillary fossa to act on a vidian nerve without acting on a portion of the sphenopalatine ganglion.

After comparing these facts with the known relations of the vidian nerve to the sphenoidal sinus, Vail thought it was logical that an inflammation in the sphenoidal sinus would be much more apt to cause an inflammatory reaction to the vidian nerve, as it is held in a bony canal, than it would in the sphenomaxillary fossa, thus indirectly acting on the ganglion. Many anatomic specimens have shown a very close relationship between the vidian nerve in its canal and the mucosa of the floor of the sphenoidal sinus. About the sphenopalatine ganglion, there is considerable areolar fatty tissue, and the ganglion is held loosely in a comparatively large space.

To explain the distribution of the painful symptoms of vidian neuralgia, Vail thought that the greater superficial petrosal nerve comes from the geniculate ganglion of the facial nerve; the greater deep petrosal is formed by a branch from the carotid plexus and the small deep petrosal from the petrous ganglion of the glossopharyngeal nerve. Thus, through the nerves uniting to form the vidian nerve, there is a close linkage between the sphenopalatine ganglion, the geniculate ganglion of the facial nerve, the superior cervical sympathetic ganglion, the glossopharyngeal nerve, and the vagus nerve. From the sphenopalatine ganglion pass orbital, nasal, and palatine branches, so that it is very easy to explain the referred pain in the eye, nose, and teeth. The explanation of the pain in the ear, a very typical and characteristic part of the vidian neuralgia syndrome, is a little more complicated. Fenton and Larsell[37] have made an intensive study of the sphenopalatine ganglion and its connections and believe that the pathway of reflex otalgia from involvements of the sphenopalatine regions was through the greater superficial petrosal nerve to the geniculate ganglion and out through the cutaneous ramus of the facial nerve to the auricular and mastoid region.

Vail believed that the pain in the ear described by sufferers with vidian neuralgia was due to impulses passing backward to the greater superficial petrosal nerve to the geniculate ganglion, and from there by either the cutaneous branch of the facial or by the tympanic nerve, while a more roundabout pathway is through the auricular branch of the vagus nerve.

The pain in the neck, back, and arm can be explained by impulses passing backward to the greater deep petrosal nerve to the superior cervical sympathetic ganglion and from there to the cervical nerves.

Differential diagnosis

A differential diagnosis should include trigeminal neuralgia, otalgia dentalis, tumors of the nasopharynx, disease of the apex of the petrous bone, and neuralgia directly due to acute or chronic anterior sinusitis.

Symptoms

Attacks of vidian neuralgia cannot be caused by any external stimulation or relieved by opiates, and they are not associated with any subjective loss of sensation. The attacks are most typically unilateral, often nocturnal, and may or may not be associated with the subjective symptoms of a nasal sinusitis. The condition, one of adult life, is most frequently found in women.

Treatment

Once the diagnosis has been made, if the case is a mild one of fairly recent duration, an injection of the sphenoidal sinus with iodized oil (Lipiodol) following the use of ephedrine, nasal douching, and colloidal silver preparations often relieve the pain, according to Vail.[35] Many acute attacks could be controlled by inserting a pledget of 10% cocaine without adrenaline in this sphenoidal recess against the front wall of the sphenoidal sinus and allowing the patient to recline with a pledget in the nose for 15 or 20 minutes.

Severe cases require a surgical procedure. This consists of a submucous resection of the septum carried back to the sphenoidal sinus, trimming the necessary part of the middle turbinate to gain full exposure of the sinus so that it may be inspected and any pathology there dealt with. This is followed by a postoperative treatment for a period of weeks to subdue the inflammation in the sphenoidal sinus. According to Vail, the prognosis as a rule is good, but it depends on the duration and severity of the symptoms, the degree to which the sphenoiditis can be eliminated, and the proximity of the vidian nerve to the sphenoidal sinus. When the vidian nerve is lying in the floor of the sinus with a very thin covering of bone, it will be affected more severely by a milder infection than a better protected nerve. Recurrences of the pain are to be expected; they come whenever there is an infection in the sinus and last as long as the infection continues. A satisfactory sphenoidal operation makes it much easier to control subsequent infections and to relieve the severe attacks by injecting a few drops of cocaine solution into the sphenoidal sinus.

There are several groups who believe that vidian neuralgia should more appropriately be placed in the atypical facial neuralgia group. The arguments for this are that it is conceivable that some patients with primary mucous membrane disease could have one or possibly two attacks of pain in the face which spread to adjacent structures. The sphenoidal sinus disease or inflammation in the region of the sphenopalatine ganglion could not explain the peculiar features demonstrated by this group of patients with so-called vidian neuralgia. Since major portions of the turbinates and adjacent mucous membrane and vascular structures receive their sensory nerve supply from afferent nerves passing through the ganglion, the application of cocaine, phenol, or alcohol to this region should dramatically stop pain, which has its source in the ganglion. However, it does not stop pain from afferent nerves that do not pass via this relatively small pathway.

Some authors seem to believe that the evidence indicates that quite different structures are involved. Because of the similarity to the group of neuralgias placed in the category of atypical facial neuralgia, it seems likely that so-called vidian neuralgia is actually a vascular syndrome involving the internal maxillary artery and especially the third portion that supplies the sphenopalatine region and the adjacent structures.

OCCIPITAL NEURALGIA

Occipital neuralgia is a disorder characterized by pain located in the cervical and posterior head regions, which may or may not extend to the orbital facial region.

Etiology

Primary occipital neuralgia is exceedingly rare. Almost invariably pain in the distribution of the upper cervical roots is secondary to irritation of the nerve by a functional derangement or disease process along its course. The most common cause for occipital neuralgia is the sustained contraction of the posterior cervical muscles in tense individuals. Additional common causes are arthritis and subluxation of the cervical spine, cervical intervertebral disk disease, traumatic neuritis resulting from whiplash injury, direct contusion of the nerve trunks, neuritis secondary to local or systemic inflammatory disease, and tumors along the course of the nerve.

Pain impulses from the posterior head regions and the neck are carried in the upper cervical posterior roots. The sensory root of the first cervical nerve is present in only 10% of individuals. The second cervical root responds to greater occipital nerves supplying the posterior scalp and appears to have the widest area of distribution. This nerve root is particularly subject to traumatic injury inasmuch as it does not have a foramen of exit but emerges unprotected between the posterior arches of the atlas and the axis. Going to this anatomic location, it is subject to crushing maneuvers that approximate these bony surfaces, for example, whiplash injury of the neck. The posterior root of the third cervical nerve supplies the postauricular region by the lesser occipital nerve. The fourth cervical posterior root is entirely cervical in its distribution.

Symptoms

According to Wolff there are three common types of headache in the back of the head and in the neck which are included in this category.[38] The first and most common is characterized by long-lasting (days, weeks, or months), more or less sustained aching of lower moderate intensity. It is commonly bilateral but may be unilateral. It is associated with stiffness of the muscles of the neck and tender points. The pain is modified by movement and manipulation of the muscles. It is not commonly associated with nausea or vomiting but may be accompanied by vertigo. The skin and underlying tissues of the neck and the head may be tender and the pain may spread to the front of the head.

The second type of occipital headache is characterized by recurrent attacks of high-intensity pain with complete freedom from pain between attacks. The headache is from 2 to 36 hours in duration, is usually unilateral in onset, but may spread to the opposite side. It is throbbing and made worse by the reclining position. Rarely it may persist for weeks. The headache is commonly associated with anorexia, nausea, and vomiting, and it is occasionally preceded by visual scotomas and paresthesias of the extremities.

Chouret[39] describes these patients as characteristically awakening in the morning with a headache. This symptom is not related to menstruation, emotional factors, physical fatigue, change in the weather, alcohol, tobacco, fruit allergies, or posture, and there is no prodrome in these patients. He said it has an occipitofrontotemporal distribution and is usually bilateral. There are no trigger zones. He says that the pain is constant, dull, and aching in character. Scalp and neck tenderness is usually present during the painful period, according to him. The frequency of attacks varies from weeks to months. The duration is variable from days to weeks. It does not occur periodically or at regular intervals. It is sometimes affected by flexion of the neck. Blurriness of vision is a constant association of the headache. This condition usually leads the patient to an ophthalmologist or an optometrist, and ocular causes for the disturbances are not found. The attack is not terminated by sleep, ergot preparations, or sedatives. According to Chouret the headache usually occurs between the second and sixth decades. It is more common in women than in men by a 2 to 1 ratio.

Differential diagnosis

Muscle tension headache is the entity most likely to be considered in a differential diagnosis. Tension headache occurs at any age and does not follow any particular pattern. It is associated with emotional tension or depression states and is relieved by psychotherapy whereas occipital neuralgia is not.

Migraine is associated with prodromal aura. It is a severe throbbing headache, hemicranial in its distribution, it has a familial tendency, and it is relieved by ergot preparations whereas occipital neuralgia is not.

Treatment

In treating occipital neuralgias, every effort should be made to relieve the underlying pathologic lesion. If the neuralgia has resulted from trauma to the cervical spine, such as a whiplash injury, conservative measures should always be given an adequate trial. These include rest, cervical traction, muscle relaxant drugs, application of moist heat, and a gentle massage. The majority of patients will improve steadily with this regimen. In some instances it is justifiable to block the greater and lesser occipital nerves of the second cervical posterior root with local anesthetics.

Anatomically the greater occipital nerve exits through the muscles and fascia of the posterior aspect of the neck and becomes superficial immediately below the occipital bone protuberance. Deep fingertip pressure over that area would elicit exquisite tenderness. At that point, an injection of 2 ml of 1% xylocaine with 3 ml of 0.6% aqueous solution of ammonium chloride will give spontaneous, complete, and lasting relief of the headache and all of its associated manifestations.

The effect is striking and dramatic. Repeated injections are rarely needed. The headache may recur and the interval between attacks varies from several weeks to several months.

The second type of occipital neuralgia described by Wolff[38] is promptly and dramatically modified by ergotamine tartrate. If the ergotamine is administered intramuscularly or intravenously soon after onset, cocaine injection into the region of the occipital artery may eliminate the headache. The interval between attacks and intensity of attacks is modified by adjustments of life situations and changes in attitudes.

Although some have had excellent results with avulsion of the greater occipital nerve, intraspinal section of the sensory root of the second cervical nerve, or combined section of the posterior root of both the second and third cervical nerves, the majority of neurosurgeons have not been too enthusiastic about these operations, inasmuch as the benefits are apt to be temporary. The pain in these patients usually returns after a period of time, and probably the cause for this is the regeneration of the nerve. On the other hand, occipital neurotomy and upper cervical posterior rhizotomy are justifiable if it can be shown that disease affecting these nerve roots is present.

PETROSAL NEURALGIA

Petrosal neuralgia is a disorder characterized by nocturnal attacks of fronto-orbitotemporal pain accompanied by lacrimation and conjunctival injection. Gardner and his associates[40] state that the syndrome they termed "petrosal neuralgia" was originally described in 1939 by Horton, MacLean, and Craig[41] as erythromyalgia of the head and later by Horton[42] as histaminic cephalalgia.

Etiology

In searching for a physiologic explanation as to how an excitation of the greater superficial petrosal nerve could cause unilateral head pain, Cobb and Finesinger[43] found that the greater superficial petrosal nerve carried secretory fibers for the lacrimal gland and secretory and vasodilator fibers for the mucous membrane of the nasal cavity. These results showed that the nerve carried somatic afferent fibers from the dura mater, internal carotid artery, and spheno-palatine ganglion to the ganglion cells in the geniculate ganglion. The most important thing that they demonstrated was that the greater superficial petrosal nerve carries vasodilator fibers to the ipsilateral cerebral hemisphere. In 1940, when Schumacher showed that cerebral vasodilation causes headaches, a chain of evidence was completed.[44]

Therefore, it appears that periodic discharges of parasympathetic impulses over the greater superficial petrosal branch of the seventh nerve should cause unilateral lacrimation, unilateral swelling, and secretion of the nasal mucosal and unilateral head pain.

Symptoms

Patients complain to the physician of a syndrome consisting of recurrent attacks of severe unilateral head pain. Associated with the pain are an intense lacrimation and conjunctival injection of the ipsilateral eye. This pain is usually sharp and stabbing in nature and it is located in the retroorbital region. These exacerbations usually occur in the early morning hours, and the attacks often awaken the patient.

Treatment

Gardner[40] reported thirteen cases of petrosal neuralgia. Three of these thirteen patients had attacks on both sides of the head. In treating these patients, he divided the greater superficial petrosal nerve seventeen times totally. Two of the patients had bilateral operations. In one patient in whom the pain recurred, the nerve was divided a second and a third time. Gardner used thiopental sodium (Pentothal) anesthesia employing the usual approach to the gasserian ganglion. The dura was elevated from the floor of the middle fossa and with the dental applicator, a bit of cotton was forced into the foramen spinosum, then the middle meningeal vessels were divided. The dura was elevated further medially until the hiatus fallopii and groove of the greater superficial petrosal nerve were exposed. The nerve could be seen leaving the hiatus and traversing the groove until it disappeared beneath the lower portion of the gasserian ganglion. The nerve was picked up on a nerve hook and divided, and a portion of it was removed.

In trying to express the value of the operation from the results of his patients, it seems fair to say that the results were excellent in 25%, fair to good in 50%, and a failure in 25%. In the failures, it was obvious that neither the efferent nor afferent impulses responsible for the attacks were interrupted. This means that the attacks of headache in these cases were not due to vasodilator impulses originating in the seventh nerve system central to the point at which the nerve was divided. Since this operation constitutes a preganglionic neurectomy, it would not be expected to relieve head pain due to discharges of vasodilator impulses if they originated in the system peripheral to the point of surgical interruption.

Gardner discussed three possible mechanisms by which this operation could relieve the head pain. The most attractive was that the operation interrupted the abnormal parasympathetic discharges which caused dilation of the cerebral meningeal and nasomucosal blood vessels. The second explanation is that the operation interrupts painful impulses coming over the geniculate somatic afferent fibers from the dura, internal carotid artery, and vidian nerve. Third, the relief might be due to the incidental interruption of the superficial temporal artery, the middle meningeal artery, or the lesser superficial petrosal nerve or perhaps to psychic factors incidental to hospitalization and operation.

As can be seen from the discussion of the symptoms of this disease, these symptoms are very similar to the entity known as histamine cephalalgia or cluster headache. The diagnosis of petrosal neuralgia is very rarely made these days, as it is commonly believed that petrosal neuralgia is the same entity as cluster headaches.

ATYPICAL FACIAL PAIN

Atypical facial pain or atypical facial neuralgia is a term used to describe an ill-defined group of craniofacial pains which do not resemble major neuralgia or pain secondary to disease of extracranial or intracranial structures. The remarkable confusion regarding atypical facial pain arises not only from the various descriptions of this disorder but also from the multiplicity of suggested causes. A distinct definition of atypical facial pain is not possible, but the term must be delimited to some degree if it is to be used intelligently. In attempting this, we can best start by stating what the term does not include. Atypical facial pain does not refer to trigeminal neuralgia, glossopharyngeal neuralgia, postherpetic neuralgia, or pains caused by obvious disease of the teeth, throat, nose, sinuses, ears, or eyes. This leaves a group of conditions characterized by pain that is deep, polylocalized, and vaguely described by the patient. The pain may be felt in regions supplied by the fifth and ninth cranial nerves and the second and third cervical nerves. The distribution of the pain is "unanatomic" in that it may involve portions of the sensory supply of two or more of these nerves and may cross the midline. In general, this pain is constant and endures for long periods, whether it be weeks or years. Trigger zones are lacking. Patients often describe the pain as boring, pressing, pulling, burning, or aching.[45]

If the pain in these patients can be relieved, the result is a most grateful patient; if the pain is unrelieved the result may be an unhappy and hostile patient. The challenge of diagnosing the etiology of the patient's pain can be a fascinating and thrilling challenge. Frequently it is not easy, especially if the referring physician has already eliminated the typical syndromes causing facial pain.

Atypical facial pain is a term like fever or convulsions. It names a symptom but does not imply a definite origin or a cause. Given a case of atypical facial pain, what are the possibilities as far as diagnosis, etiology, and treatment are concerned? In an attempt to answer some of these questions, Rushton[50] studied 100 patients initially given a diagnosis of typical facial pain who were seen at the Mayo Clinic. He found it was possible to classify the conditions of each of these patients under one of three headings: psychogenic, organic, and indeterminate. This classification was not made on the basis of any frequency of notions concerning etiologic factors or pathologic changes.[40]

Etiology

Neither the causes nor the physiologic disturbances of atypical facial neuralgia are clearly understood, but the mechanisms involved appear to be vascular, muscular, and psychogenic, alone or in combinations.

In Rushton's review of 100 patients with atypical facial pain, he found fifty-three who suffered from depressive reactions, conversive hysteria, or schizophrenia. Each of them complained primarily of facial pain. The age of onset in these patients varied from 12 to 70 years. There were forty-six women and seven men involved with this psychogenic etiology. The pain in these patients varied from 1 to 36 years in duration. Only eight of the patients had any remission of pain throughout the course of their disease. Of these eight patients, three gave no recognizable reason for remission. One had pain only with her menstrual periods, and the remaining four had noted temporary relief after minor surgical procedures on the nose, sinuses, or teeth. The other patients in this group suffered from constant pain. Thirty-three patients were unable to recognize any cause for their pain. The presumed causes offered by the remaining twenty patients were dental operations, eleven patients; being struck in the face, three patients; nervous conditions, nasal operations, parotitis, infected ear, and operation on the trigeminal nerve, one patient each.

In the second group of patients studied by Rushton, the pain appeared as a result of an actual anatomic problem such as a neoplasm or from obviously disturbed physiologic function, as in the case of vasodilating face pain. This group consisted of thirty-three patients and could be subdivided into five groups, namely those with etiology from (1) vasodilating facial pain, (2) dental disease, (3) neuritis, (4) neoplasms, and (5) miscellaneous conditions.

There were seven men and one woman who had *vasodilating facial pain* thought to be the result of dilation of arteries of the face. This pain closely resembled cluster headache, but the location was sufficiently unusual to cause some difficulty in recognition. The greatest pain was located in the lower portion of the face, in contrast to the location in the usual case of a cluster head-

ache. These attacks were brief, as in cluster headaches, and usually occurred several times within a 24-hour period. In each of these patients, treatment with ergotamine tartrate relieved the typical attack.

Six of these patients had originally been diagnosed as having trigeminal neuralgias. Various surgical procedures had been performed on these patients in an attempt to relieve the pain, including extraction of the teeth, operations on the nose and sinuses, alcohol injection, and avulsion of the branches of the trigeminal nerve and decompression of the gasserian ganglion. Each of these procedures was done to relieve the patient's pain, and each was a failure.

Dental disease was implicated as the cause in eight patients reviewed by Rushton. In each case the pain was unusual, and there was no outstanding evidence for dental disease during the early part of the illness. The pain in these patients consisted of a constant ache in the face but not the teeth, and there was a severe but intermittent ache in some patients. A few patients noted that cold food or liquids would increase the pain. Spontaneous remissions were noted in three-fourths of these patients, and analgesics were able to afford relief to the great majority of them.

The pain in the patients with dental origin of the disease was polylocalized. At no time was it localized to the offending tooth until late in the course of the illness. In five of the eight patients, final diagnosis was pulpitis, and the pain was relieved by extraction of the tooth.

It was thought that *neuritis* of some portion of the trigeminal nerve was the source of the pain in eight patients in the series by Rushton. The age of onset in these patients ranged from 24 to 73 years, and the duration of their complaints ranged from 2 months to 3 years. Presumed causes for the neuritis were trauma to the face in three patients, extraction of teeth in two, and an insect bite of the forehead in one. No cause for the pain could be recalled by the remaining two patients. In these patients, the pain is described as burning and itching, jabbing, or sticking. In each instance, it was limited to the branch of the nerve that was presumed to have been injured, and each patient had a slight but definite loss of sensation in that region.

There were three patients who had *neoplasms* as the etiology of their facial pain. Two women had suffered from pain for 5 and 6 years, before other evidence of a tumor became apparent. Each had a cylindroma, one being located in the parotid gland and one in the antrum. The third patient was a man who had an acoustic neurofibroma as the source of his aching, jabbing, and burning pain of 1-year duration.

The remaining six patients in the group with organically caused pain had a variety of *miscellaneous conditions*. The pain in each instance was unusual as a manifestation of the presumed cause, or the cause was not readily apparent. Among the conditions associated here were acromegaly, thyroditis in two women, hemiplegia after a stroke, and one man with a 22-year history of tabes dorsalis.

The third group of patients were those classified as having a pain of indeterminate etiology. This group consisted of five men and nine women. The age of onset in these patients was later than the other two groups, being over 50 years of age. The duration of pain was relatively short, as compared with that in the psychogenic pain group. The presumed causes for pain in this group as given by six patients included infections, injuries, and operations about the face. The remaining eight patients could not recognize any cause for their pain. In these patients the pain was of shorter duration and came on later in life. Remissions were common. The pain was made worse by various maneuvers, such as chewing, rubbing the face, or jarring the head. Most of these patients could obtain temporary relief of their pain with the use of ordinary analgesics. There was no reliable evidence in

any patients to indicate that the pain was psychogenic, and the character of the pain suggested the organic cause.

Kerr[46] has demonstrated that spread of pain from cervical dorsal roots to the trigeminal region may occur in humans. He did this by operating on patients under local anesthesia. In these cases, stimulation of the first cervical root gave rise to referred pain in the orbitofrontal region and the vertex. It was later shown that injections of hypertonic saline into the upper posterior cervical muscles produce pain in the frontal region. It has also been noted on occasion that stimulation of the C-2 dorsal root produced referred pain in the face.[46]

In other studies, Kerr[47] has demonstrated that there is a marked convergence of primary afferents of the first three cervical roots with those of the trigeminal throughout the subnucleus caudalis of the C-1 segment, especially in the lower half. Since the trigeminal afferents are quite sharply laminated as far as their most caudal level according to the divisions of the nerve from lateral or the ophthalmic division, to the medial or the mandibular division, and because the upper three cervical roots are not distributed evenly in this nuclear area, it follows that specific divisions are more intimately associated with individual cervical afferents. C-1 primary afferents tend to be distributed slightly more medially in the dorsal horn and are therefore related mainly to mandibular division fibers. C-2 afferents, on the other hand, converge with fibers of all three trigeminal divisions, but because C-2 fibers are distributed mainly to the lateral aspect of the C-1 segment in its upper half or ophthalmic division, afferents are present in large numbers. It is this relationship which predominates. C-3 fibers show a similar but considerably more restricted pattern of convergence with the trigeminal to that of C-2, the main difference being that the density and extent of conversions are less pronounced.

Primary afferents from C-4 have negligible relationships with trigeminal homologues, although the C-5 and lower roots do not establish any direct relationship with trigeminal primary endings. This, of course, does not exclude the possibility of functional interaction between these more caudal afferents and those of the trigeminal by way of interneurons, but this would almost certainly be at best a very weak connection, since evoked trigeminal responses cannot be recorded below the midportion of the C-2 segment, while ascending effects from stimulation of cervical dorsal roots can be recorded from the dorsal horn at most to a level of three segments above the stimulated root.

Kerr noted that pain is the first symptom in most of these patients and that the vegetative component occurs after the neurologic episode is well established. These vasomotor symptoms may be pronounced in some patients and have lead to the thought that they may be vasomotor headaches. An explanation for these symptoms cannot be given on anatomic grounds since the autonomic centers and pathways in the medulla and upper cervical cord are virtually unknown. This is particularly true for the vasomotor components.[47]

It has been maintained in the past that autonomic neurons are present in the cervical cord in the intermediate area of the gray column. If this is so it is possible that in these headaches the vasomotor component also is affected by our central convergence since in the microelectrode study referred to, convergence of both trigeminal and cervical volleys on single units in the intermediate gray matter was clearly demonstrated. However, such a vasomotor mechanism must be regarded as speculative until further anatomic and physiologic evidence can be offered regarding the autonomic function of neurons in this area.

While the etiology appears to be unknown, the underlying pain mechanism, according to Radman,[48] appears to be due to a neurovascular disturbance related to migraine. It is claimed that pain arises from distention of the internal maxillary artery and its branches, and there is often an associated pain from sustained contraction of skeletal muscles. According to Radman, the pain provoked by the distended vessels is conveyed by afferent fibers which travel by a sympathetic pathway into the spinal cord. Some of the painful impulses pass centrally to the facial, vagus, and glosspharyngeal nerves.

Symptoms

Atypical craniofacial neuralgias are characterized by not conforming to the peripheral distribution of the cranial nerves but spreading either continuously or discontinuously from one site to another. Most of the patients in this category are young or middle-aged women. Pain begins gradually or rapidly, builds up progressively over a period of 2 to 10 minutes to a maximum, lasts from 15 minutes to 6 or more hours or even days, and subsides either gradually or in some instances quite rapidly.

Pain is usually first felt in the temporal area deep behind the eyes, sometimes over the malar eminence, back up over the side of the head well within the hairline, and then in behind the ear and into the area of the posterior triangle of the cervical region. Occasionally it then extends out over the slope of the shoulder. The pain occurs more often at nighttime, in contrast to trigeminal neuralgia, which is more common in the daytime. The pain starts as a slow aching, pulling, and throbbing and will gain momentum in a crescendo fashion reaching a peak after a matter of hours. Then the patient arises and uses hot applications on the side of the head and face until the pain gradually recedes in the same slow fashion that it had at onset. The patient may then be free of pain for a period of a few days to weeks, sometimes as long as several months. The pain is never worsened by touching, eating, or swallowing. It is not deep within the ear, and it is not within the throat.

The neuralgias are strictly unilateral, although bilateral varieties have been described. The latter are much less frequent.

Vasomotor components may be prominent in such cases and any of the following or combinations thereof may be seen: nasal obstruction due to edema of the mucosa, followed often by clear, thin mucous rhinorrhea; edema of the lids; flushing of the face; lacrimation; and piloerection of the scalp. All of these are restricted to the same side as the pain syndrome and never occur contralaterally, except that the piloerection may be bilateral. They begin after the onset of the pain and disappear as it subsides. Diffuse vegetative and neurologic symptoms such as nausea, dizziness, mild vertigo, asthenia, and cold, clammy sensations may also be experienced during such episodes.

Diagnosis

The most important step, and the first one to take when seeing patients with this atypical facial pain, is to obtain a careful and very detailed history. The patient should be asked to recall his first experience with the pain and recount its exact location and character at onset. He should be questioned as to his ideas as to the etiology of it and as to what precipitates it. The subsequent course of the pain should be ascertained in an attempt to discover whether it is constant or intermittent. If remissions occur, the patient should list their frequency and duration, as well as their possible causes. It is important to discover when the pain was present, what would aggravate it, and what would relieve it. It is also important to ask these patients if the pain has remained constant in location and character or has changed throughout the course of their disease. It is also important to ask what has been used in the way of treatment—in other words, what medications have been attempted, or what maneuvers can they apply to relieve their pain.

A careful physical examination is very important in these patients, since it may reveal such conditions as thyroiditis, which will account for the pain. A good, thorough otolaryngologic examination is necessary in these patients to rule out any source of pain such as septal deviation, which may cause pressure on the nasal turbinates and therefore pain. It is often necessary to carry out dental or neurologic studies. Roentgenograms of the skull, sinuses, teeth, cervical portion of the spinal column, and temporomandibular joints may be required. In some cases special roentgenologic studies such as tomography are of value. Biopsy of any suspicious mass or region is justified in an attempt to discover the etiology of the problem.

Psychogenic aspects

Most of these patients at some time during the course of their disease have been described as having pain of psychogenic origin and their condition has been classed as a psychosomatic illness. As a group, these patients are truly distressing and unfortunate. They usually have a very long history of discomfort, and they maintain steadfastly that the pain is unbearable and incapacitating. They have a difficult time describing the pain that is bothering them, and they generally state that it is a deep pain. Accordingly, if we think of deep pain of visceral origin, it is not surprising that patients do not have the quick, disturbed reaction seen with cutaneous pain. Most of these patients have a common psychosomatic background and psychologic makeup. Because of this, and because no other strong etiologic factors have been forthcoming, it is believed that atypical facial pain is fundamentally a psychiatric disorder. A study done by Smith and associates[49] at the Mayo Clinic was undertaken in an attempt to review the psychiatric aspects of these patients with the diagnosis of atypical facial pain. Special emphasis was placed on those patients in whom no apparent or organic etiology could be found. There were twenty women and twelve men, aged 29 to 79 years, included in this study. All had undergone appropriate clinical investigations including neurologic examination before being referred for psychiatric consultation. Of the thirty-two patients, twenty-three were diagnosed as suffering from atypical facial pain, and nine were diagnosed as having trigeminal neuralgia with psychiatric features. The latter group had previously been subjected to a total of twenty-two surgical procedures, all of which failed to relieve their pain. Psychiatric diagnoses arrived at were as follows: depressive reaction, twenty patients; conversion reaction, seventeen; hysterical personality, twelve; compulsive personality, two; emotionally unstable personality, one; passive aggressive personality, one; paranoid personality, one; involutional psychotic depression, one; prolonged grief reaction, one; no psychiatric diagnosis, two patients.

As a total group, the patients were judged to be perfectionistic, striving, hypochondriacal, and depressed. Both male and female patients appeared angry and resentful, usually as a result of frustrated attempts at interpersonal relationships. The repressed anger and resentment caused both depression and facial pain.[49]

There is one disturbing feature not quite compatible with all of this—all the patients tend to give a very detailed history which is quite consistent with others who have this syndrome. Another discomforting fact is, that even though this is thought to be a psychiatric disorder, the beneficial effects of psychiatry have not been too rewarding in the treatment of this condition.

Treatment

As Friedman has mentioned, there has been no therapy completely effective in the long-term management of atypical facial neuralgias. Medical treatment is best limited to simple analgesics, sedatives, and tranquilizing drugs. For patients who are subject to depression, the antidepressants are more effective than the anxiety-reducing drugs. The number of drugs recommended in these cases is proof of the unsatisfactory status of pharmaceutical therapy.[50]

Foster[51] has recommended the use of monoamine oxidase inhibitors in these patients. For some years patients with atypical facial pain have been treated with 15 mg of phenelzine together with trifluoperazine, 1 mg three times a day, with evidence of relief. More recently, Foster recommended the use of a tricyclic compound such as imipramine, 25 mg three times a day, or amitryptyline, 25 mg three times a day.

Procedures intended to relieve pain may be of value provided they can be carried out with safety. Injection of a local anesthetic agent into the painful region or into a nerve supplying this region is of value when practical. The results of a single treatment should not be relied on, particularly when the one injection relieves the pain. In some cases injection should be repeated with sterile water to test the suggestability of the patient. Application of a solution of cocaine to painful regions in the throat or nose may relieve the pain. If relief is obtained the procedure may be repeated with a solution of quinine used as a control.

Radman[48] has recommended the treatment of these patients with one or two ergotamine tartrate tablets at the onset of their pain. This is most beneficial in patients thought to have a vasomotor or vasodilating etiology for their pain. Radical treatment in these patients consists of long-term drug therapy.

Rushton[45] has recommended the trial of histamine to induce or augment the pain or the injection of ergotamine tartrate to relieve it if the pain has characteristics suggesting that is the result of vasodilation.

The various surgical procedures described in the literature have been attended by the same absence of permanent success as medical treatment. Treatment frequently is unsatisfactory since section of one or more cranial and cervical nerves or the cervical sympathetic nerve provide only temporary relief and rarely permanent cure. Particularly when surgery has been resorted to, further distress and increased complaints may follow because, if the pain is not relieved, the discomfort of anesthesia will have been added.

For most patients with atypical facial neuralgia, the most important method of treatment is psychotherapy. Psychotherapy must be tailored to each patient and will vary with his insight, resistance, and personality structure. If the patient displays evidence of a significant emotional disorder, psychiatric consultation is of value. As a result of such study it may become apparent that the pain is the primary symptom of depression or a similar major psychiatric problem. The patient's emotional state occasionally is such that it causes him to exaggerate an organic pain which he otherwise might bear with good grace. In such cases, proper psychiatric care may so lessen the significance of the pain and it no longer presents a problem.

POSTHERPETIC NEURALGIAS

Herpes zoster involvement of the trigeminal nerve affects the ophthalmic division almost exclusively. Postherpetic neuralgia is characterized by continuous aching, burning pain that persists after the acute phase of herpes zoster has subsided.

Etiology

This condition is secondary to an inflammation of the gasserian ganglion by the herpes zoster virus. Microscopic examination during the acute phase discloses edema, hemorrhage, hyperemia, and cellular infiltration.

There is no known cause for the persistence of pain after the acute phase has subsided. This pain is not relieved by retrogasserian neurectomy, and this suggests that the pain impulses reaching consciousness may have a central origin. This would imply that the virus had extended along the secondary trigeminal pathways in the brainstem.

Symptoms

This condition usually occurs in people of middle age or older. It most commonly affects the ophthalmic division or the first division of the trigeminal nerve. The first symptom encountered in these patients is a severe burning pain in the involved area, which is followed in a few days by the characteristic cutaneous eruption. The herpetic eruption is characterized by groups of inflamed small vesicles. After the acute phase of the disease has subsided, the vesicles are replaced by punctate scars irregularly dispersed on a background of glossy hyperemic atrophic skin. This is where the term "postherpetic neuralgia" was coined. The term denotes pain persisting after the acute attack has subsided. The pain in these patients is usually a constant, burning, and aching type of pain. There may be a sharp stabbing pain superimposed on the constant pain. King[52] describes the earliest and most constant ocular sign to be conjunctival congestion on the affected side. Vesiculation and subsequent contraction generally noted in the skin are only rarely observed in the conjuctiva.

"Keratitis" appears in two forms. In the first week or two many superficial infiltrations appear. Lesions do not ulcerate, are not always associated with uveitis, and heal with little scarring. Diffuse deep keratitis starts 1 to 3 months or later after onset and is far more serious. Severe anterior uveitis, ulceration, and permanent corneal scarring may result.

Iridocyclitis may occur but is usually a benign serous type. However, large iris nodules and spontaneous hyphema may cause either troublesome glaucoma or lower intraocular tension.

Infection may paralyze the third, fourth, sixth, or seventh cranial nerve, but palsy usually is entirely gone in 2 months. If internal ocular structures are paralyzed, full recovery is rare. Involvement of the ciliary ganglion may produce total iridodplegia, or the Argyll Robertson pupil may be closely imitated. Reaction in only one eye is significant.

Optic neuritis, a rare complication of herpes, may be followed by considerable nerve atrophy. Episcleritis or acute dacro-adenitis may occur.

Vague neuralgic discomfort around the eye may be labeled psychogenic until the forehead shows diffuse patches of erythema. As a skin rash emerges, initial pain declines and gradually subsides in a few weeks.

Treatment

Medical therapy in these patients includes attempted procaine block of the nerves supplying the skin adjacent to the scarred area. Massage of the affected area for 10 to 15 minutes three or four times a day is also recommended. Some people recommend application of a mechanical vibrator three or four times daily for 10 to 15 minutes. These localized treatments combined with local anesthesia have produced considerable relief in patients. Other medical therapy such as carbamazepine and phenytoin have not given very satisfactory results. Vitamin B_{12} and intravenous procaine have also been used with little success. Local injections of corticosteroids such as hydrocortisone have been helpful in some patients. Amitriptyline, an antidepressant, has been reported to be used successfully in these patients. Twenty-five milligrams used four times a day for periods ranging from 1 to 4 months is the recommended dosage. The natural history of the condition appears to be shortened by this method of treatment. Farber[53] has recommended using chlorprothixene, which is a psychotherapeutic agent used to treat moderate to severe emotional disorders. He has used this in conjunction with carbamazepine in the successful treatment of patients with postherpetic neuralgia.

In many patients medical therapy does not afford relief from their symptoms. In these patients it has been recommended that elevation of a large flap of the painful skin or avulsion of its secondary nerve supply might provide preliminary regional anesthesia, stopping the pain. Stereotaxic trigeminal tractotomy has been recommended to afford relief from pain in patients with severe and incapacitating pain when conservative therapy has failed.

GENICULATE NEURALGIA

There are two forms of geniculate neuralgia seen in clinical practice. One is termed an idiopathic geniculate neuralgia and the other is seen secondary to an infection by a herpes virus. This is the syndrome described originally by Hunt and called the Ramsay-Hunt syndrome. We will be speaking in this section about the idiopathic geniculate neuralgia. It is often difficult to separate cases of geniculate neuralgia from glossopharyngeal neuralgia, but there is evidence that a distinct neuralgia of the intermediate nerve does occur. The intermediate nerve is usually thought of as the sensory branch of the facial nerve. Actually, it is a mixed nerve and contains autonomic efferent fibers which are part of the parasympathetic nervous system. General visceral efferent fibers arise in the superior salivatory nucleus and pass through the intermediate nerve. Most of these fibers travel with the greater superficial petrosal nerve to innervate the lacrimal gland and the glands of the nose, nasopharynx, and palate. The rest of the fibers join the chorda tympani and pass through the lingual nerve to supply the submaxillary and sublingual glands. Special visceral afferent fibers convey taste sensation from the anterior two-thirds of the tongue and they, in the nucleus of the solitary tract general somatic afferent fibers, convey sensation from the ear. It is thought that the posterior auricular branch of the facial nerve joins the auricular branch of the vagus and glossopharyngeal nerves in the cutaneous supply of the auricle and the external auditory canal.

Etiology

The cause of this disorder is not known. No one has ever described a lesion in the nerve itself or in the immediate vicinity in the few cases in which surgical treatment has been extended to the patient.

As evidence of the term "idiopathic" in the title of this disease, one must be careful not to categorize this with the Ramsay-Hunt syndrome, which is secondary to a herpetic infection of the geniculate ganglion. The symptoms are different in these two patients and, therefore, the two entities must be separated.

Symptoms

Idiopathic geniculate neuralgia develops usually in young to middle-aged adults. There have been more cases reported in women than in men, and there is no familial incidence. This neuralgia can occur on either side, with no specific preference for side. Pain is located in these patients within the depths of the ear, the auditory canal, and/or the pinna. The pain is long-lasting, occurring for several hours. Rarely there are brief paroxysms described as sharp, shooting, or burning. There is usually no trigger point to provoke the pain in these patients. However, there may be areas of localized tenderness in the region of the ear.

As mentioned, this disease can sometimes be confused with glossopharyngeal neuralgia, especially where the pain is limited to the tympanic branch. Furlow[54] reproduced the typical pain in these patients by stimulating the intermediate nerve. When the ninth nerve was stimulated, the pain was atypical in these patients, being localized in the throat, with only some radiation to the ear.

In patients with Ramsay-Hunt syndrome or pain due to herpes zoster of the geniculate neuralgia, herpetic vesicles will have been present on the auricle and in the external auditory canal. Furthermore, geniculate herpetic infections are frequently accompanied by facial paralysis and at times auditory and vestibular symptoms due to involvement of the eighth nerve.

Treatment

There has been no form of medical therapy which has afforded a great deal of success. In patients diagnosed as having this disease, a trial of carbamazepine, phenytoin, and/or mephenesin is indicated. However, the results of this therapy are often unrewarding. Treatment is similar to that undertaken in patients with trigeminal neuralgia; however, the results do not seem to be as good. Beneficial effects have increased since the beginning of the treatment with carbamazepine.

If there is intolerance to carbamazepine, the condition will respond to section of the intermediate nerve, provided the patient experiences a typical attack of pain on stimulation of his nerve as described by Furlow.[54]

SUPERIOR LARYNGEAL NEURALGIA

The superior laryngeal nerve is a branch of the vagus nerve which supplies sensory fibers to the epiglottis, the base of the tongue, and that portion of the larynx which lies about the epiglottis. The external branch of this superior laryngeal nerve carries primarily motor fibers, and the internal branch is a division which is most concerned in superior laryngeal neuralgia. This is the portion which supplies the piriform sinuses, the epiglottis, and the base of the tongue.

Symptoms

Superior laryngeal neuralgia is characterized by a number of features. Pain is severe, lancinating, and paroxysmal and is not too dissimilar from that seen in patients with trigeminal neuralgia. These patients usually state that in most cases the site of distress is the side of the neck rather than the face or ear. The pain of these patients is localized to a small region over the hyothyroid membrane on the affected side from which extension occurs, perhaps upward to the face as high as the zygoma and perhaps down to the upper portion of the thorax and medially to the midlarynx. These patients will often describe trigger mechanisms brought into play by swallowing solids, liquids, saliva, or air. These trigger mechanisms will precipitate their attacks of pain. Other movements such as yawning, stretching the neck, coughing, or palpating the skin which lies over the laryngeal nerve can also precipitate an attack in some patients. During the painful period, the patient usually does not speak, although he is able to during an acute attack. There is no evidence of any hoarseness during the duration of the symptoms. The pain may last from a few seconds to a minute or more. During the attack, a patient may have a tendency to swallow frequently, and in doing so he may manifest rather frequent belching. As soon as the attack of pain ceases, the patient immediately relaxes and resumes conversation. A variable period of refractoriness to stimulation may follow such a bout of pain.

By stimulating the internal branch of the superior laryngeal nerve, either at the plica above the piriform sinus or at its entrance to the larynx through the hyothyroid membrane, one can produce a paroxysm of pain. Application of cocaine to the piriform sinus or anesthetizing the nerve at the point where it pierces the hyothyroid membrane can actually prevent attacks of pain, but only temporarily.

The differential diagnosis in these patients with superior laryngeal neuralgia includes first of all glossopharyngeal neuralgia. In patients with glossopharyngeal neuralgia, the pain is usually located in the tonsillar region and it extends to the ear. Pain in these patients is also triggered by such mechanisms as swallowing, talking, or coughing. Trigeminal neuralgia is also dissimilar in its distribution and the trigger zones. Acute cervical fibrositis, laryngeal perichondritis, lateral bursitis, neoplasm, tuberculosis of the larynx, foreign bodies in the larynx, and laryngeal crises of tabes may be distinguished in most cases without difficulty by the objective findings. Hysteria should be considered, but direct observation of a paroxysm of pain and the absence of other hysterical signs usually suffice to eliminate this as a possibility.

Treatment

Smith[55] recommends resecting the superior laryngeal nerve. He goes about this by making an incision at the anterior border of the left sternocleiomastoid muscle. The superior laryngeal nerve is exposed and traced upward to the ganglion nodosum. Here about 0.5 cm of the nerve is resected. Immediately after the operation, pain can recur and continue in a milder, less frequent form for a few days, but during this period it is impossible to precipitate a paroxysm of pain by stimulating the piriform sinus. All pain usually ceases approximately 3 days postoperatively, and no form of stimulation can produce a paroxysm of pain thereafter.

REFERENCES

1. Lindsay, B.: Trigeminal neuralgia: a new approach, Med. J. Austr. **1:**8-13, 1969.
2. Smolik, E. A., and Hempstead, E. J.: Trigeminal neuralgia and malocclusion, Mod. Med. **21:**107-108, 1953.
3. Gardener, W. J.: Concern of the mechanism of trigeminal neuralgia and hemifacial spasm, J. Neurosurg. **19:**947-948, 1962.
4. Gardener, W. J.: Trigeminal neuralgia, Clin. Neurosurg., pp. 51-55, 1967.
5. Abbott, M., and Killeffer, F. A.: Symptomatic trigeminal neuralgia, Bull. L. A. Neurol. Soc. **35:**1-10, 1970.
6. Kugelburg, E., and Lindblom, U.: The mechanism of pain in trigeminal neuralgia, J. Neurol. Neurosurg. Psychr. **22:**36, 1959.
7. Dalessio, D. J.: A reappraisal of the trigger zones of tic douloureux, Headache **9:**74, 1969.
8. Erokhina, L. G.: EEG changes in typical trigeminal neuralgia and facial sympatheticalgias, Zh. Nevropatol. Psikhiatr. **70:**76-80, 1970.
9. Kalyanaraman, S.: Trigeminal neuralgia: a review of 331 cases, Neurol. India **18:**100-108, 1970.
10. Friedlander, A. H., and Zeff, S.: Atypical trigeminal neuralgia in patients with multiple sclerosis, J. Oral Surg. **32:**301-303, 1974.
11. Finestone, A. J., and others: Trigeminal neuralgia in diabetes mellitus, J. Med. Soc. N.J. **67:**269-270, 1970.
12. Surtees, S. J., and Hughes, R. R.: Treatment of trigeminal neuralgia with vitamin B_{12}, Lancet **1:**439-441, 1954.
13. Fields, W. S., and Hoff, H. E.: Treatment of trigeminal neuralgia with vitamin B_{12}, Neurology **2:**131-139, 1952.
14. Woodhall, B., and Otem, G. L.: Stilbamidine

treatment of tic douloureux, N.C. Med. J. **16:** 222-224, 1955.

15. Hanes, W. J.: Trigeminal neuralgia: role of allergy in etiology and treatment, Ann. Allergy **20:**635-648, 1962.

16. Dobaczewski, Z.: Treatment of trigeminal neuralgia with histamine, J. Klin. Chir. Szczekowej. Inst. Stomatol. **27:**913-915, 1972.

17. Ransohoff, J.: Surgical treatment of trigeminal neuralgia: current status: headache, Special Symposium on Facial Pain, pp. 20-24, 1968.

18. Quinn, J. H., and While, T.: Trigeminal neuralgia: treatment by repetitive peripheral neurectomy: a supplemental report, J. Oral Surg. **83:**591-595, 1975.

19. Jaeger, R.: Hot water injection into the gasserian ganglion for the treatment of trigeminal neuralgia, J. Am. Geriatr. Soc. **3:**416-423, 1955.

20. Jefferson, A.: Trigeminal root and ganglion injections using phenyl and glycerin for relief of trigeminal neuralgia, J. Neurol. Neurosurg. Psychr. **26:**345, 1963.

21. Sweet, W. H.: The trigeminal neuralgias, presented at the International Conference on Facial Pain, American Society of Oral Surgeons, October, 1967.

22. Rhoton, A. L.: Stereotaxic radiofrequency lesions for trigeminal neuralgia, J. Fla. Med. Assoc. **60:**27-30, 1973.

23. Kirschner, M.: Zur Elektrochirurgie, Arch. Klin. Chir. **167:**761-768, 1931.

24. Tew, J. M., and Mayfield, F. H.: Trigeminal neuralgia: a new surgical approach (percutaneous electrocoagulation of the trigeminal nerve), Laryngoscope **83:**1096-1101, 1973.

25. Malis, L. I.: Petrous ridge compression and its surgical correction, J. Neurosurg. **26**(Suppl.):163-167, 1967.

26. Jannetta, P. J., and Rand, R. W.: Growth description of the human trigeminal nerve and ganglion, J. Neurosurg. **26**(Suppl.):109-111,1967.

27. Weisenberg, T. H.: Cerebello-pontine tumor diagnosed for six years as tic douloureux: the symptoms of irritation of the ninth and twelfth cranial nerves, J.A.M.A. **54:**1600, 1910.

28. Harris, W.: Persistent pain in lesions in the peripheral and central nervous system, Brain **44:**457, 1921.

29. Kong, Y.: Glossopharyngeal neuralgia associated with bradycardia, syncope, and seizures, Circulation **30:**109, 1964.

30. Ryan, R. E., Jr.: Otologic etiologies of headache, presented at the Symposium on the Pathogenesis and Treatment of Headache and Facial Pain, Albuquerque, New Mexico, January 14, 1976.

31. Sluder, G.: Etiology, diagnosis, prognosis, and treatment of sphenopalatine ganglion neuralgia, J.A.M.A. **61:**1202-1205, 1913.

32. Ekbom, K., and Kugelberg, E.: Upper and lower cluster headache: brain and mind problems, Rome, 1963, Scientific Publications, pp. 482-489.

33. Lillie, H. I.: Effect of silver nitrate on the nasal mucosa of rabbits, Arch. Otol. **17:**1-7, 1933.

34. Meyer, J. S., and others: Sphenopalatine ganglionectomy for cluster headache, Arch. Otol. **92:**475-484, 1970.

35. Vail, H. H.: Vidian neuralgia, Anal. Otol. Rhinol. Laryngol. **41:**837-856, 1932.

36. Sluder, G.: The role of the sphenopalatine ganglion in nasal headaches, N. Y. Med. J. **87:**989-990, 1908.

37. Fenton, R. A.: Some observations on nasal neurology, Anal. Otol. **50:**490, 1941.

38. Wolff, H. G.: Headache and other head pain, ed. 2, New York, 1963, Oxford University Press, pp. 638-639.

39. Chouret, E. E.: The greater occipital neuralgia headache, Headache **7:**33-34, 1967.

40. Gardner, W. J., Stowell, A., and Dutlinger, R.: Resection of the greater superficial petrosal nerve in the treatment of unilateral headache, presented at the meeting of the Harvey Cushing Society, October 10, 1946, J. Neurosurg. **4:**105, 1947.

41. Horton, B. T., MacLean, A. R., and Craig, W. M.: A new syndrome of vascular headache: results of treatment with histamine: preliminary report, Proc. Staff Meet. Mayo Clin. **14:**257, 1939.

42. Horton, B. T.: The use of histamine in the treatment of specific types of headaches, J.A.M.A. **116:**377-383, 1941.

43. Cobb, S., and Finesinger, J. E.: Cerebral circulation: XIX. The vagal pathway of the vasodilator impulses, Arch. Neurol. Psychiatr. **28:**1243-1256, 1932.

44. Schumacher, G. A., Ray, B. S., and Wolf, H. G.: Experimental studies on headaches: further analysis of histamine headache and its pain pathways, Arch. Neurol. Psychiatr. **44:**701-717, 1940.

45. Rushton, J. G., Gibilisco, J. A., and Goldstein, N. P.: Atypical facial pain, J.A.M.A. **171**(5):545-548, 1959.

46. Kerr, F. W.: Atypical facial neuralgias: their mechanism is inferred from anatomic and physiologic data, Proc. Staff Meet. Mayo Clin. **36**(10):254-260, 1961.

47. Kerr, F. W.: Central relationships of trigeminal and cervical primary afferents in the spinal cord and medulla, Brain Res. **43:**561-572, 1972.

48. Radman, W. P.: Atypical facial neuralgia: a consideration in the diagnosis of oral facial pain, J. Oral Med. **26**(1):4-6, 1971.

49. Smith, D. P., and others: A psychiatric study of atypical facial pain, Can. Med. Assoc. J. **100**(6):286-291, 1969.

50. Freedman, A. P.: Atypical facial pain, Headache **9:**27-30, 1969.

51. Foster, J. B.: Facial pain, Br. Med. J. **4:**667-669, 1969.

52. King, E. F., Russell, W. R., and Rowbotham, G. F.: Facial neuralgias: symposium, Mod. Med. **26:** 233-244, 1958.

53. Farber, G. A., and Burks, J. W.: Chlorprothixene therapy for herpes zoster neuralgia, Fifth Med. J. **67**(7):808-812, 1974.

54. Furlow, L. T.: Tic douloureux of the nervus intermedius: so-called idiopathic geniculate neuralgia, J.A.M.A. **119:**255, 1942.

55. Smith, L. A., Moersch, H. J., and Love, J. G.: Superior laryngeal neuralgia, Proc. Staff Meet. Mayo Clin., pp. 164-167, March 12, 1941.

CHAPTER 8

Headache of otorhinolaryngologic origin

OTALGIA

Otalgia can be either primary or secondary. Primary otalgia describes the ear pain resulting from pathologic conditions of the ear. Secondary otalgia is pain referred to the ear from distant or adjacent nonotologic sites. Fifty percent or more of all pain experienced in the auricular region originates from another source.

Ear pain or otalgia caused by an acute inflammation of the middle or external ear is often easily diagnosed on physical examination. The symptom of earache, however, can be caused by disorders arising distant from the ear in question. When the origin of pain is remote from the area of the diseased process it is called referred pain. When a patient has an earache, particularly a mild one, he usually can indicate only that the pain is in a general area of the external ear. The patient should be asked to localize the specific site of the pain. Some patients misinterpret what is meant as ear pain and point to the temporomandibular joint, angle of the mandible, or region of the temporal artery, thereby providing the examiner with an important clue as to the cause of the pain. Patients complaining of otalgia in whom no obvious evidence of ear disease can be found must be examined for lesions other than those associated with the ear. When the source of the ear pain cannot be found on examination of the ear, the sites from which the referred pain may arise must be considered.

The fifth, seventh, ninth, and tenth cranial nerves have sensory fibers in the regions of the auricle, the external auditory canal, the tympanic membrane, and the middle ear. There is considerable overlap in the distribution of these sensory fibers. Also, the second and third cervical nerves supply sensation to the postauricular region, while the auriculotemporal branch of the fifth nerve innervates a large region in front of the auricle of the external ear and around the temporomandibular joint. Usually when examining a patient who has an earache but no inflammation in his middle or external ear, one cannot determine the precise sensory nerve distribution through which the pain is being referred until a lesion has been found. Before looking further it is imperative that the external auditory canal be examined so as not to overlook some small lesion such as a furuncle or cancer.

Primary otalgia

FURUNCULOSIS

Furunculosis represents a rather severe form of head pain. It is caused by the formation of a furuncle in the external auditory canal.

CAUSES OF PRIMARY OTALGIA

External ear
  External otitis
  Perichondritis
  Auricular abscess
  Furunculosis
  Injury
  Malignant external otitis
  Malignant or benign growth
  Fungal infection
  Foreign body
  Impacted cerumen
  Bullous myringitis
  Frostbite
Middle ear and mastoid
  Acute otitis media
  Acute mastoiditis
  Barotrauma
  Malignant or benign growth
  Acute petrositis
  Gradenigo's syndrome

Etiology. Furunculosis is most commonly seen during the swimming season. It is a circumscribed inflammation involving either the hair follicles or the sudoriferous glands. The condition has the same appearance as any other boil. Predisposing factors may be trauma to the external auditory canal, swimming, a general furunculosis, fungal infections in the external canal, or chronic eczema.

Symptoms. The most prominent symptom of furunculosis of the external auditory canal is pain, which is quite severe and constant. Severe pain is noted on any movement of the external portion of the ear. Usually it is more pronounced with movement of the jaws, such as chewing. The more the swelling, the more tension is produced on the skin in the external auditory canal, and the greater the increase in pain.

The deeper the infection goes into the tissues, the more severe the pain becomes to the patient. If the furuncle should open, the swelling is less and the tension on the skin is decreased. This, in turn, reduces the severity of the pain. There may be a slight temperature elevation with this type of ear pathology. There may be tinnitus associated with it and also a temporary conductive type of hearing loss, depending on the amount of edema and swelling of the soft tissue of the canal.

Treatment. Intramuscular penicillin is the antibiotic of choice in these patients. If the patient is sensitive to penicillin, one of the other antibiotics such as erythromycin must be employed, but their effectiveness is not nearly as good as that of penicillin. The pain may be lessened by use of one of the analgesic group of drugs such as Empirin or plain aspirin. The pain in furunculosis of the external auditory canal decreases when the furuncle ruptures and thus decreases the skin tension. Pain may be lessened by the local application of some liquid preparation into the canals, such as Otodyne, or any such preparation which contains a mild anesthetic ingredient. The ear canal should be thoroughly cleaned by the physician on each examination, and after this cleansing process a dusting powder consisting of penicillin and antisulfonamides can be employed within the canal locally.

ACUTE OTITIS MEDIA

Acute otitis media represents a low-grade acute infection of the eustachian tube in the middle ear cavity.

Etiology. Many of these conditions are seen following or during acute upper respiratory infections. The infection makes its way to the middle ear cavity by way of the eustachian tube or by way of the lymphatics or blood vessels to the mucous membrane of the middle ear cavity. Predisposing factors may be any acute respiratory condition, acute or chronic sinusitis, enlarged and infected tonsils and adenoids, or one of the childhood diseases. However, with most of these conditions, if a secondary otologic complication sets in, it is usually in the form of acute suppurative otitis media, and not the acute catarrhal form. Two common predisposing factors in this condition are nasal obstruction and hypertrophic adenoid tissue in the nasopharynx. If the normal airway of the nasal passage is interfered with by some form of nasal obstruction, there will take place a deviation from normal of the physiologic activities of the nasal mucous membrane. This will, in turn, produce an abnormality of the mucous membrane of the nasopharynx, with an increase in the possibility of extension of the infection to the middle ear cavity by way of the eustachian tube. The adenoid tissue in the nasopharynx, if it is hypertrophic, may obstruct the pharyngeal opening of the eustachian tube and thus interfere with the normal ventilation and drainage of the middle ear cavity. This will be a factor predisposing to infections of this cavity.

Symptoms. In this pathologic condition the middle ear cavity will contain serum, mucus, and epithelial debris. The tympanic membrane becomes congested to various degrees, but not as severely as in acute suppurative otitis media. The tympanic membrane may also become somewhat thickened. There may be a slight fever but it seldom goes over 100° F. The head pain is generally of the intermittent type, but in some instances it may be more constant. The patient will usually describe the pain as being of a throbbing nature, and he may notice that it throbs in a beat synchronous with his heart. In most cases the pain of acute catarrhal otitis media will be described as a dull type of ache or boring sensation. However, it may be more acute. In this condition the pain results from an inflammatory condition of the drumhead and the mucous membrane of the middle ear.

A conductive type of hearing loss is present in these cases, but it is only temporary. In some cases the fluid may be observed behind the tympanic membrane. It is referred to as the fluid level and presents itself as a darkened line, somewhat wavy, which changes position with the change of position of the head. This is not always noticeable, however, and will not be seen in cases where the tympanic membrane is either too thickened or too congested. Also, if the entire middle ear cavity is filled with fluid, the level will not be visible on examination.

Treatment. Treatment consists of two forms. One is removal of the etiologic cause and the second is treatment of the symptoms the patient is experiencing. Treatment of the etiologic factors may necessitate removing the tonsils and adenoids, but the patient's current complaint is the pain localized to the ear, which is the result of the fluid within the middle ear space. Decongestants are the best method of initial therapy in this case. These are used in an attempt to dry up the fluid from the middle ear cavity, and the decongestants in combination with antihistamine preparations often remedy the underlying causes of this problem. If a good trial is given with these medical therapeutic measures, relief of symptoms is often experienced. However, there are some cases where the fluid is not absorbed and remains present. These patients will experience continued pain and more than likely will experience some diminution of their hearing acuity. In these patients we recommend drainage of the fluid from the middle ear cavity through a myringotomy incision and insertion of a ventilation tube into the middle ear space. These ventilation tubes will fall out after a period of months, at which time the tympanic membrane will spontaneously heal.

ACUTE SUPPURATIVE OTITIS MEDIA

Acute suppurative otitis media consists of a marked hyperemia of the mucous membrane lining the middle ear cavity and the tympanic membrane.

Etiology. The most common organisms producing this condition are the streptococci, pneumococci, and staphylococci. The most virulent and dangerous of these are the streptococci, for as a rule they are more destructive to both the mastoid process of the temporal bone and the soft tissue involved. Predisposing factors may include any severe acute respiratory infection, nasal sinusitis, infected tonsils and adenoids, headcolds, chronic or acute nasopharyngitis, and acute infectious childhood diseases.

The pathologic changes which take place in the mucous membrane in these conditions may make the cilia sluggish in their movements or may completely destroy them. This will prevent the cilia from performing one of their normal functions, which is to force secretions toward the nasopharyngeal orifice of the eustachian tube.

This condition is more frequently seen in children than it is in adults, and the fact that the eustachian tube is more horizontal in children is thought to be the reason.

Acute otitis media can be brought on by attempting to do either nasal or oral surgery in the presence of acute nasal or oral inflammation such as tonsillitis and acute rhinitis. The eustachian tube connects the nasopharynx and the middle ear, which tends to make the route of infection an easy one under the proper inflammatory conditions.

Symptoms. Head pain is the most pronounced symptom of acute suppurative otitis media. This is usually in the form of ear pain and is one of the early symptoms of the disease. The pain is sharp, piercing, and often throbbing in nature. The pain is continuous. The only time the patient seems to be free from it is when he sleeps, but frequently the pain is so severe that sleep is possible only when the patient becomes completely exhausted from its effects. There may be mastoid tenderness in some of these cases if the organisms are extremely virulent. The pain is always unilateral unless both ears are involved, a condition which can occur. Often the pain may involve the entire temporal area. Along with the pain in the ear there will be an elevated temperature, a conductive type of hearing loss, a feeling of fullness in the ear, and malaise. There may also be tinnitus and vertigo.

The tympanic membrane loses its normal landmarks and becomes inflamed, edematous, and possibly bulging or pulsating. If the tympanic membrane ruptures spontaneously, it will be at the area where the bulging is most pronounced. When rupture occurs, otorrhea results. These secretions may be serous, seromucous, seropurulent, mucopurulent, or serosanguineous.

In acute suppurative otitis media the external auditory canal may become injected and edematous. This is often seen in the posterosuperior portions of the canal and produces a sagging appearance near the tympanic membrane.

Treatment. Antibiotics should be administered immediately. Penicillin is the drug of choice. If the patient is sensitive to penicillin, some other antibiotics, such as erythromycin, should be used. The patient may be relieved by using one of the analgesic group of drugs. Hot packs used when the pain is severe may tend to lessen the acuteness of the pain. Frequently a mild sedative will help in combating the acuteness of the pain in these conditions.

ACUTE MASTOIDITIS

Acute mastoiditis has become a rather rare entity with the onset of antibiotics. As a rule, acute mastoiditis is rarely a primary condition. It is usually found to be associated secondarily with the suppurative infectious disease of the middle ear. However, with the advent of antibiotics, these acute suppurative infections have come under control, and therefore we see relatively few cases of acute mastoiditis. There are a few conditions which are rather rare, in which a primary acute mastoiditis can occur, and usually in these cases the infectious process features the mastoid bone by way of the bloodstream. There is also the possibility of the patient having an acute middle ear infection which responds to treatment and which will clear up grossly. However, this may leave a residual focus in the mastoid process which can develop into acute mastoiditis at a later date.

Symptoms. These patients exhibit tenderness over the mastoid process of the temporal bone when pressure is applied to that area. This symptom manifests itself early and is usually present. A tenderness should be looked for in the area of the antrum and in the mastoid tip area.

These cases always have a purulent discharge in the ear involved, which is usually very foul-smelling and blood-tinged. In some cases there may be pulsations of the discharge which will correspond with the patient's heartbeat. This is seen in the early acute stages.

Because these patients have perforations in their tympanic membranes, there will be a conductive type of hearing loss of various degrees.

The skin over the mastoid process of the temporal bone becomes edematous and somewhat inflamed. On palpation of this skin, the physician will notice its similarity to the feel of a piece of velvet. The examination of the tympanic membrane will reveal a perforation of variable size. This perforation usually has a purulent discharge pouring from it and may be pulsating. Perforation may be central or marginal. The external auditory canal may be found to be sagging on examination. This usually occurs in the posterior wall near the tympanic membrane superiorly. This sagging condition is usually associated with the retention of the purulent material in the mastoid antrum area and the border cells. The external canal is also usually injected and inflamed.

Pain is the most common and the most pronounced symptom of acute mastoiditis. If the antrum is obstructed, the pain is even more pronounced. The pain is usually found to originate in the postauricular area and may radiate from this area to the occipital area, to the parietal area, down the neck, or even across the face and down to the area of the teeth. The pain is severe, constant, and throbbing. If there should be any involvement of the bony portion of the external auditory canal the patient will experience pain on chewing or on any movement of the jaws.

There are usually positive x-ray findings in cases of acute mastoiditis. However, the x-rays in this condition can be misleading in respect to the severity of the infectious process in the bone.

Treatment. The antibiotics should be used to combat infectious process in the bone. Again, penicillin is the treatment of choice in this type of infection. The ear should be kept as clean as possible and the discharge should be removed either by suction or by wiping with cotton wicks. Adequate drainage should be established in these cases and if the perforation in the tympanic membrane is small and not sufficient to allow for this drainage, the perforation may be enlarged by incision with myringotomy knife. If medical treatment does not bring about the desired result, surgical treatment may be needed to get rid of the infectious process. This naturally would mean a mastoidectomy.

PETROSITIS

Petrositis is not really a complication of ear infection but rather an extension of the infection into the mastoid cells surrounding the labyrinthine capsule. Except for the rather rare acute fulminating osteomyelitis of the petrosa in infants, petrositis occurs only in temporal bones with pneumatic cells in the petrous pyramid. Just as there is an inflammation of mucosal lining of mastoid air cells in every acute suppurative otitis media of any degree of severity, so there is a similar inflammation of any air cells that have developed in the petrosa. The diagnosis of petrositis is reserved for infected petrous cells with inadequate drainage causing bony changes of coalescence in the cell walls and resulting often in symptoms referable to the petrosa. In these respects, petrositis behaves exactly like acute mastoiditis in an acute middle ear infection, and the involvement of air cells in the petrous portion might simply be considered part of the pneumatic cell's involvement of acute otitis media that includes cells in the mastoid process, squama, and petrosa. In certain respects, however, petrositis differs from mastoiditis, justifying its consideration as a separate entity. These differences are:

1. The petrous pyramid is pneumatized in only a third of temporal bones past the age of 3 years, whereas the great majority of mastoid processes after the first year are pneumatized to some degree. Moreover, the petrous pyramid is never completely pneumatized. Areas of bone marrow remain adjacent to pneumatic cells, so that osteomyelitis frequently accompanies a coalescent petrositis.

2. The bony labyrinth that nearly fills the base of the petrous pyramid interposes a bottleneck between the middle ear and any petrous air cells, increasing the tendency toward impaired drainage from the cells.

3. The petrous pyramid is situated so that pus cannot find its way outward to produce a relatively harmless and easily diagnosed and drained subperiosteal abscess, as is the case of the mastoid and squama, but has a greater tendency toward intracranial extension. In the immediate preantibiotic era it became evident that the majority of cases of fatal otitic meningitis were the result of inward extension from a petrositis.

Etiology. Acute coalescent petrositis is usually associated with an acute coalescent mastoiditis and, like the latter, is due most often to beta-hemolytic streptococci or pneumococci. Chronic petrositis may be due to one of these organisms in a trapped abscess, to staphylococci with a chronic osteomyelitis of the petrosa, or, in the case of a cholesteatoma, to one of the gramnegative organisms.

Symptoms. The diagnosis of petrositis is not made frequently today and, because of unfamiliarity, sometimes missed. The diagnosis should be first suspected in any case with persistent infection and discharge after adequate treatment of otitis media and mastoiditis, or following a mastoidectomy.

The symptoms of petrositis depend on the area of the petrous pyramid affected. Air cells extend into the petrous pyramid in two main groups: a posterior group of air cells from the epitympanum and antrum that finds its way around the semicircular canals into the base of the pyramid, not infrequently extending to the apex, and an anterior group of cells from the tympanum, hypotympanum, and eustachian tube that finds its way around the cochlea into the apex of the pyramid. The posterior group of cells is present in about 30% of temporal bones, whereas the anterior group of cells is present in about 15% of temporal bones.

The two most common symptoms of petrositis are pain and persistent aural discharge following a simple mastoidectomy. In the case of a posterior petrositis the pain is occipital, parietal, or temporal and the persistent discharge is from the mastoid wound. In the case of an anterior petrositis the pain is frontal or behind the eye and the persistent discharge is from the tympanum. Diplopia due to the sixth nerve paralysis may occur when the apex is involved, the nerve being compressed by edema where it passes through Dorello's canal beneath the petrosphenoidal ligament at the tip of the petrous apex.

Diagnosis. Effective antibiotic therapy has virtually eliminated cases of acute coalescent petrositis following an acute suppurative otitis media. The few cases seen today are associated with a chronic otorrhea, rarely with a cholesteatoma, more often with a chronic osteomylitis of the petrosa or a chronic coalescent abscessed cavity in the apex.

Suppuration in the petrous portion of the temporal bones may be suspected whenever there is a persistent purulent discharge following a well-done simple or radical mastoidectomy, for after thorough exenteration of all mastoid cell tracts, the usual source for continued purulent drainage is from perilabyrinthine, peritubal, or apical petrous cells. The addition of pain around or deep to the eye, diplopia due to sixth nerve paresis, facial weakness, or vertigo, often with fever, is almost certain evidence of petrositis. Recurrence of meningitis during acute otitis media with an insufficient pathologic lesion in the mastoid to account for it and the occurrence of repeated attacks of meningitis always suggest the possibility of a petrositis, even without the other symptoms.

Radiographs should be reexamined to detect crowding and rarefaction of the petrous cells. Deep-seated ear pain accompanying the persistent discharge is an even more definite clue to the presence of petrositis.

Treatment. Acute coalescent petrositis in the preantibiotic era sometimes cleared following a complete simple mastoidectomy. Today, most cases of acute petrositis can be cured by antibacterial medication in sufficient dosage. Cases of acute petrositis requiring surgery have almost disappeared. The chronic cases due to organisms resistant to the usual antibiotics still require operation.

In some of these chronic cases a low-grade osteomyelitis is present. Surgical intervention becomes necessary when the chronic otorrhea is accompanied by pain behind the eye, intermittent vertigo, facial weakness, transient diplopia, and intermittent low-grade fever. Since it is difficult to remove every vestige of infected marrow-containing bone, surgery should be followed by antibacterial medication determined by culture taken at operation.

The treatment of persistent petrous bone infection is to provide adequate drainage by opening the diseased cell tracts to the mastoid cavity. This is best done by initial adequate mastoidectomy to visualize the involved group of cells. The posterior cells proceed immediately from Trautmann's triangle, outlining the labyrinthine capsule superiorly and posteriorly. Cells opening in the attic region may run through the arch of the superior semicircular canal or anterior to the canal over the cochlea. There may be a cell tract opening below the posterior semicircular canal running to the region below the internal auditory canal. The most difficult cell tracts to follow are those running anterior to the cochlea from the eustachian tube and the carotid region. Opening these requires a preliminary radical mastoidectomy with the sacrifice of the tympanic membrane and enlargement of the external auditory canal anteriorly. The cells are then followed by opening the medial wall of the eustachian tube just above the carotid artery.

Fortunately, this disease is rarely seen today, so that the extensive surgery described is not often needed.

Referred otalgia

As we described earlier, the fifth, seventh, ninth, and tenth cranial nerves have sensory fibers in the regions of the auricle, the external auditory canal, the tympanic membrane, and the middle ear. There is considerable overlap in the distribution of these sensory fibers. Also, the second and third cervical nerves supply sensation to the postauricular region, while the auriculotemporal branch of the fifth nerve innervates a larger region in front of the auricle of the external ear and around the temporomandibular joint. Because of this vast nerve supply the ear can be receiving pain impulses from various sources located throughout the head and neck areas. We will take each nerve involved here and discuss some of the possible etiologies which may cause pain referred to the ear.

Fifth cranial nerve. Dental disease may cause earache referred by the fifth cranial nerve. Molar impaction and infection are perhaps the most common causes of referred ear pain. Sinus inflammation or tumors in an antrum or a posterior ethmoidal sinus may cause referred otalgia through the fifth cranial nerve, although this is probably rare. Acute or chronic disturbances of the temporomandibular joint may pro-

CAUSES OF REFERRED OTALGIA

Oral cavity
  Acute glossitis
  Stomatitis
  Carcinoma of tongue
Pharynx
  After tonsillectomy or adenoidectomy
  Acute pharyngitis
  Peritonsillar abscess
  Malignant growth
  Ulceration
  Elongated styloid process
  Nasopharyngeal angiofibroma
Larynx
  Malignancy
  Ulceration
  Arthritis of cricoarytenoid joint
  Perichondritis
Esophagus
  Foreign body
  Inflammation
  Malignant or benign growth
Neuralgias
  Idiopathic geniculate
  Postherpetic
  Trigeminal
  Tympanic
  Glossopharyngeal
  Sphenopalatine ganglion
  Dental
Miscellaneous
  Thyroiditis
  Thyroid cancer
  Temporomandibular arthritis
  Mumps
  Acoustic neuroma
  Tumor of gasserian ganglion
  Injury or inflammation of C_1 to C_3

duce ear pain that is referred through the auriculotemporal branch of the fifth cranial nerve.

Seventh cranial nerve. The seventh cranial nerve can cause otalgia principally in herpetic eruptions from the viral infection of the geniculate ganglion. The pain is transient and often is overshadowed by other manifestations, particularly the seventh nerve palsy. Other lesions could touch the sensory branches of the facial nerve and

thus produce otalgia; however, this is uncommon.

Ninth cranial nerve. A lesion in the distribution of the ninth cranial nerve—the nasopharynx, eustachian tube, the region of the palatine tonsils, adjacent base of the tongue, or the lingual tonsils—may cause earache by way of the glossopharyngeal nerve. The inflammatory process of this region usually accounts for the earache that may occur in the early convalescence from tonsillectomy. Afflictions of the ninth cranial nerves, such as glossopharyngeal neuralgia, also may cause earache. The pain of glossopharyngeal neuralgia is sharp, short, and lance-like and can be precipitated either by drinking a cold liquid or by swallowing.

Tenth cranial nerve. A patient with an inflammatory or a neoplastic lesion in the upper glottis of the larynx, in the piriform sinus, or in the trachea often complains of earache on the involved side. Sometimes this is the presenting complaint to the physician. The pain is referred through the superior laryngeal branch of the vagus nerve, the tenth cranial nerve. Frequently a patient with this problem complains of hoarseness. This symptom allows the examiner to direct attention to the region that is producing referred pain to the ear.

Cervical plexus (C_2 and C_3). The second and third cervical nerves also are pathways for referred pain to the external ear and the soft tissues in the mastoid process; inflammation or mass lesions of the thyroid may produce pain to the ear. Otalgia may be an early manifestation of thyroid carcinoma, especially in children. Pain is mediated by C_2 and C_3 through the cervical plexus to the auricle. The upper cervical nerve roots supply the postauricular region. Pain due to that irritation—for example, cervical spondylosis or sternocleidomastoid myalgia—may be referred to the ear or mastoid process. There is also the possibility that otalgia may be due to an autonomic imbalance along the course of blood vessels related to these parts.

When we see a patient who has no obvious primary etiology for otalgia, we then have to think of the different etiologies for secondary or referred otalgia. In doing this we go through a checklist which we refer to as the "Ten T's." The checklist is as follows:

1. Teeth	Fifth cranial nerve
2. Tonsils	Ninth cranial nerve
3. Tongue	Ninth cranial nerve
4. Tube	Ninth cranial nerve
5. Throat	Ninth and tenth cranial nerves
6. Trachea	Tenth cranial nerve
7. Temporomandibular joint	Fifth cranial nerve
8. Tendons	C_2, C_3
9. Tics	Ninth, fifth, and tenth cranial nerves
10. Thyroid	Tenth cranial nerve, C_2, C_3

The prognosis for these patients with otalgia depends very heavily on the detection of the etiology of their pain. The prognosis depends on the location of the lesion responsible and whether or not it is amenable to further treatment.[1]

The following are a few specific examples of referred otalgia.

RAMSAY HUNT SYNDROME

Infection of the neurons in the geniculate ganglion by the virus of herpes zoster is followed by the appearance of cutaneous vesicles in the peripheral sensory distribution of the intermediate nerve. The inflammatory swelling of the ganglion produces pressure on the facial nerve and the facial canal, causing a peripheral facial paralysis.

Etiology

As mentioned, this condition represents an inflammatory condition of the geniculate ganglion caused by herpes zoster virus. It often has as predisposing factors such things as excessive exposure to cold or cold air, influenzal infections, and also tonsillar infections which would act as foci. The entire ganglion is involved, both the ascending and the descending nerves.

Symptoms

According to Hunt,[2] in his original description of this disease entity:

Clinically the cases of geniculate herpes resolve themselves into three groups. The simplest expression of the disease is a herpes of the auricle and the external auditory canal. Within this skin area is to be found the zoster zone for the geniculate ganglion. In another group of cases there is added to the aural herpes a paralysis of the facial nerve. [This he explained by pressure of the inflamed ganglion or in some cases by a direct extension of the inflammation to the nerve.] The most interesting as well as the most severe type of the disease occurs when the acoustic nerve is also involved. In this form there are with herpes auricularis and facial palsy, various auditory symptoms ranging in severity from tinnitus and diminution of hearing to the more severe forms of acoustic involvement as seen in Meniere's syndrome. [In these cases he assumed that the inflammatory process had extended to the auditory nerve which was enveloped in the same sheath and courses in the same canal as the facial nerve.]

The initial complaint of pain over the pinna in the external auditory meatus deep in the ear or throat is followed by the development of typical herpetic vesicles in the painful areas. At the same time, there is often a facial paralysis of a peripheral type with loss of taste of the anterior two-thirds of the tongue on the affected side. The pain in these patients is usually deep-seated. The eruption of the skin of the external ear is most frequently found on the anterior surface of the auricle and usually follows the terminal branches of the auriculotemporal nerve. Because this nerve does not supply the posterior surface of the auricle, it is rare to find a herpes eruption in that area. If the skin eruption is situated in the external auditory canal, it may extend to the tympanic membrane and also involve that structure.

At first the eruption is papular and then it turns into the vesicular form, containing a more or less clear serum which may become purulent. The vesicles are usually present for 3 or 4 days, and then they tend to dry up.

They may leave a crust or even form an ulcerative process as the end result.

As mentioned by Hunt,[2] along with the pain and eruption seen in this condition, there may also be a facial paralysis, tinnitus, decreased hearing, and occasionally vertigo.

As a rule, the facial disturbances and any disturbances in the labyrinth return to normal. The cutaneous lesions clear up also, but in some cases there may be a permanent loss of hearing experienced.

Treatment

These patients should be treated with adequate analgesics in an attempt to control the pain, and then a continuation of symptomatic treatment is extended. Some local topical anesthetic agent applied to the area of the vesicles may afford the patient some relief from pain. If vesicles have formed, their drying up can be hastened by draining the serum from the vesicles. If blisters have formed on the auricle, they should be protected by dressings.

Antibiotic therapy is recommended to prevent secondary infection in the external auditory canal.

Various other measures have been tried but without too much apparent success, such as vitamin B_1, radiation therapy, protein injections, and steroid injection. This treatment with steroid injection has met with some degree of success, especially recently, and may be recommended in patients with the chronic form of this disease in which the pain is unremitting.

GRADENIGO'S SYNDROME

Gradenigo's syndrome affords the otologist one of the few dramatic episodes in otologic practice and often causes no little anxiety because of what it may portend. This syndrome is relatively rare, but it occurs frequently enough to warrant inclusion of the subject in textbooks of otology and ophthalmology and facial pain. It is seldom encountered by the individual otologist, who at most may observe but a few cases in the course of practice.

Etiology

Gradenigo's[3] conclusions can be summarized as follows. The pathologic and anatomic process consists of the diffusion of pus and purulent infection of the drum cavity to the pyramidal apex through the peritubal air cells and the carotid canal. The abducens nerve is affected at the apex of the pyramid close to its passage into the dura mater. The physician has to deal with the circumscribed osteitis at the pyramidal apex and eventually with the corresponding meningitis.

Understanding of the anatomy of the region of the apex of the petrous portion of the temporal bone clarifies the probable mechanism incident to the paralysis of the external rectus muscle and the severe trigeminal neuralgia. Making its way along the base of the brain from the lower border of the pons, the abducens nerve enters the cavernous sinus by piercing the dura mater below the posterior clinoid process, where it is in contact with the periosteum at the apex of the petrous pyramid at the temporal bone for 2.5 cm as it passes over the tip of the pyramid. It becomes particularly susceptible to infection at this point. As it approaches the cavernous sinus it traverses Dorello's canal. An inflammatory process producing edema of the lining of this canal or extension of the suppurative process through the medium of a highly pneumatized petrous bone may subject a nerve to pressure with subsequent paralysis of varying degree. After it passes through the cavernous sinus, the abducens nerve enters the orbit by way of the sphenoidal fissure, where it lies between the two heads of the external rectus muscle and sends numerous small branches to the ocular surface of the muscle itself. Joining the abducens nerve are the nerve filaments which take their origin from the carotid and the cavernous plexus, from the sphenopalatine ganglion, and from the ophthalmic nerve.

It therefore becomes apparent that the sixth nerve, because of its relatively close confinement in Dorello's canal and notch in the petrous bone, is perhaps the most vulnerable of the important structures of the petrous tip in the presence of even slight derangement. It may be subject to involvement by localized meningitis, an extradural abscess, or an extension of the thrombotic process having its origin in the lateral sinus and extending into the inferior petrosal sinus which joins the cavernous sinus at the site of entry of the nerve into the wall of the sinus. Also, the fifth nerve, with its gasserian ganglion lying as it does in the Meckel's dural cavity and resting in the depression on the anterosuperior surface of the bone at its tip, can hardly escape involvement in any process in this region. The distribution of the acute pain characterizing the syndrome is explained by the intimate relation of this nerve with the tip. It is noteworthy that the pneumatic type of mastoid is more likely to be associated with the symptom complex than the sclerosed type. This phenomenon may account for the frequency with which this syndrome occurs in children, for the mastoid is predominantly pneumatized in childhood.

It has been concluded that the complications of petrositis depend on the type and degree of the pneumatization, the virulence of the infection, and the resistance of the patient. In the majority of patients, Gradenigo's syndrome is a complication of petrositis occurring otherwise as a complication of involvement of the middle ear or the mastoid such as thrombosis, extradural abscess, or abscess of the brain.

Symptoms

This syndrome is characterized by three outstanding symptoms: suppuration from the middle ear, intense pain, and loss of function of the external rectus muscle. The acute purulent otitis media extends by one of several roots to the tip of the petrous portion of the temporal bone causing localized meningitis at that point. As noted by Gradenigo, indications of retention of pus in the tympanic cavity arise because of insufficiency or complete lack of perforation; but perforation, when present, takes place usually in the anterior half of the drum. He observed that the otitis media is usually, though not always, acute and is commonly accompanied by mastoiditis. Owing to inflammation of the gasserian ganglion, extremely severe pain, generally localized in the temporoparietal region and at times in the depth of the orbit of the same side, almost always accompanies the otitis. It varies in distribution according to which branches of the fifth nerve are seriously involved, with the ophthalmic division seeming to be the most vulnerable portion. This pain, which is often agonizing, may be continuous or may abate after discharge of purulent material from the external auditory canal only to recur after 2 or 3 weeks as a precursor of the ocular complication. The movements of the eye on the affected side may likewise cause pain.

The most prominent symptom is paresis or paralysis of the abducens muscle, arising from the involvement of the sixth nerve in the inflammatory process. In most instances it is present on the side of the involved area but it may be bilateral or contralateral. Infrequently involvement of the third, fourth, seventh, and eighth nerves has been noted.

Impaired action of the external rectus muscle seems to appear unexpectedly and causes the patient to complain of diplopia because the two eyes have lost the power to coordinate properly.

The appearance of this symptom is astonishingly late, usually from 20 to 40 days after the onset of infection in the ear. Paralysis as a rule is noted a month or a month and a half after the initial symptoms of acute otitis media. There are innumerable gradations between the paresis and the paralysis. Generally, recovery is complete with gradual disappearance of the impairment. The period required for restoration of normal function varies from 1 to 3 months and rarely is as long as 5 months.

Infrequently, nystagmus may precede or accompany the paralysis. Mild photophobia is occasionally present. Vertigo has been mentioned. Pupillary reaction is normal and examination of the eye grounds gives normal results. All ocular muscles except the abducens function normally.

The clinical picture typically produced by acute purulent inflammation of the middle ear and the other cardinal symptoms of temporoparietal pain and paralysis of the abducens may in exceptional cases arise as a result of an acute exacerbation of a chronic purulent inflammation of the middle ear, according to Gradenigo. In his opinion, in about 50% of the cases of the syndrome, symptoms related to the involvement of the trigeminal and oculomotor nerves may be present.

Diagnosis

In cases of sudden paralysis of extraocular muscles, the ophthalmologist may be inclined to infer probable syphilitic origin or some toxic cause rather than to be disposed to undertake a careful search for a definite underlying cause and a definite pathologic lesion. In Gradenigo's syndrome the ocular paralysis always affects the external rectus muscle only. Treatment should be left to the otologist, for his success in treating the otitis media dictates the recovery from paralysis or paresis of the abducens muscle.

Roentgenologic study of the petrous pyramid has made possible the greatest progress in the study of this problem. Thorough roentgenologic examination, including a painstaking review of the sphenoidal sinus, and careful laboratory investigation are obviously of particular value as diagnostic aids. Among the conditions to be considered in the differential diagnosis are septic thrombosis, thrombosis of the jugular bulb, epidural abscess, syphilitic meningitis, and diffuse purulent or serous labyrinthitis.

Treatment

Recovery may take place spontaneously, or the syndrome may progress to generalized meningitis with fatal termination. Although recovery has occurred in some cases without mastoidectomy and even without myringotomy, surgical intervention is, as a rule, indicated. Some patients recover after myringotomy, and a majority recover after a simple mastoidectomy with special attention to the cells about the antrum and the zygoma. Since the syndrome is a secondary manifestation, elimination of the original focus of infection by complete exenteration of the diseased tissue in the mastoid process and middle ear permits subsidence of the pathologic changes in the petrous bone and gradual resolution of the localized meningitis with eventual restoration of the abducens muscle to normal function. Rarely has the radical procedure of exploring the petrous tip been indicated. The syndrome may develop weeks or months after a mastoidectomy, requiring reopening of the wound and further surgical measures. Complications that may occasionally be encountered in the management of this syndrome as mentioned by Gradenigo are mastoiditis, circumscribed and restricted extradural lesions of the sigmoid sinus, and also circumscribed serous or diffuse purulent meningitis with fatal termination.

Prognosis

The extradural location of the pathologic process explains the generally favorable course despite the distressing symptoms. Complete recovery usually occurs but may take place slowly, at times extremely slowly. Occasionally basilar meningitis or an abscess of the brain develops and proves fatal. Mortality is reported to be as low as 2% and as high as 20%, depending on the presence of other complications, with each case presenting an immediate prognosis that is potentially grave. With the advent of the antibiotics the instance of mortality has become even less.

ELONGATED STYLOID PROCESS

One of the first clinical cases of pharyngeal pain due to an elongated styloid process was reported by Sterling[5] in 1896. However, Eagle fully described and popularized this syndrome, which often carries his name.[6] The elongated styloid process may produce two syndromes characterized by (1) painful sensations in the pharynx, painful deglutition, and an otologic pain occurring after a tonsillectomy which may persist for years; and (2) the styloid process–carotid artery syndrome in which the symptoms are produced by impingement upon the carotid artery. Symptoms and signs are tenderness on palpation over the region of the carotid artery with parietal headaches and head pains in the area supplied by the ophthalmic artery.

Symptoms

The symptoms vary from slight throat discomfort to odontophagia, sometimes with pain radiating to the ear and a sensation of a pharyngeal foreign body. By contrast glossopharyngeal neuralgia is a sudden lancinating pain of short duration in the pharynx, usually caused by stimulation with hot or cold foods, liquids, or even tongue movements. Eagle noted that the typical patient with his syndrome had undergone tonsillectomy, and possibly scar tissue formation had stretched the sensory nerve endings made taut by the pharyngeal mucosa or the elongated styloid process. Other authors, however, have reported that only few patients with pain due to an elongated styloid process had had tonsillar operations.

The diagnosis is confirmed when the palpating finger meets a firm bony resistance in the tonsillar fossa and the patient winces from pain and declares that it is the same pain that has been bothering him. Roentgenograms merely confirm the diagnosis and are used as a guide for transpharyngeal styloidectomy. The incidental findings of an elongated styloid process seen on roentgenograms in an asymptomatic patient does not make the diagnosis of an elongated styloid process or Eagle's syndrome, for most elongated styloid processes do not cause symptoms.

Treatment

The treatment of choice for this syndrome has been transpharyngeal styloidectomy performed under general anesthesia.

Removal of the entire process is unnecessary for relief of symptoms and is indeed contraindicated due to the dangerous proximity of the facial nerve to the base of the styloid process. Also, the glossopharyngeal nerve transverses the area of excision and may be traumatized or interrupted inadvertently.

Evans and Clairmont[7] have proposed an alternative nonsurgical treatment using triamcinolone suspension and lidocaine transpharyngeal injections. They state that this is a convenient office procedure. This may be repeated as the symptoms persist. They have found this to be a successful, convenient treatment for Eagle's syndrome. This nonsurgical treatment is not suggested for the carotid artery syndrome secondary to the elongated styloid process, in which the tip deviates to cause pressure on the internal or external carotid artery, also described by Eagle. These patients will complain of head pains in the distribution of the ophthalmic artery if the internal carotid artery is involved, or pain referred to the region below the level of the eye if the external carotid artery is involved.

NASAL SINUSITIS HEADACHE

As a rule the first question a physician asks a patient on the initial visit is, "What seems to be your problem?" Many times a headache patient will reply, "Doctor, I have sinus trouble." The physician in cases such as this must then try to find out just exactly what the patient means by "sinus trouble." To many of these patients "sinus trouble" may mean nasal discharge, nasal obstruction, pain in any area of the face or head, or headache, or perhaps any combination of these symptoms.

In our estimation, more people afflicted with chronic headache attacks claim to have "sinusitis" than any other form of headache. We have noticed that many people in their initial examination claim to have sinusitis. They think their condition to be sinusitis simply because they have been suffering from attacks of chronic headaches. After a thorough history and examination of the patients, we find that only a small percentage of them actually have nasal sinus headaches; the others actually have some other form of headache problem such as myalgia, migraine, histaminic cephalalgia, or tension headache. Many of these cases which are not sinusitis at all have been treated as sinusitis by physicians for several years. Naturally, the patients have not been receiving any benefit from such treatment, and their headache attacks continue to trouble them.

To the average patient and to a surprising number of physicians, nasal sinusitis is thought to be present whenever there are any symptoms present which are referable to the head. Naturally, the mistaken diagnosis on the part of the patient can easily be explained by his lack of knowledge of what can rightfully be expected from the nose. However, the misdiagnosis by the physician has to be explained by lack of interest in the subject or, more regrettably, lack of knowledge of nasal sinusitis.

Many patients actually believe that they have nasal sinusitis merely because they have a chronic postnasal drip. However, even when a postnasal discharge accompanies head and face pain, sinusitis is much less often the cause than is generally assumed. The headache may be closely associated with objective evidence of sinus disease and lead to much unnecessary treatment.

If one were to study the sensory nerve supply of the nose and the sinuses, which is the fifth cranial (trigeminal) nerve, one would find out that when this nerve is irritated the patient may complain of pain referable to the head and eyes, the teeth, the jaw, the neck, and even the occipital area. Thus, the symptoms of nasal sinusitis are confused with the symptoms of other medical conditions.

In order to understand nasal sinusitis, we have to keep in mind the basic physiology and anatomy of the sinuses. They are air-containing cavities that develop as extensions of the nasal passages. They are lined with the same ciliated mucous membrane as the nasal passages.

Most cases of nasal sinusitis are due to changes in the structure of the lining membrane, which is very thin and normally produces a mucous type of secretion. For this membrane to function properly, the sinus must be properly ventilated and able to drain into the nasal cavities by way of the sinus ostia. Any changes which cause blockage of this ostia can produce true nasal sinusitis.

Sinusitis may be defined as an inflammation of one or more of the nasal sinuses. This inflammation is primarily in the lining mucous membrane of the nasal sinuses. Sinusitis, like many diseases, can be acute or chronic. It is rare to find severe headache from the chronic form of nasal sinusitis, but headache is extremely common in the acute type of nasal sinusitis. Therefore, it is the acute form of nasal sinusitis that we shall discuss here.

Etiology

Acute sinusitis represents an acute infection of the mucous membrane lining of any or all of the paranasal sinuses, or of their bony framework (Figs. 8-1 and 8-2). If more than one sinus is involved, a combination of symptoms results, and the condition is referred to as pansinusitis.

One of the more common conditions which can lead into an attack of acute sinusitis is a severe upper respiratory infection. Such an infection will cause an edematous condition of the nasal mucosa and may block off the natural ostium of the nasal sinus. The nasal ciliary action is also impaired by such an infection, and this impairment may help to bring about involvement of the nasal sinuses.

Certain obstructive malformations of the nasal septum, which may be either congenital or acquired, may be a predisposing factor of nasal sinusitis. Some deviations of the nasal septum may tend to block off the ostium of one or more of the nasal sinuses and in so doing can very well be an etiologic

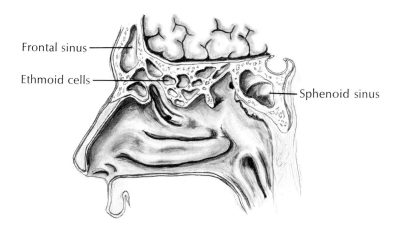

Fig. 8-1. Nasal sinuses.

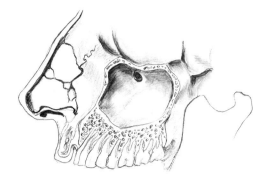

Fig. 8-2. Maxillary sinus.

factor in nasal sinusitis. If such a condition does exist, part of the treatment should consist of correcting the septal deformities by submucous resection.

Obstructive malformations of the turbinates can also play a predisposing role in the etiology of sinusitis. For example, if there is hyperplasia of the middle turbinate, there may be obstruction of the ostium of the frontal, maxillary, or anterior ethmoidal sinuses. Any form of edema of the mucous membrane of the middle turbinate can produce the same effect.

Nasal polyps can cause sinusitis conditions by acting as an obstructive mechanism, or they may aggravate an existing sinusitis, which may lead into what is known as a hyperplastic sinusitis.

An abscess or infection of the root of a tooth which happens to be located in or near the floor of the maxillary sinus may result in a maxillary sinusitis of dental origin by extension of the infection into the sinus. This is a fairly common cause of maxillary sinusitis. Such a condition causes an empyema of the antrum by infection through the dental fistula formed, or by any of the blood vessels or the lymphatics of the involved area.

Among the general predisposing causes of nasal sinusitis may be any condition which could lower the general resistance of the patient, such as infections, toxic conditions, malnutrition, metabolic disturbances, or endocrine imbalance. Certain allergic conditions which may produce a hypertrophic, edematous, boggy mucous membrane can also be predisposing factors.

Zeveleva[8] studied the indices of histamine metabolism in sinusitis and compared them with those in normal patients. He found the concentration of histamine and the content of substances endowed with an inhibitory action to histamine in the peripheral blood and blood of the nasal cavity, and and calculated the index of sensitivity to histamine. It was established that in patients with allergic rhinitis and sinusitis, histamine concentration in the peripheral blood and blood of the nasal cavity is usually augmented. The index of sensitivity to histamine rises not only at the expense of increased blood histamine level but also as the result of reduced content of substances of inhibitory action to histamine in the organism and, sometimes, the appearance of sensitizing substances (histamine stimulators).

Teisanu and Popescu-Tomus[9] report on a rarity as the cause of nasal sinusitis. They found in five patients with recurrent sinusitis that the pathologic contents of the sinuses yielded the protozoa *Trichomonas vaginalis*. Some of the patients displayed a caseous form of sinusitis. There are no other reports of sinus trichomoniasis in the literature.

May, Ogura, and Schramm[10] found that fractures of the frontal sinus can be a common factor in causing obstruction of the nasofrontal duct. Because this obstruction of the nasofrontal duct, which is so common, can lead to sinusitis as a late complication, surgical exploration of all frontal sinus fractures is recommended.

In discussing the etiology of sinusitis, Busis[11] points out that the nasal mucosa and ostia of the paranasal sinuses are particularly sensitive to pain. They are innervated by the fifth nerve, and pain may be referred to other distributions of this nerve. Persistent pain can cause muscle spasm, which may enhance the pain. The sensitivity to pain can be increased by emotional factors, poor general health, and certain environmental conditions. Tumor and infection are the main causes. Persistent bleeding, expansion of the walls of the nose or paranasal sinuses, or objective sensory changes may indicate a tumor.

D'Arcy,[12] in studying sinusitis in children, found that upper respiratory infections were the most common factor in the etiology of this condition.

In some instances a foreign body in the nasal passage may cause erosion and infection of the nasal mucous membrane and result in sinusitis. This may be done by directly obstructing the ostium of the nasal sinus, or it may be done by actually eroding through the wall of the nasal sinus. Eroding through the wall of the sinus is, of course, extremely rare, but it is worth mentioning.

Among the local predisposing causes of nasal sinusitis should be listed such conditions as hypertrophied and infected adenoids or tonsils, or both.

As mentioned previously, the most common condition which can lead into a case of nasal sinusitis is an acute upper respiratory infection. However, if such conditions are further complicated by an obstructive process, such as a deviated septum or a polyp, the possibility of a sinus infection arising becomes much greater.

Any obstructing nasal tumor may also be a local predisposing factor in nasal sinusitis if it obstructs the natural drainage of the sinus.

Let us now look at a little of the etiology of the various forms of acute nasal sinusitis.

ACUTE FRONTAL SINUSITIS

The size of the frontal sinuses does not seem to be due to diagnosed or undiagnosed infections but is probably determined by hereditary factors.

Acute frontal sinusitis may be brought about by any process that can interfere with the normal drainage of the nasofrontal duct. This interference may be either pathologic or anatomic. The pathologic conditions may include any condition that will produce edema of the mucous membrane, such as any form of allergy, polyps, hyperplasia, or an inflammatory process. It is seen in cases of deviation of the nasal septum, which will anatomically produce a blockage of the nasofrontal duct. Any excessive, hypertrophy of the middle turbinate can also produce this condition.

Acute frontal sinusitis follows certain forms of trauma, swimming, sudden exposure to high altitude, or infections ascending from either the maxillary or the ethmoidal sinuses. The bacteria most commonly causing this condition are the staphylococci, the streptococci, and the pneumococci.

ACUTE MAXILLARY SINUSITIS

Acute maxillary sinusitis may result from the direct extension of an infection in the nasal passage, through the ostium of the sinus, or it may be due to an infection of one of the tooth roots that may extend through the floor of the sinus (upper molars or premolars). It may also follow a dental extraction with the development of an oroantral fistula. When maxillary sinusitis is due to dental extraction, the symptoms usually are not pronounced for several weeks after the development of the causative process.

Such factors as septal deflection or hypertrophic middle turbinate can produce an obstruction of the ostium and result in a maxillary sinus infection. Allergy, polyps, or acute inflammatory processes may be predisposing factors to acute maxillary sinusitis.

Clinical, bacteriologic, and histopathologic studies were made in patients with persistent suppuration of the maxillary sinus. The sedimentation rate was below 50 mm per hour and the leukocyte count was only moderately increased in the majority of patients.[13]

In serum electrophoresis, total protein was within normal limits in most of the patients. The globulins were increased and albumins decreased. The most frequently cultured organism is *Streptococcus viridans,* followed by *Hemophilus influenzae, Diplococcus pneumoniae,* and *Alcaligenes faecalis.* Yellow staphylococci were also found.

Antistaphylolysis titers were increased above 1.5 in four patients. Antistreptolysin O titers were over 400 in ten patients, indicating the active role of beta-hemolytic streptococci in the early stages of the disease.

Lee[14] found that in patients with displaced roots in the maxillary sinus the roots of the maxillary first permanent molar were most commonly dislodged into the maxillary sinus (approximately 76% of patients). This high incidence of first molar involvement was believed to result to a larger extent from the intimate anatomic relationship which often exists between the root apices of this tooth and the floor of the maxillary sinus.

Lekas[15] states that while the majority of oroantral fistulas follow dental extractions, they may also result from infection, cysts, tumors of the upper jaw, or trauma or occur as a complication of surgery on the maxillary antrum.

ACUTE ETHMOIDITIS

Acute ethmoiditis is probably the most frequently found type of acute sinusitis. The ethmoidal sinuses are usually involved in some slight degree with every severe attack of acute coryza that persists for any great length of time.

ACUTE SPHENOIDITIS

The sphenoidal sinus is probably the least involved of all the sinuses. It is extremely rare to find the sphenoidal sinus involved without infection of the ethmoidal cell as well, especially the posterior ethmoidal cells.

Fruhwald and Canigiani[16] find that mucoceles in the sphenoidal sinus can result in acute sphenoditis and the headache which accompanies this condition.

Pathology

Acute infections of the nasal sinuses may be of an edematous nature, or they may be of the suppurative type. If the picture is one of edema, the mucous membrane of the sinus is found to be greatly thickened. This is due to the fact that the submucosal layer has been infiltrated with serum. The epithelial layer may at the same time be rather dry in this condition. The membrane may be swollen to a size ten times that of the normal membrane. In the submucosal layer there will be found a scattering of leukocytes. The blood vessels are dilated and very engorged, but the epithelial layer remains intact. The mucosa is greatly thickened and inflamed because of the edema present and the engorgement of the subepithelial structures.

Histologic examination of the biopsy

mucosa in chronic maxillary and ethmoidal sinusitis showed the metaplastic superficial epithelial layer with thickened low columnar cells and increased basal and goblet cells. The connective tissue revealed fibrous contraction causing atrophy of the once hypertrophied mucous glands and blood vessels surrounded by lymphocytes, plasma cells, eosinophils, and histiocytes.

If the infecting organisms are not too virulent and the general defense mechanisms of the patient's body are at a high level, resolution may take place; but if these factors are not favorable, the condition will continue on into the suppurative stage.

Any infection increases the edema, causing polyp formation, obstruction of the seromucous glands and fibrosis of blood vessels. Subsequent atrophy is responsible for the granular appearance of the sinus mucosa.[17]

In the suppurative stage, the serum and the leukocytes will escape through the epithelial lining of the mucosa where they join with the bacteria, mucus, and epithelial debris which may be present. There may be petechial hemorrhages in some cases and, if so, there will be blood mixed with the other secretions. The secretion found in these cases is at first rather thin and more or less watery. Later on, it will become rather thick and tenacious in character. This thickening is due to the coagulation of the fibrin which is present in the serum.

Resolution may then take place by the absorption of the exudate and the leukocytes ceasing to be discharged. If this resolution does not take place, the inflammation may extend deeply if the organisms are virulent or if the resistance of the patient is low. In such a case, the infection may pass into a chronic stage.

FRONTAL SINUSITIS

Initially there is a diffuse inflammation of the frontal sinus mucosa, and the nasofrontal duct becomes closed because of the edema. In the early stages there is an increase in the lymphocyte cells and the polymorphonuclear cells. Desquamation of superficial cells, with thrombophlebitis of smaller vessels and necrosis, follows. At first the exudate is serous, but it soon becomes purulent. If the process continues, the infectious condition may extend from the mucosa into the underlying bone. If the bone becomes involved, there may result either an osteitis of the floor or posterior wall of the sinus or an osteomyelitis in the anterior wall. It is through the involvement of the posterior wall that intracranial complications can become a part of the picture.

MAXILLARY SINUSITIS

In the initial stages of acute maxillary sinusitis, there is hyperemia of the mucous membrane, and a serofibrinous exudate is present. The edema produced causes an obstruction of the ostium.

Ethmoidal sinusitis and sphenoidal sinusitis do not show any distinguishing characteristics pathologically that are not found in frontal or maxillary sinusitis.

Symptomatology

Some cases of acute sinusitis may show a temperature elevation. This may be rather high, but usually a case of acute sinusitis will cause only a moderate or low-grade fever. Rarely is fever seen in cases of chronic nasal sinusitis. Various toxic symptoms, such as irritability, malaise, muscular soreness, or stiffness of the neck, may be present in acute sinusitis.

Many patients afflicted with nasal sinusitis experience some disturbances with their sense of smell. This may be seen in the form of parosmia, in which the sense of smell is perverted and the patient perceives odors which are not in evidence to a normally functioning nose. More frequently, however, these patients complain of anosmia, which is manifested by a complete loss of smell. This is temporary, however; the sense of smell tends to return to normal after the sinus infection has subsided.

Frequently these patients experience tenderness over the area of the sinus or sinuses involved. Some patients may elicit tenderness to mere palpation, whereas others may not express tenderness until actual pressure is used. This is most commonly seen in those sinuses which are superficially placed on the facial area, such as the maxillary, frontal, and anterior ethmoidal sinuses.

Sinusitis is usually short-lived and self-limited; it usually subsides shortly after the patient's head cold subsides. The discomfort and disability, if any, are brief. But when there is persistent obstruction to drainage and ventilation because of tissue changes, there may be a pathologic change in the lining membrane of the involved sinuses; the lining may become thicker and there may be an accumulation of purulent yellowish exudate.[18]

Purulent nasal and postnasal discharge is seen in most cases of nasal sinusitis. This is even more commonly seen if the condition is that of chronic sinusitis. This purulent nasal discharge is due to the empyema of the sinuses. The sinuses are commonly seen to be the focal center of such types of inflammation, far more so than the mucous membrane lining of the nasal passages. This does not mean that all patients who have a purulent nasal discharge have an actual nasal sinusitis but it does mean that it is a possibility which should be investigated. The area from which this pus is seen to be coming will help to determine which sinus or sinuses are involved. By that we mean that the anterior group of nasal sinuses drain into the middle meatus, and the anterior group of nasal sinuses is composed of the frontal, the maxillary, and the anterior ethmoidal sinuses. The posterior group of nasal sinuses is composed of the sphenoidal and the posterior ethmoidal sinuses, and these two sinuses drain into the superior meatus. Therefore, the location of the pus can show whether one of the anterior sinuses or one of the posterior group is involved, or both.

Postnasal discharge is quite prominent in cases of acute sinusitis. The patient becomes aware of this discharge when it becomes excessive, irritating, and obstructive.

Hipskind[19] points out that postnasal "drip" is not something everyone has and must live with. Nose drops are rarely beneficial and often damaging. The agent causing the nasal obstruction and discharge must be identified and controlled. Functioning tissue should not be sacrificed and radical surgery of the sinuses should be reserved for those cases in which the procedure is necessary to obtain a favorable result.

Many patients will complain of nasal obstruction. They will have difficulty in breathing properly through their nasal passages. This nasal obstruction may be either partial or complete because of a generalized edema or hypertrophy of the lining mucous membrane of the nasal passages. It may be due to the existence of nasal polyps or some other form of nasal tumor. Allergic conditions may also present the picture of nasal obstruction, by producing a boggy, edematous, hypertrophic type of nasal mucous membrane.

On the examination of the nasal passages of a patient with acute nasal sinusitis, the physician will observe the mucous membrane lining of the nasal passages to be inflamed. There may also be edema of the mucosa of the lateral nasal wall, so severe that portions of the lateral nasal wall will actually contact the nasal septum on the medial side of the nasal passage. There will be positive x-ray findings in nasal sinusitis. This, of course, is extremely helpful in establishing the diagnosis of sinusitis. It also is important in that it will help to show just what sinuses are involved.

It is impossible to tell from roentgenograms alone whether the disease in the sinus is acute or a healed and quiesent disease, if merely a thickening of the mucous membrane of the sinus is the only positive finding. The roentgenographic findings are of value only when they are correlated with the clinical findings in the symptomatology and examination of the patient. In other words, the roentgenologic examination should be looked on as a consultation, not as a complete diagnosis in cases of acute sinusitis.

Some physicians use transillumination to aid in their diagnosis of cases of sinusitis. However, we do not use it, since we do not have much faith in such a simple procedure. It can be of any significance only when it gives a negative result. It is not a true diagnostic aid, because certain anatomic variations of the sinuses may be present, and this will cause transillumination to give false results.[20] On the whole, we consider the use of transillumination to be rather amateur.

Headache, naturally, is the predominating symptom in acute nasal sinusitis. The headache is usually referable to the region of the infected sinus or sinuses. That is, if the frontal sinus is involved, the pain is usually in the area of the forehead. If the maxillary sinus is involved, the pain is in the area of the cheek on the side involved. If the sphenoidal sinus is involved, the pain may be deeply situated in the head, behind the eyes, or in the occipital area of the head. The ethmoidal sinuses, when involved, cause pain around the eyes and in the area of the bridge of the nose.

Williams[21] states that if the pressure produced in the sinuses is sufficiently great to cause pressure in the vessels of the submucosa, a referred pain will be produced. This shows the importance of taking the proper measures in relieving the engorgement of the nasal mucosa in cases of acute sinusitis.

In speaking of pain associated with nasal sinusitis, Thomas[22] states that the longer the disease runs, the more apt that the pain will be constant. In subacute and chronic cases of sinusitis, the pain may be worse in the afternoon or at night. We have rarely, if ever, seen pain to result from chronic sinusitis unless some other form of pathology is present, such as an osteomyelitis.

Headaches are less frequent at night and when the patient has been lying down for a long time; the headaches appear in the morning and may regress during the day, but not always. If the disease is of sufficient duration and intensity, pain is felt commonly in head, neck, and shoulders. The pain is only rarely referred to another region in cases of acute sinusitis, and it is usually associated with tenderness over the sinus or sinuses involved. The pain is frequently severe and incapacitating.

The patient with sinusitis most frequently complains of pain in the frontal region, as any of the nasal sinuses when infected can cause referred pain to the frontal area.

Many patients with acute nasal sinusitis note that their headache is increased in severity when they strain at stool, bend over, or stoop down. Coughing due to the postnasal drip can frequently be a part of the picture of nasal sinusitis and will increase the pain. Any jarring to which the patient might be submitted will also tend to increase the pain of the sinus attack.

The headache of hyperplastic sinusitis, in which there is the inflammatory element plus the allergic element (which may or may not include nasal polyps), may be referred to any region of the head.

Williams[23] describes the pain of acute sinusitis as burning and localized. As the disease progresses it becomes deeper and it may be referred to other areas. This occurs when the deeper structures are engorged and the purulent secretions appear as a symptom.

Sinusitis has long been considered a painful condition, and indeed in acute sinusitis there seems occasionally some basis for this contention. In acute sinusitis, if the pressure produced in the sinuses is sufficiently great to cause pressure in the vessels of the submucosa, a referred headache will be produced. However, in most instances of acute sinusitis it will be found that by relieving the congestion and contacts in the nasal chambers themselves, the headache associated with acute sinusitis will usually be completely relieved. Therefore, the headaches associated with sinusitis are usually nasal contact headaches and may be relieved by measures directed toward relieving the engorgement of the nasal mucosa.

There is a distinct form of frontal sinusitis which is due to an obstruction to the orifice of the nasofrontal duct. This causes the air of the frontal sinus to be absorbed and results in the production of a partial vacuum. The vacuum frontal headache is usually located in the frontal area and is of a low-grade intensity. This condition is characterized by the absence of purulent discharge, with no signs of pathology other than a slight redness and swelling of the nasal mucous membrane in the region of the middle turbinate. The patient with this type of nasofrontal sinusitis may elicit some slight tenderness to pressure near the floor of the frontal sinus.

The pain of nasal sinusitis is rather constant, not intermittent. The pain is not throbbing, as is the case in vascular headaches, but is a more or less dull, aching type of pain, and usually very severe.

Williams[23] states that nearly all head pains arising from the nasal and sinusal mucosa are of the deep, referred type. In the early stages of acute rhinitis and sinusitis a localized burning type of pain is present. Sensitization of the skin and other tissues of the region to which the deep pain is referred may take place. This may account for some instances of persistent pain present in patients in whom the irritating suppurative disease apparently has cleared up.

Pain of inflammatory sinal origin is usually accompanied by other nasal symptoms such as obstruction, rhinorrhea, and olfactory dysfunction as well as positive physical, laboratory, and radiographic findings. Neoplastic lesions originating from sinus mucosa may constitute a noteworthy exception. Indolent sinal pain is to be held suspect until etiology is defined.[24]

ACUTE FRONTAL SINUSITIS

The symptoms vary in direct proportion to the amount of obstruction of the naso-frontal duct. The primary symptom is a severe frontal headache. This headache is located directly over the sinus and may radiate to the vertex or behind the eyes. The pain is constant as long as there is pressure caused by the exudate being unable to drain through the nasofrontal duct. These headaches are most pronounced in the morning hours. There is tenderness to pressure in the frontal area. This is rather excessive in the area of the floor of the sinus (the roof of the orbit).

If the duct is not completely obstructed, there will be a heavy purulent discharge in the nasal passage. This may be unilateral or bilateral, depending on whether one or both of the sinuses are involved. The temperature will also vary in direct proportion to the amount of obstruction of the duct, the severity of the infection, and the patient's resistance to the infection. The more complete the obstruction, the higher the temperature will be. If the obstruction is complete, it is not uncommon to find a temperature of over 104° or 105° F.

There may be edema of the upper eyelid in cases of acute frontal sinusitis.

There will be positive radiologic findings on examination, and if transillumination is used, it will reveal opacity over the involved side.

MAXILLARY SINUSITIS

There is pain over the antral area (cheek), with an associated tenderness. The pain may radiate to the upper teeth or to the forehead area.

There is a heavy purulent nasal discharge that, on inspection of the nasal passage, is seen to be coming from the middle meatus. Along with this there is also a postnasal drip. The turbinate tissue is edematous and inflamed. The fever is in direct proportion to the virulence of the infection.

ACUTE ETHMOIDITIS

Headache is a prominent symptom of acute ethmoiditis. It is usually located between and behind the eye regions or radiates to the temporal area. The headache is constant and at times may become quite severe. The eyes are tender to pressure. The more the eyes are used, the more severe the headache becomes.

Nasal obstruction is present, and the patient is unable to breathe through the nose. This is due to the swelling of the middle turbinate. If the obstruction is severe, the patient may have anosmia.

Purulent drainage is seen in the nasal passages, coming from the middle meatus or the superior meatus or both, depending on whether the anterior or the posterior ethmoidal cells are involved. However, usually both groups of cells are involved in the average case of acute ethmoiditis. A purulent postnasal drip is also a complaint of these patients.

There may be edema of the skin between the inner canthus of the eye and the nose. The entire nasal passage is congested and the mucous membrane is edematous and inflamed; this is most pronounced in the area of the middle turbinate. A fever is usually present, along with generalized malaise and anorexia.

Positive roentgenologic findings will appear on examination. The ethmoidal cells are impossible to transilluminate.

ACUTE SPHENOIDITIS

The headache in acute sphenoidal sinusitis is usually located in the occipital area of the head, the vertex, or the frontal and eye regions. The pain may be referred from the occipital region to the mastoid area. The headache of acute sphenoiditis is constant and at times severe. These patients always seem to describe pain "behind the eye."

Vertigo may be present and may be either continuous or intermittent. A low-grade fever is usually present.

A purulent postnasal discharge is a prominent feature of acute sphenoiditis. Purulent drainage coming from the superior meatus and the sphenoethmoidal recess can be seen on examination of the nasal passages.

Sleeplessness is produced by the postnasal drip, which also causes a hacking type of cough due to irritation of the mucous membrane in the hypopharynx.

Mental symptoms such as forgetfulness, mental dullness, and inability to concentrate are often present. Ocular symptoms such as proptosis, scotomas, and enlargement of the blind spot may be found.

A characteristic radiologic feature in acute sphenoiditis is a thickening of the mucous membrane of the wall of the sinus, together with a homogeneous loss of translucency of its interior.

Diagnosis

As in any headache problem, the taking of a thorough history is essential in establishing a correct diagnosis. After the history has been taken, inspection of the nasal passages will frequently reveal the source of the nasal infection causing the headache attacks. The presence of the nasal discharge and the condition of the nasal mucous membrane are important signs for diagnostic purposes. At times, it may be necessary to use posterior rhinoscopy to locate the involved sinuses. This, of course, requires the aid of a trained otolaryngologist.

If the source of the discharge cannot be determined by the initial nasal examination, the physician should shrink the nasal mucous membrane and then employ gentle suction. This will be helpful in locating the source of the infection and will show the source of the purulent discharge.

X-ray examination of a patient in whom a sinus infection is suspected is often extremely helpful in making the diagnosis. Hallberg[25] believes that the "roentgenograms have gradually developed from the status of being merely an agent which was useful in ascertaining the size and contour of these cavities to one of considerable worth in determining the internal pathologic conditions." Any patient who gives a history of recurrent attacks of acute sinusitis should have a roentgenogram of the nasal sinuses taken (Fig. 8-3).

In many cases in which a diagnosis of some other type of organic headache can definitely be established, the physician can-

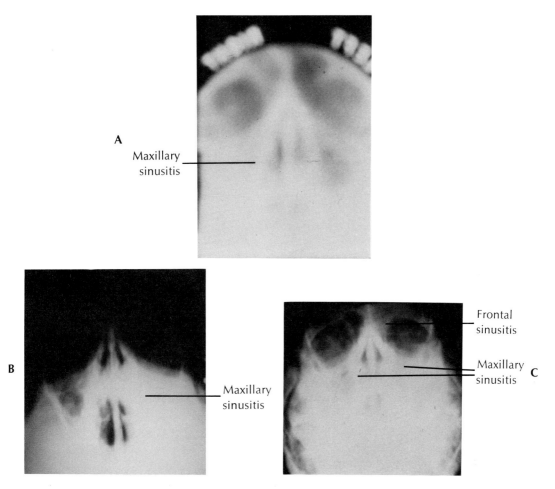

A
Maxillary
sinusitis

B

Maxillary
sinusitis

Frontal
sinusitis

Maxillary
sinusitis

C

Fig. 8-3. A and **B,** Acute maxillary sinusitis. **C,** Acute maxillary and acute frontal sinusitis.

not convince the patients that they do not have sinusitis. This may be due to the fact that previous physicians (who have not given the patient's headache problem enough time) have told these patients that they have sinusitis and have directed their treatment programs along those lines. Still others merely are determined that they actually have some other form of headache problem. In cases of this type, the taking of a sinus x-ray will aid in showing the patient that the case is not sinusitis at all, because the sinus x-rays are essentially negative.

In cases where a diagnosis of sinusitis is very obvious, the taking of sinus roentgenograms will help the physician to obtain a knowledge of the anatomic structure of the sinuses involved and the exact severity of the disease. If the headache problem is an extremely difficult one and the physician is unable to make a definite diagnosis, a sinus roentgenogram should be taken to rule out any possible sinus pathology which may not have the usual intranasal characteristics. The examination of the nasal sinuses through the use of a roentgenogram should be considered by the physician as a consultation.

If tumor formation is suspected in the case of sinusitis, tomography may be an important diagnostic aid to the physician. Radiologic demonstration of bone involvement as an indicator of tumor propagation is valuable, and tomography in more than one projection is recommended in selected patients.[26]

Another diagnostic aid in determining the function of the sinuses is rhinomanometry.[27] Airway resistance in nasal breathing can be measured with a simple inclined tube manometer. In anterior rhinomanometry (measuring one nasal cavity) the inspiratory pressure is usually 8 mm to a maximum of 20 mm H_2O; the expiratory pressure is 2 to 5 mm less. Pressures are increased in stenosis and obstruction of the nasal vestibules and valve areas; flattening of the nose with the so-called ballooning valve and atrophy of the mucosa result in decreased pressure.

By using electromanometers and a Fleisch pneumotachograph for measuring nasal pressure differences and the flow rate of the nasal air stream, it is possible to obtain more information on nasal respiratory function. Pressure recording in the maxillary sinus by rhinomanometry (even with a simple inclined tube manometer) enables the evaluation of the permeability of the natural ostium of the maxillary antrum.

Using a mask (like that of a diver) connected with a Fleisch pneumotachograph, the important technique of posterior rhinomanometry can be carried out for measuring the total nasal resistance of both sides. Also, concerning the relationship between flow and pressure of the air stream, the clinically important comparison of nasal resistance to pulmonary resistance can be made.

In some cases of sinusitis, probing, puncture, and lavage and cannulation of the sinuses will often aid in establishing a diagnosis. However, these methods are usually contraindicated in acute cases.

Complications of acute nasal sinusitis

Infection can spread and produce osteomyelitis; sterile or purulent pachymeningitis; subdural, epidural, or brain abscesses; or cavernous sinus thrombosis. Predispos-

ing factors are insufficient or inappropriate antibiotic treatment, excessively virulent organisms, and congenital body defects.[28]

The frontal sinus is anatomically closely related to the brain, the orbit, and the meninges. Therefore the complications can be quite severe. If an osteomyelitis should develop, the prognosis becomes less favorable. This can lead to a meningitis by the infection extending through the posterior wall of the sinus to the dura and the subarachnoid space. An extradural or intracerebral abscess may also develop in the frontal lobe. A subperiosteal abscess may develop above or below the eyebrow if the process extends anteriorly or inferiorly through the bone.

If the mucosa of the nasofrontal duct is partially thickened permanently by the infectious process, chronic frontal sinusitis develops; this is the most common form of complication of acute frontal sinusitis.

ACUTE MAXILLARY SINUSITIS

Acute maxillary sinusitis may "develop" into chronic maxillary sinusitis, or it may extend and cause the involvement of one of the other sinuses. An osteomyelitis of the facial bones may also result. Involvement of the maxillary sinus may also affect the eustachian tube, the middle ear, or the mastoid.

ACUTE ETHMOIDITIS

Acute ethmoiditis may extend into the sphenoidal sinus and bring about acute sphenoiditis. The acute infection of the ethmoidal sinus may turn into a chronic condition.

Cerebral abscess may be a complication of acute ethmoiditis, as may meningitis or cavernous sinus thrombosis.

ACUTE SPHENOIDITIS

Acute spheoniditis occasionally presents frontal lobe abscess as a complication. This is due to the anatomic location of the sphenoidal sinus, and it may result when the infection spreads through the body wall.

Meningeal irritation is also frequently seen with this condition, causing severe meningitis. Cavernous sinus thrombosis is another complication, as is retrobulbar neuritis.

FRONTAL LOBE ABSCESS

Frontal love abscess is actually not too common a complication of sinusitis. It may be secondary to frontal, sphenoidal, or ethmoidal sinusitis. The symptoms are chills, fever, severe headache, nausea, vomiting, and mental dullness. Increasing intracranial pressure will bring on ophthalmic symptoms such as pupil changes, optic nerve changes, visual disturbances, muscle paralysis, and papilledema. Mental symptoms include mental dullness, convulsions, personality changes, aphasia, and twitching. The terminal symptoms are coma, rapid pulse, stiff neck, high fever, delirium, twitching, hyperesthesia, paralysis, and death.

Intracranial extension or complications of suppurative sinus disease may present as a headache syndrome with subtle or dramatic flavor.[24]

OSTEOMYELITIS

Osteomyelitis is most commonly seen in the frontal sinus and rarely in the others. The symptoms consist of dull pain, low-grade fever and chills, swelling over the area involved, headache, malaise, edema of the upper eyelids, and a rapid pulse.

CAVERNOUS SINUS THROMBOSIS

Cavernous sinus thrombosis may occur with an infection of any of the paranasal sinuses. This occurs when there is extension of the infection through the venous pathways to the cavernous sinus. The symptoms occur abruptly and consist of orbital pain, exophthalmos, edema, chills and fever, nausea and vomiting, anorexia, papilledema, eye muscle paralysis, and mental dullness. The terminal symptoms are similar to those of meningitis, and the condition may be fatal.

RETROBULBAR NEURITIS

Retrobulbar neuritis occasionally appears as a complication in infections of the sphenoidal and ethmoidal sinuses. The symptoms consist of visual disturbances, which may be either sudden or gradual in onset. Retrobulbar neuritis caused by simple sinusitis of the posterior paranasal sinuses is curable, and visual disturbances will improve if the sinusitis is surgically treated early.[29]

MENINGITIS

Meningitis is seen in infections of the frontal, sphenoidal, or ethmoidal sinuses. The symptoms consist of severe headache, fever, nausea, vomiting, anorexia, neck rigidity, increased reflexes, slow pulse, prostration, Cheyne-Stokes respiration, cranial nerve involvement, papilledema, and positive spinal taps. The terminal stages are coma and death.

ORBITAL INFECTIONS

Orbital infections occur in connection with infections of the frontal, maxillary, and ethmoidal sinuses. The symptoms consist of orbital edema and pain, fever, lid edema, and headache, but no visual disturbances unless there is pus actually within the orbit.

UVEITIS

Uveitis is another conditon which can be a complication of sinusitis. It is not a common complication but it has been described in the literature.[30] Clinical evidence is offered that adequate removal of focal infection in the sinuses is possible and will cause subsidence of the uveitis with restoration of vision dependent only on the absence of previously established, irreversible changes in the ocular tissues. This applies not only to spontaneous uveitis but also to uveitis following operative or accidental trauma.

SUBPERIOSTEAL ABSCESS

The general symptoms of subperiosteal abscess are not severe. They consist of fever, edema of the inner canthus of the eye, and pain on movement of the eye. The condition, however, may lead to orbital cellulitis.

Such an abscess should be drained to prevent its spreading to either the dura or the eye. Antibiotics should also be employed.

EPIDURAL ABSCESS

Epidural abscess is often difficult to diagnose. The symptoms consist of dull, persistent, and usually nocturnal headache. There is tenderness over the involved dura. The abscess may spread to the brain or may rupture into the subarachnoid space, producing a meningitis.

• • •

Among the various types of sinusitis, maxillary sinusitis has the fewest, if any, complications. The frontal sinuses, though not present until about age 8 and developing over the following 4 years, may perforate the skull, and infection of the frontal sinuses may become complicated by meningitis and encephalitis. The same thing may occur in ethmoiditis, as the bone around it is tissue-paper thin in infants and young children. The sphenoidal sinus is encased in more solid bone, so such complications are much less frequent when this sinus is involved.

Treatment

In treating nasal sinus headache, again, we should attack the problem in a two-fold manner. That is, we should treat it prophylactically by trying to restore the nasal passages and sinuses to normal function by removing the disease present. Also, we should treat this type of patient symptomatically by relieving the headache attacks which are occurring.

PROPHYLACTIC TREATMENT

The most important feature in this phase of the treatment of nasal sinus headache is the establishment of free drainage of the sinuses. The early stage of acute nasal

sinusitis is that of engorgement and edema of the mucous membrane, according to Brown.[31] It is during this stage of acute sinusitis that head pain is an extremely prominent symptom, and treatment is primarily medical and not surgical. The reduction of this swollen, engorged mucous membrane is of prime necessity for the purpose of opening the ostia of the nasal sinuses. It is this acute inflammatory change in the mucous membrane of the nasal sinuses which is a prime factor in bringing about an intensely painful inflammatory reaction about the nerve endings of the areas involved. It is the headache which the patient experiences during this phase of acute sinusitis that the patient is interested in, for it is the symptom of pain which causes him the most discomfort, not the other symptoms which are referable to the nose and nasal passages.

Shrinkage and suction should be used in establishing drainage of the paranasa sinuses which have an existing acute inflammatory condition present. The shrinkage of the nasal mucous membrane may be brought about by using any of several different types of solutions. An isotonic solution of 1% ephedrine may be used. This solution is placed on thin pieces of cotton and applied to the area of the swollen middle and inferior turbinates to reduce the swelling. These packs can be left in the nasal passages for a 5- to 10-minute period and then removed. After removal, gentle suction applied to the nasal passages will establish drainage in most conditions. As Boies[32] states: "In an acute process, headache from tension within a sinus is common," and it will tend to "disappear as the sinus drains or the swelling subsides."

The use of the vasoconstrictor drugs in the nasal passages should not be overdone, because they can produce harmful results and become very habit-forming. A report on the microscopic changes produced by the overuse of nasal medication of this type was first published in 1946.[33] In that paper the epithelial and subepithelial tissue damage which took place when the drugs were used over a prolonged period of time was described.

When speaking of the use of the vasoconstrictor drugs in the nasal passages, Williams[34] also states that they produce a state of more and more refractory congestion and that the comfort produced by these drugs is due to their stimulation of the nerve endings for cold in the mucosa.

The vasoconstrictor group of drugs, when overused in the nasal passages, may also inhibit the normal physiologic functions of the nasal mucous membrane. It is fundamentally correct to use these drugs over short periods of time in order to establish drainage in cases of acute nasal sinusitis. However, they should not be given to the patient to use at home at his own free will, because he may overuse them and soon get into the habit of using them several times a day, every day of the year.

Applying suction in these cases should be done very gently. Prolonged suction may often prove to be harmful, and usually better results are obtained from more frequent, short applications of the suction. Any trauma from such manipulations should be avoided because in the early stages of acute sinusitis natural barriers to the infection have not been established, and, in many cases, if trauma does occur, an osteitis of the bones of the sinuses involved can possibly result.

The use of the antibiotics in cases of acute sinusitis has naturally been helpful in the treatment of acute sinusitis. For this type of condition, we generally prefer to use penicillin by the intramuscular route of administration. The concentration of the antibiotics found in nasal secretions obtained by aspiration or irrigation of the diseased sinus showed that absolutely no correlations could be established between concentrations of antibiotics and clinical parameters investigated. This lack of correlation is surprising and emphasizes the importance of further study of the pharmacodynamics of antibiotics in different organs.[35]

In treating sinusitis, Lillie[36] advocates analgesics, sedatives, antibiotics, and sulfonamides. Drainage is essential and is helped by ephedrine and gentle suction. He believes displacement to be a dangerous procedure because of contamination of the uninvolved sinuses and the eustachian tube. Hot compresses he also finds of value. In chronic cases he believes surgery to be necessary in most cases.

In speaking of the treatment of paranasal sinusitis, Moffett[37] states that drainage with the least possible destruction of tissue should be the rule. He further states that the use of antibiotics is making diagnosis more difficult in some cases. Control of allergy has cut down the need of surgery in many cases of ethmoiditis. Alfor[38] discusses the change in thinking about treating sinusitis. He believes the reasons for this change are the modern advances in chemotherapy and in the diagnosis and management of non-infectious diseases of the nose and the sinuses. Today the rhinologist has a clearer knowledge of the physiology of the nose and a respect for the integrity of the mucous membrane.

Acute maxillary sinusitis was investigated in fifty-two adults to evaluate its bacteriology and antibiotic therapy. *Staphylococcus aureus* was responsible for the infection in over 50% of the patients, and the second most common pathogen was *Pneumococcus*. Controlled study of the effect of an antibiotic (erythromycin) on the course of the infection showed that antimicrobial therapy shortened the course of illness.[39]

Gullers and associates[40] took blood samples and sinus secretions in patients with acute sinusitis who received penicillin treatment. They found that concentrations of penicillin reached in the sinus secretions were compared with severity of infection expressed by type of secretion: serous, mucous, or purulent. There were lower concentrations when the infection was severe. It was also shown that when the infection was healing, concentration of penicillin went up. It was concluded that penicillin V passes over to the sinus secretions of many patients. Under severe inflammatory conditions, however, the concentration of penicillin V is not demonstrable with the method used.

Axelsson and associates[41] took patients with acute maxillary sinusitis and placed them into four different treatment groups: (1) doxycycline (Vibramycin) plus nasal decongestant, (2) doxycycline plus irrigation, (3) spiramycin plus nasal decongestant, and (4) spiramycin plus irrigation. The patients returned after 5, 10, and 15 days of treatment for radiologic examination. They found that both doxycyline and spiramycin together with a nasal decongestant give results similar to those obtained with these same antibiotics plus irrigation; consequently, irrigation can be omitted when using these antibiotics.

On the other hand Raggio[42] believes that for relief of sinusitis treatment is directed to relief of pain, use of steam inhalation, hot applications, antibacterials, oral decongestants, and sinus lavage. The last is repeated every 2 or 3 days until the return is clear.

We can see that there is some discrepancy concerning the use of sinus irrigations.

In a study by D'Arcy[12] on maxillary sinusitis, antral washings were sent for culture and sensitivity tests. The antibiotics to which organisms were most frequently sensitive included sulfamethoxasole, followed by erythromycin and ampicillin. In 20% of the patients so much infection was revealed on lavage that it was considered wise to retain polythene tubes in the sinuses. Those patients were then subjected to twice daily lavages via the tubes until the washings were clear. Tubes were retained in the maxillary antrum for an average of 3 days.

In some cases, surgical measures may have to be adopted. If, for example, there are nasal polyps obstructing the ostium of the sinus involved, they should be removed, but this should be done after the acute phase of the condition has subsided.

Also, if a septal deformity interferes with the desired drainage of the nasal sinuses, this should be corrected by submucous resection. Again, this should be done only after the acute sinus infection has subsided. The reason for the delay in using a procedure like this to help obtain the desired drainage is, of course, to avoid any unnecessary trauma, so that any danger of osteitis may be avoided.

If surgery is considered in nasal sinusitis, Burnam[43] states that nasal physiology and, particularly, the infundibular area of the nose are most important in the pathogenesis of sinus disease. This area is the "Times Square" of the nasosinus labyrinth, and appropriate attention to its function will allow correction of the majority of sinus problems.

The basic goals of sinus surgery are as follows:

1. Alleviation of nasal and/or sinus obstruction
2. Adequate nasal and sinus ventilation
3. Eradication of chronic disease by sinus exenteration
4. Surgical drainage of sinus complications
5. Functional surgery without cosmetic deformity

The paranasal sinuses are passive appendages of the nose and will ordinarily remain disease-free when good nasal function is maintained.

If there is any allergic element present, it should be combated by trying to discover to what the patient may be sensitive and then having him avoid these elements. This can be best accomplished by the use of intradermal skin tests. The antihistamines are also helpful in allergic forms of rhinitis; however, they tend to produce a secondary side effect in many people, usually in the form of drowsiness. When this occurs, it can be counteracted by using ephedrine sulfate with the antihistamine preparation. Both will help shrink and dry up the nasal passages, and while the antihistamine is a depressant, the ephedrine is a stimulant.

When taken together, the depressant and stimulant effects are equalized.

Lillie[44] believes that for the treatment of sinusitis to be successful: "It is important that not only the disease be controlled but that the function of the nose be preserved." He adds that it is a false notion when one says, "Once sinus disease, always sinus disease."

Because most cases of sinus infections respond nicely to conservative therapy, and because of the great emotional disturbance many patients develop when confronted with the possibility of surgery, it is recommended that conservative methods be used before any type of surgical procedure is utilized. The physician's armamentarium of drug weapons can control and fight practically all such infections. However, surgery should never be denied any patient when time or other circumstances preclude an attempt at conservative therapy.

SYMPTOMATIC TREATMENT

In many cases of acute sinusitis headache, some relief can be obtained by using heat. Some physicians prefer dry heat, while others prefer moist heat. We believe that if heat is going to give the patient any relief, the best results may be obtained by using hot, wet towels, which should be placed over the painful areas. The heat in such conditions causes an increased hyperemia and leukocytosis.

Rest is essential in many cases of acute nasal sinusitis. This is true in the cases in which patients have become rather exhausted from the pain they have suffered. These patients often become irritable, and a general feeling of malaise is frequently present. Rest is often helpful to, and desired by, the patient.

The most effective agents used to dull or abort the actual pain of the acute sinus attack seem to be the analgesic group of drugs. Such preparations as aspirin, Empirin Compound, and Anacin seem to give some temporary relief from the pain produced by acute sinusitis attacks. Recently, we have obtained some good results with Fiorinal in this type of headache problem. Fiorinal is an analgesic preparation composed of 200 mg acetylsalicylic acid, 130 mg acetophenetidin, 40 mg caffeine, and 50 mg Sandoptal. Thus, it contains the same drugs as does Empirin Compound, plus the Sandoptal, which is a sedative similar to the phenobarbital group. Fiorinal helped in many of the sinus headache problems in which it was used. It certainly is as good as any of the other preparations such as Empirin Compound or aspirin.[45]

Acute frontal sinusitis. The nasal mucosa should be shrunk so that proper drainage can be established. When shrinkage has been established, gentle suction should be applied. The shrinkage can be brought about by using ephedrine or an ephedrine derivative on a cotton tampon placed in the middle meatus for approximately one-half hour.

Heat over the involved sinus, along with one of the analgesic preparations, is helpful in combating the painful element of this condition. Wet heat in the form of hot packs is usually more beneficial than the dry form of heat. However, if the pain is severe, the addition of codeine or morphine may be required. The antibiotics should be used immediately. The drug of choice is usually penicillin, if the patient does not have an allergic sensitivity to it.

Bed rest is essential in these cases, and steam inhalations are also of great benefit.

If medical efforts fail and the pain continues, or if complications set in, the treatment necessarily becomes surgical. This may be done intranasally or through an external approach. If a mucocele forms in the sinus, surgery is required. This is always done through the external approach, but mucoceles are more commonly seen in chronic cases of frontal sinusitis. If such a condition (mucocele or pyocele) exists, the acute phase of the infection should be controlled before any radical surgery is attempted.

Because of the danger of osteomyelitis

occurring, surgery is contraindicated during the acute phase of this condition, except in special instances.

SUMMARY

Symptoms

1. Frontal headache
2. Frontal tenderness
3. Purulent nasal discharge
4. Fever
5. Positive roentgenographic findings and transillumination

Treatment

1. Shrinkage
2. Suction
3. Antibiotics
4. Heat
5. Analgesics or narcotics
6. Bed rest
7. Steam inhalations
8. Surgical, if medical efforts fail

Acute maxillary sinusitis. Bed rest, with steam inhalations, is beneficial. Shrinkage of the mucous membrane and the use of gentle suction aid in establishing proper drainage. Phenylephrine will do the desired shrinking adequately, or an ephedrine or ephedrine-like preparation may be used.

The pain may be relieved by an analgesic, an analgesic plus codeine, or the use of wet heat, in the form of hot packs, applied locally to the involved area. The antibiotics, especially penicillin, are extremely helpful in cases of acute maxillary sinusitis.

If medical treatment fails, after the acute condition has subsided, an antral puncture and lavage can be used to remove the purulent material from the sinus. As a rule, this is done under local anesthesia in the average adult patient. It is important not to do it until the acute phase of the condition has subsided, because of the danger of the development of an osteomyelitis.

If this does not aid the situation, surgery will be indicated, such as making a large nasoantral window. This is done to bring about proper drainage of the sinus and to remove the diseased membrane lining the sinus. When this diseased membrane is re-moved, a new membrane will grow and take its place.

If the maxillary sinusitis is of dental origin, packing, irrigation, or manipulation of the fistulous tract are contraindicated. Many fistulas will heal spontaneously with conservative treatment. If infection ensues, antibiotic treatment is instituted according to culture and sensitivity, or a broad-spectrum antibiotic is used until the sensitivity report is available. Currettage of the fistulous tract and removal of infected granulation tissue may be carried out, followed by flap closure.

SUMMARY

Symptoms

1. Pain in cheek area
2. Tenderness in cheek area
3. Pain extending to upper teeth
4. Fever
5. Purulent nasal discharge
6. Purulent postnasal drip
7. Edematous and inflamed turbinate tissue

Treatment

1. Shrinkage and suction
2. Antibiotics
3. Analgesics, with or without codeine
4. Heat
5. Antral puncture and lavage
6. Surgery, if medical treatment fails

Acute ethmoiditis. The antibiotics should be used to attack the infection. Penicillin is usually beneficial in these cases, provided the patient does not have an allergic sensitivity to the drug. If that is the case, another type of antibiotic should be used.

The nasal passages should be shrunk, and then gentle suction should be applied. External wet heat is helpful in these cases, along with the analgesic group of drugs, to combat the pain and fever of this condition. Sometimes it is necessary to use codeine or morphine if the pain is rather severe. Bed rest is helpful, along with steam inhalations.

If the tissues do not respond to medical therapy, or when complications set in, surgery will be required.

SUMMARY

Symptoms

1. Headache
2. Tenderness in eye region
3. Nasal obstruction
4. Purulent nasal discharge
5. Purulent postnasal drip
6. Anosmia
7. Fever
8. Malaise
9. Anorexia
10. Swelling between inner canthus of eye and the nose
11. Positive roentgenographic findings

Treatment

1. Antibiotics
2. Shrinkage and suction
3. External head
4. Analgesics, with or without codeine
5. Bed rest
6. Steam inhalations
7. Surgery, if medical treatment fails

Acute sphenoiditis. Shrinkage and suction of the sinus are important. External heat in the occipital area and the analgesic drugs, with or without codeine, are successful in combating the pain of this condition. The antibiotic group of drugs is important in culminating this type of infection. Bed rest and steam inhalations are also helpful. It is extremely important to establish proper drainage in all cases of acute sphenoiditis.

If medical therapy fails, surgery may be needed. The anterior wall of the sinus is removed in order that proper drainage may be assured.

SUMMARY

Symptoms

1. Headache—occipital, vertex, or frontal area
2. Vertigo
3. Purulent postnasal drip
4. Sleeplessness
5. Cough
6. Low-grade fever
7. Mental symptoms
    a. Forgetfulness
    b. Inability to concentrate
    c. Mental dullness
8. Ocular symptoms

a. Proptosis
b. Scotomas
c. Enlargement of blind spot

Treatment

1. Shrinkage and suction
2. Antibiotics
3. External heat
4. Analgesics, with or without codeine
5. Bed rest
6. Steam inhalations
7. Surgery, if medical therapy is not effective

Case history

An example of acute sinusitis follows.

P. C., a 35-year-old white male, complained of pain over the left ethmoidal and maxillary areas over a 48-hour period. The pain was severe, dull, and rather constant. The maxillary area and the ethmoidal area on the left were both tender to pressure. He had had similar attacks in the past several years, of the same type. There was considerable nasal obstruction in the left nasal passage which was partially due to the edema and engorgement of the turbinate tissue and partially to a septal deflection to the left of a severe degree. The mucous membrane was inflamed, edematous, and boggy. There was a purulent discharge in the left nasal passage. On shrinkage with a 1% ephedrine cotton pack, the pus was seen to be coming from the left middle meatus. This patient also presented some secondary ocular manifestations in the left eye, which the ophthalmologist claimed were due to the sinusitis present. X-ray examinations revealed a cloudiness and thickness of the membranes of the left ethmoidal sinus and the left maxillary sinus. His temperature was 99.2° F.

He was treated by using shrinkage and suction, wet heat, and penicillin injected intramuscularly. His pain was relieved by using two tablets of Fiorinal. In 10 days the mucous membrane of the left nasal passage was of normal color and size, the passageway was free of any purulent discharge, the head pain had completely disappeared, the temperature was normal, and the ophthalmologic symptoms had disappeared.

Summary

A summary of the symptoms, signs, and treatment of acute nasal sinusitis headache consists of the following:

SUMMARY

Symptoms and signs

1. Nasal discharge
2. Nasal congestion and edema

3. Inflamed nasal mucous membrane
4. Tenderness to pressure
5. Temperature elevation
6. Positive x-ray findings

Pain is

1. Fairly constant
2. Dull
3. Unilateral or bilateral in area of sinuses involved

Treatment

1. Shrinkage and suction
2. Antibiotics
3. Correction of any septal deformities
4. Rest
5. Heat
6. Analgesics
7. Surgery
8. Deep x-ray

HEADACHE DUE TO NASAL SEPTUM DEVIATIONS

Deviation of the nasal septum occurs when the septum is not in the median line but is diverted more to one side of the nasal passage than the other, causing one nasal passage to be smaller than the other.

Etiology

Septal deflection is either traumatic or congenital. Some of the theories concerning the congenital aspect of this condition state that a deviated nasal septum can result from (1) faulty development of the facial bones; (2) a high arch of the hard palate, with resultant crowding of the vomer and the perpendicular plate of the ethmoid bone; (3) excessive development of the vomer; or (4) unequal development of adjacent bones, especially the turbinates.

Trauma to the external nose is a leading factor in the etiology of this condition. Since the free anterior margin of the septal cartilage lies directly under the skin of the middle of the nasal dorsum, it is easily exposed to injuries that will either split, dislocate, or bow the cartilage or bone of the septum (Figs. 8-4 and 8-5).

The nasal septum tends to protect the cribriform plate and the brain above it. Uppermost is a strong suture line built in a curve with a convexity down and forward. The front portion of this curve is formed by the end-to-end suture of the quadrilateral cartilage and the vertical plate of the ethmoid. The rear part of the suture is formed by the vomer and ethmoid bones. This is the strongest part of the nasal septum. Below this are the tongue and groove sutures formed by the cartilage fitting into the columella, the nasal crest, and the vomer. These sutures are not too strong and give way to force before the force reaches the cribriform plate and the brain.

Oddly, the trauma may have occurred without producing any noticeable symptoms other than the momentary pain from the blow, and the individual may be unaware that his nose has been broken. The

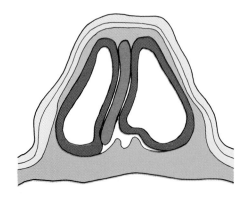

Fig. 8-4. Septal dislocation.

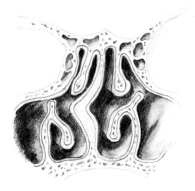

Fig. 8-5. Deviated nasal septum.

actual deviation of the septum may be discovered by examination of the nasal passages long after the trauma has taken place.

It is believed that the spurs and ridges formed on the nasal septum result from the fact that the septum is thin and flexible in childhood and, when it cannot find the proper room for its full development between the rigid hard palate below and the equally sturdy and strong nasal roof above, it merely takes the line of least resistance and buckles, thus forming spurs or ridges.

Since pain may be elicited by stimulation of the intranasal structures, it is obvious that the pressure of any swollen, hypersensitive nasal mucosa on the turbinates or septum might be a cause of headache. The configuration of the intranasal structures, such as marked hypertrophy of the nasal turbinates on the side opposite to a septal deviation, largely determines which of such patients develop headache. Compression of the middle meatus may lead to obstruction of the natural ostium of the maxillary, ethmoidal, or frontal sinuses, especially if concurrent nasal allergy or vasomotor rhinitis is present. The presence of an impacting bony spur in the region of the middle meatus predisposes the patient to blockage of the natural ostium, with the development of secondary sinusitis.[46]

Gidall[47] points out that septal deflections, spurs, or hyperplastic turbinates may cause headaches due to impingement of intranasal structures. Roydhouse[48] states that in the more severe forms of vasomotor rhinitis, there may be faceache and frontal headache, due not to any infection of the sinuses but to their becoming secondarily involved, as their small ostia are easily blocked by the nasal mucosal swelling.

Symptomatology

The chief symptom of a deviated nasal septum is nasal obstruction. This is usually unilateral. However, if the septal deformity is irregular and rather S-shaped, the obstruction can quite conceivably be bilateral. This obstruction is naturally increased when any infectious or allergic process may

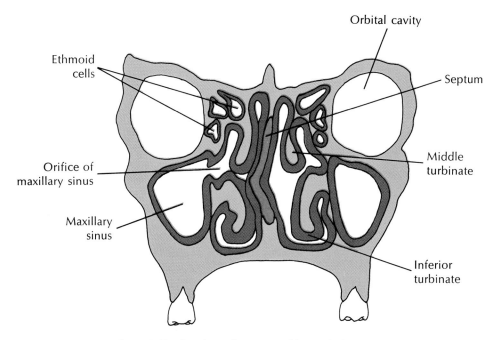

Fig. 8-6. Deviated nasal septum with nasal obstruction.

be present that will increase the size of the turbinate tissue and swelling of the mucous membrane of the nasal cavity (Figs. 8-6 and 8-7).

The deviation of the nasal septum may be in such a location that it will block the natural orifice of one of the nasal sinuses. If this occurs and infection sets in, the sinus will not be able to drain adequately, and additional trouble will be encountered.

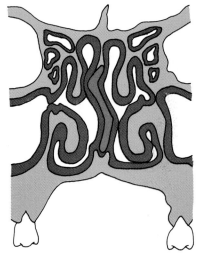

Fig. 8-7. Septal deviation with pressure on middle turbinate.

If the obstruction in the nasal passages is marked, harsh breathing will result. If so, a frequent symptom will be snoring.

Because of the disturbance in the normal nasal physiology, there may be an increase in the amount of nasal and postnasal mucous discharge. This is due to the fact that there is not enough air going through one of the nasal passages and a corresponding excess of air passing through the other nasal passage. Because of the excessive amount of air passing through the nasal passage that the septum is deviated away from, the nasal mucous membrane will try to protect itself from drying out and will, therefore, produce an excessive amount of mucus. This will usually result in a postnasal drip. If the mucosa does become dry, crusts may form. If these are picked off, bleeding may occur.

There may also be an increased susceptibility to infections of the nasal passages, because of the physiologic disturbance.

In some instances, if the septal deflection is severe, there will be a corresponding external deformity of the nose. If, by the deviation of the septum, there is pressure exerted on the lateral nasal wall in the area of any nerve, a neurologic type of headache will result (Fig. 8-8).

Williams[49] stated that pressure of the nasal septum against the middle turbinate

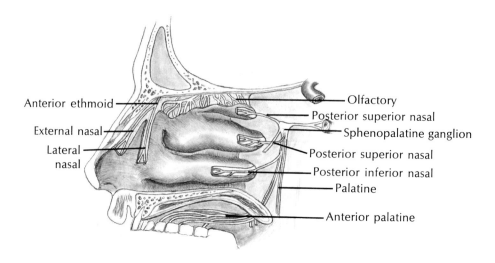

Fig. 8-8. Nerves of lateral nasal wall.

bone produces deep aching pain in the mid-forehead or eye. Complete anesthetization of contact areas relieves the discomfort, but recurrence necessitates removal of the pressing structures (see Fig. 8-7). Williams further pointed out that the temporal or malar pain caused by septal spur pressure in the sphenopalatine region is treated by operation and vasodilators.

Danforth[50] described the headache associated with nasal contact as being characteristically a unilateral headache which appears centered around the periorbital, glabella, and frontal areas. The patient describes the pain as steady and aching rather than throbbing in nature. Not infrequently the headache is preceded by an upper respiratory infection, allergic rhinitis, or vasomotor rhinitis, and the patient complains to the physician of a so-called sinus headache.

The main physical findings are usually confined to the nasal examination, where some degree of congestion of the mucous membranes is found. The nasal septum at the level of the middle turbinate may be deviated toward the side of the headache or actually come into contact with the middle turbinate, but paranasal sinus disease cannot be demonstrated.

In establishing a diagnosis of headache which is of nasal contact origin, the appearance of the nasal cavities and of the lining mucosa of the passages must be observed. This can be done easily if the soft tissues of the nasal turbinates in the lateral nasal wall have a shrinking agent applied to them. After the turbinates have been shrunk, the structural shape of the internasal region can be evaluated. In doing this there may also be some relief of the headache noted by the patient. This will be true if the shrinkage is sufficient to relieve the contact of the septal deformity with the lateral nasal wall. If this shrinkage is not enough to relieve the contact and in turn relieve the headache, the diagnosis of a headache of nasal origin may be confirmed by the relief which is obtained by cocainization of the contact area. A tampon containing a solution of 5% cocaine placed for a few minutes on the contact area will be sufficient to produce this effect.

Treatment

The only proper treatment for this condition is submucous resection or a plastic reconstruction of the nasal septum. This is done under local anesthesia. The incision is usually made posteriorly to the junction of the vestibule and the mucous membrane of the septum. The mucous membrane and the perichondrium and periosteum are then elevated away from the underlying cartilage and bone. Then the initial incision is carried through the cartilage, and the elevation of the tissue away from the cartilage and the bone on the other side is carried out. With both sides of the membrane free, the deviated bone and cartilage are then removed or replaced in a correct or better position. Sutures are then used to close the incision. The nasal passages are packed with petrolatum gauze, which is left in place overnight.

Great care should be taken not to tear the mucous membrane. If the membrane is torn in the same place on both sides, a septal perforation will result; this is undesirable.

Many surgeons prefer to combine this procedure with a plastic reconstruction of the nasal septum; in such cases removal of the septal cartilage and bone is avoided.

The modern concept of the physiology of the nose requires a rigid septum with sufficient cartilage to prevent atrophic changes. This may mean leaving in position large pieces of cartilage and preventing their displacement at a later date. The cartilage must be kept partially attached to one of the mucosal flaps. The retained cartilage should be attached to the convex side. Successful treatment may result from intranasal surgery to correct the structural deformity of the septum or from the use of vasoconstrictors to place the offending vessels in spasm.

In treating this condition Thomas[51] says that if septal deformities are present, they should be corrected surgically. If infection and hyperplasia are present they should also be treated and kept under control.

Successful surgical correction of a nasal deviation not associated with recent trauma usually depends on proper management of the accompanying septal deformity. Selection of the proper septorhinoplastic technique must be critically evaluated with regard to the type of septal deviation encountered and to the surgeon's technical ability. Rigid rules cannot be made governing whether rhinoplasty can be performed simultaneously with septal surgery or whether it should be carried out as a staged separate procedure.[52]

Ergotamine tartrate is an effective agent in management. An aerosol oral inhalant (Medihaler-Ergotamine) is useful in the diagnosis of headaches of vascular origin, assuring a rapid method of providing blood levels of ergotamine via the transpulmonary route. A significant number of patients in whom this type of headache was either suspected clinically or diagnosed by a previous response to an anticephalalgic (Cafergot) or to nasal cocainization have responded promptly following the diagnostic use of this oral inhalant.[50] We have never found this to be very successful in cases of headache with this type of etiology.

The headache associated with this nasal abnormality is usually successfully treated by the use of one of the analgesic group of drugs.

OTHER PATHOLOGIC CONDITIONS OF THE NASAL SEPTUM PRODUCING HEADACHE

Besides nasal septum deviation, there are a few other pathologic conditions of the nasal septum which present headache as one of their symptoms. While these conditions are not as frequently seen as septal deviations, they do exist and deserve mentioning.

Septal abscess

Septal abscess formation represents a collection of pus beneath the mucous membrane of the septum.

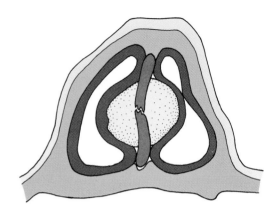

Fig. 8-9. Septal abscess.

Etiology. Septal abscess is usually due to an infection of a septal hematoma that has been caused by trauma. Occasionally an abscess of the septum is seen in such conditions as typhoid fever, measles, or furunculosis of the columella (Fig. 8-9).

Symptoms. Swelling, redness, and edema of one or both sides of the septum are present. This may also extend to the external nose. If the perichondrium becomes involved, the cartilage may become destroyed. Nasal obstruction will result from the swelling, and this is accompanied by pain, tenderness, fever, and malaise. Frontal headache is also associated with this condition.

The headache associated with septal abscess is a constant, severe, throbbing type of pain. It is chiefly brought about by the pressure, which the abscess produces on the structures of the lateral nasal wall.

Treatment. As soon as pressure is relieved the headache will subside, so the treatment should be chiefly centered around treatment of the abscess itself. The analgesic type of drugs will usually be sufficient to help relieve the severity of the headache.

As far as the treatment of the abscess itself is concerned, the abscess should be incised in its most dependent portion. This should be done under local anesthesia but may require a general anesthetic in children. After incision the pus should be removed by gentle suction. The use of a drain

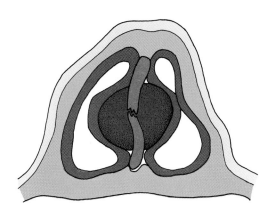

Fig. 8-10. Septal hematoma.

may be required in some cases. Drainage may also be maintained by excising a segment of the mucous membrane bordering the incision. Hot saline packs are useful in keeping the incised abscess open for drainage.

Antibiotics should be used immediately, both systemically and also locally, in the form of ointments, when crusting is present.

Complications. Necrosis of the cartilage may result, causing a fall of the dorsum of the nose. Thrombosis of the cavernous sinus is another complication of this condition.

Septal hematoma

A septal hematoma is a collection of blood beneath the mucous membrane of the nasal septum (Fig. 8-10).

Etiology. Septal hematoma is usually traumatic in origin. It is seen in such conditions as contusions and fractures of the septum, and it can also occur following nasal septal surgery.

Symptoms. Nasal obstruction is produced by the swelling and is accompanied by a feeling of pressure in the nose. Fever to a mild degree and a dull frontal headache are often associated with this condition.

The headache associated with septal hematoma is produced by the same pathologic mechanism as the headache of septal abscess. That is, it is due to the swelling pro-

duced by the hematoma which results in pressure upon the structures of the lateral nasal wall. The pain is constant, throbbing and at times quite severe.

Treatment. Relief of the headache resulting from septal hematoma will actually not completely occur until the pressure produced by the swelling of the hematoma is relieved. The analgesic group of drugs will reduce the pain of this condition, but as long as the swelling exists the pain exists to various degrees.

For treatment of the hematoma itself, small hematomas may be aspirated with a sterile needle and syringe. Large hematomas will require incision near their inferior portion. This is done under local anesthesia. The blood and the clot should be removed by using gentle suction. A thin petrolatum gauze packing, left in place overnight, may be required to approximate the mucous membrane and perichondrium and prevent further bleeding. This also compresses the space produced by removal of the blood clot. Antibiotics may be employed to prevent complications such as septal abscess.

Nasal synechia

Nasal synechia is probably much more commonly seen than either nasal septum abscess or nasal septum hematoma; however, it is less likely to produce headache than either of these conditions. Nasal synechia constitutes a band of connective tissue covered with mucosa, which results in a bridge of tissue from the medial to the lateral nasal wall.

Etiology. Synechiae are adhesion bands of scar tissue that result from the loss of epithelium from two adjacent areas of the mucosa. This can be due to trauma, nasal surgery, cautery, or lacerations.

Pathology. Two ulcerative areas are found in the nasal passage, and granulation tissue forms over the ulcerative areas and unites. This gradually becomes epithelialized and forms scar tissue, in a type of band.

Symptoms. Sometimes this condition is asymptomatic. Obstruction can be produced if the synechiae are large enough. The synechiae may block the ostium of a nasal sinus and may produce symptoms of sinusitis, including headache.

The headache associated with nasal synechia is a dull type of pain, and usually besides the presence of the synechia there is present some other associated pathologic condition, such as nasal allergy or nasal infection, which tends to temporarily enlarge the soft tissue of the lateral nasal wall. This soft tissue engorgement results in sinus blockage and resultant headache.

If the area does not completely epithelialize, some bloody secretions may be present as a nasal discharge.

Treatment. The adhesive processes should be removed. This may be done under local anesthesia. The adhesions are cureted or scraped away and the raw ends cauterized with silver nitrate solution. A petrolatum gauze pack should be left in place overnight to help prevent the reformation of the process. This procedure may have to be repeated to obtain satisfactory results.

Another procedure that can be used following the surgical separation of the adhesive bands is to place a piece of Teflon film between the two raw surfaces. This is put into place and then secured anteriorly by a suture through the vestibular skin. The Teflon is left in place until the area involved is completely healed.

The analgesic group of drugs is usually sufficient to bring about relief from the headache of this condition. If any other pathologic condition is found to accompany the nasal synechia such as allergy or infection, this should also be treated.

Nasopharyngitis

While the nasopharynx is not actually a portion of the nasal septum, anatomically it is situated at the posterior end of the nasal septum. The nasopharynx actually begins superiorly at the choanal end of the septum and extends downward to the oral pharynx. This is a difficult area for anyone but a trained otolaryngologist to examine. It is examined by using either a small nasopharyngeal mirror or a pharyngoscope. Examination is made through the oral cavity.

Headache may be one of the symptoms of nasopharyngitis. If the posterior surface of the soft palate, which is the anterior surface of the nasopharynx, is inflamed, the headache is usually in the frontal area. If the posterior surface of the nasopharynx is inflamed, the resultant headache is usually in the occipital area or the back of the neck. This would include inflammation in the adenoid area and has occasionally been referred to as Thornwald's headache. If the side of the inferior nasal meatus or the posterior half of the inferior meatus is the site of the inflammation, the corresponding headache, if it occurs, will be in the temporal area.

Naturally, the treatment program should be directed primarily to the pharyngitis by using antibiotics and local treatment to the area involved.

Relief of the headache itself in this condition is usually obtained by merely using one of the analgesic group of drugs.

SUMMARY

SEPTAL ABSCESS

Symptoms	Treatment
1. Swelling	1. Drainage
2. Redness	2. Suction
3. Edema	3. Hot saline packs
4. Nasal obstruction	4. Antibiotics
5. Pain and tenderness	5. Analgesics
6. Fever and malaise	
7. Frontal headache	

SEPTAL HEMATOMA

Symptoms	Treatment
1. Nasal obstruction	1. Aspiration
2. Fever	2. Incision and drainage
3. Frontal headache	3. Antibiotics
	4. Analgesics

NASAL SYNECHIA

Symptoms	Treatment
1. Asymptomatic	1. Surgical removal under local anaesthesia
2. Nasal obstruction	2. Analgesics
3. Headache	

NASOPHARYNGITIS

Symptoms	Treatment
1. Soreness of throat	1. Antibiotics
2. Headache	2. Local medications
3. Fever	3. Analgesics
4. Malaise	

REFERENCES

1. Kern, E. B.: Referred pain to the ear, Minn. Med. **55**:896-898, 1972.
2. Hunt, J. R. H.: Herpetic inflammations of the geniculate ganglion: a new syndrome and its complications, J. Nerv. Ment. Dis. **34**:73-96, 1907.
3. Gradenigo, G.: Sulla leptomeningite circoscritta E: sulla paralisi dell' abducente di origine otitica, Gior. Accad. Med. Torino **10**:59, 1904.
4. Knauer, W. J.: Gradenigo's syndrome, Arch. Otolaryngol. **46**:303-316, 1946.
5. Sterling, A. W.: Bony growths invading the tonsil, J.A.M.A. **27**:734-735, 1896.
6. Eagle, W. W.: Elongated styloid process: report of two cases, Arch. Otolaryngol. **25**:584-587, 1937.
7. Evans, J. T., and Clairmont, A. A.: The non-surgical treatment of Eagle's syndrome, Eye Ear Nose Throat Mon. **55**(3):94-95, 1976.
8. Zeveleva, Z. A.: Some indices of histamine metabolism in patients with different forms of chronic rhinitis and sinusitis, Vestn. Otorinolaringol. **32**:24-28, 1970.
9. Teisanu, E., and Popescu-Tomus, D.: Trichomoniasis of paranasal sinuses, Otorinolaringolgie **16**:265-269, 1971.
10. May, M., Ogura, J. H., and Schramm, V.: Nasofrontal duct in frontal sinus fractures, Arch. Otolaryngol. **92**:534-538, 1970.
11. Busis, N.: Headache as viewed by an otolaryngologist, Trans. Pa. Acad. Ophthalmol. **22**(2):69-72, 1969.
12. D'Arcy, F.: Chronic sinusitis in children, J. Irish Med. Assoc. **67**:456-458, 1974.
13. Palva, T., and others: Chronic maxillary sinsitis, Acta Otolaryngol. **54**:159-175, 1962.
14. Lee, F. M. S.: Displaced root in maxillary sinus, Oral Surg. **29**:491-504, 1970.
15. Lekas, M. D.: Odontogenous maxillary sinus involvement, R. I. Med. J. **53**:681-683, 697-698, 1970.
16. Fruhwald, H., and Canigiani, G.: Mucoceles of sphenoidal cavities, Monatschr. Ohrenheilkd. **105**:25-33, 1971.
17. Laskiewicz, A.: Pathology of paranasal sinuses: allergic factors, Acta Otolaryngol. (Stockh.) **54**:502-510, 1962.
18. Richards, L. G.: "Sinus trouble doctor," Consultant **2**:14-16, 1962.
19. Hipskind, M. M.: Postnasal drip and sinusitis, Minn. Med. **46**:15-21, 1963.
20. Thornell, W. C.: Symptoms and methods employed in diagnoses of sinusitis, Proc. Staff Meet. Mayo Clin. **19**:470, 1944.
21. Williams, H. L.: Headache from the standpoint of the otolaryngologist, J. Iowa Med. Soc. **37**:45, 1947.
22. Thomas, E. C.: Obscure sinus infections, Med. Times, pp. 199-206, February, 1960.
23. Williams, H. L.: Somatic head pain from the standpoint of the rhinologist, otologist, and laryngologist, Lancet **74**:22-26, 1954.
24. Lederer, F. L., Tenta, L. T., and Tardy, M. E.: Otolaryngologic aspects of headache and head pains, Headache **11**:19-32, 1971.
25. Hallberg, D. E.: Roentgenologic aspects of the paranasal sinuses, Proc. Staff Meet. Mayo Clin. **19**:472, 1944.
26. Dorph, S., Oigaard, A., and Jensen, J.: Tomography in diagnosis of tumors in paranasal region, Adv. Ororhinolaryngol. **21**:40-46, 1974.
27. Ey, W.: Rhinomanometry in functional diagnosis of inflammatory diseases of nose and sinuses, H.N.O. **22**:254-255, 1974.
28. Blumenfeld, R. J., and Skolnik, E.M.: Intracranial complications of sinus disease, Trans. Am. Acad. Ophthalmol. Otolaryngol. **70**:899-908, 1966.
29. Fujita, Y., and others: Retrobulbar neuritis caused by mucopyoceles and sinusitis of posterior paranasal sinuses, J. Otolaryngal. Jpn. **74**:23, 1971.
30. Lubart, J.: The association of uveitis and sinuses, Eye Ear Nose Throat Dig., pp. 13-18, June, 1962.
31. Brown, H. A.: Pathologic changes in sinusitis, Proc. Staff Meet. Mayo Clin. **19**:468, 1944.
32. Boies, L. R.: Headache and neuralgia of nasal origin, Chicago Med. Soc. Bull. **53**:83, 1950.
33. Ryan, R. E.: The histologic effect of repeated applications of certain nose drops on the nasal mucous membrane of rabbits, Ann. Otol. Rhinol. Laryngol. **56**:46, 1947.
34. Williams, H. L.: The treatment of sinusitis, Proc. Staff Meet. Mayo Clin. **19**:474, 1944.
35. Axelsson, A., and Brorson, J. E.: Concentration of antibiotics in sinus secretions—ampicillin, cephradine, and erythromycin estolate, Ann. Otol. Rhinol. Laryngol. **83**:323-331, 1974.
36. Lillie, J. C.: Diagnosis and office treatment of sinusitis, Clin. Med., pp. 1263-1266, October, 1957.
37. Moffett, D. B.: Surgery of the paranasal sinuses, South Med. J. **50**:1221-1223, 1957.
38. Alfor, V. R.: Sinusitis: diagnosis and office management, South. Med. J. **50**:1223-1227, 1957.
39. Reynolds, R. C., Catlin, F. I., and Cluff, L. E.: Bacteriology and antibiotic treatment of acute maxillary sinusitis, Bull. Johns Hopkins Hosp. **114**:269, 1964.
40. Gullers, K., Lundberg, C., and Malmborg, A. S.: Penicillin in paranasal sinus secretions, Chemotherapy **14**:303-307, 1969.
41. Axelsson, A., and others: Treatment of acute maxillary sinusitis: doxycycline and spiramycin with

and without irrigation, Ann. Otol. Rhinol. Laryngol. **82:**186-191, 1973.

42. Raggio, T. P., and others: Sinus problem: practical approach, J. Med. Soc. **114:**315-318, 1962.
43. Burnam, J. A.: Rational approach to surgery of paranasal sinuses, J. Fla. Med. Assoc. **60:**23-26, 1973.
44. Lillie, H. I.: Symposium on diseases of the paranasal sinuses, Proc. Staff Meet. Mayo Clin. **19:** 481, 1944.
45. Ryan, R. E.: Fiorinal—a new agent for the treatment of non-vascular headache, Med. Times, p. 259, April, 1952.
46. Graham, J. K.: Headache of nasal origin, J. La. Med. Soc., **122**(2):375-379, 1970.
47. Gidall, S. H.: The distal symptoms of nasal and paranasal involvement, Clin. Med., pp. 479-485 March, 1961.
48. Roydhouse, N.: Sinusitis: symptoms and treatment, N. Z. Med. J. **61:**306-310, 1962.
49. Williams, H. L.: Somatic head pain from the standpoint of the otologist and laryngologist Lancet **74:**22-26, 1954.
50. Danforth, H. B.: Nasal vascular headache. Laryngoscope **74:**115-121, 1964.
51. Thomas, W. C.: Schluder's headache and allied neuralgias, J. Med. Assoc. Ga. **48**(2):64-68, 1959.
52. Parisier, S. C.: Correction of deviated nose, Arch. Otolaryngol. **92:**60-65, 1970.

CHAPTER 9

Headache of ophthalmic origin

WALTER R. STAFFORD

Our knowledge of the basic mechanisms responsible for headache leaves much to be desired. The patient does not often describe the pain associated with the eye well. Careful questioning is usually necessary in order to determine where the pain is: in the eye, in the orbit, in the face, in the head, and so on. The following outline of the history is useful in the examination for headache of ophthalmic origin:

A. What is the age of patient?
B. Where are the headaches? Be precise, where do they begin?
C. How long have the headaches been present? Are they becoming:
   1. Better or worse?
   2. Longer or shorter?
   3. Less or more severe?
   4. Less or more frequent?
D. How frequent are they?
E. Are they always the same type? If not, the history on each one may be needed separately. Describe the type of pain (sharp, dull, ache, throbbing, constant).
F. When do the headaches begin?
G. Is the onset sudden or gradual?
H. Are there any associated autonomic symptoms?

I. Are there any associated neurologic symptoms?
J. Is there a family history of headaches?
K. Is there any past history of injury?
L. Does the headache have any known precipitant?
M. What is the duration without therapy?
N. What gives relief?
   1. Relieved by sleep
   2. Relieved by short nap
   3. Remedies used
      a. How long before relief?
      b. How much medication used?
   4. Relieved by not using eyes
O. What makes the headache worse?
   1. Use of eyes in distant vision
   2. Use of eyes in near vision
   3. Watching moving objects
P. If the patient wears glasses:
   1. When did he first start to use glasses?
   2. Why? If for headaches, were they the same type?
   3. Were they relieved?
   4. How old are present glasses?
   5. Were the glasses verified with the prescription?

We will discuss ophthalmologic headache under the following headings:

1. Eyestrain
2. Increased intraocular pressure (glaucoma)
3. Organic ocular disease
4. Nonocular causes of ocular headache
5. Headaches due to bone diseases
6. Migraine
7. Ophthalmoplegic migraine
8. Ocular findings in nonocular headache
9. Psychogenic headaches

EYESTRAIN
Etiology

The importance of refractive errors and muscle imbalance in producing ocular discomfort and headaches has received disproportionate emphasis in ophthalmologic quarters. The time-honored term "eyestrain" was introduced by S. W. Mitchell,[1] who attributed it to Tyrrell of England. The term "eyestrain" seems to depict clearly what appears to be fundamental in producing certain types of headaches. It is commonly accepted by both the public and many medical authorities that headaches are often produced by uncorrected refractive errors. The mechanism of the headache is said to be sustained and forced contraction of the ciliary muscle, leading to its vascular engorgement. Pain impulses are thought to be referred through the ciliary ganglion to the nasociliary nerve and then via the supratrochlear and supraorbital branches of the frontal branch of the first division of the trigeminal nerve. Ciliary muscle contraction and relaxation are automatic and continuous as eyes are focused at various distances.

It is not possible to state dogmatically that errors of refraction or abnormal motility are the entire basis for the production of ocular headache, even when the correction of these errors provides relief. Some people with only slight errors of refraction or slight muscle imbalance cease to complain of headache when a proper prescription for glasses has been given. Other people with more pronounced errors of refraction or muscle imbalance do not complain of headache and even may prefer to go without glasses in spite of the improvement in their vision when wearing them. This apparent contradiction has been explained on the grounds that those patients with slight errors are constantly trying to overcome the difficulty, thereby accounting for tiring and straining the ciliary muscle. Those with greater errors are said not to make such efforts and thereby avoid ciliary muscle strain. Several studies show that although this explanation covers some cases, it does not explain all cases. From such studies it appears that headaches are relatively uncommon in people who accommodate more than normally. However, a significant proportion of people who have headaches on doing close work can be helped by wearing glasses. This can be explained if it is accepted that contraction and relaxation of the ciliary muscle are involuntary continuous processes during waking moments and that they do not in themselves produce headaches.

Headaches of eyestrain origin are apparently caused by the contraction of the extraocular muscles attached to the globe and the so-called accessory muscles of accommodation, which are situated in the eyebrows and forehead. These muscles through traction on the epicranial aponeurosis result in occipital headaches. When the excessive accommodation brought into play when focusing on small objects becomes difficult is neutralized by glasses, there follows relaxation of the scalp and neck muscle tension and hence relief of the headache.

Ocular headache due to eyestrain usually comes on after the eyes have been used in some particular task. The headache usually commences as a sensation of heaviness which slowly becomes more acute. Some headaches are described as dull, others as throbbing, bursting, sharp, and so on. The discomfort around the eyes may spread even to the posterior occiput, although the forehead and temples are more frequent sites. Except for the frontal region generally and accompanying tired sensations of the eyes, headaches associated with eyestrain are rarely localized with any degree of exactness by the patient. The typical eyestrain headache usually appears some hours after the eyes have been used and then gradually increases in severity if continued efforts are made to go on with the visual work at hand.

Diagnosis

The diagnosis of ocular headache due to eyestrain is largely dependent on a careful history (see outline, p. 279). With a good history the diagnosis is frequently obvious. Without an adequate history it is often not possible even after a complete ocular examination. Some of the symptoms have been described already. Very few children below school age complain of headaches as a result of eyestrain. In school-age children and adolescents there is the possibility that the headaches form a basis for escape from school work. In older individuals the complaints may be based on a form of neurosis. Adults in the age of presbyopia complain of ocular discomfort but rarely genuine headaches. Their eyes tire and print becomes blurred.

Headaches due to eyestrain generally come on in the afternoon or evening. Those awakening the patient from sleep are almost never due to eyestrain. Headaches beginning in the morning after sleeping are seldom due to eyestrain, unless there was some prolonged visual task the night before and the individuals retired with a headache. Headaches which occur at widely spaced intervals are unlikely to be related to eyestrain.

Headaches which have been present only a few days should not be blamed on eyestrain without a reasonable waiting period. It is true that the patient's compensating mechanisms for his refractive error may suddenly fail and allow the headache, but in the vast majority of such patients the headache is not due to eyestrain. A patient should never be forced into the possibly needless use of glasses for many years simply because he has had a headache for a few days. A headache lasting only a second or several seconds is not likely to be due to eyestrain. Headaches of constant severity lasting many days and headaches not increased or decreased by use of the eyes are very unlikely to be due to eyestrain.

If the patient wears glasses, he should be asked when he started wearing them and why. If headaches were the reason for the patient obtaining glasses, and especially if the headache was of the same type as he has now, it would be important to know whether the glasses seemed to relieve the headache. Patients who have many sets of glasses from many reliable sources and who have had no relief from wearing any of them require either an extraordinary eye examination or, much more likely, investigation of other possible causes of headaches. If the patient's glasses seem to be causing the headache, or if they give no relief, one must be certain that the glasses are correct.

Treatment

In the treatment of eyestrain as an ocular cause of headache the prescribing of lenses, including prismatic corrections particularly for vertical imbalance, depends on conclusions based primarily on the history and secondarily on findings in refraction. Prescribing lenses for the relief of headache solely on the basis of refractive or motor errors is quite likely to be unproductive unless the history has pointed to eyestrain as a factor. The relief of eyestrain headaches by the use of lenses designed to equalize retinal image size differences (aniseikonia) has received a great deal of attention in the United States during the past few years. My experience, and that of others, with such lenses indicates that they rarely accomplish the purpose for which they are prescribed. A majority of the individuals who are given such lenses are also neurotic. There are no absolute or normal values in refraction, visual acuity, muscle imbalance, convergence power, accommodative power, and general visual performance on which the physician can depend. An error in refraction in one patient may be the cause of numerous important and even incapacitating symptoms, while another patient who has the same refractive error and who uses his eyes in the same manner may have no symptoms at all. The visual act is such an extremely complicated one that defects in any part or at any level of the visual apparatus may readily be compensated for by adjustments at other levels. In addition, patients are also extremely variable in their physical and sensory makeup.

In the normal eye there is no danger to the eyesight in not correcting errors of refraction. Many patients are extremely concerned that eyestrain will produce eye disease. Most often their symptoms are immediately alleviated or even stopped by the assurance that going without glasses will lead to no harm to the eyes. A responsible ophthalmologist, therefore, does not order glasses for the refractive error alone, but largely for the relief of symptoms or complaints. As long as the patient is able to satisfactorily compensate for a refractive error, glasses are not necessary. On the other hand, there are many patients who have true eyestrain headaches which are relieved with proper glasses correction.

INCREASED INTRAOCULAR PRESSURE (GLAUCOMA)

Glaucoma is an eye disease whose complete clinical picture is characterized by increased intraocular pressure, excavation and degeneration of the optic disc, and typical nerve fiber bundle damage, producing arcuate defects in the field of vision. Eyes with narrow anterior chamber angles and shallow anterior chambers have symptoms caused by blockage of the pupil or of the angle itself by the iris. The abrupt rise of intraocular pressure caused by sudden angle occlusion stretches the corneal lamellas and destroys their optical interrelationships, resulting in corneal haze. The patient notices foggy or hazy vision with rainbow-colored halos around lights. Often

the pressure level is not high enough to cause ocular congestion and severe pain and produces only mild to moderate discomfort and one-sided headaches. The headache is orbital or supraorbital in location and steady in nature. All of the symptoms may subside in 30 minutes to 2 hours if the blockage is relieved. The longer the period of blockage, the more congestion will occur and the more likely it is that permanent damage to the angle will be done. A very narrow angle is ready for closure and it is only a matter of time before one of these transient attacks becomes a permanent closure.

When angle closure has been established the symptoms of the intermittent attack become much more severe and permanent. The cornea will appear steamy and has a ground-glass appearance. The patient will experience blurred, foggy vision with colored halos around lights. The pupil will assume a vertically oval, mid-dilated, and fixed position. The eye will become very congested as the conjunctival vessels dilate. The pain will vary from a feeling of discomfort and fullness around the eye to one of the most severe of all pain. Usually the more congested the eye, the more severe the pain. This pain follows the trigeminal nerve distribution and may be limited to the eye or may spread reflexly to the forehead, ear, sinuses, and teeth. In some unfortunate patients teeth have been mistakenly extracted because of this severe referred pain. Autonomic stimulation may occur. Nausea and vomiting usually accompany the acute attack and may so overshadow the pain and dim vision that the patient may be treated for any of a number of abdominal disorders ranging from "stomach flu" to intestinal obstruction. Not a few patients have had sinus operations and occasionally even a laparotomy because of severe nausea, vomiting, and shock. In addition the oculocardiac reflex produces a bradycardia, and there is often profuse sweating.

Glaucoma producing uncontrollable pain is a common cause of enucleation and has an unhappy way of becoming bilateral. In a patient who has an artificial eye, the history of orbital or supraorbital pain about the remaining eye may be the clue that this eye is now suffering from glaucoma.

The diagnosis will be made by the signs and symptoms and the finding of an elevated intraocular pressure. Therapy for acute angle closure glaucoma is useful only as a prelude and preparation for surgery. The principal aim of medical therapy is to pull the iris away from its contact with the angle, thus avoiding permanent damage. The more quickly this can be accomplished, the better, for synechias to the angle may become permanent in a few hours. All medical measures should be used simultaneously by the ophthalmologist. The necessary surgery can be performed much more safely if the pressure is normalized. Miotics, such as pilocarpine, are used to pull the iris away from the peripheral angle. Carbonic anhydrase inhibitors, such as Diamox, to inhibit the production of aqueous, are commonly used. Osmotic agents, such as glycerin or mannitol, dehydrate the vitreous and reduce the intraocular pressure.

The best general rule to follow is that surgery is indicated in all cases of pupillary block and angle closure glaucoma. Exceptions can be made, but it is still the best general rule to follow. Until an iridectomy provides a bypass for aqueous flow, the pupillary block remains as a continuing threat to the eye even if the pressure has been normalized and the angle can be temporarily held open by miotics. Almost 50% of eyes whose fellow eyes had suffered an attack of angle closure previously have themselves developed angle closure within a period of 5 years even though treated with miotics. When the patient was not faithful with the miotics, the incidence of acute attack rose to 89%. Iridectomy is the operation of choice in an eye with pupillary block and angle closure. This provides a bypass for aqueous flow, breaks

the pupillary block, and allows opening of the obstructed angle.

ORGANIC OCULAR DISEASE

Inflammatory affections of the eye and orbit frequently account for pain in the eye or in the region surrounding the eye. The surface structures, conjunctiva, and cornea are extremely sensitive to touch, and pain is noted under a variety of circumstances. The deep ocular structures are insensitive to pain.

Conjunctivitis

Inflammation of the conjunctiva is the most common of all eye diseases in the Western Hemisphere. Most cases are caused by microorganisms, but other causes include viruses, allergens, foreign bodies, chemicals and other irritants, fungi, and parasites. The conjunctiva contains many blood vessels and mucous-producing cells, but relatively few pain fibers. This accounts for the marked inflammatory response without severe pain, which is characteristic of conjunctivitis. Conjunctivitis causes tearing, exudate, injection, itching, or a mild to moderate pain or ache. The discomfort is localized to the external eye region and, in many cases, may be bilateral. Conjunctivitis must be differentiated from the other causes of a red or injected eye, such as iritis, acute glaucoma, or corneal disease. The diagnosis is made from the signs and symptoms, which in turn depend on the etiology of the conjunctivitis. The treatment varies with the cause of the disease and may depend on the results of a laboratory culture.

Blepharitis

Inflammation of the eyelids is the most common lid disorder. Its causes are similar to those of conjunctivitis. Save for the hordeolum (stye) and chalazion, blepharitis rarely causes significant ocular or periocular pain. The hordeolum and chalazion, or internal hordeolum, are common infections of the eyelid glands usually due to a staphylococcal infection. They are characterized by a localized, red, swollen, and acutely tender area in the lid, depending on which of the glands have become infected. They are essentially abscesses in the lid. Pain is the primary symptom, and the intensity of the pain is in direct proportion to the degree of lid swelling. Cellulitis of the lid may be a complication. Treatment may include warm compresses and topically applied antibiotics. Some may require incision and drainage.

Keratitis

Inflammation of the cornea may be caused by foreign bodies, abrasions, allergic reactions, and ulcers. Corneal ulcers may be the result of bacteria, viruses, fungi, allergy, vitamin A deficiency, exposure, chemical and other irritants, neurotrophic disorders due to fifth cranial nerve lesions, and other unknown causes. Since the cornea has many pain fibers, most superficial corneal lesions such as corneal foreign bodies, abrasions, or many ulcerations will cause pain and photophobia. The pain is so characteristic as to be frequently described as a foreign body sensation. It is augmented considerably by the movement of the lids over the cornea, particularly the upper lid. It differs considerably from the deep-seated neurologic pain of iritis or iridocyclitis. The pain from a corneal foreign body or abrasion is accompanied by profuse tearing, photophobia, injection of the conjunctiva, blepharospasm, and radiation of pain to the forehead. The foreign body sensation is frequently not referred to the cornea, but instead is often interpreted as a localized scratching sensation beneath the upper lid. Since the cornea serves as the window of the eye and refracts light rays, corneal lesions cause some degree of blurred vision. The blurring is greater if the lesion is centrally located. The diagnosis is made from the signs and symptoms which depend on the cause of the keratitis. The treatment is directed toward the etiology.

Uveitis

Inflammation of the uveal tract may involve any or all of the three divisions. Anterior uveitis involves the iris (iritis) or ciliary body (cyclitis) or both (iridocyclitis). Posterior uveitis involves the choroid (choroiditis) and frequently the retina as well (chorioretinitis). Inflammatory disorders of the uveal tract are usually unilateral and are more common in the young and middle-age groups. In most cases the etiology is not known. Inflammation of the uveal tract has a multiplicity of causes and may involve any portion singly or any two or all three portions simultaneously. Two major types of uveitis may be distinguished on clinical as well as pathologic grounds: nongranulomatous and granulomatous.

The first is the more common of the two. Because pathogenic organisms have not been found in the nongranulomatous type and because this type responds to steroid therapy, it is often thought to be due to an immune sensitivity phenomenon. Granulomatous uveitis usually follows active invasion of the tissues by the causative organism—bacterial, viral, fungal, parasitic, or other. Nongranulomatous uveitis tends to be localized in the anterior portion of the uvea, hence the iris and ciliary body are most commonly involved. Granulomatous uveitis is more diffuse and tends to involve the posterior portion of the uvea, hence the choroid and retina tend to be involved.

The pain of anterior uveitis (iritis or iridocyclitis) can be severe but is usually less overwhelming than that of acute glaucoma. It is frequently referred widely, and patients may complain of earache, pain in the teeth, or pain over one of the sinuses. Pain is usually described as throbbing or neurologic in character and is often associated with photophobia, which may be severe enough to overshadow other aspects of the pain. Excessive lacrimation and blepharospasm are often observed. The eye is likely to be tender to palpation.

The onset is usually acute and the deep throbbing pain is usually worse at night and in the early morning hours. Vision is blurred, the pupil is small, and a circumcorneal flush caused by dilated blood vessels about the limbus is present. In granulomatous uveitis the onset is usually slow and more insidious. Pain is minimal or absent and photophobia is much less severe. Vision is blurred, but the eye is only mildly red and injected.

The diagnosis can be difficult and complicated and is usually left to the ophthalmologist. The treatment includes dilation of the pupil (cycloplegia and mydriasis), topical or systemic antibiotics where indicated, and topical or systemic steroids.

Optic neuritis

Optic neuritis is a general term used to describe involvement of the optic nerve as the result of any inflammation, demyelination, or degeneration of the optic nerve. The optic neuritis may begin near the surface of the nerve, in the core of the nerve, at the nerve head, or as far posteriorly as the optic chiasm. A wide variety of diseases can cause optic neuritis, including demyelinating diseases, local extension of inflammatory diseases, toxic and metabolic causes, blood dyscrasias and vascular diseases, avitaminosis associated with generalized infectious diseases, malignant invasion of the nerve, and many others. Loss of vision is usually of a marked degree and may be total. There is frequently pain in the region of the eye, especially on movement or palpation of the globe. Some forms of optic neuritis produce swelling of the disc tissues and surrounding retina.

Confusion with papilledema is the most common differential diagnostic problem. The patient's history, visual acuity, field defects, and ophthalmoscopic examination tend to make the diagnosis. Ideally the treatment is directed toward the cause. If the cause cannot be treated or is not known, the treatment is less often satisfactory.

Orbital pseudotumor

Orbital pseudotumor is a relatively rare inflammatory reaction which clinically resembles a neoplasm. It is a diagnosis of exclusion since the etiology is not known. Inflammatory pseudotumor is characterized by exophthalmos, restriction of ocular movement, and swelling of the lids. Pain and diplopia are present in about half of cases. The onset is usually gradual. The pain, when present, varies in intensity and is rarely severe.

The resemblance of psuedotumor to neoplasm usually necessitates an exploratory surgical procedure with biopsy. The tissue usually reveals only signs of chronic inflammation. Treatment is not satisfactory and includes steroids systemically in very high doses and in some cases radiation therapy.

Ocular and retrobulbar pain without ocular disease

The complaint of mild to moderate localized pain in an eye or immediately behind the eyes when no obvious ocular disease exists is a common problem to ophthalmologists. In many cases the symptoms seem to be magnified by the patient's unfounded anxiety regarding glaucoma, impending blindness, or brain tumor. Some patients describe stabbing pains, others dull, continuous pain, and others a feeling of pressure in the eye. Few of these pains herald the onset of any ocular or even intracranial disease, and only rarely is it possible to find any plausible explanation. A sympathetic, reassuring physician and routine analgesics are, in most cases, all that the patient requires.

NONOCULAR CAUSES OF OCULAR HEADACHE

Pain of nonocular origin also may be referred to the eye and its surrounding area if there is distortion or inflammation of other structures supplied by the ophthalmic division of the trigeminal nerve.

Diabetes

Diabetic oculomotor palsy is often associated at its onset with severe pain in the eye or on the homolateral side of the head. The pain varies in intensity but may be very severe. This is an occasional complication of diabetes and may be a first evidence of the disease. Usually the diabetes is not severe and the patient is an older adult. The third and sixth nerves are affected about equally and the fourth nerve is rarely affected. The palsies are unrelated to the severity of the diabetes. One of the puzzling features of this condition is the almost universal recovery in 1 or 2 months at most. The recovery seems to occur regardless of the control of the diabetes.

Giant cell arteritis

Giant cell arteritis, also known as temporal or cranial arteritis, is a polysymptomatic disseminated disease of the aged. It frequently begins with low-grade fever, anorexia, malaise, and weight loss, followed in a week or two by severe unilateral or bilateral frontotemporal or occipital head pains, scalp tenderness, and, in 30% to 40% of cases, devastating bilateral visual loss. Although the disease is usually self-limited, lasting for several months, occasionally the patient dies from cardiac or cerebral ischemia. The ischemic optic neuropathy produced by this disease is one of the major causes of rapidly developing bilateral blindness in the patient over 60 years of age. The etiology is unknown; however, the condition is usually classified with the collagen diseases. Visual loss in one or both eyes is frequently the symptom which changes the patient's nonspecific and often puzzling medical problem into a readily recognized disease. Often the patient experiences transient loss of vision for a few days before sight is completely lost. The loss of vision is frequently abrupt. One eye is usually affected first, the other eye being involved at an interval of from 1 to 10 days. Occasionally both eyes are affected simultaneously.

The diagnosis is aided greatly by a high degree of suspicion in cases with the symptoms already mentioned. The erythrocyte sedimentation rate is abnormally high in over 90% of patients with giant cell arteritis. It is rarely essential to perform temporal artery biopsy for diagnostic purposes since the nature of the disease is often not in serious doubt. Nevertheless, having histologic proof of a diagnosis is always satisfying. The inflammatory arteritis is a patchy phenomenon, and a negative biopsy does not exclude the diagnosis. A diagnosis of temporal arteritis calls for immediate and prolonged steroid therapy. Visual loss, once established, does not recover.

Intracavernous carotid aneurysm

Aneurysms arising from the internal carotid artery as it traverses the cavernous sinus behave differently from aneurysms arising elsewhere in the skull by virtue of their position. These aneurysms arise from a large artery as it traverses a venous sinus. Because of their ocular symptoms, patients are frequently referred to an ophthalmologist. This aneurysm is a relatively uncommon type of cerebral aneurysm. The onset of symptoms is sometimes abrupt, but usually it is slow and progressive, with episodes of activity during which there may be severe pain in the region of the eye. At these times paresis of ocular muscles may occur on the affected side. Pain behind the eye and in the forehead on the involved side is sometimes a prominent symptom. The pain tends to be severe and lancinating, but it may occur at intervals, leaving the patient relatively free of symptoms in between. The diagnosis is made on neurologic evidence, and the treatment is in the realm of the neurosurgeon.

Aneurysms of the carotid–posterior communicating artery junction

Aneurysms, of the carotid–posterior communicating artery junction are of interest to the ophthalmologist since they are one of the principal nontraumatic causes of isolated total third nerve palsies. Prior to subarachnoid hemorrhage, ipsilateral frontal head pain located behind the eyes and above the brow occurs in about 25% of cases. The pain may occur intermittently for months or even years before the aneurysm ruptures or even produces an oculomotor palsy. The pain can assume a migrainous pattern and is usually of the boring type which the patient very readily distinguishes from any ordinary headache. The diagnosis and treatment are in the neurosurgeon's field.

Painful ophthalmoplegia (Tolosa-Hunt syndrome)

Painful ophthalmoplegia is thought to be due to a chronic inflammation of the cavernous sinus. The pain may precede the ophthalmoplegia by several days or may not occur until some time after. The pain behind the eye and in the brow is characterized as steady and frequently described as "boring" or "gnawing." Neurologic involvement of the third cranial nerve is most common, but the fourth and sixth may also be involved, as well as the ophthalmic division of the trigeminal nerve. The symptoms may last for days or weeks and spontaneous remission, sometimes with residual neurologic deficit, occurs. At intervals of months or years attacks recur. The diagnosis is made on the signs and symptoms, and steroid therapy usually results in prompt improvement.

Occlusion of the posterior cerebral artery

Most patients in whom occlusion of a posterior cerebral artery occurs experience no pain. Exceptions to this have been reported by Knox and Cogan.[2] They noted that a very distinct pain in the eye may be reported by patients with vascular accidents in the region of the ipsilateral posterior cerebral artery. The pain may be moderately severe in the eye and supraorbital region and may be associated with nausea. They believed that the pain was referred from tentorial branches of the ophthalmic division of the trigeminal nerve.

Histaminic cephalalgia

Of all the painful syndromes of the head histaminic cephalalgia, or migrainous neuralgia, is one of the most distinctive. This headache is principally due to dilation and distention of cerebral arteries. The histaminic headache is characterized by frequent, short attacks of severe unilateral head pain occurring once or many times daily in clusters of several weeks or months. In most patients the clusters are separated by pain-free intervals of a few months or perhaps several years. Individual paroxysms of pain may last from 10 minutes up to 1 or 2 hours. They are usually accompanied by vasomotor symptoms consisting of ipsilateral tearing, conjunctival injection, rhinorrhea and nasal congestion, flushing, sweating, and even occasionally Horner's syndrome. Histaminic cephalalgia is the most strikingly periodic of all periodic diseases. Individual attacks may occur at the same time of day or night, and the clusters may occur with equal regularity. The onset is usually in persons in their thirties or forties and rarely in children or after age 60.

The diagnosis is made by the findings of the distinctive signs and symptoms; the treatment is discussed elsewhere.

HEADACHES DUE TO BONE DISEASE

Periostitis and osteomyelitis of the bones of the skull and face may produce headache. Syphilitic periostitis or osteitis is now uncommon. It frequently involves the bones of the orbit in middle age. Frequently in inflammatory involvement of the bones of the skull and orbit there is localized pain and generalized headache. Malignant disease of bone may similarly account for pain in the region of the lesion and generalized headache as well. Osteitis deformans and oxycephaly are frequently associated with generalized headache.

Migraine

Migraine is a common, periodic malady of unknown etiology and varied symptomatology, the most prominent feature of which is intense recurrent unilateral headache associated with visual disturbances and vomiting. The disorder has a strong familial tendency, being directly transmitted in half the cases, most usually through the mother. The disorder involves the cranial and cerebral microvascular regulatory systems, but the etiology remains unknown. A classic attack is preceded by prodromal symptoms—drowsiness, lassitude, hunger, constipation, or other generalized disturbance. The episode itself is frequently ushered in by an aura typically characterized by visual disturbances and occasionally by aphasia, paresthesias, and pareses. Visual disturbances are the most characteristic and usually are quite striking. They consist of brilliantly colored, shimmering spectral lights and scotomas with homonymous distribution. Many varieties of visual disturbance occur and usually last 15 to 20 minutes, gradually fading over the next 10 or 15 minutes. Thereafter the headache usually begins.

The headache, the most characteristic symptom of migraine, typically commences as a localized boring pain and spreads in a cumulative, expansile fashion to involve the whole side of the head and sometimes the neck. All varieties of headache occur from slight to very severe and may last for several days. Nausea may occur at any time in the attack and may lead to vomiting, which may afford some relief. The treatment is discussed elsewhere.

OCULAR FINDINGS IN NONOCULAR HEADACHE

Clues to nonocular causes of headache may be discovered on ocular examination brought about by the presence of a headache. These include the recognition of papilledema and its differential diagnosis, including pseudopapilledema caused by hyperopia and elevated disc anomalies, particularly buried drusen in the nerve head. Other forms of disc edema, including central retinal vein obstruction, venous stasis retinopathy, ischemic papillopathy, and papillitis, must be recognized. The recognition of optic nerve and chiasm compression, as well as various visual field defects, is also necessary.

PSYCHOGENIC HEADACHES

Headaches of functional origin commonly occur and are frequently brought to the ophthalmologist's attention. While they are most typical of the affective neuroses, they may also have a hysterical origin, such as the person who develops a headache to escape a distasteful duty. The neurotic headache may assume a bewildering variety of types. It may be characterized by a feeling of pain, constriction as of a band around the skull, numbness, or emptiness or alternatively a feeling of fullness in the head. It may vary considerably in site, being frontal, temporal, occipital, or referred to the back of the eyes. It is usually very vividly described as being intolerable or overwhelming, expansile, or bursting, or histrionically described, as if a vise or a skewer were torturing the brain. Yet, unlike organic headaches, a psychogenic headache rarely interferes with the patient's activities (unless the activities are not pleasant), as much as the patient's description would suggest otherwise. It is rarely affected by physical factors such as stooping, straining, or coughing but rather is affected by emotional and environmental influences. It is less persistent but respond poorly to analgesics.

Headaches associated with the ocular neuroses are common. In patients with these headaches a frank discussion of the particular problem and prescribing of the necessary glasses are the proper treatment. Cooperation of the patient with the ophthalmologist is usually all that is needed in such a case if the patient is intelligent. Psychiatric consultation is usually unnecessary.

Pain on exposure to excessively bright light is called photophobia. This represents a referred type of pain through close association of cephalic and sensory centers.

Some individuals complain of severe pain in the eyes and headache after exposure to ordinary light. During examination they seem to tolerate well the lights of the examiner. There is no appreciable error of refraction or muscle imbalance. Such persons are often described as suffering from retinal asthenopia or retinal irritation. The term is one which means nothing as regards positive findings. Ophthalmoscopically visible changes are not present. The majority of these patients suffer from an ocular neurosis, and their treatment is very difficult. The normalcy of their eyes should be emphasized. Sometimes tinted lenses make these patients happy, and neutral density filters may be useful in patients who complain of severe glare.

REFERENCES

1. Mitchell, S. W.: Headaches from eyestrain, Am. J. Med. Sci. **71:**363-375, 1876.
2. Knox, D. L., and Cogan, D. G.: Eye pain and homonymous hemianopsia, Am. J. Ophthalmol. **54:**1091-1093, 1962.

CHAPTER 10

Headache of dental origin

EDWARD J. HEMPSTEAD

The initial appointment with the new patient should consist of what may be designated as the interview[1] as well as the preliminary examination. The chief complaint should be ascertained, and questions pertaining to the medical and dental histories should bring to the fore, among other things, the mood, manner, and anxiety of the patient.

The language of pain is spoken in many ways. It can be caused by trigeminal neuralgia, arthritis, traumatic injury, infecion malignancy, temporomandibular joint disorders, and dental occlusion interferences. All represent a substantial segment of the facial pain problem.

As long as the mouth continues to be an organ of gratification and aggression, patients will suffer from psychologic disease of the oral cavity and temporomandibular joint dysfunction.[2] However, the treatment of facial pain and mandibular dysfunction *cannot* be limited to one organ.[3]

HISTORY

Historically,[4] the literature on the treatment for persons suffering from facial pain dates back to about the year 1773, when Fothersgill wrote "on the subject of a painful affliction of the face." He stated that the etiology of the disease was unknown and that the pain was associated with trigger zones. He also stated that the pain occurs:

1. In patients over 40 years of age
2. More often in women
3. In edentulous patients and during movements of the mandible, such as eating, talking, or sneezing

In 1821 Charles Bell of England demonstrated that the trigeminal nerve and not the facial nerve supplied sensations to the face.

Only after the report in 1934 of James Costen,[5] an outstanding otolaryngologist, did medical and dental theories on facial pain merge and receive attention. Costen and Ernst[6] contributed nonoperative techniques through their combined study of the head and neck anatomy, subjective symptoms, and uniform radiographic technique.

TREATMENT OF FACIAL PAIN

The problems of pain[7] are amenable to therapy from many specialties in the medical and dental professions. One approach

290

can be made by way of the organ systems, such as the nervous, osseous, and muscular ones, and many other related tissues.

A second approach is to study the abnormal physiology of pathologic conditions as they relate to the organ systems—that is, ways in which abnormal growth, congenital anomalies, or injuries, no matter how inflicted, induce pain and provide additional information about the phenomenon of pain.

Still another approach exists: study at the cellular level. It is inevitable that great progress will be made by this approach to produce additional knowledge toward diagnosis.

TRIGEMINAL NEURALGIA

In our treatment of "facial pain patients," we must consider the vast domain of the fifth cranial or trigeminal nerve, in conjunction with the facial (seventh), glossopharyngeal (ninth), and vagus (tenth) nerves, cervical nerves 1 to 6, and the osseous-muscular structures.

In an article on trigeminal neuralgia and mandibular joint dysfunction, Smolik and I reported on the results of fifty-four patients treated for trigeminal neuralgia.[8] By careful elicitation of the history and examination of the dental condition, together with proper conservative construction of the mechanics of the temporomandibular joint, relief was achieved in fifteen cases of major neuralgia with four failures, and in twenty-one cases of minor neuralgia with seven failures. Three patients who had posterior rhizotomy did not respond; one chose suicide. Others still had occasional episodes of comfort.

ORAL DYSFUNCTION

Since our efforts are directed to the patient affected by a dental malocclusion or oral dysfunction, we must consider this affliction and its effects.

Extraorally, the direction of movements as used in oral function should be noted.[9] A dental malocclusion with tooth support on one side, and due to loss of function on the opposite side, causes a structural deviation with changes in the suspensory musculature and condylar function. This results in mandibular deviation and an acquired occlusion with painful effects.

Deficiency occurs when force cannot be applied to the area and evenly distributed over every minute section of that area. The direction of force must be such that over time, wear or function will continue to maintain the original condition of support in the underlying structures.

The acceptable (not *normal*) maxillomandibular relationship or occlusion of natural teeth and artificial dentures is that static and functional relationship of the teeth which permits the anatomic and physiologic structures influenced by the closure to exist in a state of equilibrium.[10] It is virtually impossible to ascertain the occlusion on patients exhibiting any degree of severity of pain-dysfunction symptoms until those symptoms have been nearly alleviated by the use of reversible means, such as the mandibular repositioning splint.[11] Investigators use the modern techniques of electromyography, cinefluorography, pantographic recordings, and mandibulography to analyze the jaw in the rest position and in various movements.[12]

PHYSIOLOGY OF OCCLUSION

To establish an understandable and workable method of evaluating the discrepancies in an off-bite caused by malocclusion, we must understand the normalcy of the composite of maxillomandibular relationship.[9] We cannot judge something to be wrong unless we can fathom what is right. Having done so, we can then proceed to reverse the degeneration process into a norm that is within the patient's range of living tolerance and functional efficiency. This does not occur immediately. Often muscles must readapt and proprioception alter.

Rehabilitation of the head and neck anatomy, based on the previously mentioned causes of malocclusion, must be a part of the treatment planning.

Before starting any replacement, we are interested in the correction of malocclusion to alleviate pain. The edentulous patient will require more rearrangements of dental occlusion, since the artificial denures depend on alveolar and cancellous bone for function and direction of forces.

TEMPOROMANDIBULAR JOINT

The temporomandibular joint problem is extremely complex. Not all facial pain is associated with the temporomandibular joint per se, but it involves the musculature associated with the movements of the mandible and the stability of the head on the vertebral column.

Many theories and techniques have been expounded in literature, clinical reports, and textbooks on temporomandibular joints. For example, Costen[13] reported in 1951 many techniques that were used to relieve patients of painful neuralgia. Included were the manner and method of palpation of the muscles and mandibular joint intraorally. He also discussed "splinting the mandible to prevent painful movement of the condyle, as well as to an urgency of careful study of impacted third molar teeth in young patients as revealed by their related trismus."

Patients having subjective symptoms of mandibular dysfunction and facial pain present diagnostic problems to the dental practitioner.[14] These symptoms consist of the inability to chew without pain, clicking of the joint, headaches, pounding of the ear, lack of confidence when speaking, and affection of the eustachian tube. Diseases of the temporomandibular joints are commonly undiagnosed or misdiagnosed because they mimic many different disorders and have such a variety of symptoms.[15]

PSYCHOLOGIC EFFECT OF PAIN

Physical pain may blend with the reaction of the human organism as a whole to pain.[16] Psychologic disturbances and emotional tension may be associated with the clinical picture. Therefore, it is important that the professions persist in their associated efforts through consultations, evaluation of symptoms, and physical and dental examinations using specialized studies or diagnostic aids.

CASE HISTORIES

Atypical (minor) trigeminal neuralgia and temporomandibular joint dysfunction

A male patient, age 88, was examined in consultation for evaluation of facial pain and oral cavity discomfort. He complained of headaches, cracking sounds within the ears, and inability to chew food or even talk without pains across the lip and along the lower jaw.

The patient had undergone many types of treatment, but the dental history was most significant. Several years previously, all natural teeth, infected gum tissue, and bony irregularities were extracted to treat the pain. Artificial dentures were fabricated and occlusion corrected. However, the pain was not entirely interrupted. Additional medication and oral intervention through injections of anesthetics followed.

Temporomandibular joint radiographic interpretation, with the facial profile of the patient including the lines of facial muscle markedness, along with a prior history of unsuccessful treatment, proved a basis for our treatment.

Using an indicated technique including the Boos pressure bimeter, emergency therapy was instituted using the same dentures. However, temporary metallic splints were used to predict the results of the principles, for this patient's acceptable maxillomandibular relativity and *not* normal occlusion was our goal toward alleviation of subjective symptoms. This procedure, used as a last approach, did reduce the intensity and frequency of patient's pain.

After sufficient time for trial with adjustments and evaluation of results, additional denture changes were made.

There were some changes in the myositis and myospasms with diminished contractions.

The patient had difficulty with the increased opening of his mouth; however, the diet was modified and he was freed from his original subjective symptoms.

Bilateral neuralgia pain with trigger zones

A 54-year-old female patient was examined for facial pain after referral by a neurosurgeon. She complained of pain when her lip was touched, glossodynia, and headaches involving the whole left side of her face and neck area. She had suffered from this pain for 2 years and had been treated with vitamin B_{12}, vitamins, and the usual commercial headache remedies. Several posterior teeth had been removed, but the pain continued. There were no replacements for the missing teeth. Temporomandibular radiographs showed the right condyle to be slightly narrow in the anteroposterior dimension, and the fossa space seemed worn or smaller. The pain was diagnosed as arising from the second division of the fifth nerve on the left side of the face.

Emergency injections were administered to alleviate pain and conservative treatment was continued. Partial splinted dental appliances were designed and results were good. Pain recurred, however, during the process of permanent dental treatment, and alcohol injections had to be used.

At this writing, this patient has not had any neurosurgery or therapy other than the dental approach and medication along with injections as mentioned, and she is still not edentulous. By wearing the removable splints, which are altered to compensate for facial changes, she is comfortable.

Acute dislocation and dysfunction of the temporomandibular joints

A 25-year-old woman was referred to my dental office in February, 1964, for emergency treatment of dislocation of both temporomandibular joints.

The patient had been hospitalized and treated unsuccessfully for the dislocation by manipulation and reduction under general anesthesia. The patient described her symptoms and their onset as follows: "Two evenings ago, while at a movie, my jaws locked during the act of laughing. I was unable to close my mouth or lower my jaw."

The patient was able to open her mouth only several millimeters, and the action was accompanied by facial pain through the tension of the musculature, or contraction of the external pterygoid muscles. Maxillary and mandibular posterior teeth were missing without replacements. There was no mandibular occlusal plane; the maxillary left canine was impacted. An acquired malocclusion, attributable to factors of heredity and habit, was noted.

Diagnosis was facial muscle spasms and limitation of both temporomandibular joints with an acquired occlusion and, of course, the dislocation.

Initial treatment was given as rapidly as possible. The maxillomandibular relativity was registered by gently forcing the mouth open. Metallic onlay splints were prepared for the mandibular posterior teeth to the height required by the occlusal plane. These were inserted, together with the removable maxillary splint. These corrective appliances adjusted the occlusion and the splints, which allowed limited opening of the jaws, were accommodated painlessly. Oral functions could now be performed without pain, but the patient was able to discard the appliance only for the time necessary for oral hygiene before extreme discomfort was experienced.

Two years later, fixed crown and bridge restorations for the mandibular posterior teeth were designed according to the height and contour of the metallic onlay splints to provide permanent restorations. In the process of the designing and fitting of the prosthesis under local anesthesia, problems were caused by the patient's inability to sustain mouth opening. Icebags were frequently held to the face to counteract the pain experienced, and several treatment sessions were terminated prematurely because of the patient's extreme discomfort. However, treatment gradually became less painful for the patient because of adaptation of the nerve receptors to the repeated stimuli.

Maxillary impressions were taken and an immediate maxillary denture was also fitted without alveolar surgery. The prosthesis was fitted without labial flange or extension.

Some years later, the denture cracked and was repaired immediately while the patient waited in the dental office; she experienced severe pain while the denture was outside her mouth. A spare denture was made subsequently.

The most recent follow-up (1976) confirmed that the patient was comfortable and happy with the treatment and the function of the prosthesis.

Dental pain or dysfunctional temporomandibular joints

A patient, age 52, complained of pain within the pathways of the second and third divisions of the fifth nerve on the left side of face and was referred by a neurosurgeon. The patient had no physical health problems other than the facial pain, the inability to chew, and headaches.

The patient had received dental fillings many times and only recently had undergone dental extractions on the affected side of face to eliminate the pain. However, there was no relief. The patient was referred to a physician who, after examination with negative results, sought consultation from the neurosurgeon. The patient was then sent to my office.

Panorex films showed an absence of all posterior teeth on the left side of mouth. The natural teeth on the right side were restored.

An evaluation of the dental experiences was made and removable dental splints were designed to afford the indicated occlusal plane pathways. Coverage of the edentulous areas resulted in an acceptable neuroosseous muscular balance of the head and neck anatomy.

The patient had extensive dental rehabilitation after the pathologic occlusion had been corrected. She has been free from original pain complaint for several years.

Temporomandibular joint dysfunction and prognathic acquired occlusion

The patient, age 62, was referred by internist to neurosurgeon and then to our office for bilateral pain of a neuralgia type, deep and almost constant. This discomfort was increased when trying to talk, chew, or even smoke a pipe or cigar.

During a checkup by his internist, the patient stated that removable partial dentures had just been made. Shortly after beginning to wear them, the deep neuralgia pain started.

My attention was directed to an acceptable occlusion or maxillomandibular relativity, which I obtained without appliances.

Through various techniques, I was able to eliminate many of the symptomatic disorders and afford function.

SUMMARY

In my experience as a copractitioner with the medical profession in the examination of over 1,400 private practice patients, I have noted several things.

Those patients afflicted with oral facial pain tolerate one of the most excruciating pains known.

Through time, many diagnostic aids and specialized skills continue to appear in the realm of therapy. However, practitioners must include their own brand of explanatory psychotherapy for patients.

As far as dentistry is concerned, no set scheme of occlusion or articulation has proved superior, except that preferred by the individual practitioner.

There is a need for adequate follow-up to reevaluate the patient's condition, both from the original complaint and toward continued dental maintenance to meet the patient's needs.

Certainly the exchange of techniques, seminars, and literature between the professions is necessary for teamwork to help the patient.

REFERENCES

1. Kornfeld, M.: Mouth rehabilitation, ed. 2, St. Louis, 1974, The C. V. Mosby Co., p. 21.
2. Freese, A. S., and Scheman, P.: Management of temporomandibular joint problems, St. Louis, 1962, The C. V. Mosby Co., p. 99.
3. Schwartz, L.: Disorders of the temporomandibular joint, Philadelphia, 1959, W. B. Saunders Co., pp. 24, 128.
4. Smolik, E. A., and Hempstead, E. J.: Trigeminal neuralgia and mandibular joint dysfunction, Postgrad. Med. 12(5): 419, 1952.
5. Costen, J. B.: A syndrome of ear and sinus symptoms dependent upon disturbed function of the temporomandibular joint, Ann. Otol. Rhinol. Laryngol. 43(1):1, 1934.
6. Ernst, E. C., and Costen, J. B.: X-ray study in relation to the mandibular joint syndrome, Radiology 30(1):68-75, 1938.
7. Costich, E. R.: Research horizon, facial pain, Philadelphia, 1968, Lea & Febiger, p. 269.
8. Smolik, E. A., and Hempstead, E. J.: The dolorous tic, Newsweek 38(21):62, 1951.
9. Guzay, C.: American Academy for Functional Prosthodontics, Chicago, Illinois: Personal communication.
10. Frank, C., American Academy for Functional Prosthodontics, Chicago, Illinois: Personal communication.
11. Roth, R. H.: Angle Orthodontist 43(2):136-153, 1973.
12. Mahan, P. E.: Research in physiology of significance to dentistry, J. Am. Dent. Assoc. 72(6): June 1966.
13. Costen, J. B.: The present status of the mandibular joint syndrome in otolaryngology, Trans. Am. Acad. Ophthalmol. Otolaryngol., p. 819, Nov.-Dec. 1951.
14. Schwartz, L.: Diagnosis of temporomandibular joint disorders, Dent. Radiogr. Photogr. 36(4):84, 1963.
15. Morgan, D. H.: The great imposter, J.A.M.A. 235(22):2395, 1976.
16. Weinberg, L. A.: Temporomandibular joint function and its effect on concepts of occlusion, J. Prosth. Dent. 35(5):553-566, 1976.

CHAPTER 11

Psychogenic headache

Psychogenic headaches probably represent one of the most difficult phases of the entire headache field. There are many reasons for such a statement. We feel certain that there are far more real pathologic headache problems which are at first thought to be psychogenic than there are actual psychogenic headache cases which are at first thought to have an organic basis. By that we mean that too often a physician who has not made a thorough examination and taken a thorough history will pass off the patient's complaints as being neurotic or psychogenic and not pay enough attention to them. Many cases of this nature are later found to have a pathologic etiology and not be psychogenic at all. We have seen many cases of headache of various types which were handled elsewhere by merely giving the patient a sedative, a tranquilizer, an analgesic, or any combination of these types of drugs. This treatment is usually due to lack of attention on the part of the physician to actually investigate the problem thoroughly. It is much rarer to find a psychogenic headache which has been receiving treatment for other disorders, such as sinusitis, myalgia, migraine, or some other type of head pain; at least we have found this to be so in our experience in the field of headache treatment.

However, the diagnosis of psychogenic headache should not be put off until all physical causes of the pain have been ruled out. The physician should be conscious of the general characteristics of the pain of psychogenic origin. Among these are continuous headache during the entire day but no involvement with sleep. The disturbance frequently involves several areas of the head. In the conversion depression type of headache the patient often complains of multiple headache symptoms.

In dealing with this type of headache, many conditions have to be investigated. Among these are depression, psychoses, neuroses, hypochondria, psychosomatic disorders, psychasthenia, and anxiety.

ETIOLOGY

The average patient with a psychogenic personality has failed to adjust to his surroundings and his environment. At times, this may reach such an extreme that it gives him an antisocial personality, or at least an asocial one. His pain is often in the form of a delusion or hallucination; it is actually very real to him, whereas it is false to everyone around him.

Many people are found to be hypersensitive and excessively irritable. We have found many patients with psychogenic headaches to be extremely self-centered.

They will often do anything to get their way or sometimes to get attention. An example of this is that they will complain of a severe headache attack merely to get the attention or the sympathy of their mates or their friends. While many patients are self-centered, they are not necessarily selfish. To put it bluntly, many of these individuals simply crave attention, and they use the complaint of headache as a means of obtaining it. If the patient is unable to obtain this attention he will become quarrelsome and irritable.

The patient is quite frequently found to be shy, and some times he has characteristics of impatience. Most of these individuals are found to feel keenly and resent what they might erroneously think is neglect.

Another characteristic often found in the personality of the patient with a psychogenic headache is that he often exaggerates his complaints. This may go to such an extreme that the functional elements is obvious from the very onset of the case history obtained from the patient. This is one of the very common features of the patient.

Anxiety is often the most common symptom of the patient with a psychogenic headache complaint. The anxiety at times may be vague and indefinite, in the form of a fear that he is going to have a headache attack. While there is not any actual physical pain experienced by these patients, some may have actual psychic pain from believing that they have headaches. They think they have pain, and they are so convinced that they do that they actually suffer mental pain of an anxiety nature. This can be very distressing to the patient mentally, but there is no actual physical pain. However, it is often difficult to convince these patients that their pain is functional and not pathologic. The state of anxiety may either arise from some emotional upset or be spontaneous. The emotional upset which can bring this anxiety about may often be some insignificant stimulus which would probably be ignored by the average personality.

Headache is one of the most common symptoms of anxiety. Patients may complain of their pain in any area of the head. Many patients will seek the advice of a physician because of problems which are entirely based on anxiety. Psychogenic headache often has its source primarily in a state of anxiety and may arise through a conversion process.

Depression is also a common etiologic factor in psychogenic headache. Depression is found more often in these patients when there is an inhibited state present; as the depression increases, the headache will also increase. When depression is the etiologic factor, the patient will also usually complain of other symptoms such as difficulty in sleeping, loss of appetite, giddiness, or even cardiac symptoms. The depressive psychogenic headache usually occurs at regular intervals, and patients frequently complain of multiple painful symptoms, not headache alone.

If the physician is confronted with a headache problem which does not have an organic basis, this frequently indicates that the patient may have a personality disturbance or is subjected to some form of environmental stress. This stress may be occupational, social, or domestic. This personality disturbance may be actually a matter of insecurity.

Many patients show a need for love and affection. The patient may often, in this respect, have a Dr. Jekyll and Mr. Hyde personality. By that we mean that he may be extremely affectionate and still very resentful at the same time. While he is in search of and in need of love and affection, this type of person is often found to be incapable of loving very deeply anyone or anything but himself. Many times these individuals take extreme delight in hurting the very people whom they actually love the most.

Another characteristic seen frequently in this patient is the feeling of jealously or envy. Often these patients will be envious or jealous of people whom they do not even know or associate with. Some women may be envious of the affection the nextdoor neighbor shows his wife, and in order to obtain this affection or attention from her own husband she may complain of severe headaches. This is very obvious to everyone except the husband.

In many patients afflicted with psychogenic headache, the basic cause for personality maladjustment is a feeling of insecurity. Some women patients may feel insecure in their home surroundings, and they often think that by attracting attention or gaining sympathy from those around them they become more secure. This is often accomplished, in their way of thinking, by complaining of some form of illness or disturbance. It seems that headache is all too frequently chosen as the disturbance to complain about in many of these cases.

Thus, psychogenic headache may actually be said to be the result of a defense mechanism in a frustrated personality. These patients are actually seeking a way to escape the problems they have. Of course, worry and frustration play a major role in the development of many of these cases of psychogenic headache. This is commonly seen in women at the menopausal age; in men whose business is not running smoothly; in children doing poorly in their schoolwork; in families in which there are poor marital relationships; in persons who do not have anything to think about but themselves; and in persons who have too much mental inactivity.

Because the routine general physical examination, otolaryngologic, neurologic, and ophthalmologic examinations, routine laboratory tests, and x-rays are all essentially negative, the psychogenic headache problem has to be diagnosed from the subjective statements of the patient and from a survey of his general behavior during examination and during the time he is giving the physician his case history. The examinations mentioned are essential in that they will tend to rule out any possibility of an organic basis for the headache attacks. Therefore, the history of the psychogenic headache

problem and an observation of the general characteristics of this type of patient, along with his behavior, are extremely important. While of great importance in all headache problems, they are probably even more significant with this type of patient.

Quite often we may find some family history of psychogenic headache, but, on the other hand, a family entirely sound, mentally and physically, may have one individual case of psychoneurosis manifest itself in the form of a psychogenic headache problem.

All psychogenic problems may be either congenital or acquired. A person may be constitutionally inferior from birth and only need some form of external stimulus to bring forth some type of psychoneurosis, such as psychogenic headache attacks. On the other hand, a psychoneurosis may be acquired by a mentally and physically sound person experiencing some form of severe external psychic trauma. Most patients who are correctly diagnosed as having psychogenic headaches simply do not have a nervous system which can cope with the ordinary demands of everyday life. Because of this strain there is a breakdown and the psychoneurosis appears. This may occur at practically any stage in life from childhood on through adulthood.

Psychogenic headache may, therefore, be brought about from a variety of causes. The chief factors to bear in mind in these cases are anxiety, depression, hypochondriasis, fatigue, and hysteria (conversion).

With all of these etiologic factors one thing is apparent: emotional factors play an important part in the production of this type of headache. Emotional instability is the thing to look for in dealing with this type of headache problem.

SYMPTOMATOLOGY

In all cases of psychogenic headache patients are rarely, if ever, inconvenienced by the headache attacks. They will often say they had had severe headaches all day but they dressed in the evening and went to a party, movie, or some form of entertainment; then when they came home later that evening the headache attack again was so severe that they could hardly stand it. On questioning, they will state that they had a perfectly enjoyable evening while they were out and were not bothered or inconvenienced by the headache at all. Some will state that the headache went away and then came back as soon as they were on the way home. It is rather difficult to find an organic type of headache that will act as conveniently as this.

These individuals will demonstrate in their histories that the pain of their attacks never seems to interfere with their work, their sleep, or their play. A psychogenic headache history will usually reveal that the patient states that he had had severe headache all evening and went to bed and had a good night's rest; however, on awakening in the morning, the headache returned. This again is hard to visualize in any severe form of organic headache attacks, because often the pain is so severe that patients lie awake at night, toss and turn for many hours, and finally get to sleep through sheer exhaustion. We have seen some psychogenic headache patients who claim that sexual intercourse helps to relieve their headache; others get relief by playing golf; others find relief by wining and dining in some nightclub; and still others can end their attacks by having a severe quarrel with those around them (as they put it, they "let off steam"). These things sound and actually are ridiculous; they merely show that this type of patient does not let his headache interfere with his work or play.

Psychogenic patients do not appear to be unhappy. They may be giving the physician a case history of their headache attacks and be smiling from ear to ear. However, if the physician interrupts and asks them the question, "Are you having any headache at the present time?" they may often change their facial expressions from a smile to a severe frown and state that they are in utter misery. This is another clue which often helps

to diagnose the psychogenic headache problem.

Psychogenic headaches are frequently found to be severe, and often the patient will complain of a sensation of having a tight band around his head, which seems to get tighter and tighter. Some may complain of a feeling of having a heavy weight on the top of the head, which seems to get heavier and heavier and at times feels as if it might press through their very skull. Some patients will complain that their pain is dull, while others will complain of a throbbing or a knife-like pain which they can "hardly tolerate." If the psychogenic headache patient is of a hysteric nature, he will complain of an intense, agonizing type of head pain which tends to drive him to exhaustion. Some may state that the sensation they experience is not exactly one of pain, but it is an unpleasant feeling or sensation in their head which they cannot accurately describe. They usually claim their headache to be intense, rather than mild, especially if headache is their chief complaint. In other words, their complaints are often very bizarre. They may give a picture which could not possibly fit into any headache pattern and one which may vary from day to day and never have any definite form or consistency. This bizarre pattern of the headache problem may be quite confusing initially. However, it eventually is a great aid in making the final diagnosis of psychogenic headache. The reason for this variance in the description of the headache attack by these patients is that when pain does not actually exist it can be described in one manner by one patient, and in another manner by other patients.

The pain of a psychogenic headache problem may be in any location and of any type. Some may complain of the pain as being chiefly in the frontal region of the head; some, in the occipital area; some, in the vertex of the head; and still others, of a generalized type of head pain. Therefore, the location of a psychogenic headache is not important; it may be anywhere.

The psychogenic headache is usually of

variable duration, from several hours to several days.

If anxiety is present, vertigo may result from hyperventilation. This is frequently a conditioned reaction to stress. With recurrent anxiety and excessive emotional tension, anorexia is common. Chronic anorexia with weight loss is usually a result of fatigue due to stress and to overactivity. Aerophagy occurs most frequently in the slightly debilitated, tense patient, and it is prone to become rather habitual.

Patients may present several symptoms at one time, but usually one will be the predominant feature, and this is most frequently found to be headache.

Any change in the nature of the pain or the pattern of the pain of the typical psychogenic headache patient is important, for it may be an indication that some actual organic type of headache may be starting within the patient.

The timing of the headache is often a good diagnostic symptom. Monday morning headaches in the school child or a working man often indicate unhappiness in school or working conditions. The housewife having her headaches when the husband and the children are at home for any length of time (such as the weekends) may also be diagnostic of this type of headache.

These patients are easily irritated and, more frequently than not, the pain is found to be more severe when they are confronted with some form of emotional disturbance or some form of stress or strain, whether mental or physical. In many of these cases, mere trifling incidents which the average person would not even notice may excite or annoy the person with a psychoneurosis of the psychogenic type.

If the psychogenic headache problem is in a child, it is usually found to be in the oldest child of the family. He is usually the one who is in the greatest need for attention in the average family, for more attention is generally focused on the younger children by the parents. Frequently his drives are not understood by the parents, and he is frequently unable to adequately express himself. In many families, the oldest child is also required by the parents to accept certain responsibilities within the family group which are actually beyond his limitations because of his age. On the other hand, the younger child or children in the family are not free of the possibility of being prone to psychogenic headaches, because they are more likely to be afflicted by the power of suggestion. In children, another factor which may be a precipitating factor for psychogenic headache is insecurity. This may develop in a child if the parent himself is a chronic complainer, is chronically ill, or is dead.

The psychogenic headache problem may, therefore, be difficult to diagnose if the physician fails to spend enough time in taking a thorough history of the case, for it is truly from the history that the diagnosis must be established, since all tests and examinations are essentially negative as far as the headache problem is concerned.

DIAGNOSIS

Diagnosis requires differentiation of the psychogenic type of headache from any type of organic headache. This should not be a matter of exclusion alone. The diagnosis in this type of case depends on a very careful case history and close observation of the patient's expressions and behavior. The general routine examination will reveal nothing of value, since it will be essentially negative insofar as the headache attacks are concerned. The other examinations, such as otolaryngologic, neurologic, and ophthalmologic, will also be essentially negative in respect to the headache attacks. The routine laboratory tests and skull and sinus x-rays will also lend little or no help in solving the problem because they also will be primarily negative in relation to the headache attacks.

However, it is absolutely essential in all of these cases that a complete and thorough examination be given the patient before arriving at a diagnosis of psychogenic headache. This must be done so that the physician may be absolutely certain that there is no organic pathology present. It is a dreadful thing for a physician to diagnose a case as one of psychogenic headache and later find that some organic condition had been producing the headache all along. This is especially true in the case of a patient of this type who has a fear of such things as a brain tumor or cancer. It is also advisable to reexamine these patients at various intervals, because even a psychogenic personality can develop a real organic condition in time.

The diagnosis, therefore, depends a great deal on the history, and through the history the physician will discover the presence of the psychogenic factors in the headache problem.

A physician should not have any fear of diagnosing a headache problem as being psychogenic if he or she has completely exhausted the possibility of any organic basis through thorough history-taking, examinations, and observations of the patient. But this type of diagnosis should *never* be stamped on a patient unless he has been thoroughly and completely studied, both physically and psychologically.

These patients are usually very willing to talk about their headache problem, and the physician should be equally willing to listen. While listening to the patient tell his story the physician should be observant for any emotional overtones present in the patient's response to questions and the manner in which he gives his history of the case. Many patients may be chiefly concerned that they make a good impression on the physician. If the patient is depressed, he is usually slow in his response to questions.

Actually each psychogenic headache patient is an individual, and it is rare to find two of these headaches exactly alike.

TREATMENT

The treatment program used in psychogenic headache problems may be psychotherapy, pharmacotherapy, or a combination of the two.

The successful treatment of a psychogenic headache can either be quite difficult and nearly impossible, or it can be a rather simple matter. Success often depends on a true appreciation of the nature of the condition on the part of the physician. The treatment should be directed toward the etiologic factors which cause the psychogenic imbalance, just as it should in an organic headache problem.

These patients require a complete personality adjustment. The basic maladjustment in the patient's life must be identified, and his personality should be modified so that he can overcome his maladjustment and cope with the average, everyday problems of life. This in reality may be termed "psychologic therapy." Every psychotherapeutic method which might bring favorable results in these cases should be used. The physician will find that use of psychotherapy will require very delicate handling and tact. These patients have to be handled carefully. They should not obtain from the physician the idea that their headache attacks are imagined. In order to direct a good treatment program in a case of psychogenic headache, the physician must gain the cooperation and the confidence of the patient. This may very well take a considerable amount of time and patience on the part of the physician and perhaps also on the part of the patient.

Quite often the success of the treatment of a psychogenic headache problem depends on the personality of the physician. The physician must take a gentle, kindly attitude toward the patient and his problem. He must have an understanding attitude toward the situation and, above all, patience. The physician cannot expect to get anywhere in these cases by adopting a somatic attitude.

In dealing with the psychogenic headache problem, certain pitfalls are to be avoided. The intelligence of the patient should not be insulted by merely telling him that there is nothing wrong with him, as no organic condition or disease exists, and that he is just imagining that he is ill. This should be guarded against because many of these patients would have snapped out of their troubles long ago if they could have, and they would obviously, therefore, not have consulted the physician at all. Each patient visits the physician either out of his own concern or the concern of someone else over his symptoms.

The patient must be given insight into his condition before there can be any attempted adjustment of his personality. The physician will find that there are many factors, both social and environmental, which are beyond control. This fact will also tend to make the therapy program more difficult and will be a real test of the physician's patience, because the effects of these factors have to be overcome. There will be many inner conflicts which the physician will find difficult to "pry loose" from the patient, and these conflicts also tend to complicate the treatment of these cases.

The physician has to handle each case with a considerable amount of diplomatic skill. Each case may require a different technique, as the patient's psychologic individuality has to be considered in each case. In other words, the physician must determine the patient's mentality; this can be done while the physician is taking the patients's history and observing his behavior.

The physician must convey the idea to the patient that his problem is of extreme importance to the physician. Above all, the physician must not convey the idea that the patient merely imagines that he has headaches; still, on the other hand, he must be convinced that no pathologic condition exists. This is where real tact and skill are required.

To obtain results in the treatment in psychogenic headache cases, a prime necessity is that the patient have a true desire to be cured of his headache attacks. The patient must be taught self-control and also shown how he may overcome his emotional imbalances. The pain that a patient with a psychogenic headache has is as real to him as if he actually had some form of organic headache. It is utterly useless, therefore, for the physician to tell the patient that there is nothing the matter with him. Many of these patients fear brain tumors, cancer, or insanity. For this reason they should not be told that their trouble is imaginary or that "nothing is the matter with you." This type of answer from the physician will only make the problem more difficult on the part of the patient.

The patient can be told that he is unduly nervous and upset and that this may be the basis for his headache attacks. He should then be shown that he, and he alone, will be able to overcome this nervous attitude. This will tend to help the physician gain the confidence of the patient, help save the patient's self-respect, relieve the patient's mind of fear concerning any existing tumor, cancer, or insanity, and, above all, greatly help the physician in obtaining results in the treatment program. The patient should be advised to avoid any situation or individuals which might upset him, at least for some period of time.

Some patients experience relief from their headache attacks by the use of biofeedback. This form of headache therapy seems to work better in the psychogenic headache patient than it does in any other form of headache problem in which its use is indicated, as far as we are concerned, for it is a form of psychotherapy.

The physician should assume the role of an unprejudiced, stable, and understanding listener. If the physician can succeed in accomplishing this, handling this type of headache problem will be much easier. These emotional problems should be managed by giving the patient the proper guidance and correcting any unhealthy situations and attitudes which may exist.

In some cases of psychogenic headache, medications are found to be helpful. For example, if the individual is extremely nervous, emotionally upset, and tense, a mild sedative is often of value. However, the better the physician carries out the psychotherapy portion of the treatment program, the less use there will be for medications. Sedatives should be used only on a temporary basis, because it is too easy for them to become habit-forming. The patient is told that he has no organic basis for his headaches; therefore, if he is given too much in the line of medications, he will begin to wonder if there actually is something organically wrong with him, because he will instinctively realize that medications are not generally used in nervous or psychogenic conditions. This will cause the patient to lose faith in the physician's primary approach of personality adjustment. Prescribing medication will often tend to assure the patient of the physician's interest in his headache problem. This will in turn usually encourage this type of patient to cooperate to a greater extent with the physician.

The analgesic group of drugs seems to be as good as any to use symptomatically in this type of headache problem. Needless to say, the narcotic or habit-forming type of drug should never be used in this type of headache patient. If the patient is depressed, a mood elevator such as amitriptyline (Elavil) or protriptyline (Vivactil) may be required in the treatment program. If the patient has tension or anxiety in the background of the case, a mild tranquilizer may be of benefit, such as diazepam (Valium) or meprobamate (Equanil). Some cases also are relieved by such preparations as Bellergal, which is a combination of belladonna alkaloids, ergotamine tartrate, and phenobarbital.

Frequently a placebo will afford these patients symptomatic relief of their headache pain. This is not hard to understand, for after all this is psychogenic pain, not organic pain. There are many patients who merely "like to take medicine" and, therefore, psychologically they may obtain some relief if medications are given for a short period of time along with the psychotherapy of personality adjustment and reassurance.

It may appear strange to state in one place that some patients should be given medications for the psychic value they might provide and in another place to that medication should not be given, because of the poor psychologic effect it might produce on the patient. However, this merely shows that every case of psychogenic headache is an individual and different problem, a study in itself. Since there may be no two psychogenic headache problems exactly alike, each patient should be studied thoroughly and treated as an individual, and not merely treated on a pattern basis.

There is no product available on the drug market which will be as beneficial to the psychogenic headache patient as will be removal of etiologic factor which is causing it.

These cases, if handled properly, can be helped by the physician; it is generally not necessary for patients to receive psychotherapy from a trained psychiatrist. The physician should remember that "essence of patience and tincture of time" are necessary to achieve desired results in these cases.

CASE HISTORY

D. D., a 19-year-old female, had complained of headaches for as long as she could remember. They usually occurred in the frontal regions, bilaterally, almost daily, and would last throughout the day. There was no association of her attacks with her menstrual periods or any other associated manifestations. However, on further questioning it was found that her attacks would usually begin in the mornings and fade out in the late afternoons. She was a college student and on questioning admitted that she disliked school. School was over around 3:00 P.M. or 4:00 P.M., and soon after school was out her headaches would disappear. Her pain was dull and did not bother her at home, at play, or when she was out socially. She has no nasal, gastrointestinal, or ocular disturbances with the headache attacks. There was no tenderness over the areas involved. She often found temporary relief with aspirin or some form of analgesic. She had no disturbances of her sleep or appetite from the headache attacks.

During the history-taking phase of her case, she did not show any evidence of pain. Her entire examination failed to show any abnormalities. Her sinus x-rays were negative, her blood pressure was within normal limits, and her entire physical picture was that of a normal 19-year-old female. Vasoconstrictor and vasodilating drugs failed to produce any change in her headache pattern.

This case was diagnosed as a psychogenic headache

problem on the basis of an unhappy school life. She was reassured that there was no organic basis to her condition, and psychotherapy was instituted. She became interested in extracurricular activities, and her grades improved in general. Her headaches, needless to say, became a thing of the past.

SUMMARY

Symptoms and signs
1. The patient is not inconvenienced by the headache.
2. Pain does not interfere with work, sleep, or play.
3. Patient is not unhappy.
4. Patient is tense and has an apprehensive personality.
5. Coomplaints are bizarre.
6. Pain may be of any type or in any location.
7. Pain is more severe with emotional disturbances, stress, or strain.

Negative

1. Physical examination
2. Fundi examination
3. Blood pressure
4. Neurologic examination
5. X-rays of head and sinuses

Treatment
1. Personality adjustment
2. Analgesics
3. Mild tranquilizers
4. Reassurance
5. Antidepressants
6. Biofeedback

CHAPTER 12

Headache of systemic origin

ROBERT S. KUNKEL, Jr.

In other areas of this book, the basic mechanisms involved in the etiology of headache are discussed. There are a limited number of ways that systemic illnesses can produce headache. Vasodilation of the extracranial and larger intracranial vessels, traction on the great vessels and pain-sensitive structures at the base of the brain, inflammation of the extracranial and intracranial vessels, and sustained contraction of skeletal muscles of the scalp and neck are the basic causes of headache, no matter what the underlying etiology. Diseases of other organs in the head such as the eyes, ears, nose, and teeth can, of course, cause headache and are discussed elsewhere.

In discussing some of the more common systemic conditions which may be associated with headache, one should remember that the cause of the head pain is due to one of the above-mentioned basic mechanisms. Therefore, there is no specific pain pattern associated with any particular illness. One must take a very detailed history and perform a complete physical examination in order to arrive at the diagnosis of some underlying disease process which might be implicated in the causation of the headache. Underlying systemic causes of

headache should be searched for in all patients who have had a recent onset of headache, and in those persons whose headache does not fall into a specific pattern of migraine, cluster, or muscle contraction headache.

It would be impossible to list and discuss all of the possible systemic disorders which may be associated with headache. Various categories of diseases, along with the more common clinical entities in each broad disease category, are discussed.

HEADACHE AND INFECTION

Systemic infections can involve the structures within the cranium and be the cause of headache. Local infectious processes are discussed elsewhere in this book. Infection of the cranial structures can arise from extension of infection from local adjacent areas such as the sinuses, ears, and skull, or it may develop as the result of a hematogenous spread of infecting agents from a distal portal of entry or distant site of infection in another organ system. Fever from infection anywhere in the body without any direct central nervous system involvement is a common cause of headache.

Although infection in the brain is usually

304

categorized according to whether the involvement is primarily in the meninges (meningitis) or the brain parenchyma (encephalitis), the inflammatory process often involves both areas. The head pain accompanying intracranial infection is probably secondary to the inflammatory reaction of the infection. This lowers the pain threshold in the nerve endings about the vessels and dura at the base of the brain.[1]

Acute meningitis

Acute meningitis can result from infection of the meninges by almost any pathogenic bacteria. The bacteria may reach the meninges from adjacent structures by way of the bloodstream or be introduced through a skull fracture or even a lumbar puncture. The signs and symptoms of acute meningitis are similar, no matter what infecting organism is present.

Etiology. The most common etiologic agents causing acute purulent meningitis are *Meningococcus, Hemophilus influenzae, Pneumococcus,* and *Streptococcus.*[2] Although the history of the illness and some specific clinical findings may enable one to suspect a specific bacteria to be present, the symptomatology is similar regardless of the etiologic agent. These infecting agents cause inflammatory changes with exudate formation and thickening of the meninges. This causes traction and pressure on the pain-sensitive structures in the cranial vault. Meningococcal infection may occur in epidemics.

Symptomatology. Acute meningitis is accompanied by chills and fever. There may have been a preceding infection elsewhere in the body. The headache is quite intense. It is constant, generalized, and tends to be throbbing. It often is more severe in the occipital area. Photophobia is common. The pain is made worse by any jolting or movement such as walking, shaking the head, bending, or stooping. Lying down flat usually will decrease the intensity of the pain. Stiffness of the neck is usually present

and may be severe. This rigidity occurs because of involvement of the upper cervical roots in the inflammatory process.[1] Nausea, vomiting, stupor, and even coma are not infrequent. Focal neurologic deficits are rare, however.[2] Irritability, accompanied by fever, may be an early symptom, especially in children.

Diagnosis. The diagnosis of meningitis is made with certainty only by isolation of the organism from the cerebrospinal fluid. Meningitis can be strongly suspected, however, when the typical clinical symptoms and signs are present. Findings such as stiffness of the neck, positive Brudzinski and Kernig signs, and fever, along with the recent onset of a severe headache, should make the physician highly suspicious. A petechial skin rash along with the other signs and symptoms would suggest meningococcal meningitis. Leukocytosis is common. Cerebrospinal fluid shows an elevated pressure, is purulent with many cells, contains predominantly polymorphonuclear leukocytes, and has an elevated protein content and low sugar content. Organisms may be seen and cultures will identify the infecting organism with certainty.

Treatment. The headache of acute meningitis will respond to treatment with the appropriate antibiotic. Analgesics and often narcotics are needed to control the pain until the infection is treated. Fluid and electrolyte management is necessary, and occasionally removal of cerebrospinal fluid with subsequent lowering of the intracranial pressure is helpful in reducing the intensity of the headache.

Subacute meningitis

Subacute meningitis is usually caused by tuberculosis or other fungal infections.

Etiology. Tuberculosis of the meninges is always secondary to tuberculosis elsewhere in the body. It is often characterized by intense inflammatory reaction with thickened fibrotic tissue about the base of the brain. Fungal meningitis can be caused by *Cryptococcus neoformans,* histoplasmosis, mucormycosis, blastomycosis, actinomycosis, aspergillosis, and *Candida,* as well as other agents.

Symptomatology. Tuberculous meningitis tends to be a more indolent process than acute bacterial meningitis. The headache is a dull generalized aching and occasionally a throbbing sensation is noted. Fever is usually present, but of a low grade nature. Lethargy, apathy, and confusion are common symptoms. Stiffness of the neck, nausea, and vomiting are common. As the illness progresses, stupor and coma are not uncommon. Because of the intense reaction in the basal area of the brain, cranial nerve deficits may be present.

Fungal infections cause symptoms similar to tuberculous meningitis. One should suspect a fungal etiology if the patient has been taking long-term antibiotics, corticosteroids, or immunosuppressive agents or if he suffers from some chronic disease such as a hematologic disorder and develops headache along with fever and mental aberrations.

Diagnosis. The diagnosis of tuberculous or fungal meningitis depends on isolating the organism from the cerebrospinal fluid. This is sometimes difficult, however, and one may have to wait many days or weeks for the cultures to confirm the diagnosis. Typical cerebrospinal fluid findings in tuberculous meningitis include elevated protein, low sugar, and a moderate pleocytosis with predominantly lymphocytes being present. Cranial nerve involvement as well as other neurologic abnormalities are often evident on examination.

Treatment. Since tuberculous meningitis can be a fatal disease, treatment should be started if the suspicion is high, even though bacteriologic proof is not available. Three major drugs should be used for central nervous system involvement with tuberculosis. Isoniazid, rifampin (or streptomycin), and ethambutol are the currently preferred drug regimen. The headache may have to be treated with mild narcotics while awaiting the effects of the antituberculous therapy, but if possible, narcotics and sedatives should be

avoided because of the possible interference with evaluating the mental status. Treatment of fungal meningitis is not very satisfactory, although amphotericin B has sometimes brought about a cure. Some newer antifungal agents may soon be available.

Aseptic meningitis

Aseptic meningitis is an irritation or inflammation of the meninges caused by a viral agent or some other irritant. It is the most common central nervous system viral syndrome.[3]

Etiology. Many different viral agents can cause meningeal symptoms and signs. The most common viruses include Coxsackie B, mumps, echo, lymphocytic choriomeningitis, and polio viruses. Aseptic meningitis is usually a self-limited and benign condition, with most persons recovering without sequelae within 10 days.

Symptomatology. Stiffness of the neck, fever, headache, and photophobia are common symptoms. Patients with aseptic meningitis are usually not as ill as those with bacterial meningitis. Meningeal symptoms often accompany or follow systemic symptoms of viral infections involving other organ systems.

Diagnosis. The cerebrospinal fluid typically shows a mild pleocytosis predominantly of lymphocytes and mild elevation of the protein, but with a normal sugar content. If chronic inflammatory symptoms of the central nervous system develop, one should consider fungal or tuberculous infection to be present.

Treatment. No good treatment for aseptic or viral meningitis exists. However, treatment is usually unnecessary. Symptomatic treatment with mild analgesics to relieve the headache may be indicated.

Encephalitis

Encephalitis is inflammation of the brain parenchyma which may accompany a systemic illness. Headache is usually a predominant symptom.

Etiology. Encephalitis is usually caused

by viral agents, and many viruses have been implicated. Rickettsial organisms and syphilis also commonly cause encephalitis. Inflammation of the brain parenchyma as well as perivascular inflammation and meningeal irritation cause symptoms.

Symptomatology. Generalized steady headache, fever, and stiffness of the neck are common symptoms. The headache may be quite severe, and like other conditions with increased intracranial pressure, the headache will be increased with exertion, bending, stooping, or coughing. Because of parenchymal involvement, seizures, confusion, and altered states of consciousness, along with focal neurologic deficits, are common in encephalitis, whereas they are not commonly seen in meningitis. Sore throat, myalgia, headache, and gastrointestinal symptoms commonly precede the neurologic symptoms.

Diagnosis. The diagnosis of encephalitis is suspected from the symptoms. Cerebrospinal fluid findings are similar to those of aseptic meningitis, with mild increase in pressure, pleocytosis, mild elevation of protein, and normal sugar. Serologic tests as well as recovery of the virus from the cerebrospinal fluid prove the diagnosis. The various serologic tests should be paired and show a rise in titer in the convalescent sample. The diagnosis is also aided by knowing whether other cases of viral encephalitis have been reported in the area.

Treatment. The treatment of viral encephalitis is not satisfactory. There are no specific agents available to treat viral encephalitis except for perhaps herpes simplex. The headache should be controlled with analgesics, and antiseizure medications may be necessary.

Syphilis

Syphilis is considered here by itself since its involvement of the central nervous system can take several forms. Neural syphilis can be asymptomatic, with only cerebrospinal fluid abnormalities, or may involve primarily the meninges, vasculature, or parenchyma. A recent case report demonstrates that syphilis must still be considered as an etiologic agent in headache.[4]

Etiology. *Treponema pallidum* usually invades the central nervous system during the secondary stage of syphilis. The symptomatic forms include meningeal, vascular, and parenchymal involvement. Symptoms often are delayed months and even years from the time of infection. The fever which accompanies systemic dissemination may play a role in causation of the headache.

Symptomatology. The symptoms, of course, depend on the principal area of involvement. Meningeal involvement often causes cranial nerve palsies.[2] The headache in the meningeal form is diffuse, nonlocalized, and tends to be throbbing. It may be influenced by positional changes and may awaken the patient at night. The pain is usually intermittent and severe. Vascular neurosyphilis is characterized by endarteritis with thrombosis giving focal neurologic signs. Meningoencephalitis usually accompanies the vascular type. The headache may be a steady pain or of a pulsatile quality. Focal neurologic deficits accompany the headache that is of recent onset.

Diagnosis. The diagnosis is confirmed with a positive test for syphilis in the cerebrospinal fluid. If gummatous lesions are present, they may be demonstrable on a brain scan. Often the diagnosis is not suspected until a routine blood serology shows positive.

Treatment. Treatment of neurosyphilis is procaine penicillin in a total dosage of 9 to 12 million units. Analgesics may be used to treat the pain, and as with any involvement of the brain, narcotics should be avoided if possible.

SUMMARY

Symptoms and signs
1. Fever
2. Mental aberrations
3. Neurologic deficits
4. Worsening with position or exertion
5. Dull ache in character

Treatment
    Treatment of underlying infection

HEADACHE DUE TO ENDOCRINE DISORDERS

Several abnormalities of the endocrine system may be associated with headache. Although the mechanisms of the pain occurring with the various endocrine disorders are not well understood, it appears that vasodilation and vascular mechanisms usually play a dominant role. Hypoglycemia occurring with many various conditions seems to be the most common triggering mechanism. Tumors of the pituitary or hypothalamic areas are often associated with endocrine disorders and may cause headache from pressure and traction on pain-sensitive structures within the cranium.

Hypoglycemia

Low blood sugar is a precipitant of migraine headaches in many persons.[5] The headache that frequently occurs when the migraineur skips meals may be due to hypoglycemia. In susceptible persons, functional hypoglycemia occurring during a glucose tolerance test will precipitate a vascular headache. Hypoglycemia may be of the "functional" or organic variety.

Etiology. Hypoglycemia, like hypoxia, acidosis, and other metabolic derangements, affects the neurons. Vasodilation occurs in response to this stress on the neurons. Hypoglycemia can be due to many causes. Probably the most common etiology is the so-called functional or reactive hypoglycemia which occurs 3 to 4 hours after eating and is demonstrated during the third to fifth hour of a glucose tolerance test. Blood sugar levels must be under 50 mg/100 ml to cause hypoglycemic symptoms. Many persons with functional hypoglycemia have many psychosomatic complaints, and the headache may be on that basis rather than the actual low blood sugar level. Merely skipping a meal may cause enough hypoglycemia to induce a headache in persons susceptible to vascular headaches.

Hypoglycemia due to an islet cell tumor of the pancreas, liver disease, insulin reactions, or impending insulin shock in diabetic individuals may induce a headache. This headache is due to organic hypoglycemia and usually occurs before meals and often in the early morning hours. It is aggravated by exercise and continued fasting. Other endocrinopathies such as hypothyroidism, hypopituitarism, and adrenocortical insufficiency may be accompanied by hypoglycemia of such a degree as to cause headache. There is a growing list of nonpancreatic neoplasms being reported which have been associated with hypoglycemia.[6] The hypoglycemia with these tumors may be due to several different causes.

Symptomatology. The headache of hypoglycemia is usually of a vascular type with a pulsatile or throbbing character. The pain may be bilateral in the temples or unilateral and indistinguishable from that of a typical migraine attack. Nausea and vomiting occur in most every case, whether the headache is unilateral or bilateral.[5] Other symptoms of hypoglycemia such as palpitations, diaphoresis, weakness, fatigue, tremor, hunger, and dizziness may often accompany the headache. Convulsions and coma may occur in those with organic hypoglycemia.

Diagnosis. The diagnosis of a hypoglycemia-induced headache depends on the history of the pain pattern from the patient and the finding of a blood sugar level under 50 mg/100 ml, either on the glucose tolerance test or in the fasting state. Hypoglycemia as an etiology of the headache can be suspected when the sufferer notes that the headaches occur when he skips meals or occur regularly 3 to 4 hours after a meal heavy in sugar content. Organic causes of hypoglycemia, such as pituitary, thyroid, or adrenal insufficiency, should be considered. Hypoglycemia due to hyperinsulinism from an islet cell tumor will typically occur in the early morning hours, several hours after eating.

Treatment. The treatment depends on the cause of the hypoglycemia. For the functional or reactive hypoglycemic patient, a diet with a high protein content and multiple small feedings should eliminate the hypoglycemia. Psychotherapy may be needed if many other complaints are present. If endocrine deficiencies are found, they should be treated with replacement therapy. Regular meals are important for the migraineur who has hypoglycemia-induced migraine. Migraine may be almost eliminated in some by strict observance of diet. Adjustment of the insulin dosage, of course, will eliminate the hypoglycemia due to excessive insulin. Surgical removal of an islet cell adenoma is curative of the headache due to this organic type of hypoglycemia.

Thyroid disease

Thyroid dysfunction may be associated with headache. Both overactivity and underactivity of the thyroid gland may be associated with headaches.

Etiology. The etiology of the headache in hypothyroidism may be related to hypoglycemia accompanying the hypothyroid state. It may also be of the muscle contraction type since myalgia and muscle symptoms are very commonly seen in the person with hypothyroidism. Hyperthyroidism with its increased metabolism, anxiety, and tension may be accompanied by tension headache. It is imperative to determine whether the thyroid disorder is primary or secondary. A pituitary lesion, in addition to being the cause of hypothyroidism, may in itself be causing some headache. Thyroid dysfunction may be associated with hypothalamic or pituitary lesions. Inappropriate response of the hypothalamus to stress and other stimuli has been postulated as the basic mechanism present in migraine.[7,8] Thus, the hypothalamus may be a common site of vascular as well as endocrine instability and dysfunction.

Symptomatology. The headache of hypothyroidism or hyperthyroidism is nonspecific. It is usually a dull throbbing pain with some vascular features. It is generally constant and persistent as opposed to the peri-

odic headache of migraine, hypoglycemia, and other vascular headaches. The many symptoms associated with hypo- and hyperthyroidism are also present and usually are more disturbing to the patient than the headache. Cervical myalgia and muscle contraction headaches may be seen in the patient with hyperthyroidism who is anxious and tense. Cervical myalgia may also be seen in those patients with hypothyroidism who have muscle symptoms.

Diagnosis. The diagnosis of thyroid dysfunction is much easier now with the many tests available, some of which are quite specific. One can no longer stop with merely testing the thyroid function, however. Pituitary and hypothalamic function should be evaluated.[9] A primary intracranial process may be the cause of the thyroid dysfunction and may in itself cause headache by local pressure. X-rays of the skull, visual field examinations, and laboratory tests for thyrotropin and other pituitary hormones should be done to exclude intracranial lesions.

Treatment. Treatment is relatively simple in the hypothyroid state. Replacement therapy with thyroid cures the headache as well as the other symptoms. The patient, of course, has to be told that he needs to take thyroid the rest of his life. Radioactive iodine and surgical therapy are used for the hyperthyroid state unless a pituitary lesion needs treatment. The treatment of the headache of thyroid dysfunction is the treatment of the basic underlying thyroid abnormality, although simple analgesics may be necessary until the thyroid condition is controlled.

Adrenal insufficiency

Headache may be present in the person with adrenal insufficiency.

Etiology. The periodic hypoglycemia of adrenal insufficiency, as well as the hypotension, are probably the basic causes of the headache in Addison's disease or other causes of adrenal insufficiency. The headache, therefore, is usually vascular in origin. The adrenal insufficiency may be primary, secondary to pituitary disease, or iatrogenic due to prior treatment with exogenous corticosteroids. The last is probably the most common cause of adrenal insufficiency at the present time. Etiology of primary adrenal failure may be infectious, hemorrhagic, or idiopathic.

Symptomatology. The headache tends to be periodic but has no characteristic pattern. It is generalized rather than unilateral or localized and is a throbbing, pulsatile pain. Other typical symptoms of adrenal insufficiency such as nausea, vomiting, weakness, diarrhea, anorexia, weight loss, and syncope may be present.

Diagnosis. The diagnosis depends on eliciting a history compatible with adrenal insufficiency. Hypotension and hypoglycemia, as well as electrolyte abnormalities, are found on examination. Confirmatory laboratory studies are low levels of adrenal steroids in the blood and urine which are unresponsive to ACTH stimulation in primary adrenal failure. Adrenal insufficiency secondary to pituitary failure can also be diagnosed readily, by demonstrating a response to ACTH stimulation.

Treatment. Treatment with corticosteroid replacement should restore the patient's well-being with a normalization of the blood pressure and blood sugar. The headache and the other abnormalities, if they are due to the adrenal insufficiency, should be relieved with correcting the underlying problem.

Hyperparathyroidism

Neurologic symptoms and headache are not uncommon in primary hyperparathyroidism.[10]

Etiology. Neuromuscular abnormalities secondary to the hypercalcemia and other metabolic derangements such as magnesium deficiency in hyperparathyroidism may play a role in the causation of headache. Hypertension, frequently present in hyperparathyroidism, may also be a factor in the etiology of headache.

Symptomatology. Headaches in primary hyperparathyroidism tend to be a steady dull pressure type of pain and nonlocalized. Lethargy, confusion, and depression may be seen with high serum calcium levels. Muscle weakness may be quite profound with hypercalcemia. Renal calculi and gastrointestinal symptoms are also quite common in hyperparathyroidism.

Diagnosis. The diagnosis is suggested by the finding of elevated serum calcium levels. With automated laboratory tests in most hospitals now being done routinely, elevated serum calcium levels are being found much more commonly. Parathyroid hormone levels are confirmatory of primary hyperparathyroidism if available. Other conditions causing hypercalcemia such as immobilization and malignancy should be excluded.

Treatment. The treatment of primary hyperparathyroidism is surgical removal of the adenoma. Treatment of other underlying diseases causing hypercalcemia may be indicated. Lowering of the serum calcium may bring about dramatic improvement in the clinical symptoms seen with hypercalcemia.

Pituitary lesions

Etiology. Pituitary tumors can cause headache by the direct effect of their growth on surrounding cranial structures or by the dysfunction of the various endocrine glands under pituitary influence. Headache is quite common in acromegaly and often occurs with craniopharyngioma and pituitary adenomas.

Symptomatology. The headache of intracranial tumor is discussed elsewhere. It is usually diffuse and not well localized. Symptoms pointing toward endocrine abnormalities may also be present.

Diagnosis. Visual symptoms or defects on visual field testing may be present. X-ray demonstration of enlargement of the sella and various endocrine deficiencies lead to the diagnosis.

Treatment. Depending on the type of pituitary lesion, surgery or irradiation therapy may be indicated.

SUMMARY

Symptoms and signs

1. Hypoglycemia
2. Vascular headache
3. Myalgias and muscle contraction headache
4. Primary or secondary endocrinopathy

Treatment

Replacement therapy

HYPERTENSION AND HEADACHE

Headache is often thought of as a frequent symptom of hypertension. It is important to realize that the hypertension has to be quite significant, with diastolic readings in the 120 to 130 mm Hg range, in order to cause headache. In a group of patients with malignant hypertension, however, headache was present in 77% of those with neurologic symptoms and 74% of those without neurologic symptoms.[11] Most headaches in the mildly hypertensive patient are not due to hypertension. Such factors as anxiety, tension, and other psychogenic factors are believed to play a role in causing the headaches seen in people with hypertension. The exact relationship of headaches to the level of hypertension in the individual patient continues to be debated in the literature.[12] Migraineurs are the exception in that very mild elevations of blood pressure can greatly increase the frequency and severity of migraine attacks. It is also important to realize that certain antihypertensive agents in common usage, such as reserpine and hydralazine, can in themselves be a cause of headache.

Sustained hypertension

Hypertension may be caused by many different factors such as renal artery disease, renal parenchymal disease, endocrinopathies, blood disorders, and intracranial disease. Most frequently, however, hypertension falls into the "essential" category in which no specific etiology has yet been discovered. One should also remember that when first seeing a patient with a rather severe headache, the blood pressure may be elevated secondary to the patient's response to pain, and, therefore, would not be the primary problem causing the headache.

Etiology. The cause of head pain in the hypertensive patient is thought to be due to the dilation of intracranial and extracranial arteries.[1] Digital pressure on the carotid and superficial temporal arteries and the use of ergotamine will reduce the intensity of the pain, as is seen in other vascular headaches. Studies have demonstrated that there is often no direct correlation between the headache intensity and the immediate blood pressure levels.[13]

It has been postulated that vasodilating substances are released possibly from the kidney to counteract the vasoconstrictive effects of hypertension. These substances (possibly prostaglandins) are believed to cause the vasodilating headache during the early morning hours or other periods of relaxation when headache often occurs in the hypertensive individual.[14] Hypercapnia of sleep may cause vasodilation and increased intracranial pressure, which may be another factor causing the typical early morning headache pattern.[15]

Symptomatology. The headache of sustained hypertension, whatever the etiology, tends to follow a characteristic pattern. The discomfort tends to be dull, throbbing, and nonlocalized, although the occipital area seems to be the most frequent location of discomfort. Typically, the headache begins in the early morning hours, reaching a peak when the patient awakens. The pain generally diminishes as the patient gets up and moves about during the day. The patient may find less discomfort by sleeping with the head elevated. Activity which increases blood pressure or intracranial pressure, such as bending, stooping, coughing, straining, or exertion, may aggravate the headache.

Many persons with hypertension seem to have a headache which is quite typical of muscle contraction headache, and yet the pain seems to ease with treatment of the hypertension. The scalp is often tender and sore to touch. Whether or not the muscle contraction headache is due to anxiety and tension alone or is related to the hypertension is uncertain.

If the headache is related to hypertension, other symptoms associated with hypertension may be present. These include fullness in the head, dizziness or true vertigo, flushing, insomnia, and restlessness. Unless the patient has migraine with hypertension, the common symptoms of migraine are missing, even though the headache is of the vascular nature. Visual, neurologic, and gastrointestinal symptoms so common in migraine are absent. Hypertension headache is believed by some to be more common in persons who have previously had migraine.[16]

Diagnosis. As already discussed, the exact relationship of headache to hypertensive levels is uncertain. With significant hypertension or malignant hypertension, one can assume that the headache is at least in part related to the hypertension. In the migraineur with mild hypertension, one can assume that the blood pressure level may be playing a role in the frequency and severity of the migraine attacks. In the mildly hypertensive patient, the blood pressure should certainly be treated, even though one cannot say for certain that the headache is directly related. Needless to say, blood pressures should be taken in any patient who is being examined and checked for a headache evaluation.

Treatment. The treatment of the headache of hypertension is essentially treatment of the elevated blood pressure. If a recognizable etiology is found, such as renal artery stenosis or primary aldosteronism, surgery may be indicated. In the overwhelming number of cases, however, medical management is appropriate. Today there are many antihypertensive medications available. As previously stated, one should be alert to the fact that reserpine, probably by way of serotonin depletion, may in itself cause a vascular headache and that hydralazine and other vasodilating or ganglionic blocking drugs may aggravate vascular headache. Analgesics may be needed to control the pain while blood pressure is being brought under control. Small doses of ergotamine tartrate may be very effective in controlling the headache, but caution should be used to avoid aggravation of the blood pressure itself. More recently, biofeedback training has been found useful in the treatment of hypertension and headache with or without hypertension.[17]

Paroxysmal hypertensive headache

In addition to the headache seen with sustained hypertension, certain conditions causing sudden paroxysmal rises in the blood pressure can cause severe headache. These headaches are caused by the acute expansion and dilation of cranial arteries secondary to the sudden rise of blood pressure.

ORGASMIC AND EXERTIONAL HEADACHES

Orgasmic and exertional headaches are probably more common than realized. The former can be quite severe and provoke much fear. Both headaches are very brief and of high intensity. The pain is usually bilateral, throbbing in the occipital and vertex areas. Orgasmic headache in the past has evoked concern about the possibility of an intracranial aneurysm being present, but most now believe that this is usually a benign condition not associated with structural vascular abnormalities.[18]

Treatment consists mainly of reassurance and explanation. Occasionally, prophylactic ergotamine may be helpful. Indomethacin has been said to be useful in the exertional type of headache.[19]

PHEOCHROMOCYTOMA

Probably the best known paroxysmal vascular headache is that induced by a pheochromocytoma.

Etiology. The headache of pheochromocytoma is vascular in origin. The sudden rise in blood pressure with the paroxysmal attack causes distention and dilation of the intracranial and extracranial arteries as manifested by a throbbing, pounding headache of severe intensity. Release of levarterenol, an alpha-receptor stimulator, causes arterial and venular constriction. Secretion of epinephrine, primarily a beta-receptor stimulator, causes arteriolar dilation and venular constriction.[20]

Symptomatology. The headache of pheochromocytoma is bilateral, usually throbbing in nature, and of short duration. The headache is usually located in the frontal and occipital areas, but may be anywhere. The pain is usually severe and hits abruptly, occurring along with other symptoms of the typical paroxysm of pheochromocytoma. In most patients, the paroxysm of symptoms including headache lasts less than 1 hour.[21] The headache reaches peak intensity within minutes and often awakens the patient in the early morning hours. Nausea commonly accompanies the headache, along with perspiration, palpitation, and pallor.

Diagnosis. The diagnosis of pheochromocytoma depends on eliciting the history of the typical paroxysmal attack with all of its various symptoms. The diagnosis may be confirmed by performing provocative tests with histamine or tyramine or alpha-receptor blockade with pentolamine in persons with sustained hypertension. Elevated urinary levels of vanillylmandelic acid, metanephrines, and catecholamines are confirmatory. These levels may be more evident if collected following provocative testing.[20]

Treatment. Surgical removal of the tumor or tumors is the treatment of choice in a patient with pheochromocytoma. Medical treatment for the most part has been unrewarding.

Malignant hypertension

Malignant hypertension with hypertensive encephalopathy is associated with numerous neurologic symptoms, in addition to headache. Headache occurs in about 75% of persons with malignant hypertension.[11]

Etiology. The exact etiology of malignant or accelerated hypertension is unknown. It is associated with renal failure. A malignant phase of hypertension may develop in one who has had essential hypertension for years. The headache is believed to be due mainly to cerebral edema.[1] There is marked vasoconstriction of cerebral vessels leading to ischemia and localized edema. Extreme hypertension itself may lead to vasoconstriction with subsequent ischemia, edema, and even necrosis of the arterial wall.[22] Focal or massive cerebral hemorrhage may also play a role in the causation of symptoms.

Symptomatology. The headache in malignant hypertension may be of a vascular type with a pulsatile throbbing character which varies with position and activity. It may occur mainly in the early morning hours. It is more likely, however, to be a rather constant, dull, steady pressure type pain because of the cerebral edema and intense vasoconstriction rather than vasodilation. The headache may be occipital or frontal in location. The headache may become increasingly severe many months before hypertension enters the malignant phase and may be a good warning sign of this event.[23]

Other symptoms are quite common in malignant hypertension and are usually those seen in renal failure. Confusion, dementia, and impairment of consciousness are common. Seizures and dizziness are also frequently seen. Focal ischemic lesions or cerebral hemorrhage may cause focal neurologic symptoms and signs. Papilledema and retinal hemorrhages are commonly seen.

Diagnosis. The diagnosis of malignant hypertension, or the malignant phase of essential hypertension, is made when hypertension becomes accelerated and is accompanied by papilledema. Vascular changes occur in many organs leading to dysfunction of those vital organs and increasing renal failure. Retinal hemorrhages, in addition to the papilledema, may be present.

Treatment. Very aggressive antihypertensive therapy is necessary to reverse the extremely high mortality rate seen in malignant hypertension. Analgesics not containing phenacetin may be used. The headaches should ease as the blood pressure is lowered. Vasoconstrictor medications should be avoided. Propranolol would seem to be a useful drug in this situation, but would not likely be an effective drug by itself in controlling the blood pressure. A combination of medications is usually needed to control the hypertension. Since organ damage is occurring, it is essential to lower the blood pressure rapidly.

SUMMARY

Symptoms and signs

1. Throbbing, pounding headache, occurring in early morning hours, worse with exertion, occipital in location, bilateral
2. May aggravate migraine
3. May be associated with tension

Treatment

1. Lowering blood pressure
2. Analgesics

HYPOTENSION AND HEADACHE

Hypotension is blamed by many patients and physicians alike as causing headache, as well as a myriad of other symptoms. Since hypotension is prevalent in asthenic persons with many psychogenic and functional complaints, it is very difficult to ascribe the headache or other symptoms to the hypotension alone. Postural hypotension with a significant drop in the blood pressure may cause a vascular type of headache. The symptoms of headache should be correlated with the positional change and assuming the upright position.

The treatment of significant symptomatic hypotension consists of using vasoconstrictive agents, along with elastic tights or other garments.

HEMATOLOGIC DISORDERS AND HEADACHE

Diseases of the blood may be associated with headache. The headache usually is of a vascular etiology. It may be due to hypoxemia secondary to anemia with resultant dilation of the cranial arteries, or the vessels may be dilated and congested because of the increased blood volume of polycythemia. Leukemia and lymphoma often involve the central nervous system and may be accompanied by headache.

Anemia

Etiology. Anemia of any type, if severe enough, will result in cerebral hypoxia. Hypoxia is a cause of cerebrovascular dilation. If the hypoxia is accompanied by an increase in carbon dioxide tension in the blood, the dilation of the cerebral vessels, especially the arteries and arterioles, is quite profound.[1] Acute blood loss may be accompanied by headache, even if the hemoglobin is not severely depleted. Chronic blood loss will be accompanied by headache if the hemoglobin is quite low. Hemolytic anemias such as acquired or congenital hemolytic anemia, sickle cell disease, paroxysmal nocturnal hemoglobinuria, and anemias due to sensitivity to drugs may also cause headache and should be considered in the differential diagnosis of anemia.

Symptomatology. The headache of anemia is a generalized throbbing discomfort. It is usually not localized. The pain tends to be constant but can be intermittent, and on occasion it may even be unilateral, just as in the migraine syndrome. Factors influencing vasodilation such as exertion, fever, straining, or bending will aggravate the headache of anemia. Other symptoms of anemia such as lightheadedness, fatigue, and even syncope may be present. The craving for ice or cold water may be a clue that the person is suffering from anemia.

Diagnosis. The diagnosis is made by the finding of a low hemoglobin level in one with a recent onset of headache. The cause of the anemia should be investigated and remedied if possible. As already stated, there is nothing specific about the headache of anemia.

Treatment. The treatment of the headache of anemia is to restore the hemoglobin to normal by the use of iron if needed and by treating the cause of the anemia. The headache itself can be controlled with mild analgesics. It would not be wise to use strong vasoconstrictive agents in one with severe anemia. This may potentiate ischemia caused by the hypoxia secondary to anemia.

Polycythemia

Polycythemia vera frequently presents with headache as an early symptom. Around 40% of patients with polycythemia, primary or secondary, present with headache.[24]

Etiology. Vascular distention, increased blood viscosity, and increased intracranial pressure account for the headache of polycythemia vera.[25] In secondary polycythemia due to lung disease, high altitude sickness, or other hypoxic states, low oxygen content also plays a role in the occurrence of headache. Carbon dioxide retention in chronic pulmonary disease with or without polycythemia may cause vasodilating headache.

Symptomatology. The headache in polycythemia, whether primary or secondary, is usually a generalized dull, throbbing, pounding headache. Factors such as bending, stooping, or straining, which increase central venous and cerebral pressure, will aggravate the discomfort. Vertigo, dizziness, visual symptoms, paresthesias in the extremities, and tinnitus are frequent neurologic symptoms occurring in polycythemia, although headache is the most common neurologic symptom.[24] Focal neurologic abnormalities often occur secondary to thrombosis in the person with polycythemia.

Diagnosis. The diagnosis of polycythemia is made from the blood count. Secondary polycythemia usually does not have the leukocytosis and thrombocytosis seen in polycythemia vera. Blood volume studies are often helpful. Since polycythemia may be present for a long time, the headache may not be of recent onset, but more of the chronic type. There is nothing specific about this or any of the headaches secondary to disease states. Blood gas measurements and pulmonary function studies may be necessary to determine the cause of secondary polycythemia.

Treatment. Polycythemia may be treated with repeated phlebotomies alone. A phlebotomy will, of course, ease the headache temporarily. Chemotherapeutic agents are often indicated for long-term control of polycythemia. If the polycythemia is of the secondary type, treatment of the primary disease state may control the polycythemia and, therefore, control the headache. Often, however, the underlying disease is not easily treated. Simple analgesics can be useful, but vasoconstricting agents should not be used and narcotics should be avoided.

Leukemia

Neurologic symptoms frequently occur with leukemic involvement of the central nervous system. Acute or chronic leukemia may involve the central nervous system in several ways, so that the etiology of symptoms may be quite different.

Etiology. Hemorrhage, both parenchymal and subarachnoid, occurs most often in granulocytic leukemia whereas meningeal infiltration with leukemic cells is the most frequent central nervous system lesion in lymphocytic leukemia.[26] Meningeal leukemia occurs during complete remission and is more likely to develop in the long-term survivers.[27]

Parenchymal hemorrhage seems to be most related to the level of leukocytosis, with 25% of persons with white cell counts over 50,000 per cubic millimeter having significant parenchymal brain hemorrhage.[26] Blood viscosity may also play a role in the neurologic symptoms and may result in vasodilation because of decreased flow and tissue hypoxia. Thrombocytopenia also plays a role in cerebral, subarachnoid, or subdural hemorrhage. Alterations in the immune mechanim by the disease or by the chemotherapeutic agents may also cause infectious meningitis in leukemia patients and may be a factor in the causation of headache.

Symptomatology. Focal neurologic symptoms and signs frequently occur with leukemic involvement of the central nervous system. Infiltration, hemorrhage, and vascular thrombosis may all play a role in the symptoms. However, symptoms of increased intracranial pressure, such as headache, vomiting, lethargy, and seizures, are more common than the focal symptoms or signs.[26] Headache tends to be diffuse, generalized, and nonthrobbing. There should be no scalp muscle tenderness. The headache rarely is present without other neurologic signs. Fever is usually present.

Diagnosis. The diagnosis is suggested by finding neurologic symptoms and signs in the leukemic patient. Hemorrhages in other areas of the body may be a clue to neurologic involvement. Spinal fluid analysis in meningeal leukemia usually shows pleocytosis, increased protein, increased pressure, and hypoglycorrhachia. Central nervous system involvement may be present when the disease seems to be controlled. Electroencephalographic abnormalities or an abnormal brain scan may be helpful clues as to the central nervous system involvement.

Treatment. If headache is present due to involvement of the brain with leukemia, there is usually extensive involvement and the prognosis is grave. Chemotherapeutic agents, administered systemically or intrathecally may be helpful. Likewise, local brain irradiation may be beneficial in alleviating some of the symptoms. Analgesics and narcotics, if necessary to control pain, are indicated while attempts at treating the underlying disease process are made.

Lymphoma

Infiltration of the brain or meninges by Hodgkin's or non-Hodgkin's lymphoma may cause headache.

Etiology. Distortion of pain-sensitive structures by space-occupying lesions or involvement of cranial nerves by the disease may be the cause of symptoms. Involvement of the skull or cervical vertebrae may also be the source of pain.[28,29] Fever, which often accompanies these diseases with or without infection, may also be a source of headache. Central nervous system infection, along with the lymphomatous process, may also add to the complex etiology of headache.

Symptomatology. If the headache is chiefly due to fever, the pain will be of a vascular nature. The discomfort will be generalized, throbbing, and pounding in character. Intracranial mass lesions will be accompanied by a more persistent pain which will vary with body position and activity. Involvement of the cranial nerves may cause a neuralgic type of pain. Central nervous system lymphomatous involvement is usually manifested by alterations in mental status with confusion, somnolence, personality change, stupor, and coma. Focal neurologic and multiple cranial nerve findings are common.[29]

Diagnosis. Abnormal cells in the cerebrospinal fluid may be present with central nervous system lymphoma. Low cerebrospinal fluid glucose and elevated protein values are common. The brain scan, electroencephalogram, and skull films are frequently abnormal. Bone marrow involvement is almost always present in patients with central nervous system involvement by lymphoma.[29]

Treatment. Aggressive therapy with chemotherapeutic agents used intrathecally and radiation may control central nervous system lymphoma. The headache should be treated with nonnarcotic analgesics and the fever, if present, should be treated.

SUMMARY

Symptoms and signs

Anemia
1. Hypoxia
2. Vascular dilation
3. Diffuse throbbing

Leukemia, lymphoma
1. Fever
2. Generalized headache, related to position and activity
3. Neurologic symptoms and signs common
4. Hemorrhages common

Treatment

1. Restoration of the blood count to normal
2. Treatment of the cause of anemia
3. Chemotherapeutic agents
4. Irradiation
5. Analgesics

COLLAGEN VASCULAR DISEASE AND HEADACHE

Many disorders which have been grouped in the broad category of collagen vascular disease are associated with inflammatory involvement of blood vessels. The term "connective tissue disease" has been used to describe many of the same conditions which involve many different tissues and organ systems and are often associated with a vasculitis. It is believed that immune complex injury may account for the vasculitis, as well as the underlying disease process in these conditions. Diseases in this category include giant cell (temporal) arteritis, periarteritis nodosa, rheumatoid arthritis, scleroderma, dermatomyositis, polymyositis, allergic vasculitis, and systemic lupus erythematosus. Temporal arteritis, discussed elsewhere in detail, has been shown to be an immune disorder.[30]

Etiology. The most frequent cause of headache in this group of diseases is the vascular injury that occurs as part of a vasculitis. Release of vasoactive substances such as histamine, serotonin, kinins, prostaglandins, heparin, and perhaps others leads to inflammatory changes in the vessels and increased vascular permeability. Many of these same substances have recently been extensively studied and implicated as playing a major role in the migraine syndrome.[31]

Small cerebral vessels have no perivascular nerves and are probably in themselves not the cause of painful sensations. Inflammatory changes with edema and structural damage or distortion of surrounding tissues may be a factor. In a study of patients with systemic lupus erythematosus, which affects primarily small vessels, no association between headache complaints and disease activity, unless neurologic symptoms were present, could be demonstrated.[32] Periarteritis nodosa and giant cell arteritis, which affect larger arteries, are often associated with headache. Other factors which play a role in the causation of vascular type headaches in any of these conditions are hypertension, which often occurs in these conditions, and fever, also a common finding when any of these diseases are active.

Muscle contraction type headaches may be present with or without a vascular component in polymyalgia rheumatica, which is often associated with giant cell arteritis. Polymyositis may also be associated with a muscle contraction type headache. Of course, muscle ischemia secondary to vascular insufficiency, occurring with the vasculitis of any of these conditions, may be the source of a more steady and constant pain in the scalp or neck muscles. The tightening of the scalp in scleroderma may be a factor in the headache found in this condition.

Symptomatology. The headache in any of the disorders of the collagen vascular group is nonspecific. Vascular involvement is usually believed to be present and the pain usually is a pulsatile, throbbing sensation. It tends to be constant and unremitting but may be intermittent, similar to attacks of migraine. Factors which affect vascular headaches, such as the Valsalva maneuver and activity, will aggravate this type of headache. There will be symptoms of other organ involvement. Fever, weight loss, fatigue, malaise, arthralgias, myalgias, and other systemic symptoms will likely be present. Focal neurologic deficits may be present from cerebrovascular involvement. With an active vasculitis, skin lesions may be present and offer a clue to the underlying disorder.

Muscle contraction headache with constant tightness and pressure sensation may also be present in some of these conditions. Tenderness of the scalp muscles and blood vessels may be present. Painful neck and shoulder motion may also be found.

Raynaud's phenomenon has been described in almost all of the collagen vascular diseases. An association between Raynaud's phenomenon and migraine has also been noted.[14]

Diagnosis. Recent onset of headache, along with various systemic symptoms, should suggest the presence of one of these conditions. The diagnosis of any of these diseases may be difficult. Laboratory tests reflecting acute inflammation will be elevated during activity of the disease. Some specific tests like the L.E. test, antinuclear factor, and muscle enzymes may be helpful. Muscle biopsy with examination of the muscles and blood vessels may give typical findings in certain diseases. Often there is overlap among the various conditions and one can only diagnose the condition as a mixed connective tissue disease.[33]

Treatment. Treatment of the headache with any of the vasoconstrictive agents should be avoided because of the vascular involvement with inflammation and the danger of promoting ischemia distal to the disease. Simple analgesics or mild narcotics, if necessary, should be used while treatment of the underlying condition is accomplished. Corticosteroids or immunosuppressive agents or both should bring relief from the headache if the underlying condition responds. If hypertension is present, that should also be treated.

SUMMARY

Symptoms and signs

1. Throbbing, pounding
2. Tenderness of the scalp
3. Fever
4. Systemic symptoms
5. Neurologic deficits
6. Skin lesions

Treatment

1. Avoidance of vasoconstrictive drugs
2. Treatment of underlying disorder

CEREBROVASCULAR DISEASE AND HEADACHE

In addition to the inflammatory involvement of the cranial arteries, which is discussed elsewhere, arteriosclerotic involvement of the carotid and basilar artery systems may be associated with headache. Headache is not an uncommon symptom in cerebrovascular disease. It is seen in transient ischemic attacks, whether associated with embolic phenomenon or thrombosis of the internal carotid artery. Completed stroke also is commonly associated with headache, and headache is one of the typical symptoms of carotid artery thrombosis.[1] Headache just before, during, or after a transient ischemic attack has been noted to occur in approximately 45% of patients.[34]

Etiology. The exact etiology of the headache seen in cerebrovascular disease, regardless of the disease process present, is unknown. It has been postulated that dilation of the collateral vessels accounts for the pain present in thrombosis of arteries.[35] It should be remembered, however, that only the larger intracranial vessels are supplied with pain fibers. Inflammatory changes, edema, and hypoxia may also play a role in the headache of ischemia. Intense vascular type headache has been reported to follow carotid endarterectomy.[36]

Symptomatology. The headache of carotid thrombosis or cerebral embolus may occur hours before other neurologic symptoms, or after a completed stroke. It usually is on the same side as the vascular event. It is usually not severe and lasts from a few minutes to several hours. The pain may be pulsatile or a nonspecific pressure type sensation. Recurring headaches of similar type may occur with recurring transient ischemic attacks. Symptoms of transient ischemic attacks, especially if accompanied by headache, may mimic the migraine syndrome. Recurrent attacks of a short headache which precedes, rather than follows, the onset of neurologic symptoms suggest the diagnosis of transient ischemic attacks. With carotid thrombosis, the neurologic symptoms and findings are evident and suggest the diagnosis. Discovery of a carotid bruit on examination in one with the recent onset of headaches should suggest that significant carotid artery disease might be present and warrants further investigation.

Treatment. In the patient with transient ischemic attacks, surgical removal of an ulcerated plaque or an endarterectomy of the stenotic lesion may be indicated. Antithrombotic drugs such as aspirin, dipyridamole, or sulfinpyrazone may be helpful. In the patient with carotid thrombosis, the headache will usually subside in a few days and no further treatment for the headache is necessary. It is very important to make the proper diagnosis of this condition in order that one might avoid using vasoconstrictive agents such as one would use in the vascular headache of the migraine type. Reliance on simple analgesics for pain relief should be the rule while tackling the underlying vascular problem.

SUMMARY

Symptoms and signs

1. Vascular pain
2. Transient neurologic deficits
3. Carotid bruit

Treatment

1. Antithrombotic measures
2. Surgery

CARDIAC DISEASE AND HEADACHE

Headache may be associated with arteriosclerotic heart disease and valvular lesions of the heart. Angina due to arteriosclerotic heart disease may be manifested as pain in the face, jaw, or neck. Occasionally, patients with angina present to the dentist because of recurring jaw pain.

Ischemic heart disease

Etiology. The etiology of this type of pain is myocardial ischemia, with referral of pain to the neck and face.

Symptomatology. The pain may be of a burning, pressure, or aching quality. It typically will occur with exertion and ease with rest. Occasionally, it will occur at night without exertion, but one should also get the history of a direct correlation with exertion. The pain typically is worse with exertion in cold temperatures. Diaphoresis, nausea, and breathlessness are often symptoms which accompany the anginal pain. The pain may be located in the jaw, neck, shoulder, back, or arm, with or without pain in the typical anterior chest location.

Diagnosis. The diagnosis is made strictly from the typical history relating the pain to exertion. Electrocardiographic evidence of ischemic heart disease will be helpful in arriving at the diagnosis. Stress testing and coronary angiography may be necessary to confirm the diagnosis.

Treatment. Treatment consists of the use of vasodilators and avoiding precipitating factors. Exercise and other exertion that causes pain should be avoided. Coronary artery surgery may be indicated. Vasodilating drugs used for angina may in themselves cause a vascular type of headache and aggravate migraine. Propranolol might be a very useful addition if vasodilator drugs induce headache.

Valvular heart disease

Aortic insufficiency may be associated with vascular headaches and neck pain.

Etiology. The etiology is unknown, but presumably in susceptible persons, the thrust of a large volume of blood throughout the carotid arteries causes the pulsatile discomfort because of stretching of the carotid sheath. Pharyngitis with inflammation of cervical lymph nodes may also play a role in the carotid tenderness and discomfort.

Symptomatology. In a study of a large number of patients with aortic insufficiency, carotid artery tenderness and pain were present transiently in several patients.[37] Throbbing sensations in the head, abdomen, and neck were also common. The pain seems to be intermittently present.

Diagnosis. The typical murmur of aortic insufficiency, along with a wide pulse pressure, should suggest the diagnosis if other factors have been excluded. Tenderness over the carotid arteries is often demonstrated.

Treatment. Simple analgesics or mild narcotics for the painful discomfort may be necessary. The pain may continue even after aortic valve surgery corrects the insufficiency.

Bacterial endocarditis

Headache is a common symptom of subacute bacterial endocarditis.

Etiology. The etiology of headache in bacterial endocarditis may be due to the arteritis that develops from septic emboli or the embolic phenomenon itself, or the headache may be merely a manifestation of the fever accompanying this disease. When headache is the only neurologic symptom of subacute bacterial endocarditis, there seems to be a temporal relationship to fever.[38]

Symptomatology. The headaches in patients with subacute bacterial endocarditis are vascular in origin and usually of a pulsating character. It is generalized rather than unilateral in location. Fever is almost always present. Focal neurologic deficits due to ischemia may also be present.

Diagnosis. The diagnosis depends on suspicion of the condition. The presence of a heart murmur, fever, anemia, and peripheral signs of embolic phenomenon are characteristic. The diagnosis is confirmed by positive blood cultures.

Treatment. The headache can be treated with simple analgesics until the infection is controlled. Vasoconstrictive agents should, of course, be avoided.

RENAL DISEASE AND HEADACHE

Acute and chronic renal disease can be associated with headache. Chronic renal failure with azotemia may or may not be associated with accelerated or malignant hypertension. Malignant hypertension is discussed elsewhere.

Acute glomerulonephritis

Etiology. Headache is frequently a symptom of acute glomerulonephritis. The infec-

tion preceding the nephritis may be a cause of the headache. Acute hypertension may also play a role in the headache. Electrolyte abnormalities and fluid retention, if present, may be contributing factors.

Symptomatology. The headache tends to be generalized and pulsatile and is usually constant, rather than intermittent and unilateral as seen in migraine. If fluid retention is extreme and there is acute renal failure, the headache may become more of a constant and steady pressure due to cerebral edema. Other symptoms of acute renal disease such as edema, nausea, and malaise may be present.

Diagnosis. Recent onset of headache suggests an underlying disease. Pharyngitis with continuing malaise and edema would suggest that glomerulonephritis might be present. Glomerulonephritis can be diagnosed by typical urinary findings and renal biopsy. The headache accompanying the disease as noted is quite nonspecific.

Treatment. The headache itself should be treated with simple analgesics. Treatment of high blood pressure, if present, will be helpful. Treatment of the glomerulonephritis should reduce the blood pressure and result in easing of the headache.

Chronic renal disease

Etiology. Chronic renal failure may be due to glomerulonephritis, pyelonephritis, nephrosclerosis, or a manifestation of some systemic disorder such as an arteritis or amyloidosis. The brain itself may be directly affected by a systemic disease which also affects the kidneys. The headache and other neurologic symptoms may, therefore, be due to the underlying disease and not a complication of the renal involvement. No matter what the etiology of the primary renal disease, the neurologic symptoms of chronic renal failure with azotemia are similar.[39] Electrolyte abnormalities and azotemia undoubtedly play a role in the neurologic symptoms of chronic renal disease. The headache itself is probably mainly due to cerebral edema.[1]

Symptomatology. The headache in persons with renal failure and azotemia tends to be a rather steady, constant pressure type sensation. It is generalized and not localized. It is not usually influenced by activity or position. Meningeal signs such as nuchal rigidity and Kernig's sign are not uncommon in uremic states.[40] Other symptoms of cerebral dysfunction occur as the condition progresses. Alterations in alertness, mental clouding, confusion, and delirium may occur as the condition worsens. Hypertension is usually present and may play an additional role in the causation of headache.

Diagnosis. The diagnosis is made with the findings of mental abnormalities and the demonstration of decreased renal function with azotemia and electrolyte abnormalities. With chronic renal failure, anemia usually is present and may be another factor in the causation of cerebral symptoms, including headache.

Treatment. Correction of the electrolyte abnormalities and treatment of azotemia with fluids and low protein intake may be helpful in improving the cerebral symptoms. Hypertension should also be treated. Diuretic agents and hyperosmolar solutions, such as mannitol, may reduce the cerebral edema and thereby ease the headache. In the appropriate case, renal transplantation may be indicated. The headache itself should be treated with simple analgesics. Since the underlying condition is chronic, avoidance of narcotics, if at all possible, is indicated. In the event of severe renal failure, dosages of analgesics may have to be reduced.

ELECTROLYTE DISORDERS AND HYPOXIA
Electrolyte abnormalities

Electrolyte disturbances may be associated with headache and other cerebral symptoms. The electrolyte imbalance may be the result of excessive intake, retention, or excessive loss. Many acute and chronic diseases are associated with electrolyte abnormalities.

Etiology. Hyponatremia causes chronic headache, probably secondary to cerebral edema.[41] Likewise, states of dehydration or excessive loss of electrolytes by way of diarrhea, vomiting, fistulas, or injury may be associated with headache. Fever, often associated with systemic illnesses and electrolyte abnormalities, undoubtedly contributes to the headache often seen in disorders of electrolyte imbalance.

Symptomatology. The headache will be quite variable but usually of a steady nature because of the cerebral edema. If fever is present, the pain may take on a vascular character. Symptoms of mental dysfunction such as confusion, lethargy, and altered state of consciousness may also be present. Edema and low hematocrit secondary to fluid retention may be present and may be an additional factor in the causation of headache.

Diagnosis. Serum electrolytes should be routinely checked on anyone with headache. They are often clues to an underlying disease state.

Treatment. Treatment consists of correction of the abnormal electrolyte levels and treatment of the underlying disease. The type and source of fluid loss should be used as guidelines in fluid replacement.

Hypoxic states

Cerebral hypoxia, whatever the etiology, is a frequent cause of headache. Carbon dioxide elevation also causes vascular dilation and headaches. Carbon dioxide retention occurs in many conditions which are also associated with hypoxia.

Etiology. Carbon dioxide retention in the blood causes vascular dilation of cranial vessels. Chronic pulmonary insufficiency causes both hypoxia and carbon dioxide retention, a potent combination as far as causing headaches is concerned. High altitude exposure before acclimatization is also associated with hypoxia and frequent headaches. Secondary polycythemia occurring in those living in high altitudes with decreased oxygen available also plays a role in the headache. Restrictive ventilation from other pulmonary disease or massive obesity can also be the cause of carbon dioxide retention.

Symptomatology. The headache of hypoxia is of the pulsatile, throbbing type, characteristic of vascular dilation. It is a generalized pain. The headache tends to be daily and rather constant. Other symptoms of hypoxia, such as lethargy, tremor, and impairment of consciousness, may be present. Dyspnea and cyanosis secondary to chronic pulmonary disease may also be evident. Headache secondary to obesity and restrictive pulmonary disease may be worse in the early morning because of hypoventilation and carbon dioxide retention during sleep.

Diagnosis. Laboratory studies will show a low oxygen saturation and high carbon dioxide content. Secondary polycythemia may also be present in chronic pulmonary disease and exposure to high altitudes. Pulmonary function studies may show obstructive changes or findings suggestive of restriction with hypoventilation.

Treatment. Treatment consists of improving pulmonary function. Bronchodilators, intermittent positive pressure breathing, and antibiotics may be indicated. Phlebotomy may be helpful if polycythemia is present. Oxygen should be given cautiously, if at all, because of the danger of eliminating the hypoxia which is stimulating the respiratory center. Adaptation to high altitudes or returning to lower altitudes may be helpful in cases where this plays a role.

HEADACHE CAUSED BY EXPOSURE TO CHEMICAL AGENTS AND TOXINS

Many agents inhaled or ingested will cause headache in susceptible persons. The etiology of the headache is usually vascular and may be due to hypoxia or direct vascular dilation.

Carbon monoxide poisoning

Carbon monoxide poisoning causes many deaths yearly. Chronic exposure to carbon monoxide may be a source of chronic headache. Automobile exhausts, poorly ventilated furnaces and other heat-ing devices, and industrial exposure are common sources of carbon monoxide.

Etiology. The cause of headache in carbon monoxide poisoning is hypoxia. Carbon monoxide binds to hemoglobin with an affinity of 250 times that of oxygen. It displaces oxygen from the hemoglobin molecule and also interferes with release of oxygen from hemoglobin at the tissue level. Cerebral edema and focal hemorrhagic lesions also are common.[42]

Symptomatology. Headache is an early and common symptom of carbon monoxide poisoning. It is diffuse, nonlocalized, and constant. It may be throbbing or of a steady aching character. Dizziness, nausea, weakness, muscular irritability, mental clouding, confusion, and coma are other common symptoms. Focal neurologic findings may be present. It is believed that chronic neurologic and perhaps cardiac deficits may exist after treatment of the acute episode if exposure to carbon monoxide has been of some duration.[42]

Diagnosis. History of exposure and symptoms suggest the diagnosis. The carbon monoxide level in the blood will be high. Arterial blood gases may be misleading because oxygen tension may be near normal since the carbon monoxide impedes release of oxygen from the hemoglobin.[43]

Treatment. Immediate use of 100% oxygen is indicated and should be continued until the carbon monoxide level is below 5%. Occasionally, positive pressure by respirator is necessary, and, if available, hyperbaric oxygenation is very useful. The headache will ease as the carbon monoxide is removed, but neurologic residuals may remain.

Nitrites and monosodium glutamate

Exposure to nitrites causes vascular dilation, and in susceptible individuals it will cause headache. Nitroglycerin and nitrates used for ischemic heart disease are well-known causes of severe throbbing headaches in certain persons and may actually be intolerable. Persons working in the manufacture of dynamite regularly suffer from headaches.[44] The nitrite is absorbed through the skin. Nitrites used as food coloring and as preservatives in processed meats such as frankfurters, bacon, cold cuts, and ham have been shown to cause vascular headaches in certain persons. The "Chinese restaurant syndrome" has been shown to be due to sensitivity to monosodium glutamate used in the preparation of Chinese and other Oriental foods.[45]

Etiology. Although the exact etiology of the headache due to nitrite and monosodium glutamate exposure is unknown, the headache secondary to dynamite exposure is most certainly due to vasodilation. Vasodilation probably is the most significant factor in the headache due to nitrite ingestion, but the exact biochemical changes involved have not been worked out.[45,46] The symptoms produced by monosodium glutamate seem to be related to the amount ingested and occur only in certain susceptible individuals.

Symptomatology. The headache of nitrite exposure is a pulsatile, throbbing type of headache, usually bilateral, and may be accompanied by facial flushing. Sensitivity to monosodium glutamate may cause several different types of symptoms. It may cause a burning sensation in the chest, spreading to the neck, shoulders, arms, and abdomen; throbbing and pressure in the frontal and malar areas; or a pressure sensation in the chest.[45] The symptoms last 30 to 60 minutes and usually begin 15 to 30 minutes after oral ingestion of monosodium glutamate. The symptoms are quite suggestive of the paroxysmal attack seen in pheochromocytoma except hypertension is absent. Nausea is also absent.

Diagnosis. The diagnosis of sensitivity to nitrite or monosodium glutamate depends entirely on the history of ingestion of the offending agent prior to the onset of symptoms. The sufferer may or may not have had vascular headaches previously.

Treatment. Once the etiology of the headache is recognized, the cure of the condition is avoiding exposure. Amphetamines and caffeine have been suggested as helpful in controlling the nitrite headache due to dynamite exposure.[44]

Lead poisoning

Headache may be part of the clinical spectrum seen in lead encephalopathy, although seizures and mental aberrations are much more common.

Etiology. Exposure to lead in industry, by pica, or, as now frequently seen, by ingestion of moonshine leads to chronic encephalopathy. Cerebral edema is the prominent pathologic picture. Anemia is commonly present also.[47]

Symptomatology. Headache, diffuse or localized, but nonthrobbing, may accompany the neurologic symptoms. Seizures, focal or generalized, are common. The anemia may be severe and be the cause of fatigue. Confusion, hypertension, and azotemia are also common symptoms.

Diagnosis. Basophilic stippling of the erythrocytes may be spotted in the peripheral blood smear. Elevated levels of urinary lead, especially after intravenous EDTA, are diagnostic of lead intoxication.

Treatment. Removal of lead by the use of chelating agents is the treatment of choice. Elimination of exposure will hopefully prevent recurrence. The headache itself should be treated with mild analgesics, and because of the mental symptoms, narcotics or sedatives should be avoided if possible.

Other chemically induced headaches

Methemoglobinemia and sulfhemoglobinemia, which may develop from excessive amounts of acetanilid, sulfonamides, aniline compounds, nitrates, and phenacetin, may cause headache because of cerebral hypoxia secondary to the abnormal hemoglobin. Acute poisoning from carbon tetrachloride, benzine, arsenic, and anticholinesterase insecticides may cause headache.

Many drugs will cause headache. Some of the more common are the nitrates, hydralazine, papaverine, chlorpromazine (Thorazine), and clofibrate (Atromid-S), which cause headache because of vasodilation. Reserpine, probably because of serotonin depletion, may also cause chronic vascular headache. Indomethacin may aggravate or cause a vascular headache. Its probable mode of action is in causing vasoconstriction, which is then followed by a rebound vasodilatory phenomenon in a few hours.

GYNECOLOGIC HEADACHE

Headaches are frequently associated with the menstrual cycle. There is no specific type of headache that is related to the menstrual cycle, though migraine seems to be most commonly associated with the menstruating female. Muscle contraction and psychogenic headaches, however, may also occur in relation to the menstrual cycle. There are also some women who begin to have headaches at the time of menopause for the first time in their life. Many women thus present themselves to the gynecologist because of the apparent relationship of their headaches to the menstrual cycle.

Premenstrual and menstrual headache

Etiology. Many factors are involved in the headaches associated with the menstrual cycle. Muscle contraction, psychogenic, and migraine headaches may all be related.[48] Fluid retention undoubtedly plays a role in exacerbation of menstrual migraine and is associated with the premenstrual tension syndrome in which muscle contraction headache is also a prevalent symptom. It is believed that a disproportion between estrogen and progesterone levels underlies the fluid retention associated with the menstrual cycle.[49] Sodium retention secondary to estrogen is a prominent feature associated with the fluid retention. Fluid retention in muscles and even cerebral edema may cause the headache seen with premenstrual fluid retention. Psychogenic factors associated with the menstrual cycle, sexual problems, and pregnancy may be of paramount importance in the causation of headache associated with the menstrual cycle.

It has been found that falling estrogen levels in the immediate premenstrual period is probably the major triggering mechanism in inducing migraine headaches at the time of menses.[50] In those experiments, it was possible to postpone the onset of a migraine attack by giving exogenous estrogens. The migraine occurred when the estrogen support was withdrawn.

Symptomatology. Headaches associated with the menstrual cycle are often of the typical migraine type, either classic or common, and occur regularly just prior to the onset of the period or during the actual flow. Migraine may also occur midcycle at the time of ovulation. Any or all of the typical migraine symptom complex may be present. Generalized vascular headache without localization or nausea and vomiting, such as seen in the typical migraine attack, may be present. Very often, the migraine seen with menses will disappear during pregnancy, only to return following delivery. Typical migraine occurring with menstrual periods often subsides with menopause.

Muscle contraction headache may also occur on a regular periodic basis associated with the menstrual period. Premenstrual tension symptoms, such as irritability, weight gain, abdominal distention, and breast engorgement, seem to be more prevalent in the woman with menstrually related headaches, whether of the migrainous or muscle contraction type. Typical muscle contraction headache with tightness and stiffness in the neck and the feeling of a tight constricted band around the head may be associated with the anxiety and irritability accompanying the menstrual period.

Diagnosis. The classification of any headache as menstrually related depends on the history of headache occurring with menses or at midcycle on a regular, periodic basis. The type of headache is diagnosed according to the symptoms present and the characteristics of the headache. Menstrual migraine is a typical migraine headache occurring in association with the menstrual period. A typical muscle contraction headache or headaches on a purely psychologic basis may also be diagnosed according to the symptoms present.

Treatment. If weight gain and fluid retention are prominent features, sodium restriction and diuretic therapy may lessen the intensity of the headache, whether of the muscle contraction or migraine type. Diuresis and fluid restriction alone usually do not alleviate the headaches completely, but may modify the severity of the symptoms. The other symptoms of fluid retention will also be lessened. Vasoconstrictive agents, such as ergotamine tartrate, may be used in the treatment of menstrual migraine. Sometimes prophylactic medications for migraine can be used intermittently at the time of menses in an effort to prevent the periodic occurrence of menstrual migraine. Since the medication would be used intermittently, one need not fear using short intermittent courses of methysergide or powerful prophylactic drugs. Regular periodic migraine attacks can often be completely prevented by the intermittent use of one of these prophylactic agents such as methysergide, propranolol, cyproheptadine, or even ergotamine tartrate on a regular daily basis for a short time.

Analgesics may be helpful in any of these menstrual headaches. Relaxants and tranquilizers on a regular or intermittent basis may be beneficial. Progesterone used for a few days prior to menses may reduce many of the symptoms including headache associated with the premenstrual tension syndrome.[49] Androgens have also been shown to markedly reduce the premenstrual symptoms. Psychotherapy may be indicated in certain persons with severe emotional problems related to menses. Hysterectomy or oophorectomy, which have been performed in the past in an effort to control migraine, are not helpful and are no longer recommended as measures to control the menstrual migraine headache.

Menopausal headache

A few women begin having recurring headaches when they go through menopause. They have not had a problem with headaches previously.

Etiology. Vasomotor instability with hot flushes, palpitations, sweats, and headache may be related to estrogenic deficiency. Anxiety and depression are also important factors in the menopausal headache and other menopausal symptoms.

Symptomatology. The vasomotor symptoms of menopause are present along with the headache. Many of these women never have had problems with headaches in prior years. The headache may be a throbbing vascular type of headache, either localized or generalized, or may be a more constant steady pressure type sensation such as seen in the depressed patient. Early morning awakening typical of depression is common. Profuse sweating, flushing, and warmth are common menopausal symptoms.

Diagnosis. Onset of headache, whether vascular, tension, or psychogenic in origin, during the menopausal time can be labeled as a menopausal headache. There is no characteristic type of menopausal headache.

Treatment. Addition of estrogens, which so often aggravate migraine, may be very beneficial in the woman with menopausal headache and may control the other vasomotor symptoms. Estrogen should be cycled. They should be taken for 3 weeks and then stopped for 1 week on a regularly monthly schedule to avoid stimulation of the endometrium. Sometimes testosterone in small doses will also be beneficial. Tranquilizers as well as psychologic help and support can be very beneficial to women with menopausal symptoms. If the headache is quite typically vascular or migrainous, the usual migraine medications should be tried.

SUMMARY

Symptoms and signs

1. Vascular, muscle contraction, or psychogenic headaches, associated with menstrual period
2. Fluid retention
3. Irritability
4. Relief during pregnancy
5. Relief with menopause

Treatment

1. Diuretics
2. Fluid restriction
3. Ergotamine
4. Tranquilizers
5. Analgesics

BONE DISEASE AND HEADACHE

Any disease of the bone which affects the skull or upper cervical region may cause headaches. Bone diseases are not a common cause of headache, however.

Etiology. Some bony conditions involving the skull are Paget's disease (osteitis deformans), fibrous dysplasia, eosinophilic granuloma, multiple myeloma, hyperostosis frontalis interna, oxycephaly, and the various lymphomas. Any of these bony abnormalities may at times be associated with headache. Many are found incidentally when skull films are taken as part of the headache workup and their importance in the causation of headache is uncertain. Some are manifestations of other conditions such as malignancies and some are developmental abnormalities. The etiology of headache is usually displacement of cranial structures or compression of cranial nerves.

Symptomatology. Headache may or may not be associated with any of the bony conditions discussed. The malignant diseases such as myeloma, lymphoma, and eosinophilic granuloma are usually manifested by localized pain and tenderness over the specific area of involvement and the bony defect.

Paget's disease, the most common of these conditions, may cause symptoms by compression of intracranial content or nerve roots. The headache associated with Paget's disease, therefore, may be constant and aching, or have more of the characteristics of a neuritic type of pain. Cranial nerve palsies often occur. Deafness due to compression of the auditory nerves is common.[1] Fibrous dysplasia may be indistinguishable from Paget's disease on x-ray or by symptoms. Oxycephaly due to premature closure of sutures is often accompanied by a low-grade steady headache with papilledema due to increased intracranial pressure.

Diagnosis. The diagnosis of these various bony conditions may be suggested by the typical appearance on x-rays of the skull. A biopsy may be needed to determine the exact etiology of a lytic lesion seen on the x-rays. Paget's disease, multiple myeloma, and hyperostosis frontalis interna may be diagnosed by their x-ray appearance. The alkaline phosphatase is usually elevated in Paget's disease. Anemia may be present in some of the neoplastic conditions.

Treatment. The neoplastic skull lesions are treated by surgical excision, radiation, or chemotherapy. Paget's disease, if symptomatic, may be treated with calcitonin or cytotoxic drugs. Occasionally, decompression of nerves that are compressed by the bony overgrowth in Paget's disease or fibrous dysplasia may relieve the pain. In oxycephaly, decompression may be needed to alleviate the intracranial pressure.

GASTROINTESTINAL DISEASE AND HEADACHE

Bilious headache is a term that has been used in the past. Over the years, many causes of migraine have been postulated. Gallbladder disease, probably because of the severe nausea and vomiting accompanying migraine, has been implicated as a cause of migraine. In the past, cholecystectomy, like hysterectomy, has been performed in an effort to alleviate headaches. Neither operation is indicated and has no scientific basis in controlling headaches.

Inflammatory bowel disease

Inflammatory bowel disease such as regional ileitis or ulcerative colitis may be associated with headache. Both of these conditions are accompanied by fever and persons with these diseases are often quite toxic. This may be the cause of a vascular type of headache. It should be remembered that severe emotional problems are prevalent in persons with chronic inflammatory bowel disease, and these emotional problems may in turn be the actual cause of the headache accompanying such diseases.

Constipation

Headache is quite a common symptom in persons who have chronic constipation.

Etiology. It is unclear whether the headache of chronic constipation is due to fecal retention, which may result in absorption of toxic substances, or is due to reflexes initiating in the distended colon. It is known that bladder distention in persons with spinal cord lesions may cause acute rises in blood pressure resulting in a vascular headache.[1] Chronic constipation and other gastrointestinal symptoms are commonly seen in persons with emotional problems and nervous tension. Straining, by increasing intracranial pressure, may cause headache of a vascular type.

Symptomatology. The headache of constipation is a generalized throbbing pain which is worse with straining, bending, stooping, coughing, or sneezing. Fatigue, malaise, and abdominal discomfort are usually common symptoms occurring in the person with chronic constipation. Visual or neurologic symptoms such as seen in migraine are absent. The headache tends to be of low-grade intensity and is not disabling.

Treatment. Treatment consists of adequate hydration, stool softeners, or laxatives to combat constipation. Establishment of regular bowel habits should be attempted. Emotional problems should be treated with either psychotherapy or medications and psychotherapy. The headache itself should be treated with mild analgesics. Narcotics of any kind should be avoided. Antidepressant medications, which are so commonly used for treatment of emotional disorders, very often will cause constipation and aggravate chronic constipation. This often becomes a difficult problem in bowel management.

DIALYSIS HEADACHE

Headaches occur quite frequently in association with hemodialysis for chronic renal disease. Most of the work in this field has been done by Dr. John Graham and his associates in Boston.[51-53] Approximately 70% of patients undergoing dialysis have headache during the actual dialysis procedure.[52] Dialysis headache is considered here as a separate entity because it involves several factors such as chronic renal disease, electrolyte abnormalities, fluid abnormalities, and emotional factors.

Etiology. The exact cause of the headache occurring during hemodialysis is unknown. There seems to be a correlation between the headache occurring and the decrease in serum sodium during dialysis, but there are likely many other factors involved.[53] Low renin levels have also been found in persons who are experiencing headache during the hemodialysis procedure.[51] Altering the duration of dialysis and the concentration of the dialysis bath does not seem to affect the headache. The alteration in the blood urea level likewise apparently does not play a major role in the causation of headache during hemodialysis.

Since there are so many changes occurring in the electrolytes, blood urea, and other substances, as well as the movement of fluid in and out of the vascular space during dialysis, it would be very difficult to pinpoint any one specific cause of the headache. Elaboration of various vasoactive substances by the kidney has been postulated as important in the causation of the dialysis headache.[53]

Symptomatology. Persons with migraine are prone to have migraine attacks during dialysis. These may be very typical migraine headaches with unilateral throbbing pain accompanied with nausea and vomiting. They may also have a generalized vascular type headache. Nonmigraineurs also frequently have a vascular type of headache with bilateral throbbing pains in the temples occurring after being on the artificial kidney for a few hours. Nausea and vomiting may also accompany these vascular headaches. The headaches tend to occur at approximately the same time during each dialysis cycle and usually diminish a few hours after completion of dialysis. Muscle contraction headaches due to acute anxiety and generalized emotional upset also occur with increased frequency during the dialysis cycle.[53] Depression undoubtedly also plays a large role in the causation of headaches in one undergoing dialysis, but the headache due to depression will be more a persistent headache, occurring daily, even on days when the patient is not undergoing dialysis.

Diagnosis. The occurrence of headache during the period of dialysis, whether present prior to renal failure or not, suggests that the dialysis procedure itself is related to the etiology of the headache. One can be quite certain that the dialysis procedure is related to the headache when the headache occurs at approximately the same time during each dialysis cycle. The term "dialysis headache" should be restricted to those headaches occurring during the actual dialysis procedure and not be used to describe the chronic headache in the depressed patient with renal failure who is undergoing dialysis.

Treatment. Changing the concentration of the sodium in the dialysis fluid may affect the severity of the headache.[53] The speed of fluid exchange does not seem to influence the development of headache, nor does the blood urea concentration.

The patient should be treated with medication prior to the time of onset of the headache; this will often lessen the severity of the pain. Analgesics taken prior to the onset of the headache may reduce the intensity of the headache. Ergotamine taken prior to the onset of migraine or other vascular headaches may also control the headache. The ultimate treatment of this type of headache, of course, would be nephrectomy with renal transplantation. This will eliminate the need for dialysis and reduce the frequency of headache. After nephrectomy many persons are taking immunosuppressive drugs and corticosteroids, which in themselves will dampen the intensity of vascular headaches.

REFERENCES

1. Dalessio, D. J.: Wolff's headache and other head pain, ed. 3, New York, 1972, Oxford University Press.
2. Merritt, H. H.: A textbook of neurology, ed. 5, Philadelphia, 1973, Lea & Febiger.
3. Meyer, H. M., Johnson, R. T., Crawford, I. P., Dascomb, H. E., and Rogers, N. G.: Central nervous system syndromes of "viral" etiology, Am. J. Med. 29:334, 1960.
4. Parnes, L.: Headache rounds, return of an old imposter, Headache 15:111, 1975.
5. Wilkinson, C. F.: Recurrent migrainoid headaches associated with spontaneous hypoglycemia, Am. J. Med. Sci. 218:209, 1949.
6. Chandalia, H. B., and Boshell, B. R.: Hypoglycemia associated with extrapancreatic tumors, Arch. Intern. Med. 129:447, 1972.
7. Graham, J. R.: The natural history of migraine: some observations and a hypothesis, Trans. Am. Clin. Climat. Assoc. 4:1, 1952.
8. Sicuteri, F.: Migraine, a central biochemical dysnociception, Headache 16:145, 1976.
9. Kunkel, R. S., and Black, A. V.: Pituitary tumor and myalgia, Cleve. Clin. 43:17, 1976.
10. Karpati, G., and Frame, B.: Neuropsychiatric disorders in primary hyperparathyroidism, Arch. Neurol. 10:387, 1964.
11. Clarke, E., and Murphy, E. A.: Neurological manifestations of malignant hypertension, Br. Med. J. 2:1319, 1956.
12. Editorial: Headache and blood pressure, Lancet 1:896, 1976.
13. Sutherland, A. M., and Wolff, H. G.: Experimental studies on headache: further analysis of the mechanism of headache in migraine, hypertension and fever, Arch. Neurol. Psychiatr. 44:929, 1940.
14. Graham, J. R.: Headache related to medical disorders. In Appenzeller, O., editor: Pathogenesis and treatment of headache, New York, 1976, Spectrum Publications, Inc.
15. Hinsdale, H. B.: Headache in vascular disease and hypertension, Headache 13:85, 1973.
16. Walker, C. H.: Migraine and its relationship to hypertension, Br. Med. J. 2:1430, 1959.
17. Blanchard, E. B., and Young, L. D.: Clinical applications of biofeedback training, Arch. Gen. Psychiatr. 30:573, 1974.
18. Paulson, G. W., and Klawans, H. L.: Benign orgasmic cephalgia, Headache 13:181, 1974.
19. Diamond, S.: Exertional headache, J.A.M.A. 237:580, 1977.
20. Kirkendall, W. M., Leichty, R. D., and Culp, D. A.: Diagnosis and treatment of patients with pheochromocytoma, Arch. Intern. Med. 115:529, 1965.
21. Thomas, J. E., Rooke, E. D., and Kvale, W. F.: A neurologist experience with pheochromocytoma, J.A.M.A. 197:100, 1966.

22. Byrom, F. B.: The pathogenesis of hypertensive encephalopathy and its relation to the malignant phase of hypertension, Lancet **2:**201, 1954.

23. Kincaid-Smith, P., McMichael, J., and Murphy, E. A.: The clinical course and pathology of hypertension with papilloedema (malignant hypertension), Q. J. Med. **27:**117, 1958.

24. Silverstein, A., Gilbert, H., and Wasserman, L. R.: Neurological complications of polycythemia, Ann. Intern. Med. **57:**909, 1962.

25. Williams, W. J., Beutler, E., Erslev, A. J., and Rundles, R. W.: Hematology, New York, 1972, McGraw-Hill Book Co., p. 205.

26. Phair, J. P., Anderson, R. E., and Nanuki, H.: The central nervous system in leukemia, Ann. Intern. Med. **61:**863, 1964.

27. Schwartz, J. H., Canello, J. P., Young, R. C., and DeVita, V. T., Jr.: Meningeal leukemia in the blastic phase of chronic granulocytic leukemia, Am. J. Med. **59:**819, 1975.

28. Bunn, P. A., Schein, P. S., Banks, D. M., and DeVita, V. T., Jr.: Central nervous system complications in patients with diffuse histiocytic and undifferentiated lymphoma: leukemia revisited, Blood **47:**3, 1976.

29. Fein, S. B., and Newill, V. A.: Cerebral Hodgkin's disease, Am. J. Med. **17:**291, 1954.

30. Dalessio, D. J., and Tan, E. M.: The immunological basis of temporal arteritis, Proceedings of the International Headache Symposium, Basel, Switzerland, 1971, p. 58.

31. Dalessio, D. J.: Vascular permeability and vasoactive substances: their relationship to migraine, Adv. Neurol. **4:**395, 1974.

32. Atkinson, R. A., and Appenzeller, O.: Headache in small vessel disease of the brain: a study of patients with systemic lupus erythematosus, Headache **15:**198, 1975.

33. Mixed connective tissue disease, Bull. Rheum. Dis., **25:**829, 1974.

34. Medina, J. L., Diamond, S., and Rubino, F. A.: Headaches in patients with transient ischemic attacks, Headache **15:**194, 1975.

35. Fisher, C. M.: Headache in cerebrovascular disease. In Viken, P. J., and Bruyn, G. W., editors: Handbook of clinical neurology, Amsterdam, 1968, North-Holland Publishing Co., p. 124.

36. Leviton, A., Caplan, L., and Salzman, E.: Severe headache after carotid endarterectomy, Headache **15:**207, 1975.

37. Harvey, W. P., Segal, J. P., and Hufnagel, C. A.: Unusual clinical features associated with severe aortic insufficiency, Ann. Intern. Med. **47:**27, 1957.

38. Jones, H. R., Siekert, R. G., and Geraci, J. E.: Neurologic manifestations of bacterial endocarditis, Ann. Intern. Med. **71:**21, 1969.

39. Raskin, N. H., and Fishman, R. A.: Neurological disorders in renal failure, N. Engl. J. Med. **294:** 143, 1976.

40. Madonick, M. J., Berke, K., and Schiffer, I.: Pleocytosis and meningeal signs in uremia, Arch. Neurol. Psychiatry. **64:**431, 1950.

41. Maxwell, M. H., and Kleeman, C. R.: Clinical disorders of fluid and electrolyte metabolism, ed. 2, New York, 1972, McGraw-Hill Book Co., p. 635.

42. Beck, H. G., Schulze, W. H., and Suter, G. M.: Carbon monoxide—a domestic hazard, J.A.M.A. **115:**1, 1940.

43. Larkin, J. M., Brahos, G. J., and Moylin, J. A.: Treatment of carbon monoxide poisoning: prognostic factors, J. Trauma **16:**111, 1976.

44. Schwartz, A. M.: The cause, relief, and prevention of headaches arising from contact with dynamite, N. Engl. J. Med. **235:**541, 1946.

45. Schaumburg, H. H., Byck, R., Gerstl, R., and Mashman, J. H.: Monosodium L-glutamate: Its pharmacology and role in the Chinese restaurant syndrome, Science **163:**826, 1969.

46. Henderson, W. R., and Raskin, N. H.: "Hot dog" headache, individual susceptibility to nitrite, Lancet **2:**1162, 1972.

47. Whitfield, C. L., Ch'ien, L. T., and Whitehead, J. D.: Lead encephalopathy in adults, Ann. Intern. Med. **52:**289, 1972.

48. Kashiwagi, T., McClure, J. N., Jr., and Wetzel, R. D.: The menstrual cycle and headache type, Headache **12:**103, 1972.

49. Greene, R., and Dalton, K.: The premenstrual syndrome, Br. Med. J. **1:**1007, 1953.

50. Somerville, B. W.: The influence of progesterone and estradiol upon migraine, Headache **12:**93, 1972.

51. Bana, D. S., and Graham, J. R.: Renin response during hemodialysis headache, Headache **16:**168, 1976.

52. Graham, J. R., and Yap, A. U.: Headache and hemodialysis: natural history and epidemiology, Proceedings of the International Headache Symposium, Elsinore, Denmark, 1971, p. 79.

53. Yap, A. U., and Graham, J. R.: Biochemical changes in patients suffering headache during renal dialysis, Proceedings of the International Headache Symposium, Elsinore, Denmark, 1971, p. 85.

CHAPTER 13

Headache of neurologic origin

NINAN T. MATHEW

INTRACRANIAL PAIN-SENSITIVE STRUCTURES AND MECHANISMS OF HEADACHE

The majority of intracranial structures are insensitive to pain. These include the brain parenchyma, ependymal lining of the ventricles, choroid plexuses and much of the dura and pia-arachnoid covering the convexity of the brain. We owe our present knowledge about the pain-sensitive structures of the head to the work of Ray and Wolff.[1,2] The intracranial pain-sensitive structures include (1) large veins and venous sinuses, (2) dural arteries (anterior and middle meningeal), (3) large arteries at the base of the brain (proximal 20%) leading to and coming from the circle of Willis, (4) the dura in the anterior and posterior fossa and parts of the dura in the middle cranial fossa (those in the vicinity of the middle meningeal artery), (5) the fifth, ninth, and tenth cranial nerves, and (6) the upper cervical nerves. All the structures of the scalp are pain-sensitive.

Innervation of the pain-sensitive structures can be broadly divided in two. Pain from the upper surface of the tentorium and the anterior and middle cranial fossa is transmitted by undefined pathways in the trigeminal nerve. The pain is felt in the frontal, temporal, or anterior parietal areas on the same side. The inferior surface of the tentorium and the whole of the posterior fossa are supplied chiefly by the upper three cervical nerve roots and so refer pain to the upper part of the neck and back of the head. Since the ninth and tenth cranial nerves also supply the posterior fossa, pain may sometimes be referred to the ear or throat. Thus the pain is felt close to its intracranial origin with certain exceptions. A recurrent branch of the trigeminal nerve arises from the ophthalmic division near its origin and supplies the posterior half of the tentorium and the falx. Pain from the posterior half of the sagittal sinus and upper surface of the transverse sinus is felt commonly in the retroorbital region, because of the transmission through this nerve.

The spinal tract and nucleus of the trigeminal nerve play an important part in head and neck pain. Ramifying sensory fibers from the upper three cervical dorsal roots pass through this pathway, and this permits referral of pain from the upper neck to the head and vice versa. Stimulation of the first cervical posterior root constantly gives rise to frontal and dorsal pain in humans.[3] Pain from the lower cervical spine may rarely be referred to frontal and retro-orbital area. The mechanism of this referred pain is not clear. One explanation is that pain may be secondarily produced in the overacting upper neck muscles and then referred anteriorly through the spinal tract and nucleus system of the trigeminal nerve.

A classification of intracranial conditions causing headache is as follows:

A. Meningeal irritation
  1. Subarachnoid hemorrhage
  2. Meningitis
  3. Meningoencephalitis
  4. Postpneumoencephalographic reaction
B. Traction or displacement of intracranial pain-sensitive structures
  1. Space-occupying lesions
    a. Brain tumors, cysts
    b. Brain abscess
    c. Hematomas
      (1) Extradural
      (2) Subdural
      (3) Intracerebral
  2. Increased intracranial pressure
    a. Secondary to space-occupying lesion
    b. Secondary to obstruction of cerebrospinal fluid pathways (hydrocephalus)
    c. Benign intracranial hypertension
  3. Reduced intracranial pressure
    a. After lumbar puncture
    b. After ventriculoatrial and ventriculoperitoneal shunt
    c. Posttraumatic and postsurgical tear of meninges and cerebrospinal fluid leakage
C. Simple intracranial vasodilation
  1. Medications
    a. Nitrites
    b. Histamines
  2. Circulating toxins
    a. Acute infectious febrile illness
    b. Foreign protein reactions
    c. "Hangover" headache
    d. Caffeine withdrawal
  3. Metabolic
    a. Hypoxia
      (1) Chronic pulmonary insufficiency
      (2) High altitude
    b. Hypercapnia
      (1) Chronic pulmonary insufficiency
      (2) Pickwickian syndrome
      (3) Extreme obesity
    c. Hypoglycemia
      (1) Insulin induced
      (2) Spontaneous
  4. Postconcussional
  5. Postconvulsive
  6. Acute cerebrovascular insufficiency—transient ischemic attacks
  7. Acute hypertensive reactions
    a. Acute nephritis
    b. Pheochromocytoma
    c. Tyramine ingestion by a patient taking monoamine oxidase inhibitors
    d. Hypertensive encephalopathy
  8. Headache in hypertensive patients
  9. Cough headache and effort or exertional headache of benign etiology
D. Cranial nerve disorders
  1. Compression of cranial nerves
  2. Trigeminal and glossopharyngeal neuralgia
  3. Extreme stimulation (ice cream headache)

HEADACHE DUE TO CONDITIONS CAUSING MENINGEAL IRRITATION
Subarachnoid hemorrhage

Etiology. The most common cause of subarachnoid hemorrhage is rupture of an intracranial aneurysm. The other common causes include rupture of an arteriovenous malformation, cranial trauma, and bleeding into the subarachnoid space secondary to a spontaneous intracerebral hemorrhage in a hypertensive individual. Blood dyscrasias, hemorrhage from a malignant brain tumor, and some forms of vasculitis are other less frequent causes of subarachnoid hemorrhage.

Symptomatology. The headache due to rupture of an intracranial aneurysm resulting in subarachnoid hemorrhage usually starts suddenly and dramatically, like a blow on the head. Physical exertion and sexual intercourse are common precipitating events for a rupture of aneurysm. A severe unilateral headache soon becomes generalized and spreads to the back of the neck. The headache is accompanied by severe photophobia and in some cases there may be gradual or rapid alterations in the level of consciousness. Neck stiffness and Kernig's signs invariably develop. There may be focal or generalized seizures. Focal neurologic deficits such as dysphasia, monoparesis, or hemiparesis may develop if a middle cerebral artery aneurysm ruptures, producing an intracerebral hematoma as well. Third nerve palsy with dilated fixed pupil is common in rupture of posterior communicating artery aneurysm. Various combinations of third, fourth, fifth, and sixth nerve involvement may be seen in association with internal carotid artery aneurysms. If the internal carotid artery aneurysm ruptures into the cavernous sinus it becomes a caroticocavernous fistula, resulting in a pulsating exophthalmos with cranial nerve palsies (third, fourth, and sixth) and bruit over the eye and temples. Subhyaloid hemorrhages may be seen in the ocular fundi, and papilledema may develop within a few days in less than 15% of patients. The majority of patients with ruptured intracranial aneurysms appear to be hypertensive during the acute phase of the subarachnoid hemorrhage, and some of them may show electrocardiographic and cardiac rhythm changes which may be mistakenly attributed to primary heart disease. Bleeding from an arteriovenous malformation can be precipitation by minor trauma to the head. The subarachnoid hemorrhage from arteriovenous malformation is less explosive than that due to rupture of aneurysm, but it could recur more frequently. Focal seizures and focal motor or sensory deficits are more common in arteriovenous malformation.

Diagnosis. When subarachnoid hemorrhage is suspected, spinal puncture has to be done for confirmation of the diagnosis. A uniformly blood-stained cerebrospinal fluid is found in the first few days after bleeding, and xanthochromia develops thereafter to last for up to 30 days. Cerebrospinal fluid protein may be elevated and a lymphocytic cellular reaction may be found.

Computerized axial tomography of the brain is useful in making a diagnosis of the presence of blood in the subarachnoid space, expecially if the amount of blood in the space is large. This also helps to rule out intracerebral hemorrhage or hematoma.

Patients with subarachnoid hemorrhage develop many complications[4] such as cerebral vasospasm, acute hydrocephalus, rebleeding (usually in the second week), cerebral edema, metabolic complications such as inappropriate antidiuretic hormone secretion, secondary infection such as pneumonia, and cardiac arrhythmias. These patients should be transferred to a neurologic center with intensive care facilities as soon as possible. If the patient's general condition permits, an emergency cerebral arteriography is indicated.

Treatment. Neurosurgical treatment for an aneurysm depends on the site, the number, the general condition of the patient, the patient's age, and the adequacy of the cerebral circulation as a whole to develop collaterals in the event a major artery such as the common carotid artery is to be ligated. Cerebral vasospasm demonstrable in the arteriogram may delay surgery for a number of days.

Medical treatment includes complete bed rest and antihypertensive and antifibrinolytic agents like ϵ-aminocaproic acid (EACA). EACA prevent fibrinolysis and hence stabilizes clot formation, helping to prevent rebleeding. Hypotensive therapy is recommended by some. Dexamethasome is helpful in reducing cerebral edema. The role of anti–cerebral vasospasm drugs such as alpha-adrenergic blocking agents or beta-adrenergic stimulants is not adequately established.[4]

If no aneurysm or arteriovenous malformation is found, the patient is confined to bed for 4 to 6 weeks and resumes normal activities gradually.

UNRUPTURED INTRACRANIAL ANEURYSM

Headache is not a usual symptom of an unruptured intracranial aneurysm. The incidence of history of migraine in patients with subarachnoid hemorrage due to rupture of aneurysm varies from 5% to 6%[5,6] and is not very different from that of the general population. Wolff[7] found that seven out of forty-six patients with subarachnoid hemorrhage had suffered from migraine and twelve had periodic recurrent headaches. However, the side of the aneurysm did not always relate to the side of the headache, and Wolff considered that the headache was independent of the presence or absence of aneurysm. Giant unruptured aneurysms of the internal carotid artery may occasionally be present as unilateral recurrent headaches.

CEREBRAL ARTERIOVENOUS MALFORMATIONS AND MIGRAINES

It remains uncertain from the published statistics whether there is an increased association between migraine and cerebral arteriovenous malformations. The majority of series show an incidence of 5% of cerebral arteriovenous malformations presenting as classic migraine. In a patient in whom attacks of migraine habitually affects the same side of the head in association with visual disturbances in the opposite half of the body, special effort should be made to listen for intracranial bruit. An intracranial bruit is a fairly reliable sign of an arteriovenous malformation. If the hemiparesis outlasts the headache by a number of hours or focal seizures develop in the opposite side of the body, the chance of finding an arteriovenous malformation is high. Under such circumstances, computerized axial tomography (CAT scan) of the brain after infusion of contrast media, followed by cerebral arteriogram, will be diagnostic. Some patients with arteriovenous malformations have repeated small subarachnoid hemorrhages which may be mistaken for migraine attacks. Parietooccipital areas are a common site of arteriovenous malformations,

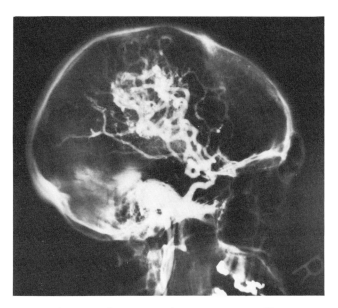

Fig. 13-1. Arteriogram showing a large parietal arteriovenous malformation in a patient who also has recurrent symptoms of classic migraine.

and patients may have episodic symptoms which may be indistinguishable from an attack of classic migraine (Fig. 13-1).

Meningitis and meningoencephalitis

Etiology. Awareness of the antecedent conditions which might lead to development of meningitis is important in making an early diagnosis. Middle ear infections with mastoiditis and paranasal sinus infection lead to direct spread of pyogenic bacterial infection to the meninges. Hematogenous spread occurs mainly from pneumonia. In the postoperative period (following craniotomy, spinal surgery, ventriculoatrial or ventriculoperitoneal shunting) there is a high risk of infection. Other predisposing situations prolonged immune suppression with therapeutic agents for malignant disease after renal transplantation. People with traumatic or spontaneous cerebrospinal fluid rhinorrhea are prone to get recurrent meningitis.

Invasion of the meninges by malignant cells and subsequent infiltration results in the condition known as meningitis carcinomatosa. In this condition early involvement of cranial nerves with facial pain and cranial nerve palsies is not uncommon.

Symptomatology. Headache is a prominent symptom when the meninges is inflamed as a result of bacterial, viral, parasitic, or fungal infections. Pyogenic and viral infections generally develop over a period of a few days but on occasions appear so acutely as to resemble a subarachnoid hemorrhage. Parasitic, fungal, and tuberculous infections are chronic in nature and the onset is insidious. Continuous severe headache is an early prominent feature of most cases of bacterial, viral, and tuberculous meningitis. The pain is bilateral, extends down the neck, and is made worse by head movements. The associated features are photophobia, fever, and irritability. Neck stiffness and Kernig's sign are important physical findings in acute cases. In chronic tuberculous and fungal meningitis cranial nerve palsies (usually sixth and

third) may be encountered, and intracranial pressure with papilledema may also be found. In herpes simplex encephalitis, fever, altered sensorium, and focal or generalized seizures are common. Focal neurologic electroencephalogram, brain scan, and CAT scan abnormalities pointing to specific affections of temporal lobe may be seen in some cases of herpes simplex encephalitis. Such cases are mistaken for brain abscess clinically.

Diagnosis. Lumbar puncture is essential in the diagnosis. The cerebrospinal fluid contains an excess of cells, mostly polymorphonuclear leukocytes in pyogenic infections and in the acute phase of some cases of viral encephalitis. A purely lymphocytic pleocytosis usually indicates a viral infection but may be found in some cases of tuberculous or cryptococcal meningitis. A low cerebrospinal fluid glucose usually indicates that the infecting organism is metabolizing glucose and may suggest a pyogenic, tuberculous, or cryptococcal infection. The same is true of carcinomatous meningitis also. Cerebrospinal fluid Gram stain, cultures, India ink preparations, animal innoculations, and special antibody techniques are needed for specific diagnosis.

Postpneumoencephalographic reaction

Introduction of air, oxygen, or contrast media into the subarachnoid space for diagnostic studies may result in a sterile inflammatory reaction with lymphocytic pleocytosis of the cerebrospinal fluid. This results in headache, photophobia, and neck stiffness. The natural post–spinal puncture headache is compounded by the inflammatory reaction of the meninges in these cases. The differential diagnosis, of course, is a true meningitis introduced at the time of the lumbar puncture. The headache is diffuse and worse the day after the procedure but may continue for a number of days. If severe headache, neck stiffness, and fever persist beyond a few days, a second spinal puncture to exclude a bacterial meningitis is in order. For headache due to sterile inflammatory reaction the patient should be kept flat on the bed and given plenty of fluids and simple analgesic medications.

HEADACHE PRODUCED BY TRACTION OR DISPLACEMENT OF INTRACRANIAL PAIN-SENSITIVE STRUCTURES
Space-occupying lesions
BRAIN TUMORS AND CYSTS

Pathophysiology. Brain tumors produce headache by local traction or a displacement of the pain-sensitive intracranial structures and by distant traction related to displacement of the brain. Distant traction may be related to the tumor mass directly or indirectly, when internal hydrocephalus or ventricular obstruction occurs. Generalized increased intracranial pressure itself produces headache. Headache is usually occipital when the tumor is located in the posterior fossa. Supratentorial tumors produce headache which is felt mainly anteriorly.

Symptomatology. Unless a tumor or a cyst occupies a strategic position along the line of the cerebrospinal fluid pathway of the ventricles, it is able to attain considerable size before causing headache. Infiltrating gliomas which remain intracerebral may attain large size and occupy a major portion of a cerebral hemisphere without causing headache, because the pain-sensitive structures may remain undisturbed. These tumors are more likely to produce focal or generalized seizures, focal paralysis, or progressive intellectual impairment or other neurologic deficit than headache in the initial stages of the disease. A sudden onset of severe headache with worsening of already existing neurologic deficit or development of neurologic symptoms for the first time may be seen in some of the tumors like glioblastoma multiforme, because of bleeding into the tumor area or thrombosis of a major cerebral vein with subsequent cerebral infarction.

Localized swelling and tenderness can be seen at the site of a meningioma. The mastoid area may show slight swelling and tenderness in case of a cerebellopontine angle tumor. The headache produced by an intracranial mass lesion is usually a steady, deep, nonthrobbing, dull ache which may be paroxysmal to start with but which becomes continuous later as the lesion expands and intracranial pressure increases. When it is severe it may be associated with nausea and vomiting. It tends to be worse on awakening. However, headaches due to brain tumor form only a small percentage of headaches which appear on awakening, the most common being a headache associated with depression. In the beginning the pain may be of some localizing value, although it is often referred to another part of the head. When unilateral, the headache tends in most cases to be on the side of the tumor. When intracranial pressure increases, the pain is usually generalized and is of no localizing value.

In certain tumors of the third ventricle the headache may come on paroxysmally. In such cases, changes of the position of the head, particularly bending over or lying down, may initiate severe headache. This has been explained as due to the ball-valve action of the tumor.[8]

In posterior fossa tumors headache is a prominent early symptom and is referred to the occipital region and posterior aspect of the neck. However, intramedullary tumors of the brainstem, especially brainstem gliomae, may progress with other neurologic signs and without headache.

Headache is an early manifestation of tumors of the upper brainstem region, especially pinealomas. This is due to early obstruction of the aqueduct of Sylvius and development of increased intracranial pressure.

Tumors in and around the pituitary gland usually cause bilateral frontoretroorbital and temporal headache which may initially be mild and intermittent. As the tumor expands it may become continuous and bursting in character. Usually endocrine changes, visual impairment, optic nerve changes, and plain x-ray changes in the sella turcica make the diagnosis fairly easy.

Occipital lobe tumors can give rise to headache associated with vomiting and visual hallucinations in the homonymous visual field, simulating migraine. A careful neurologic examination will reveal that there is a persistent homonymous visual field defect between attacks, and serial examinations will reveal the progressive nature of the problem, unlike migraine.

Intracranial cysts are usually congenital, posttraumatic, or associated with brain tumors. Congenital cysts like arachnoid cysts are very slowly expanding and may remain without producing symptoms or signs for a number of years. Headache and other neurologic signs may develop gradually. Posttraumatic cysts are usually secondary to severe cerebral damage due to cerebral laceration and brain necrosis and are associated with neurologic deficit. Headache is not a usual symptom, except when the cysts are loculated and expand rapidly with fluid accumulation.

Brain tumors associated with cyst formation are craniopharyngioma, cystic astrocytoma of the cerebellum, and some glioblastomas. The clinical behavior of these cysts depends on their parent neoplasm. In general the intracranial cysts produce clinical symptoms indistinguishable from those of tumors.

BRAIN ABSCESS

Etiology. Brain abscesses form as a result of local spread of infection from extracerebral sources or by hematogenous spread. The most common causes are otitis media, mastoiditis, frontal sinusitis, local scalp infections, and open head injury, especially gunshot wounds. Hematogenous spread occurs from pneumonia or other systemic or localized areas of infection. Acute or subacute bacterial endocarditis with resultant cerebral embolism may lead to multiple cerebral abscess formation. Children with cyanotic congenital heart disease are prone to get cerebral abscesses.

Symptomatology. The symptoms of cerebral abscess are essentially the same as those of any expanding lesion of the brain. Headache is an early symptom. Fever, nausea, vomiting, and focal convulsions are frequent. Increased intracranial pressure with papilledema may develop in a few days.

Because of the extensive cerebral edema associated with the development of a cerebral abscess, electroencephalographic abnormalities in the nature of focal slow waves develop early. This is helpful in suspecting a cerebral abscess.

EXTRADURAL HEMATOMA

Etiology and pathology. Extradural hematomas are almost always of traumatic origin and are invariably associated with fracture of the skull. The bleeding which results in the hematoma is arterial, usually due to rupture of the middle meningeal artery which runs its course very close to the bone. Acute extradural hematoma develops rapidly and results in compression and shift of the brain. Herniation of the medial aspect of the temporal lobe through the tentorial hiatus is common and results in compression, distortion, and secondary vascular changes producing infarction of the upper brainstem.

Symptomatology. Severe headache associated with progressive alteration in the level of consciousness is characteristic of extradural hemorrhage. After the initial period of altered sensorium due to brain concussion, there is usually a lucid interval before the patient starts showing signs of progressive brain herniation. During the lucid interval headache may be the only symptom. But eventually dilation of the ipsilateral pupil, progressive deterioration of level of consciousness, third nerve paralysis, and pyramidal tract signs develop. If proper surgical intervention is not undertaken as an emergency, the condition is fatal.

Diagnosis and treatment. X-ray of the skull is extremely useful and is a must in all patients suspected of having an extradural hematoma. A fracture involving the temporal and parietal bones is invariably seen in patients with extradural hematomas. A shift of the calcified pineal gland or choroid plexes shadow in the opposite direction may indicate a space-occupying lesion. A CAT scan of the brain is diagnostic as it shows high-density areas close to the bone with shift of the midline structures to the opposite side. The distinction between acute extradural and acute subdural hematoma is almost impossible based on CAT scan alone. But associated fracture of the skull bone and the rapidly deteriorating clinical course are suggestive of extradural hematoma. Cerebral arteriogram invariably confirms the presence of an extradural hematoma by showing an avascular area close to the bone with shift of the midline structures. There have been reports of extravasation of the arteriographic contrast media into the extradural space through the ruptured middle meningeal artery.

Acute extradural hematoma is one of the most important neurosurgical emergencies. The patient should be surgically treated as soon as possible. If there is any delay in obtaining the appropriate tests to confirm the diagnosis in a patient with typical clinical features and fracture of the skull, surgical intervention should be done as an emergency since further delay may prove dangerous. Use of intravenous mannitol or urea is indicated to reduce the intracranial pressure both preoperatively and postoperatively.

SUBDURAL HEMATOMA

Etiology. A history of head trauma is obtained in the majority of patients with subdural hematomas. But unlike the case in extradural hematoma, the trauma could be minor. At times the trauma might seem so insignificant to the patient that he forgets to mention it. Spontaneous subdural hematomas, or those precipitated by very minor head trauma, are seen in elderly individuals, chronic alcoholic persons, patients receiving anticoagulation therapy, and those with blood dyscrasias and bleeding tendency.

Pathology. The majority of subdural hematomas are due to venous hemorrhage and hence are not as explosive as extradural hematomas. Subdural hematomas can be divided into acute and chronic varieties pathologically and radiographically. In the acute variety the fluid contained in the subdural space is predominantly fresh blood, and the dura and the arachnoid membranes do not show much of pathologic reaction. As the hematoma becomes chronic, the size becomes larger, possibly due to osmotic absorption of fluid by the high protein-containing blood elements in the subdural cavity. In addition, a thick membrane forms around the hematoma as a result of pathologic reaction. The fluid in the cavity is no more fresh blood but a chocolate-colored fluid.

The pathologic effect of a subdural hematoma on the brain is similar to that of extradural hematoma, the only difference being the speed with which these effects occur. As the size of the hematoma increases, progressive herniation of the medial part of the temporal lobe through the tentorial hiatus takes place, resulting in changes in the third cranial nerve as well as upper brainstem.

Symptomatology. Headache is the most common symptom of subdural hematoma. It may be ipsilateral to the hematoma in some cases. Alteration in the levels of consciousness is the most important symptom accompanying the headache. In the elderly patient with subdural hematoma, confusion and disorientation may be the most striking symptoms and headache may not be a prominent problem.

Papilledema may be found in the chronic variety. Signs of brain herniation such as dilation of the ipsilateral pupil, ipsilateral paresis of the third cranial nerve, and contralateral or ipsilateral hemiparesis may be seen, depending on the stage of the patient. The third nerve, which crosses from midbrain to the cavernous sinus, is stretched by the herniating medial aspect of the temporal lobe. The cerebral peduncles are also compressed against the tentorium. Signs of a third nerve paresis (ptosis, enlarged pupil, failure of the eye to adduct or elevate fully) or hemiparesis are therefore indications for immediate action.

Diagnosis. An electroencephalogram is a useful test in the diagnosis of subdural hematomas. The general experience has been that about 90% of patients with subdural hematoma have abnormal electroencephalograms.[9,10] Correct lateralization of a single hematoma is possible in better than three-fourths of the patients with abnormal tracings. However, diffuse abnormalities occur with unilateral hematoma. Serial electroencephalographic examinations may be necessary to pick up abnormalities due to subdural hematoma in a patient complaining of headache following a severe head injury.

X-ray of the skull might be of diagnostic value if there is a shift of the calcified pineal gland across the midline. Even though computerized axial tomography is extremely helpful in detecting the presence of intracranial hematoma, it may sometimes prove to be falsely negative for subdural hematoma after the initial weeks of a head injury because the hematoma may become "isodense" with the brain parenchyma, making it difficult to be recognized.[11] Associated shift of the midline structures or deformation of the ventricles should be an indication for an arteriogram. After the isodense period the hematoma becomes less dense and thus is easily spotted. A cerebral arteriogram is highly diagnostic of subdural hematoma, especially the chronic variety. An avascular area with concavity toward the bone, which is usually well visualized in the later phases of an angiogram, is highly characteristic. In addition, there may be shift of the midline vessels.

Treatment. Surgical evacuation of the hematoma is the treatment of choice in the majority of cases. With surgical treatment the headache invariably disappears. There have been few advocates of conservative nonsurgical treatment for subdural hematoma, which consists of measures to reduce intracranial pressure such as intravenous mannitol, urea, or glycerol.[12]

INTRACEREBRAL HEMATOMA

Etiology and pathology. The majority of intracerebral hematomas or hemorrhages are spontaneous and result from hypertensive small vessel disease. Traumatic intracerebral hematoma is usually associated with cerebral laceration or contusion. Other etiologic factors include blood dyscrasias, especially thrombocytopenia and disseminated intravascular coagulation. Arteriovenous malformations may result in intraparenchymal hemorrhage.

The most common sites of intraparenchymal hematomas are (1) near the external capsule and thalamic region, (2) the pons, and (3) the cerebellum, in decreasing order of frequency. The supratentorial hemorrhages result in rapid development of pressure effect, shift of the midline structures, and eventual brain herniation. The hemorrhage may also dissect down into the upper brainstem, accounting for rapid loss of consciousness. The cerebellar hemorrhages result in upward herniation of the vermis of the cerebellum and herniation of the tonsils through the foramen magnum.

Symptomatology. Excruciating headache of sudden onset is invariably the presenting symptom of a spontaneous intracerebral hemorrhage in a hypertensive individual. The headache is followed by rapid development of paralysis, usually a dense hemiplegia in a massive supratentorial hematoma. Signs of brain herniation become evident soon. Milder focal neurologic deficits such as dysphasia occur in small hematomas. In cerebellar hemorrhage the initial headache is suboccipital. This is usually followed by paralysis of eye movements, abnormal dyskinetic eye movements, and paralysis of limbs. Abnormal respiratory patterns may ensue. Patients

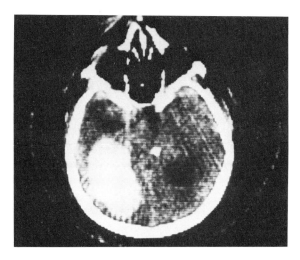

Fig. 13-2. Computerized axial tomography of the brain showing large intracerebral hematoma with displacement of midline structures and enlargement of ventricle.

with pontine and cerebellar hematoma become rapidly comatose.

Diagnosis. Computerized axial tomography has proved to be the most useful test in detecting an intracerebral hematoma. A high-density area with surrounding low-density zone is characteristic of an intracerebral hematoma with cerebral edema (Fig. 13-2). A CAT scan is the best test for detecting a cerebellar hematoma.

A spinal tap may show a blood-stained cerebrospinal fluid, and if there is bleeding into the ventricles the cerebrospinal fluid will be grossly bloody.

Treatment. Prognosis of an intracerebral hemorrhage is generally poor. The pontine hemorrhages are fatal in about 75% of cases, and conservative treatment is all that is possible. Cerebellar hematomas are also fatal if proper surgical treatment is not undertaken rapidly. An early diagnosis and evacuation of the cerebellar hematoma, in experienced hands, result in fair recovery, but the patient may be left with a residual disabling neurologic deficit. A supratentorial hematoma may be evacuated if there is an impending brain herniation. But in the majority of cases medical treatment to reduce cerebral edema and other general medical measures are adequate. Residual neurologic deficits are invariable in patients recovering from cerebral hemorrhage.

Increased intracranial pressure

Headache is the most common symptom of an increase in intracranial pressure. Increased intracranial pressure may be due to (1) space-occupying intracranial lesions such as tumors, cysts, or hematomas (discussed previously), (2) obstruction of cerebrospinal fluid pathways producing a hydrocephalus, and (3) benign intracranial hypertension.

OBSTRUCTION OF CEREBROSPINAL FLUID PATHWAYS

Etiology. Any lesion which obstructs the flow of cerebrospinal fluid from the lateral ventricle through the foramen of Monro, third ventricle, sylvian aqueduct, fourth ventricle, and its exit foramina or prevents the passage of cerebrospinal fluid over the cortex to its absorption sites will cause a rapid increase in intracranial pressure so that headache becomes the main presenting symptom. Cysts of the third ventricle, especially colloid cysts, tumors encroaching the posterior part of the third ventricle such as pinealomas, congenital stenosis of the aqueduct, and obstruction of the aqueduct and fourth ventricle by tumors arising from the fourth ventricle, such as an ependymoma, are usual causes of hydrocephalus. Adhesive arachnoiditis due to chronic meningitis obstructing the exit foramina and the subarachnoid space near the sylvian areas and congenital malformations in the posterior fossa, such as Dandy-Walker syndrome and Arnold-Chiari malformation, produce obstruction to cerebrospinal fluid pathways.

Stenosis of the aqueduct is usually a congenital malformation which does not produce any symptoms until some systemic infection causes proliferation of its ependymal lining, which then blocks the canal and produces an acute internal hydrocephalus.[13] Communicating hydrocephalus may form following subarachnoid hemorrhage, head injury, and some forms of meningitis due to obstruction of cerebrospinal fluid pathways near the cerebral convexities.

Symptomatology. Headache is the most common presenting symptom. Headache is more or less constant and usually worse on awakening. It is diffuse and is aggravated by coughing or sneezing. As the intracranial pressure increases, nausea, vomiting, and visual disturbances may develop. Diplopia due to paralysis of unilateral or bilateral lateral rectus muscle is seen in severe cases. Sixth nerve paralysis is usually a false localizing sign in these cases. Papilledema develops fairly early in obstructive hydrocephalus and, if untreated, will go on to secondary optic atrophy, resulting in permanent visual impairment. Ataxia of gait is a common sign of rapidly developing hydrocephalus. Restriction of upward gaze may also be seen in some cases as a nonspecific sign, even though it is considered pathognomonic of a pinealoma. The clinical manifestation of a congenital aqueductal stenosis may occur for the first time in adult life when a patient presents with a progressive headache.

Diagnosis. X-rays of the skull are helpful because of the changes in the sella as a result of increased intracranial pressure. The sella enlarges in size with demineralization of its processes and walls, and eventual destruction. Changes are also observed in the cranial vault. Separation of the sutures

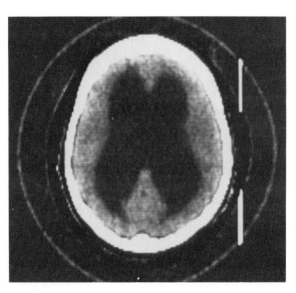

Fig. 13-3. Computerized axial tomography of brain showing enormous enlargement of lateral ventricles in patient with acute obstructive hydrocephalus.

is invariably seen in children with internal hydrocephalus. A CAT scan is diagnostic in internal hydrocephalus (Fig. 13-3). One may have to resort to a pneumoencephalogram in some cases in order to arrive at an etiologic diagnosis of the hydrocephalus. This is especially true in some cases of third ventricular obstruction, aqueductal stenosis, obstruction to the exit foramina of the fourth ventricle, and obstruction to the passage of cerebrospinal fluid to the convexity of the brain.

Treatment. Once the diagnosis is made, the treatment is neurosurgical. Usually a shunt is put in to divert the cerebrospinal fluid circulation. Either a ventriculoatrial or ventriculoperitoneal shunt is used. If a specific entity, such as a tumor, is found causing the obstruction, surgical excision or irradiation or both is indicated, depending on the situation and type of tumor.

Following a cerebrospinal fluid shunt operation a patient may come back with headache and other neurologic symptoms, which result from complications such as blockage of the shunt and development of subdural hematoma. Blockage of the shunt is more frequently seen in patients with high cerebrospinal fluid protein. Headache may reappear as a result of a chronic low cerebrospinal fluid pressure after the shunt operation.

BENIGN INTRACRANIAL
HYPERTENSION

Pseudotumor cerebri and otitic hydrocephalus are synonyms for this condition.

Etiology. Even though this condition was originally described in children with thrombosis of the lateral sinus, it was later recognized that a number of different conditions can lead to development of benign intracranial hypertension. Changes in all three intracranial fluid compartments—namely, the cerebrospinal fluid, the brain parenchymal fluid, and the blood volume—may contribute to this condition. The following outline gives the known associations of benign intracranial hypertension.[14]

A. Interference with cerebral venous outflow and disorders of cerebral vascular dilation
  1. Intracranial venous sinus obstruction
    a. Mastoiditis
    b. Otitis, sinusitis
    c. Trauma
    d. Blood dyscrasias with thrombosis
    e. Oral contraceptives
  2. Extracranial cerebral venous obstruction
    a. Thrombosis of superior vena cava
    b. Block dissection of neck
    c. Mediastinal tumor
  3. Cerebral venous stasis
    a. Oral contraceptives
    b. Endocrine dysfunction as in pregnancy and menarche
  4. Cerebral vascular dilation due to carbon dioxide retention
    a. Extreme obesity, pickwickian syndrome
    b. Chronic obstructive pulmonary disease
    c. Respiratory paralysis
B. Disordered membrane transport mechanisms
  1. Endocrine dysfunction
    a. Obesity
    b. Pregnancy
    c. Menarche
    d. Addison's disease
    e. Hypoparathyroidism
    f. Steroid therapy and its withdrawal
  2. Hypervitaminosis A
  3. Tetracycline therapy
  4. Postinfectious state
C. Dysfunction of the arachnoid villi
  1. Blockage by increased protein in cerebrospinal fluid
    a. Guillian-Barre syndrome
    b. Spinal cord tumor

Symptomatology. The condition is referred to as benign intracranial hypertension because of the relatively benign course of the disease and the relative well-being of the patient. The majority of the patients are young or middle-aged, moderately obese females with some menstrual irregularities. Apart from constant, unremitting headache, the patient does not usually have any other complaints. On neurologic examination papilledema is invariably present without any focal neurologic abnormalities. The patient generally looks healthy and well. If left untreated, the papilledema can lead to secondary optic atrophy and consequent visual loss. Occasionally sixth nerve paresis may develop.

Even though in the majority of cases it is a self-limiting disease a chronic form is well recognized.

Diagnosis. A patient who presents with headache and papilledema should be examined thoroughly to exclude other intracranial processes. In benign intracranial hypertension the skull x-rays and the electroencephalogram are normal. The next step is a CAT scan of the brain, which usually reveals a relatively small ventricular system without any other abnormality. No enlargement of ventricles or displacement is found, unlike other causes of intracranial hypertension. Pneumoencephalography and arteriography reveal a "pinched" appearance of the lateral ventricles without any other abnormality. Obstruction to the lateral or sigmoid venous sinuses can be detected in the last phases of cerebral arteriogram. Once a space-occupying lesion is excluded, a spinal tap can be done safely, which will reveal a very high intracranial pressure, usually in the order of 300 to 400 mm H_2O. Cerebrospinal fluid cell count and chemistry are normal, and cerebrospinal fluid is sterile.

Treatment of the condition is mainly aimed at reducing the intracranial pressure. Furosemide (Lasix), acetazolamide (Diamox), and other diuretics have been used. Corticosteroids are preferred by others. Long-term use of oral glycerol is recommended by some. If medical treatment fails, and if there is a threat of a secondary optic atrophy developing, a subtemporal decompression may be indicated. Some neurosurgeons prefer a lumbartheco-peritoneal shunt.

Reduced intracranial pressure

Etiology. Reduced intracranial pressure following lumbar puncture, ventriculoatrial

and ventriculoperitoneal shunt, and cerebrospinal fluid leakage from traumatic or surgical tear of meninges can cause headache. Puncture of subarachnoid space for the introduction of air, anesthetic, radiographic contrast material, radioactive materials, or steroids may produce headache. Leakage of the cerebrospinal fluid through the dural-arachnoidal puncture hole brings about a dilation of intracranial vessels and traction on the blood vessels.

Symptomatology. Headache frequently occurs within hours following lumbar puncture. About 32% of patients develop headache following spinal puncture.[15-16] The headache after spinal puncture varies with postural changes. It is most severe when the patient is upright and it is relieved when he lies down. The headache is bifrontal or bioccipital in location, but may involve the entire head. Headache usually begins 6 to 48 hours after the spinal puncture and may last for a number of days. There were cases where it lasted for 2 to 3 weeks. The size of the needle used, amount of fluid withdrawn, and multiple punctures are factors predisposing to the development of post–lumbar puncture headache.

A sterile meningitis which rarely occurs after lumbar puncture is another less common cause of headache following this procedure. The pain usually begins within a few hours of the tap and may occur while the patient is horizontal. A repeat cerebrospinal fluid examination shows a sterile fluid with slight pleocytosis and slightly elevated pressure.

Treatment. Frequency of headache following lumbar puncture may be reduced by using a fine gauge needle, having the patient lie prone for 4 hours after lumbar puncture, and maintaining bed rest for 24 hours afterward. Lying flat in bed and drinking large quantities of fluids are the treatment of choice for this type of headache. Analgesics may not be of much help. The intravenous injection of caffeine in doses of 7.5 gm may give temporary relief. Epidural injection of blood has been suggested as a form of treatment by some, but has not gained widespread acceptance yet.

HEADACHE DUE TO INTRACRANIAL VASODILATION
Postconvulsive headache

Generalized headache is a fairly common postictal phenomenon of cerebral seizure disorder. This appears soon after recovery of consciousness and may last for several hours. The mechanism of the postseizure headache is presumed to be due to generalized cerebral vasodilation due to lactic-acidosis which results from an enormously increased cerebral metabolism under relatively hypoxic conditions induced by a grand mal seizure.

Acute cerebrovascular insufficiency and transient ischemic attacks

Thrombosis of a major artery such as the internal carotid artery may cause gross uni-lateral cerebral edema and displacement of intracranial vessels and headache of the affected side (Fig. 13-4). Headache may be an associated symptom in transient ischemic attacks. In transient ischemic attacks of the internal carotid territory the headache is felt in the frontal region, and the occipital region may be the main site of headache in transient ischemic attacks of the vertebro-basilar system.[17] Approximately 25% of the patients with transient ischemic attacks may have associated headache.[18] It should, however, be emphasized that complicated migraine such as the hemiparetic or the basilar artery type may simulate a transient ischemic attack. The profile of the attack, the age group involved, and the previous history of long-standing migraine including family history will help an early differentiation between the two. The mechanism of headache accompanying transient ischemic attacks is not known. It is possible

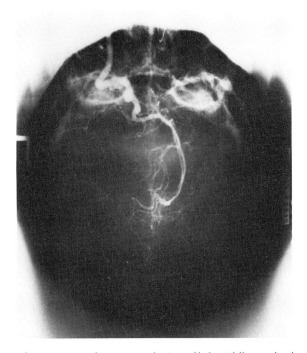

Fig. 13-4. Left carotid arteriogram showing occlusion of left middle cerebral artery, subsequent cerebral edema, and extreme displacement of anterior cerebral artery across the midline to the right.

that sudden dilation of collateral channels in response to the sudden demand made on them may be playing a part in the production of these headaches.

Hypertension headache

The incidence of headache in hypertension may not be different from that of the general population. The headaches commonly seen are either migraine or muscle contraction headaches. However, in severe hypertension, especially if the diastolic pressure is above 120 mm Hg or more, a special form of headache may develop. Early morning headache on awakening which lasts for 2 or 3 hours thereafter is typical of severe hypertension. The headaches are predominantly occipital. In most patients the headache reduces in intensity and frequency as the blood pressure is reduced by treatment. Many hypertensive individuals almost never have headaches, and the headache on awakening is not pathognomonic of hypertension. In my experience, chronic scalp muscle contraction headache which is associated with depression is the most common cause of headache on awakening.

A sudden extreme rise in systemic blood pressure such as occurs in pheochromocytoma, acute nephritis, and patients taking monoamine oxidase inhibitors who ingest tyramine-containing substances and those taking sympathomimetic drugs causes severe headache. In pheochromocytoma the headache is experienced in the early phase of the attack but may disappear when symptoms of blanching, sweating, and tachycardia are well established, possibly because of the constriction of cranial vessels by circulating catecholamines. The symptoms of pheochromocytoma vary with the proportion of adrenaline and nonadrenaline produced by the tumor. If pheochromocytoma is suspected, appropriate chemical and pharmacologic tests should be done to prove the diagnosis.

Hypertensive encephalopathy occurs in patients with malignant hypertension. Headache invariably accompanies hyper-

tensive encephalopathy. It is a severe, generalized, throbbing headache, which may tend to localize in the occipital region. The blood pressure reaches a level of 150 to 160 mm Hg diastolic. Confusion, lethargy, obtundation, and focal or generalized seizures may accompany the process. Hypertensive retinopathy and, most characteristically, papilledema are found. Focal neurologic signs such as transient monoparesis may also be seen.

Hypertensive encephalopathy is due to failure of cerebral autoregulation which results in a "breakthrough" of cerebral circulation, producing cerebral edema with traction or displacement of pain-sensitive structures and increased intracranial pressure.[19] These in turn cause the headache in hypertensive encephalopathy.

Treatment is urgent. Strong antihypertensive agents have to be used to bring down the blood pressure. Medications such as mannitol which bring down the intracranial pressure are also helpful in reducing the severity of the headache.

CRANIAL PAIN DUE TO CRANIAL NERVE DISORDERS
Compression of cranial nerves

Any lesion compressing the fifth, seventh, ninth, or tenth cranial nerves can cause pain referred in the face, ear, or throat. The pain is usually constant, with more severe paroxysms at intervals. The severe paroxysmal pain is that of acute lancinating type simulating an idiopathic trigeminal or glossopharyngeal neuralgia. Careful neurologic examination is essential in all cases of cranial neuralgias. Impairment of sensation over the distribution of fifth cranial nerve, in the external auditory meatus, or over the posterior pharyngeal wall supports the diagnosis of a lesion of the fifth, seventh, or ninth cranial nerves, respectively. Corneal reflex is extremely sensitive and may be affected very early in compressive lesions of the fifth nerve. Other neurologic signs such as involvement of neighboring motor cranial nerves, long tract signs, or cerebellar signs should definitely point to compressive lesion as the cause of the cranial pain. Appropriate tests are warranted to rule out tumors, aneurysms, and abscesses.

HEADACHE OF CERVICAL ORIGIN

Etiology. A number of conditions affecting the cervical spine and related structures can cause recurrent headaches. These include (1) traumatic fracture or dislocation of cervical spine, (2) degenerative cervical spondylosis and cervical disk disease, (3) rheumatoid arthritis, and (4) whiplash injury.

The mechanism of headache seen in association with cervical conditions is not entirely clear. Some of the possible explanations are given in an earlier section on mechanism of headache. In rheumatoid arthritis degeneration of the upper cervical vertebral joints are common with resultant atlantoaxial dislocation. Compression of the upper cervical nerve roots causes pain. Signs of spinal cord compressions are also found in these cases.

Cervical spondylosis most commonly affects the lower cervical spine and the mechanism of headache in this condition is not clear. While stimulation of the upper cervical nerve roots may refer pain to the trigeminal distribution, there is no known means of referral of pain to the head from the lower cervical spine.[20] Headache is not an invariable accompaniment of cervical spondylosis. When headache is a symptom of a patient with cervical spondylosis, the clinical features of the headache are usually those of muscle contraction headache. It may be initiated by the patient's concern over the neck condition or may be independent of it.

A vascular mechanism has been postulated for headache arising in association with cervical spondylosis. It is hypothesized that the cervical spondylosis may damage the periarterial nerve plexus of the vertebral artery by osteophytes impinging on it, thus setting up a diffuse headache.

Symptomatology. In headache of cervical origin, pain is usually unilateral but sometimes becomes bilateral. The headache is nuchal and occipital in location. The pain is commonly along the trapezius muscle, radiating up to the occipital area over the top of the head toward the ipsilateral side of the head. The headache is usually worse in the morning. It is described as a dull ache or a stabbing pain. However, it is sometimes described as throbbing, especially when it is retroorbital. Pain may last for a number of days and is aggravated by movements of the neck. Another feature is repeated attacks of painful stiffness of the great muscles of the neck.

In patients with cervical spondylosis and diskogenic disease, other neurologic symptoms and signs of radiculopathy and spinal cord compression may be apparent. In rheumatoid arthritis, generalized arthritic disease is evident. The movements of the cervical spine are greatly limited and very painful. Sudden atlantoaxial dislocations and quadriparesis may occur.

The part played by whiplash injury of the cervical spine is difficult to assess in the absence of definite radiologic changes. The majority of post–whiplash injury headaches have features in common with chronic scalp muscle contraction headache. The majority of patients show some degree of anxiety and depression.

Diagnosis. In a person having nuchal and occipital headaches for the first time after the age of 50, cervical spondylosis may be considered as one of the possible causes. A plain x-ray of the cervical spine is very informative in this respect. However, roentgenographic evidence of cervical spondylosis is very common in asymptomatic individuals above the age of 50. Careful neurologic examinations are essential to detect features of radiculopathy or spinal cord compression. Electromyographic and myelographic examination may be necessary in some cases.

Treatment. Because of the resemblance of these headaches to chronic muscle contraction headache, the general approach to treatment is similar to that of muscle contraction headache. Cervical traction may help some patients. Application of heat and massage of neck muscle may give temporary relief.

Surgical treatment is indicated only if medical therapy is unsuccessful, and then only when significant arm pain is present with an associated neurologic deficit which can be demonstrated on examination and recorded electromyographically. Surgery should not be used for pain alone, particularly for posterior occipital headache which so often accompanies cervical spondylosis. Another indication for surgery is progressive myelopathy, particularly with evidence of spinal cord compression. Two major surgical approaches are posterior laminectomy and anterior fusion.

REFERENCES

1. Ray, B. S., and Wolff, H. G.: Experimental studies on headache: pain sensitive structures of the head and their significance in headache, Arch. Surg. **41**:813, 1940.
2. Wolff, H. G.: Headache mechanisms, Int. Arch. Allerg. **7**:210, 1955.
3. Kerr, F. W. L.: A mechanism to account for frontal headache in cases of posterior fossa tumors, J. Neurosurg. **18**:605, 1961.
4. Mathew, N. T., Meyer, J. S., and Hartmann, A.: Diagnosis and treatment of factors complicating subarachnoid hemorrhage, Neuroradiology **6**:237-265, 1974.
5. Blend, R., and Bull, J. W. D.: The radiological investigation of migraine. In Smith, R., editor: Background to migraine, London, 1967, William Heinemann Medical Books, p. 1.
6. Davis, E.: Subarachnoid hemorrhage, Med. J. Austr. **2**:12, 1967.
7. Wolff, H. G.: Headache and other head pain, London, 1963, Oxford University Press.
8. Fulton, J. F., and Barly, P.: Tumors in the region of the third ventricle, J. Nerv. Ment. Dis. **69**:18, 1969.
9. Friedlander, W. J.: The electroencephalographic findings in 39 surgically proven subdural hematoma, Electroencephalogr. Clin. Neurophysiol. **3**:59-62, 1951.
10. Sullivan, J. F., Abbott, J. A., and Schwab, R. S.: The electroencephalogram in cases of subdural hematoma and hydroma, J. Neurosurg. **13**:449-454, 1956.
11. Amendola, M. A., and Ostrium, B. J.: Diagnosis of isodense subdural hematoma by computed tomography, Am. J. Roentgenol. **129**:693-697, 1977.
12. Bender, M. B., and Christoff, N.: Nonsurgical treatment of subdural hematoma, Arch. Neurol. **31**:73-79, 1974.
13. Russell, D. S.: Observations on the pathology of hydrocephalus, M.R.C. Special Report No. 265, London, 1949.
14. Mathew, N. T., Meyer, J. S., and Ott, S.: Increased cerebral blood volume in benign intracranial hypertension, Neurology **25**:646-649, 1975.
15. Davenport, K. M.: Post puncture reactions, N.Y. J. Med. **60**:881, 1964.
16. Tourtellotte, W. W., Haerer, A. F., Heller, G. L., and Somer, J. E.: Post lumbar puncture headaches, Springfield, Ill., 1964, Charles C Thomas, Publisher, p. 6.
17. Fisher, C. M.: Headache in cerebrovascular disease. In Handbook of clinical neurology, vol. 5, Amsterdam, 1968, p. 124.
18. Grindal, A. B., and Toole, J. F.: Headache and transient ischemic attacks, Stroke **5**:603-606, 1974.
19. Skinhoj, E., and Strandgaard, S.: Pathogenesis of hypertensive encephalopathy, Lancet **1**:461-462, 1973.
20. Lance, J. W.: The mechanism and management of headache, ed. 2, London, 1973, Butterworth & Co.

CHAPTER 14

Temporal arteritis

Temporal arteritis was initially described by Horton, Magath, and Brown[1] in 1934. This condition represents an inflammatory lesion of the temporal artery. However, the disease is not strictly confined to the temporal arteries, any of the cranial arteries may be involved, as well as many arteries elsewhere in the body. This condition is self-limited and benign. In the literature this condition is occasionally referred to as giant cell arteritis, Horton's syndrome, cranial arteritis, or granulomatous giant cell arteritis. Temporal arteritis may be defined as an inflammation of collagen or fibrous tissue which occurs in elderly people. It starts slowly and runs a progressive course.

ETIOLOGY

Temporal arteritis is the name given to a local and systemic symptom-complex which is usually found in older patients. It is rarely found in patients who are younger than 55 years of age. However, because of the severe attendant morbidity of the disease, the diagnosis of temporal arteritis should not be excluded solely on the basis of the age of the patient. The peak age incidence seems to be around the seventieth year.

Temporal arteritis is actually a disease of unknown etiology. This condition seems to affect both sexes equally and is found fre-

quently in the patient with atheromatous degeneration or arteriosclerosis with or without hypertension. Analogous findings may be caused by arteriosclerosis in elderly patients in whom the clinical characteristics of histaminic cephalalgia appear even without the inflammatory or thromboangitic aspect of the process.

Temporal arteritis is a distinct clinical entity which is usually characterized by local inflammatory changes along the course of one or more of the cranial arteries. The temporal arteries are the most frequently involved, but the arterial involvement may be widespread throughout the body.

PATHOLOGY

Temporal arteritis is a systemic vascular disease, originally of the tunica media. The pathologic picture is usually characterized by either a complete or a partial obliteration of the lumen of the vessel by connective tissue and round cells. The intima becomes greatly thickened because of the proliferation of young fibroblasts in a mucoid matrix. Foci of subacute inflammatory cells occur in opposition to areas of medial necrosis.

The media is usually infiltrated with round cells or plasma cells, lymphocytes, and eosinophils, and focal necrosis can be seen along with giant cell formation. This produces a picture of a granuloma near the elastic lamella. Occasionally an intramural aneurysm may be present. In the acute zone of the media there is an inflammatory reaction present along with zonal necrosis. Foci of interstitial hemorrhage along with scattered eosinophils are also observed.

The elastica is fragmented or folded. In the internal elastic lamella there is focal necrosis, and attempts at reduplication are frequently observed. There is also some calcification in this layer, and some giant cells are usually seen.

Smith,[2] using the electron microscope, found the characteristic histologic feature of temporal arteritis to be a giant cell reaction with a disruption of the internal elastic lamina. The most prominent feature of the affected artery was the large number of multinucleated giant cells along the junction of the media and intima, areas where the intimal elastic lamina was absent. No evidence of microorganisms or virus particles was found, and the results were considered to be compatible with an immunologic reaction.

In the adventitia there is a spotty perivasculitis. On some occasions a contract phlebitis of the venae comitantes may be observed. The edema present is usually due to a fibrous hyperplasia around the blood vessels and the nerves. This also is responsible for the patient's pain. In some cases a thrombus will be found.

On the whole temporal arteritis presents a pathologic picture of a granulomatous process. The lesion is a subacute or chronic arteritis and periarteritis with an infiltration of lymphocytes, monocytes, and leukocytes, with scattered eosinophils and giant cells predominating.

SYMPTOMATOLOGY

The symptoms of temporal arteritis may often be nonspecific at the onset of the disease and may be limited for several weeks or even months to systemic reactions, such as fever, chills, general malaise, weakness, anorexia, and weight loss. This stage is usually followed by severe headaches.

A patient with temporal arteritis usually experiences a severe, boring type of headache in the temporal area. This may be unilateral or bilateral, depending on whether one or both of the temporal arteries are involved. The pain is usually found to be more severe during the sleeping hours. The pain generally will persist throughout the day and it may migrate from the temporal area to the neck regions.

The head pain of temporal arteritis is usually aggravated by such things as straining, sneezing, coughing, and chewing. Headache is a prominent feature of temporal arteritis because of the involvement of the cranial vessels and the contiguous nerve fibers.

The skin over the temporal vessels may appear to be inflamed. The temporal blood vessels seem to be enlarged and are usually extremely tender. Pressure on these vessels will usually make the headache more severe. These arteries should be palpated by the physician in order to determine whether or not they are still pulsating. This is an important diagnostic aid in temporal arteritis.

It is interesting that most patients often find it extremely painful to chew. Horton[3,4] concluded that these patients have an intermittent claudication of the jaws, found only in this type of patient.

Radiologic examination of patients usually fails to give the physician any diagnostic help.

Laboratory findings usually show a leukocytosis. Throughout the entire course of the disease there is an increased sedimentation rate. The electrophoretic protein of the blood serum fibrinogen level is often raised, as is the blood platelet level. There may be an increased ratio of alpha$_2$ and gamma globulin.

Lubbers and Edelhoff[5] state that the main aspect of temporal arteritis consists of inflammation of the temporal arteries, which appear as swollen, indurated strands of the temples and may show no pulsation, and the skin over the pencil-sized arteries may be reddened. They believe that infections may be the etiologic factor in many of these cases. Resection of the temporal artery is their choice for relief of headache of this type. They believe that in many cases this resection may also help to preserve the eyesight. They think that such a resection interrupts the pain-conducting centripetal fibers of the sympathetic nerves involved. Cortisone and corticotropin are advocated for the medical treatment of this condition.

Some cases of temporal arteritis present what is termed "skip lesions."[6] Skip lesions are said to be present when one or more sections of a temporal artery have the appearance of typical arteritis while other sections from the same artery have none of the characteristic features. An artery with skip lesions, therefore, can contain sections with and without arteritis. This shows the importance of the biopsy of long segments of the artery and of examining multiple histologic sections. It also points to the importance of a contralateral temporal artery biopsy when the examination of the first side might be normal.

The most serious complication of temporal arteritis is occlusion of the central retinal arteries, which will result in the sudden loss of vision. It is because of the ocular symptoms that many patients initially consult an ophthalmologist. Actually about half of patients have visual defects which are generally due to the disease.[7] The most common local cause of the loss of vision is acute ischemia of the optic nerve. Other causes are ischemic retinopathy, occlusion of a central artery or a central artery and vein, residual optic nerve or retinal lesions, and paresis of ocular muscles. Some patients may become blind even without apparent involvement of the temporal arteries. Involvement of the eyes occur in 30% to 50% of patients.[8]

In temporal arteritis, three types of changes have been reported—retinal ischemia, as seen in cases of occlusion of the central retinal artery; ischemia of the optic papilla with overlying exudate; and

functional vascular abnormalities, which may involve blood vessels in any part of the visual tract and suggest a descending atrophy of the optic nerve. Any artery in the body may show the same pathology changes as the temporal arteries.

Suspicion that ocular lesions are a part of the syndrome of temporal arteritis may be heightened if the patient gives a history of general malaise, weakness, anoxeria and weight loss.

Permanent loss of vision is usually preceded at times by attacks of brief transient loss. The anatomic basis of lesions of the optic nerve, the retina, and the ocular muscles is giant cell arteritis involving the ophthalmic artery or its branches. Blindness is the most distressing sequel of this disease. However, with early diagnosis of the condition and the institution of prompt and adequate treatment, the incidence of blindness may be greatly reduced.

Temporal arteritis may occur in an occult form in which blindness is the presenting symptom.[9] Classic symptoms and signs including those referable to the temporal artery may be totally absent or may follow the onset of bilateral blindness. Also the symptoms may be so misleading that they obscure the correct diagnosis.

The term "occult temporal arteritis" is used to describe the form of temporal arteritis where these factors obscure true diagnosis. Occult temporal arteritis should be considered when adult and elderly patients lose the vision in one eye without any apparent cause.[10] Visual loss may occur in the second eye within a few days. Thus temporal arteritis may initially be manifested by its complications.

Some patients may also have hypertension, arteriosclerosis, or occipital arteritis. These patients sometimes have involvement of the tongue. A case has been reported in which the anterior two-thirds of the tongue was atrophied from the temporal arteritis.[11]

Skin lesions of the scalp associated with temporal arteritis are rare but do occur.[12]

These lesions are thought to be ischemic in origin. Other organs found to be involved with temporal arteritis are the salivary glands, the pharynx, the occipital and cervical portions of the head, and occasionally the axilla and the extremities.

The belief that polymyalgia rheumatica is a manifestation of temporal arteritis has not been disproved.[13] The reason for this belief is that the microscopic examination shows a disseminated giant cell arteritis of the aorta and some of the large vessels arising from the aorta.

The symptoms of temporal arteritis may vary widely, according to the region affected. There may be symptoms of cerebral involvement, such as melancholia, disorientation, and occasional signs of more permanent cerebral injury. In other cases the symptoms may be cardiac, gastrointestinal, or genitourinary in origin. The otolaryngologic, neurologic, and general physical examinations of these patients may be entirely negative.

Temporal arteritis tends to involve the temporal artery first and then other cervical and extracranial arteries. Smith and Dalessio[14] suspect a relationship between wearing glasses and the development of temporal arteritis.

Wagner and Anweiler[15] found atypical features of temporal arteritis which consisted of violent occipital pain, localized loss of hair, scalp necrosis, facial neuralgic pain, and trophic disorders of the oral cavity and the nose.

Reuther and Betz[16] found occasional ischemic manifestations in the skin and mucosal surfaces of the head and also ischemic necrosis of the tongue. They say, however, that these conditions are indeed rare in cases of temporal arteritis.

Schalit and Podoshin[17] point out that the symptoms of a typical case of temporal arteritis may be masked temporarily by other causes of pain such as severe acute nasal sinusitis.

Schutz[18] believes that because temporal arteritis almost always affects persons in the older age group, it may represent a geriatric form of autoimmune vasculitis. He further states that there is a relatively good prognosis, provided irreversible complications are avoided by early diagnosis and appropriate therapy.

DIAGNOSIS

The diagnosis of temporal arteritis may be suspected in patients 55 years of age or older who have a history of malaise, weakness, fever, and anorexia. If the temporal artery is involved the sedimentation rate will be elevated. This is also true if only the ophthalmic artery is involved. A biopsy of the temporal artery should be made if the sedimentation rate is increased.

If temporal arteritis is present, this biopsy will show the classic findings of granulomatous arteritis. Of course, before this biopsy and sedimentation rate are taken, the history of the patient and the examination (palpation of the temporal and occipital arteries) should be positive for temporal arteritis. Careful palpation of the temporal arteries and its branches is essential. When these vessels are the seat of arteritis, the arterial wall is increased several times in thickness by virtue of the subintimal proliferation of connective tissue and the swollen state of the media. As a result, when the affected vessel is compressed against the underlying cranium, the vessel cannot be flattened to the point of disappearance or of obliteration. Instead, a firm pipe-like vessel persists and can be felt by palpation.

Often an initial finding of anemia of undetermined origin is a clue to diagnosis of temporal arteritis. Although most patients with temporal arteritis have mild nonspecific complaints, more than 60% have normochromic, normocytic anemia and a greatly increased sedimentation rate.[19]

TREATMENT

No type of treatment is specific for temporal arteritis. However, if the condition is recognized early and steroids are administered promptly, the ocular complications can be avoided or at least minimized. The steroids will control the arteritis as long as it endures and thus safeguard the vision which remains.

Once the diagnosis has been established, patients should be hospitalized so that the steroid dosage can be controlled and the patient can be observed frequently. An initial dosage of 300 mg of cortisone or its equivalent should be given the first day and reduced in accordance with the changes in the sedimentation rate. The steroid therapy may have to be continued for weeks or months, depending on the disease.

Relief of the headache of temporal arteritis may be obtained in some cases by resection of a portion of the temporal artery involved.[20] However, this is not always successful, and it is done only as a last resort. It is theorized that resection of a portion of the artery counteracts the pain by interrupting the pain-conducting centripetal fibers of the sympathetic nervous system.

To relieve the pain, a simple analgesic is not enough. Such agents as codeine, morphine, and meperidine (Demerol) are usually required.

Chambers[21] believes that the pain of temporal arteritis can be relieved by injecting procaine along the course of the temporal artery.

Frassineti and Rizzini[22] report on a case of temporal arteritis in which the outcome was fatal. This patient complained continuously of bitemporal headaches along the course of the superficial temporal arteries. The headache decreased with periarterial infiltration with procaine, but a slight headache appeared in the back of the neck, which they attributed to involvement of the vertebral arteries. About 3 months following the initial onset of the condition, this patient suddenly died. This was attributed to the fact that the arteritis process had involved an encephalic, probably a bulbar, vessel. In this case the histologic specimen showed periarteritis, mesoarteritis, and endarteritis of a chronic granulomatous productive type, with the presence of giant cells and the absence of eosinophilia, which are typical of temporal arteritis.

Retrobulbar repository steroid injections with systemic steroid therapy were found to give prompt, prolonged improvement of vision in cases of temporal arteritis complicated by occlusion of the central retinal artery or optic neuropathy. Retrobulbar steroid injections can be tried in patients with severe loss of vision and when the prognosis is poor.[23] Many other drastic forms of therapy for temporal arteritis have been tried, primarily because the prognosis for vision in patients with temporal arteritis is usually bad.

Rygvold and Funchald point out that when using steroid therapy in temporal arteritis, great care must be taken not to reduce the dosage too rapidly.[24] They found relatively common recurrences during and after the therapeutic period if too rapid a reduction in dosage or too brief a period of treatment was given the patient.

SUMMARY

Symptoms and signs

1. Patient usually over 55
2. Malaise
3. Anorexia
4. Weight loss
5. Enlarged, tender, rigid temporal vessels
6. Increased sedimentation rate
7. Ocular disturbances (visual decrease or loss)

Pain is

1. Temporal area or generalized
2. Severe
3. Boring
4. Unilateral or bilateral
5. More severe at night during sleep
6. Constant
7. Aggravated by
   a. Chewing
   b. Sneezing
   c. Coughing
   d. Straining
8. May migrate to neck

Treatment

1. Cortisone
2. Procaine injections
3. Surgery

REFERENCES

1. Horton, B. T., Magath, T. B., and Brown, G. E.: Arteritis of the temporal vessels, Arch. Intern. Med. **53**:4000, 1934.
2. Smith, K. R., Jr.: Electron microscopy of giant cell (temporal) arteritis, J. Neurol. Neurosurg. Psychiatry **32**:348-353, 1969.
3. Horton, B. T.: Symposium: head and face pain; medicine, Trans. Am. Acad. Ophthalmol. **49**:23, 1944.
4. Horton, B. T.: Temporal arteritis, Proc. Cent. Soc. Clin. Res. **19**:78, 1946.
5. Lubbers, P., and Edelhoff, J.: Clinical aspects and therapy of temporal arteritis, Chirurg **26**:443, 1955.
6. Klein, R. G., Campbell, R. J., Hinder, G., and Carry, J.: Skip lesions in temporal arteritis, Mayo Clin. Proc. **51**:504-510, 1976.
7. Wagener, H. P., and Hollenhorst, R. W. The ocular lesions of temporal arteritis, Am. J. Ophthalmol. **45**:617-630, 1958.
8. Panter, K.: Recent studies on symptomatology of temporal arteritis with special reference to the literature since 1949 and 2 case reports, Dsch. Z. Nervenheilkd. **176**:219-232, 1957.
9. Simmons, R. J., and Cogan, D. G.: Occult temporal arteritis, Arch. Ophthalmol. **68**:8, 1962.
10. Gutrecht, J. A.: Occult temporal arteritis, J.A.M.A. **213**:1188-1189, 1970.
11. Brearley, B. F., and McDonald, J. G.: Temporal arteritis resulting in infected gangrene of the tongue, Clin. Med. **69**:2477-2478, 1962.
12. Barefoot, S. W., and Lund, H. Z.: Temporal (giant-cell) arteritis associated with ulcerations of scalp, Arch. Dermatol. **93**:79, 1966.
13. Hamrin, B.: Polymyalgia rheumatism with arteritis, Lakartidningen **63**:3877-3891, 1966.
14. Smith, R., and Dalessio, D. J.: Temporal arteritis—why the temporal artery? Headache **12**(1): 18-19, 1972.
15. Wagner, A., and Anweiler, J.: Temporal arteritis a frequently misdiagnosed disease, Taegl. Prox. **13**: 1-6, 1972.
16. Reuther, R., and Betz, H.: Temporal arteritis with ischemic necrosis of the scalp and tongue, Nervenarzt **43**:257-262, 1972.
17. Schalit, M., and Podoshin, L.: Temporal arteritis masked by contralateral pansinusitis, Int. Rhinol. **9**:153-157, 1971.
18. Schutz, R. M.: Temporal arteritis, Kreisl **5**:284-287, 1973.
19. Whitaker, J. J., Hagedorn, A. B., and Pease, G. L.: Anemia in temporal arteritis, Postgrad. Med. **40**:35-39, 1966.
20. Lubber, P. and Edelhoff, J.: Clinical aspects and therapy of temporal arteritis, Chirurg **26**:443-450, 1955.
21. Chambers, W. R.: Experiences in severe intractable headache, South. Med. J. **47**:741, 1954.
22. Frassineti, A., and Rizzini, V.: Temporal arteritis: fatal case, Sett. Med. **42**:565, 1954.
23. Schimek, R. A., and Newsom, S. R.: Restoration of vision in temporal arteritis by retrobulbar injections of steroids, Am. J. Ophthalmol. **62**:693-696, 1966.
24. Rygvold, O., and Funchald, P.: Temporal arteritis, T. Norske Laegeforen **93**:690-692, 1973.

CHAPTER 15

Allergic headache

The topic of allergic headache is always a subject of great controversy. Allergists are quick to say that allergy plays a significant role in the production of headache. However, this is merely theoretical and is far from proved. However, it is only fair to state that the allergic factors should be thoroughly investigated in cases of chronic headache, especially those in which the diagnosis is difficult.

Headache and allergenic predisposition have a known relationship that is older than the present concept of allergy itself. More than a century ago, the medical literature noted that sensitivity to a particular food might cause a specific type of headache.[1] Other early writings showing the existence of such a relationship include a paper published in 1873,[2] in which the frequency of headache among asthmatic patients was shown, and a report in 1892,[3] which demonstrated blood eosinophilia in patients during headache attacks.

Allergy is a form of hypersensitivity affecting various tissues. The term "allergy" denotes the specific change in the reactivity of an organism toward an allergenic substance (proteins of certain foods, bacteria, pollen, and so on), as a result of contact with that substance.

The occurrence and intensity of allergic reactions, and possibly the development of allergy itself, are significantly affected by psychic, nervous, climatic, endocrine, and metabolic factors. Accurate diagnosis of the allergic state is a delicate task.

Within the past several years there has been a considerable amount of discussion by allergists concerning the etiology of migraine. They often have stated that migraine is due to allergy. However, this idea has been generally disproved. There is, however, such a headache as an allergic headache. It is difficult, however, to show the exact relationship of allergy to headache because, in an allergic individual, not all coexisting disease syndromes need be of allergic origin. Furthermore, even if some allergenic material can produce a headache in a given patient, the same headache can also, under different conditions, be elicited by other factors.

In 1931, a group of recurrent allergic headaches was described by Eyermann.[4] These, however, did not follow the recognized migraine pattern. In many of these cases nasal obstruction and discharge were present, and the headache was often diffuse and bilateral. Many of the cases described by Eyermann presented headache in the frontal region of the head, and the pain would often migrate from the frontal region and spread out over the entire head. The patients underwent skin tests and were found to be sensitive to certain foods and pollens, different patients being sensitive to different things. These headaches were called allergic headaches, and not migraine, by Eyermann.

Later, in 1932, Goltman[5] reported a group of unusual cases of headache. He found that many of his patients were not relieved by the avoidance of foods and that skin reactions were positive to certain inhalants, such as pollens, orrisroot, hairs, and danders. Satisfactory relief was obtained in these cases by hyposensitization. It was further found that this group of patients had nasal and respiratory symptoms of a local nature.

Zussman[6] states that most of the problems of recurrent headaches seen in practice are of the allergic frontal and occipital type, and only 5% to 10% of headache fall into the classic migraine type of vascular headaches. He also says that allergic headaches are always associated with other allergic manifestations, usually of the respiratory type, such as hay fever, allergic rhinitis, and bronchial asthma. He found a high incidence of familial allergy and headaches in the patients' histories and noted that sensitization to pollens and inhalants plays the major role in patients with recurrent allergic headaches.

Sanders[7] states that allergy is a frequent cause of headache, so frequent that the possibility of allergy should be considered in all patients with headaches. On the other hand Friedman[8] concludes that allergic headaches are not a common form of headache. With this we totally agree.

It seems that allergists think that allergic headache is a common form of headache and nonallergists think it is not.

ETIOLOGY

Many years ago, Ogden[9] found that house dust was one of the etiologic features of headache. He presented several cases of frontal headache and stated that this type of pain followed a rather definite pattern. It could be shown to be due to an inhalant allergen, house dust. He believed that the full importance of house dust had been neglected and that this was the reason for many unsatisfactory results in the treatment of headache.

Some types of headache may be caused by inhalant substances and foods. If so, we find positive skin reactions to certain foods, relief of symptoms following avoidance of foods or inhalants, and subsequent recurrence of symptoms after eating the foods or after exposure to various inhalants. It is conjectured that the basic change is an edema of the meninges and the causes leading to this change are the offending foods or inhalants, a factor in the etiology.

Unger[10] believes that food allergies can cause headache. He states that among the many causes of headache, food allergy is one. Its discovery is a laborious, time-consuming, and complicated business, through elimination diets and trial feeding. The elimination diet test consists of 2-week periods in which the patient does not take a particular food item or a combination of up to five items. Trial feeding is exactly the opposite. In the selection of food items for these tests a detailed history is of prime importance. The most frequently reported alimentary causes of headache include chocolate, pork, coffee, wheat, milk, eggs, chicken, nuts, oranges, spices, legumes, and drugs.

Foods are perhaps more important in allergic headache than inhalants, although the shock tissue may be present anywhere in the body, regardless of the offending allergen. The vascular reaction produces edema in various parts of the brain. This is reflected by varying symptoms, depending on the area involved. Increased capillary permeability and dilation of the arterioles are usually present.

Allergy may be the cause of "migraine-like" headaches. Notice the term "migraine-like" is used. Many headaches that do not meet the requirements of migraine are diagnosed or classified as migraine. Migraine is considered a clinical entity, but we do not know its cause. It more than likely has something to do with the endocrine system. By the same token allergy can be influenced by the endocrine system. This is demonstrated by the frequent change in the shock organ at the various stages of life. The skin is the common shock organ in infants. Between the stage of infancy and childhood the upper respiratory tract may become the shock organ. The lower respiratory tract may take over at puberty with the appearance of asthma. During the menopause the shock organ may again change, this time affecting the gastrointestinal tract, mimicking gallbladder disease. It is not uncommon to see gastrointestinal symptoms in older patients disappear while they are being treated for nasal allergy. Pregnancy often influences (usually improves) the existing allergy. Those phenomena occur too frequently to be coincidental.

Another type of headache in the allergic group is accompanied by peripheral edema, polydipsia, weight gain several days preceding the attack, and polyuria with weight loss heralding the culmination of the attack. The head pain is generalized and is associated with a feeling of pressure, dizziness, and mental confusion. This type of headache, as described by Hansel, occurs in allergic individuals and is frequently related to other allergic manifestations such as urticaria, angioedema, atopic dermatitis, or gastrointestinal allergy.[11]

Patients with headache due to involvement of the nose and paranasal sinuses also fall into this category. Most of these patients have symptoms of chronic nasal allergy and probably belong in the group having frontal headache, as described by Ogden.[12]

Uzkaragoz and Saraclar[13] believe that allergic headache may be classified into primary and secondary types. The primary type is caused by the direct action of ''H'' substance on the cerebral arteries and may vary from a simple frontal headache to typical migraine. The most common secondary allergic headache is the sinus headache, which is frequently associated with allergic rhinitis. The secondary type often occurs in patients experiencing emotional difficulties and is associated with other manifestations of an allergic reaction. The authors conclude that the mechanism of allergic headache is based on the immunologic characteristics of the individual who is affected by both internal and external factors. The internal factors are allergens, infections, emotion, endocrine changes, and exertion. The external factors are climate changes, odors, and irritants.

Speer[14] believes that the causes of migraine should include allergy. With this we cannot agree. He lists allergic causes of migraine to be inhalants and foods. Unger and Cristol[15] are other allergists who believe migraine to be an allergic type of headache caused by one or more foods.

We strongly agree that there is such a headache as an allergic headache. However, we definitely do not believe it to be a very common type of headache. We strongly disagree with the theory that migraine has an allergic etiology; we are sure that it does not. However, since all of the theories of the etiology of migraine are at the present time theoretical, anyone is entitled to an opinion.

Other vascular mechanisms of pain may play a role during the so-called allergic headache. When the branches of the anterior meningeal artery, which supplies the nasal mucosa, become dilated and produce a certain degree of pressure change in the walls, the previously described pathway of pain is initiated. The pain may also occur because of mucosal edema with pressure on the nerve endings surrounding the blood vessels in this area, which in turn become dilated and thus also produce pain. The mucosal edema may produce the initial pressure or the vasodilation may occur initially. When the headache occurs in the frontal area the frontal branch of the supraorbital artery, which is also a branch of the ophthalmic artery, is visibly dilated during the acute stage of the headache. The anterior and posterior ethmoidal arteries also play a role in producing pain when the ethmoidal sinuses are involved. These branches are also present in the frontal sinus and in the nasal mucoperiosteum.[16]

Swinny[17] reported cases of allergic headache due to absorption of lanolin. Thus, the physician is warned that the mechanism of allergic headache can occur through the absorption of substances through the skin.

To be correctly classified as an allergic headache, the headache should, therefore, appear after the ingestion of certain foods or the exposure to certain other specific allergens; positive skin tests should show some specific hypersensitivity; and good results should be obtained from either desensitization or elimination diets. Usually these patients also have some other form of allergic pathology along with the headaches.

Haywood and McGovern[18] have made a simple classification of allergic headache:

1. Primary allergic headache (vascular type, resulting from direct action of chemical mediator substances on cerebral microcirculation)
2. Secondary allergic headache (of which there are three types, each resulting from changes secondary to the allergic reaction itself)
   a. So-called sinus headache
   b. Pressure-referred headache (pain referred from another area where allergic edema exists)
   c. Somatopsychic-psychosomatic complex (psychophysiologic allergic tension-fatigue syndrome with headache)

Allergic patients with headaches often have special interrelated problems. Allergic rhinitis, for example, often is complicated by sinusitis and associated so-called headaches of nasal vasomotor reaction (sinus headaches). Atopic patients frequently are noted to have significant emotional overlay, and muscle contraction headaches (tension headaches) are common in this group. Finally there is some evidence that vascular headaches (migraine) frequently are associated with, or even initiated by, hypersensitivity mechanisms.[19]

Haywood and McGovern[18] state that the term "allergic headache" denotes headache that results from a pathophysiologic response initiated by an antigen-antibody reaction. Once the specific reaction of antigen (allergen) with homologous antibody (reagin) occurs, there may occur a variety of physiochemical phenomena resulting in so-called target tissue changes and headache in the predisposed individual.

Current knowledge of basic immunologic mechanisms leading to pathophysiologic changes which produce hypersensitivity reactions and certain true allergic headache would bring about a four-stage reaction:

1. Antigen-antibody activity at a "cellular" level or at a "humoral" level (immunologic or enzyme basis)
2. Resultant cullular damage that leads to the outpouring of histamine and the other "H" substances
3. The physiopharmacologic action of these "H" substances on the so-called shock tissues, including parts of the macrocirculation and microcirculation
4. The response of these "shock" tissues whose reaction pattern causes the physical symptoms observed[19]

SYMPTOMATOLOGY

In most cases of allergic headache there are usually some symptoms present which are referable to the nose. Usually there is some nasal obstruction and congestion, a watery rhinorrhea, and sometimes sneezing. On examination, the nasal mucosa is found to be pale, which is commonly seen in cases of allergic rhinitis, and the mucosa is hypertrophic and rather edematous. Normally the mucous membrane of allergic rhinitis is bluish-gray. This does not mean that all nasal allergy patients also have allergic headaches, but the reverse is true; most patients with allergic headache do have some allergic symptoms which are referable to the nose.

Ogden[20] stated that if nasal symptoms are associated with headache, it is obvious that many of these cases are primarily due to nasal allergy. Therefore, attention must be directed to a correct etiologic diagnosis. Usually skin-testing procedures are employed, with special emphasis on inhalant allergy.

Swelling of the nasal turbinates secondary to allergy leads to pressure against the septal or lateral nasal walls and may produce headache by irritating the nerve ganglia in the nasal passages. This may result in pain in any part of the head as well as radiated pain into the neck, back, shoulders, and upper extremities. Pain may be referred through known neuronal pathways or at times does not appear to have any particular spinal reference.

Allergic headache of sinus origin is most commonly due to pressure on nerves from swollen mucosa about the sinus ostia. This type of cephalalgia may be associated with either hay fever, in which there is a seasonal incidence of symptoms corresponding to peak periods of specific pollination, or more often with perennial allergic rhinitis, wherein symptoms are of chronic or semichronic, intermittent, or nonseasonal character.[18]

Allergic headaches are usually periodic. They occur only when the patient comes into contact with the allergen causing the trouble, whether it be an inhalant or food. In these individuals one usually does find a positive family history of allergy, a past history of allergic disease, and association of headache with definite concurrent and recurrent allergic symptoms. The allergic symptoms as well as the headaches in some of these individuals may be precipitated by exposure to offending allergens and occasionally to physical agents (for example, cold or heat) and relieved on their withdrawal.

Usually the allergic type of headache is bilateral and frequently more pronounced in the frontal area, the vertex, or the occipital area. However, Sanders,[21] in speaking of the location of allergic headache states that it may be situated in one discrete area, confined to one side of the head (occiput or frontal area), or generalized. The headache may produce or simulate an increased intracranial pressure. Sometimes the patient complains of pressure behind the eyes.

Ogden[22] concludes that allergy is frequently a cause of headache, especially that found in the frontal area.

Eyermann[4] stated that while true allergic headaches are usually frontal in nature, they may also be atypical and may be generalized. Both frontal and generalized headaches may result from dilation of branches of the internal carotid artery.[18] Vascular pains may appear on any part of the head.

Allergic headaches caused by a sensitivity to foods do not necessarily follow any pattern as to location, onset, or severity. They mimic all types of headache.[21]

So we see there is a considerable amount of disagreement concerning the location of the pain of allergic headache.

Since the duration of the attacks may vary from less than an hour to several days, there is nothing characteristic about this.

Some may add to the severity of the symptoms by reingestion of the causative agent. The degree of sensitivity and the rapidity of elimination of the allergen must play some part in the duration of the symptoms.

The onset of the headache may be minutes after the ingestion of the allergen or hours later, depending on the sensitivity of the person as well as the type of reaction—that is, immediate or delayed. The onset of the headache may vary even in the same person. Probably more headaches develop 4 to 6 hours after absorption of the allergen than any other time. This is more noticeable in the patient who awakens in the early morning, 2 to 4 A.M., with a severe headache after ingesting a sensitizing food. If the patient is highly sensitive to a food and any extracranial or intracranial structures are the shock organ, headache is more likely to appear immediately. If the patient is not extremely sensitive to a food, symptoms might not appear unless the food is eaten at frequent intervals such as two to three times a day or 2 or more days in succession. The frequency of the food ingestion seems to be of more importance than the amount of the food ingested.

There may be some mild gastrointestinal symptom in the allergic type of headache. If so, it is usually nausea, but it is not severe and in many cases it is not even present.

As a rule, allergic headaches are seen in adults; only rarely are they present in children. A family history of allergic headache is quite common, just as is a family history of other types of allergic disturbances.

As for severity of the headache, this tends to vary considerably. It depends a great deal on the threshold of pain of the patient. Also some patients have a habit of complaining much more easily than do others. This depends a great deal on the mental attitude of the patient.

TREATMENT

Certain factors are needed to call a headache attack an allergic headache. Either the attack must follow the ingestion of certain foods, or it must follow exposure to certain inhalant antigens. If either of these two factors can be established in taking the history from the patient, the patient should be given skin tests. If positive skin tests can be obtained they would indicate that the patient has a specific hypersensitivity toward these substances. If these are obtained, the patient should then be desensitized against the antigens which were found to give the positive skin reactions. Along with the desensitization program, the patient should be placed on a diet free from any of the foods giving a positive skin reaction. If this form of treatment abolishes the headache attacks, then the diagnosis of allergic headache certainly can be established.

Shapiro and Eisenberg[23] believe that specific therapy should be given to the allergic headache patient. They say that specific therapy includes control of home environment, elimination of offending foods, or hyposensitization, depending on the allergen. No single symptomatic remedy is reliably effective. Early in an episode, attacks may be aborted by an injection of 0.5 ml of aqueous epinephrine 1:1,000. In headaches arising from blocked sinus ostia, packing the nose with a large cotton wick saturated with decongestant solution brings relief.

A complete allergy study is necessary for the correct diagnosis and treatment of this condition. Hyposensitization, elimination diet, and symptomatic therapy are valuable in preventing the recurrence of these headaches. Avoidance of the offending allergens is very important. When feasible, surgical treatment of any chronically infected area, including the removal of polyps, may be of additional assistance.

Grater and associates[24] found allergic headache, which was associated with nasal symptoms, to be benefited from the use of Sinutab. This product contains drugs which counteract the symptoms of nasal allergy. In other words, they directed their attention toward the nasal allergy, and when this was controlled, the allergic headache was correspondingly controlled. They further concluded that this drug was of benefit only in cases of allergic headache with these associated nasal allergies. Similar findings are reported by Flohr, Grater, and Baldwin.[25]

As with all types of recurrent headaches, a thorough knowledge of the patient is desirable, for the patient must receive sympathetic support and understanding care if his own insights are to be heightened, if the intervals between the attacks are to be lengthened, and if relief is to be obtained. Great benefit can accrue from a few talks together that may lead to modification of living habits, goals, stressful situations, and certain reaction patterns to stress.[18]

When these measures have failed to keep an individual's allergic headache under control, the advisability of a thorough allergic study should be considered. This must then include a detailed allergy history, indicated skin testing, and hyposensitization to offending airborne allergens, in addition to other selected diagnostic and antiallergic therapeutic modalities as well as those previously mentioned. For severe recurrent or protracted allergic headaches not relieved by other medications, a short "blocking period" with corticosteroids may be of distinct help for symptomatic relief.

In allergic headaches complete avoidance or removal of offending allergens (usually inhalants or ingestants) is the ideal. Unfortunately, this is usually impossible, although much can be gained by practical elimination procedures. Also, a positive program for proper use of symptomatic medication as outlined by the physician will give the patient confidence in his ability to cope with acute episodes of headache.

The antihistamines are also helpful in the treatment of allergic headache. We find tripelennamine (Pyribenzamine) and chlorpheniramine (Chlor-trimeton) to be the most helpful. These drugs act by inhibiting the stimulating action of histamine on smooth muscle and the formation of edema. We like to give the average patient with allergic headache 50 mg of tripelennamine every 4 hours or 12 mg of Chlor-trimeton Repeatab twice a day. These antihistamine drugs very frequently will have side effects, usually in the form of drowsiness. Sometimes they will produce vertigo, dryness of the mouth, concentrated urine, and mental dullness.

CASE HISTORY

Mrs. R. R., a 35-year old female, complained of headaches during the past 12 years. She admitted that they were not of such severity that she could not stand the attacks, but they had been present irregularly over such a long period of time that they were exceedingly annoying. The headaches were bilateral and quite often generalized throughout the entire head. They were present for various lengths of time. On some occasions they would persist for several days. There were no gastrointestinal, ophthalmologic, or rhinologic symptoms associated with the attacks. However, on careful questioning she stated that there was some nasal obstruction present with most of the headache attacks.

The headaches were not associated with her menstrual periods and she stated that they were not "sick headaches." The attacks were not postural and there was no tenderness associated with the headaches. The headaches were not of the migratory type. Throbbing in nature, her attacks would begin rather suddenly and end in a like manner.

There were no associated manifestations except for the fact that she did think that the attacks were more frequent and more pronounced during the winter season. She complained of a violent headache attack two evenings before her first visit to the office. This attack came on rather suddenly, not long after she had started dancing, and became so severe she had to leave the dance floor. In less than 1 hour after she had left the dancing party, her headache had completely cleared without any medication. This patient also noticed that every time she would go to a beauty parlor she would get a severe headache.

The otolaryngologic and general physical examinations were negative. Her neurologic, ophthalmologic, and fundus examinations were also all of a negative nature.

This headache problem did not fit into the exact pattern of a vascular headache. It was decided that this patient should be given skin tests. Her skin tests were all negative except for one item; orrisroot gave a positive reaction. When this positive reaction was found, the history became much clearer. She had noticed the headaches to be present always when she went to the beauty parlor. Naturally, she came into contact with orrisroot in such an establishment. She had noticed that the headaches were much more severe in the wintertime than they were during the summer season. The explanation here was that during the summer months she became very tan because of repeated sunbathing and therefore, did not wear any make-up except for a little lipstick. Thus, she was not using products with orrisroot in any great quantities or so frequently in the summer as she did in the winter months.

The third interesting point in this case is the fact that she had such an extreme, intensive headache while at a dancing party. On questioning the person at the country club who was in charge of the dining room where the dance was being held, it was found that to make the dancing more enjoyable, the entire dance floor had been sprinkled with talcum powder. The talcum powder brought this patient into contact with the orrisroot and thus produced a typical allergic headache attack.

This patient was instructed how she could stay away from cosmetics and how she could use cosmetics which were orrisroot-free. She was told to avoid beauty parlors as much as possible. The antihistamines in this case produced only fair results. The patient showed remarkable improvement by avoiding the causative agent, the orrisroot products, as much as possible.

SUMMARY

As stated before, we do not believe that migraine is of an allergic etiology. However, there are some headaches which are due to allergy, but these two types of headache should not be confused.

Too many things today are referred to as being due to an allergy or a virus simply because we are not exactly sure of the etiology. These expressions offer "a way out" for the physician. Perhaps this may be the case also in trying to place the blame for migraine onto allergy.

As was pointed out by Ogden,[9] an allergic survey can be made only after a proper diagnostic approach has been used, and only after the functional and organic nonallergic headaches have been definitely ruled out. If this is undertaken, the diagnosis will be made much more readily.

In most patients with any type of allergic headache, properly conceived and adequately administered therapy in accordance with the principles outlined usually is productive of good to excellent relief of symptoms.

REFERENCES

1. Feinberg, S. M.: Allergy: facts and fancies, New York, 1951, Harper & Row, Publishers.
2. Trousseau, A.: cited in Schwartz, M. S.: Is migraine allergic disease? J. Allergy 23:426, 1952.
3. Neusser, E.: cited in Vaughan, W. T.: Allergic migraine, J.A.M.A. 88:1382, 1927.
4. Eyermann, C. H.: Allergic headache, J. Allergy 2:106, 1931.
5. Goltman, A. M.: Unusual cases of migraine with special reference to treatment, J. Allergy 4:51, 1932.
6. Zussman, B. M.: Allergy associated with severe migraine-like headache, South. Med. J. 58:1542, 1965.
7. Sanders, S. H.: Headaches of allergic origin, Eye Ear Nose Throat Mon. 41:829-830, 1962.
8. Friedman, A. P.: Headache and allergy, Am. J. Nurs. 64:117-120, 1964.
9. Ogden, H. D.: Inhalant sensitization in allergic headaches, South. Med. J. 41:931, 1948.
10. Unger, A.: Food allergies may cause headache, Am. Allergy 8:534-538, 1950.
11. Hansel, F. K.: Clinical allergy, St. Louis, 1953, The C. V. Mosby Co.
12. Ogden, H. D.: Frontal headache, New Orleans Med. Soc. J. 104:326, 1952.
13. Uzkaragoz, K., and Saraclar, Y.: The mechanism of allergic headache, Hagettepe Bull. Med. Surg. 3:53-68, 1970.
14. Speer, F.: Allergic factors in migraine, Mod. Med. 39:101-106, 1971.
15. Unger, L., and Cristol, J.: Allergic migraine, Am. Allergy 28:106-109, 1970.
16. Meyer, L., and Kaufmann, M.: A review of the headache problem in allergy, South. Med. J. 52:1495-1507, 1959.
17. Swinny, B.: Headache due to absorption of lanolin, South. Med. J. 52:168-169, 1959.
18. Haywood, T., and McGovern, J. P.: Allergic headache, Headache 9:141-146, 1969.
19. McGovern, J. P.: An etiologic mechanism and a new classification of allergic headache, Headache 4:205-216, 1964.
20. Ogden, H. D.: The treatment of allergic headache, Am. Allergy 9:611-615, 1951.
21. Sanders, S. H.: Headache of allergic origin, Eye Ear Nose Throat Mon. 41:936-938, 1962.
22. Ogden, H. D.: The relationship of allergy to headache, Headache 1:14-24, 1961.
23. Shapiro, R. S., and Eisenberg, B. C.: Allergic headache, Ann. Allergy 23:123, 1965.
24. Grater, W. C., Haywood, T. J., and McGovern, J. P.: Diagnostic and therapeutic application of drug therapy in allergic patients suffering from headache, Headache 2:160-164, 1962.
25. Flohr, L., Grater, W. C., and Ballwin, J.: Combination drug therapy for headaches: evaluation by an internist, allergist, and otorhinologist, Eye Ear Nose Throat Dig., pp. 23-26, May 1961.

CHAPTER 16

Alcoholic headache

Depending on how it is used, alcohol can be considered to be either a drug or a food. When it is used as a drug it may be called on to produce sedative, tranquilizing, hypnotic, or anesthetic effects. This all depends on the dosage. Caution must be used, however, for the ingestion of this substance can lead to addiction or dependence. In fact, alcoholism is one of the most prevalent types of drug addiction in the civilized world. When used as a food it supplies 7 calories per gram, but these are really empty calories because alcohol contains no essential elements even though it supplies heat and energy.

Alcohol differs from ordinary foods because it is not stored by the body; the major portion of ingested alcohol is metabolized by the liver. The rate of metabolism is constant and is not influenced by either high or low blood levels.

Graham[1] states that alcohol is not stored by the body; 80% to 90% of its oxidation occurs via obligatory hepatic metabolism without regulatory control over the rate of ethanol metabolism. The extrahepatic metabolism of ethanol and its excretion in the urine, breath, and sweat are of minor importance in its elimination, but the constant relationship between the blood ethanol level and the amount of expired ethanol is responsible for the popular breath test used to detect legal intoxication.

Dalessio[2] stated that alcohol is almost entirely metabolized in the liver. Only a little is excreted unchanged in the urine, perspiration, or tears. The concentration of alcohol depends to some extent on the type of alcohol ingested. If one drinks gin and vodka, a sharp rise in blood alcohol is appreciated, sharper than if one takes wine or beer.

Alcohol is ordinarily metabolized in the body at a relatively constant rate.[2] It is possible, however, to modify this rate by eating foods, especially those containing the common sugar fructose. Experimental studies show that mean blood alcohol levels are lower after the ingestion of fructose, using the subject as his own control. Thirty grams of fructose will increase the rate of metabolism of alcohol by 15% to 30%. No other sugars have this effect on alcohol metabolism including glucose, galactose, and sucrose. Ingesting large amounts of vitamins, including the B-complex vitamins, vitamin C, vitamin E, and the like, will not affect the rate of alcohol metabolism in the healthy human. But fructose will make alcohol burn in the body considerably faster than it would be burned otherwise.

Etiology

Alcohol is probably the most frequently consumed substance of all those exogenous substances which are toxic to the brain. Many individuals who develop the alcoholic habit and become chronic alcoholics will actually become psychogenic problems. A functional psychoneurosis will develop which actually arises from an emotional immaturity. Emotional maturity is not attained by these persons, frequently because it is blocked unconsciously by too much parental dominance or love during the individual's childhood or adolescence. Therefore, when these persons reach the age when social maturity is needed, they are unable to grasp it thoroughly. They have a feeling of inferiority and a natural unconscious desire for regression to childhood days when they had less responsibility. There are many ways in which these individuals can effect this regression, but the easiest and quickest way is to turn to the abusive use of alcohol. This is because alcohol is so easily obtainable and society does not frown on its use, but it does frown on its overuse. The emotionally immature patient is thus easily susceptible to alcoholism. These individuals will usually develop a guilt complex which they are also unable to handle properly. This merely drives them more to the alcohol, for they will employ it in greater quantities to relieve themselves of this new guilt complex.

Alcohol is very soluble in water. Its absorption is through the stomach directly into the bloodstream by simple diffusion. Alcohol is distributed into the body tissues and body fluids proportional to their water content. Alcohol enters the brain tissue at a very rapid rate and may even be found in the cerebrospinal fluid.

Alcohol has a tendency to increase the volume and the flow of urine and because of this a resultant dehydration may occur.

Granerus and co-workers[3] found that the histamine content of various alcoholic drinks was estimated by purification on an ion-exchange column and subsequent bioassay. The red wines and sherries investigated contained large amounts of histamine (208 to 1,506 μg free histamine base per 100 ml); white wine, beer, and port occupied an intermediate position (2.6 to 19 μg free histamine base per 100 ml); and whisky and brandy, which are distilled, showed no histamine activity. They concluded that the headache and flushing sometimes experienced after drinking alcohol may be partly due to the histamine content, and that it is difficult to state whether histamine is primarily or secondarily involved in such reactions.

ACUTE ALCOHOLISM
Symptomatology

When a large quantity of alcohol is consumed, the influence is found to be chiefly on the nervous system and is evidenced by muscular incoordination, mental disturbances, and headaches. The headaches frequently appear after the individual is home and in bed, or even on arising the morning following the drinking. These alcoholic headaches are usually constant and throbbing. Any straining, such as coughing, stooping, and straining at stool, will tend to make these headaches much more severe. Head movements of any excessive type will increase the severity. Usually these headaches are worse if the head is on a horizontal plane with the rest of the body. Individuals obtain some slight relief by propping up their heads with a few pillows. The alcoholic type of headache is vascular and is due to the dilation of the cerebral vessels and the blood vessels of the scalp. Therefore, any factor which might conceivably tend to increase the intracranial pressure will also make these headaches much more severe.

Other symptoms of acute alcoholism are deep and slow respirations, full pulse, flushed face, dilated pupils, and alcoholic breath. Symptoms arising from alcohol ingestion are those associated with intoxication or with withdrawal and, in general, are related to the blood alcohol level.

Symptoms are increased as the blood alcohol level changes, and they tend to improve at constant blood alcohol levels.

At times, such factors as emotional stress and physical exhaustion may be associated with the onset of alcoholic headache.

Alcohol may produce pain in the occipital area in patients with chordoma.[4]

Dogadakis and Ziefer[5] describe headache produced by alcohol in a case of urticaria pigmentosa of the maculopapular type.

Treatment

The headache of acute alcoholism may be relieved by rest and ice packs, and the analgesic group of drugs (Empirin Compound, Fiorinal, and aspirin) may give some relief. Some individuals receive considerable relief the morning after from the caffeine in coffee. Acute alcoholism usually requires little treatment unless acute alcoholic coma occurs.

It is sometimes possible to reduce the intensity of a hangover by employing fructose, either therapeutically or prophylactically. Fructose is particularly plentiful in honey and it is also present in vegetables and vegetable extracts such as tomato juice. A slice of toast well spread with honey, taken prior to bedtime after an evening of considerable drinking, is a simple and effective remedy for hangover. The ingestion of vegetable juices during the hangover hours may be helpful in hastening the metabolism of whatever alcohol remains in the body to be metabolized. Thus, the standard morning-after cocktail of tomato juice with some added spices may be more therapeutically sound than suspected previously.[2]

CHRONIC ALCOHOLISM
Symptomatology

Chronic alcoholism may have certain nervous system effects, such as muscular unsteadiness, mental dullness, irritability, forgetfulness, peripheral neuritis, tremors, thickness of speech, visual hallucinations, insomnia, stupor, and delirium tremens. Gastrointestinal symptoms of chronic alcoholism may consist of poor appetite, constipation, stomach dilation, cirrhosis of the liver, furred tongue, and avitaminosis. Headache is not so common a feature of chronic alcoholism as it is in acute alcoholism.

After prolonged alcohol ingestion alcohol withdrawal syndromes may occur.[1] These withdrawal syndromes can be classified into diagnostic groups of increasing severity: (1) the tremulous state, (2) alcoholic hallucinosis or the tremulous state plus hallucinations without disorientation, and (3) delirium tremens. Although overlap occurs, most patients can be conveniently catalogued into one of the three groups.

Treatment

Chronic alcoholism requires the care of a well-trained psychologist, and even then many of these patients cannot be helped. Eventually the patient should be referred for some form of group therapy, perhaps Alcoholics Anonymous.

Sometimes specific medical therapy can help the alcoholic stop drinking. Disulferam (Antabuse) is a medicine which interferes with the metabolism of alcohol.

REFERENCES

1. Graham, D. Y.: Alcohol and alcoholism: acute and chronic sequelae, Tex. Med. **71**:71-76, 1975.
2. Dalessio, D. J.: Alcohol, alcoholism, the social drinker and hangover, Headache **13**:173-176, 1973.
3. Granerus, G., Sevensson, S. E., and Wetterovist, H.: Histamine in alcoholic drinks, Lancet **1**(7609): 1320, 1969.
4. Peekin, G. D.: Alcohol induced pain in chordoma, Br. Med. J. **3**:478, 1973.
5. Dogadakis, C., and Ziefer, I.: Flushes, freckles, and headache, Headache **16**:91-95, 1976.

CHAPTER 17

Myalgia of the head

Myalgia of the head represents a type of headache which arises from the musculature. It is very frequently not diagnosed, and this is most unfortunate because it is a very common form of headache. Besides being a common form of headache, the diagnosis is quite simple if the symptomatology is known. Relief from the pain of this condition is also easily given to the patient.

Many patients who actually have myalgia of the head complain to their physician that they have "sinus trouble" or "sinus headaches." Examination of these patients reveals tender areas in the musculature about the head and the neck.

Williams and Elkins,[1] in defining myalgia of the head, state that it may be divided into two categories. "In the first category, the myalgia process may exist in the postural muscles inserting into the cranial bones. In the second category, the muscles having their origin from the bones of the skull are involved, particularly the occipitofrontalis and the temporal muscles." They further state that "when one of the muscles originating from or inserting into the cranial bones is involved in myalgia, then there is a circumscribed region of tenderness which may or may not be, but usually is, the seat of a spontaneous pain during an attack." Pressure on the region of tenderness may produce referred pain.

Pain referred to the musculature of the head is a very common complaint encountered by the physician. Unfortunately, this condition throughout the years has been given numerous different terms which sometimes is rather confusing. Myalgia of the head has also been referred to as fibrositis, myositis, myofascitis, myofascial pain syndrome, fibromyositis, and numerous other entities.

Myalgia of the head is frequently seen by the physician during the seasons of the year when there is frequent and sudden temperature change. Actually myalgia of the head belongs under the field of intrinsic or physical allergy.

ETIOLOGY

The present concept of the etiology of myalgia of the head is that it is due to a physical type of allergy. Physical allergy is a syndrome which clinically may be very difficult to differentiate from the antigen-antibody type of allergy. In the physical type of allergy, we find the patient to be very sensitive to any type of sudden temperature change. He may have an attack precipitated by drafts, air conditioning, electric fans, any sudden change from hot to cold or cold to hot, changes in the atmospheric pressure, or even changes in the humidity.

There are two physical reactions, as described by Duke.[2] The first is what Duke believes to be contact reactions, in which symptoms are produced at the site directly exposed to the action of the physical agent. The second purely physical reaction Duke describes is the reflex-like reaction in which the phenomena occur in tissue not directly exposed to the action of a physical agent; this may be confined to one site or to one structure, or it may be generalized.

Duke further described physical allergy as a syndrome clinically indistinguishable from the antigen-antibody or immunologic type of allergy, the existing agents being heat, light, cold, mechanical irritation, changes in the atmospheric pressure, and changes in the humidity, along with emotional disturbances.[2] Thus a physical or intrinsic form of allergy depends on a different physiologic stimulus from that found in the antigen-antibody type of allergy.

Using the method devised by Code[3] in a group of cases of physical (intrinsic) allergy, Rose[4] pointed out that the histamine content of the circulating blood was likely to increase after exposure to an appropriate stimulus, while, on the other hand, the histamine content of the blood of a group of normal patients tends to remain fairly constant.

Lewis, Grant, and Marvin[5] showed that following the stimulation of the skin of patients who had been sensitized by physical agents, a condition of partial or complete refractoriness to further stimulation of the same type was established. They believed that the production of a painful condition, such as myalgia, by physical stimuli was a phenomenon similar in nature to the cutaneous reaction produced by physical agents. Lewis and Grant[6] further showed that in the skin of human beings sensitized by exposure to physical irritants, further exposure to such irritants after a latent period will produce a reaction indistinguishable from that produced by the injection of histamine.

Williams pointed out that the funda-mental reaction of allergy, whether of an antigen-antibody or a physical type, is a reaction of the peripheral arterial bed.[7] In certain areas arteriolar constriction with capillary and venular dilation and atony may lead to local tissue anoxia, increased capillary permeability, increased interstitial fluid, and release of toxic substances such as histamine, heparin, and the like, depending on the type of cell injured. There is evidence that such reactions occur in individuals who have a tendency toward dysfunction of the autonomic nerves, specifically cholinergic hyperactivity.

Areas of hyperactivity of the cholinergic nerves are more apt to appear in the head and cervical region, because these are the areas which show the emotional reactions transmitted by the autonomic nerves, that is, the site of the flushing and paling to emotional perturbations. This seems to result in a special autonomic instability in these regions.

Some investigators believe that the general idiosyncratic disposition toward intrinsic allergies is based on a hereditary factor. The hereditary factor is probably far more important in the occurrence of the physical allergy type of case than are such external influences as local sensitization, inflammation, or trauma.

Lewis[8] and Kellgren[9,10] established the condition of myalgia of the head on an experimental basis. These men demonstrated that the pain present in an attack of myalgia of the head is the same type of pain experienced when a muscle is forced to exercise under ischemic conditions. They further concluded that pain from a given muscle is felt over certain definite regions and that it seems to follow a certain definite, segmented type of pattern. Lewis concluded that the pain from a given muscle is determined by a chemical or a physiochemical stimulus which is developed in the muscle mass. He calls the stimulus the "P" factor. He further states that the process is rapidly reversible in the presence of oxygenated blood. These studies lead to the conclusion that, possibly, local vaso-constriction in the arterial end of the capillaries might lead to a deficit in oxygen, and this may be the basic physiologic abnormality in these cases.

The fact that an abnormality may be present in the vasomotor nervous system of patients afflicted with a physical allergy is brought forth by White and Smithwick[11] when they state that, according to the evidence available, the parasympathetic system never reacts with a diffuse discharge to natural stimuli.

Myalgia almost always appears as the result of the action of physical or emotional stimuli, although some physicians wish to incriminate food allergy in certain instances. A demonstrable antigen-antibody mechanism associated with myalgia is rare. Myalgia may be initiated by an acute or sometimes even chronic infection, since it has been shown that physical sensitization takes place more readily in the presence of infection.

Rose[4] believes that it is possible to distinguish between the antigen-antibody type of allergy and the physical type of allergy. He is of the opinion that evidence points to the fact that histamine is released in the physical type of allergic reaction.

Duke[2] believes that specific hypersensitivity to physical agents could be the result of the development of a chemical substance in certain tissues. Following such sensitization, stimuli from the vasomotor system will release the chemical substance and will result in either a general or a localized reaction.

Some persons advocate the theory that the muscular pains experienced in cases of myalgia are due to certain allergic disturbances. This is based on the fact that the blood of some allergic individuals is deficient in sugar and a diet that corrects this deficiency is required. When this deficiency is corrected by dietary methods, these muscular pains leave. The form of diet advocated is one that eliminates foods that overstimulate insulin production and cause hypoglycemia. It is low in starches, free of refined sugars, and high in vegetables, unsweetened fruits, eggs, meat, and other proteins. There seems to be very little evidence in the medical literature to back up this theory of myalgia.

Selye[12] has stated that whenever the organism is placed in a critical situation, it meets the crisis with a typical tissue defense reaction. He believed that at least some of the symptoms of the alarm reaction are due to the liberation of histamine from various tissues of the body. He concluded from his study that one of the functions of the adrenal glands is to counteract or detoxify this metabolite. Exposure to variable surrounding temperatures and excessive fatigue are among the agents likely to act as alarming stimuli.

Williams[13] concludes that "a fundamental, inherited, localized cellular abnormality occurs which results in some change in the permeability of the cellular structure and a concomitant release of histamine when the deficient cell is affected by stimuli which obtain little or no response from the normal cell. The disorganization which is produced as a result of the stimulus is an injury response of the cell which in turn causes the release of the histamine with subsequent vasodilation and pain." Williams further states that there is evidence to show that the sympathetic and the parasympathetic action may not be normal in these patients.

Any condition which tends to produce increased tension in the muscles of the body, such as is present in anxiety tension states, tends to precipitate an attack of myalgia of the head in patients who are prone to it.

In any discussion of the etiology of myalgia of the head, it seems certain to the experienced observer that the symptom complex of myalgia may be initiated or at least profoundly affected in many cases by the emotional state of the patient. The observant physician cannot help but be impressed by the rather high percentage of patients with this syndrome who show evidence of a tension state.

Boies[14] states that in his opinion "the most acceptable theory of the etiology of myalgia is that it results from a spasmodic contraction of the arterial limbs of capillaries with a localized release of histamine and its vasodilating effects."

Williams[15] states that pharyngeal myalgia is caused by a tender superior constrictor muscle on the involved side of the pharynx. When patients afflicted with this disorder swallow, they experience a severe, deep, usually unilateral pain which is referred to the vertex of the head.

In conducting electromyographic examination of the muscles of the neck and the temporal area, Pozniak-Patewicz[16] found that no muscle action potentials were found provided the control subjects were relaxed. The majority of headache patients, though voluntarily relaxed, showed continuous electrical activity in muscles resulting from sustained spasm. This phenomenon seems to be characteristic for headache patients and was termed "cephalalgic" spasm of the head and neck muscles. Cephalalgic spasm is further thought to be a consequence rather than a cause of headache.

Robarb[17] has shown that severe muscular pain and fatigue of the muscle can result when the duration of the rest period after exercise is inadequate to permit elimination of the pressured catabolite. He further states pain in the musculature does not summate.

SYMPTOMATOLOGY

Myalgia of the head and neck is characterized by the recurring presence of isolated firm and tender areas in the bodies of certain muscles of the head and neck. It is characteristic for these tender regions to recur in the same locations. In attacks of myalgia these regions become increasingly tender and produce pain referred to a distance in a distribution not that of the cutaneous nerves but rather of myotomes. The pain is of the deep type, rises slowly to a crisis, and slowly subsides.

As is usual with allergic headaches myalgia tends to be unilateral but in rare instances may be bilateral. When this is the case, however, the pain tends to be more severe and the signs more definite on one side or the other. The pain suffered by the patient experiencing myalgia of the head is rather characteristic of the type of pain which is commonly seen to be of muscular origin. The pain attacks come on very gradually and gradually increase until they reach their maximum, and then the pain fades out in the same manner. It is not the sudden type of pain that is seen in histaminic cephalalgia, for example.

The pain is often referred to a distance from the circumscribed tender regions which are characteristically associated with myalgia of the head. If the pain is referred to other areas, these areas do not have the tenderness that is seen in the original areas.

As a rule, myalgia is more commonly seen in the third decade of life or later. It is common to see myalgic conditions following some form of acute infection. At least it is safe to say that sensitization to physical agents is much more readily accomplished in the presence of acute infections.

Myalgia of long duration does not usually tend to produce any secondary structural changes, but we may often find associated with myalgia of the head some forms of neuralgia of one or more divisions of the trigeminal cranial nerve. If this does occur, it is always seen on the same side as the involved tender areas.

The pain of myalgia of the head can easily be precipitated by anything which might tend toward the production of any increased tenseness in the postural group of muscles. This may be brought on by such conditions as nervous tension or anxiety states.

In myalgia, stiffness is not increased on disuse of the muscle, and symptoms are not relieved by mild exercise. In fact, the contrary is true. The symptoms are not increased by fatigue or greatly relieved by rest or food, and there is no marked diurnal variation in symptoms. Salicylates, which give so much relief from fibrositis, produce little or no relief from myalgia.

In some cases of myalgia of the head, such nasal disturbances as mucoid nasal and postnasal discharge are present. This may be accompanied by paroxysmal attacks of violent sneezing. It is suggested that this is due to the occurrence of vasodilation. This may tend to suggest that there may be suppression of the normal sympathetic influence through the superior cervical sympathetic ganglion.

Tinnitus and vertigo, symptoms referable to the ears, may be present in cases of myalgia of the head.

Williams[13] pointed out the association of myalgia with vasodilating (vasotonic) pain, endolymphatic hydrops, and vasomotor rhinitis and the fact that together they form the syndrome of physical allergy of the head.

The tissue changes which are commonly seen in rheumatic conditions do not occur in myalgia of the head. These tissue changes consist of hyperemia, inflammatory proliferation of the connective tissues involved, and the formation of serous exudates. Both macroscopically and microscopically, the tissue areas involved fail to show any definite pathologic change.

The pain of a myalgia patient is said to be similar to that produced experimentally by exercising a muscle which is in an ischemic condition.

In discussing which muscles or groups of muscles show a tendency toward myalgia, Williams[18] states:

They are: (1) the upper border of the trapezius and its insertion; (2) the insertion of the splenius capitis into the mastoid process and that portion of the muscle just distal to the insertion; (3) the upper third of the sternocleidomastoid muscle; (4) the styloid process, the stylohyoid muscle, and the anterior belly of the digastric muscle; (5) the styloglossus muscle and its insertion into the tongue, with a sense of entire freedom from tenderness of the remainder of the tongue; (6) the superior constrictor of the pharynx (when the superior constrictor of the pharynx is involved, swallowing occasionally will produce a pain in the ear which is so severe that it might very easily be confused with the pain of glossopharyngeal neuralgia); (7) the cricoarytenoideus posterior muscle (involvement of this muscle may frequently produce pain on talking);

patients who are experiencing a case of myalgia of the cricoarytenoideus posterior muscle will quite often consult a physician in regard to their sore throat only to be greatly annoyed by the statement that no evidence of sore throat is present; (8) the temporalis muscle; and (9) the occipitofrontalis muscle.

This does not mean that the muscles mentioned in the previous paragraphs are the only muscles which may be affected, but they are, by far, the muscles most commonly attacked by myalgic conditions. The involvement of any muscle in myalgia of the head is almost always of a unilateral nature; however, one muscle alone, or several muscles together, may be involved in one single attack of myalgia of the head.

The importance of palpation of the structures of the head and pharynx in the diagnosis of myalgia was pointed out by Lewis,[8] one of the first in the United States to stress the importance of this condition.

Some patients afflicted with myalgia of the head may have so-called trigger areas whose existence may be entirely unknown to the patient. A trigger area is actually a physical sign discovered on physical examination. It is a localized spot of deep tenderness, with a lowered deep pain threshold as measured by the Hardy algesiometer. When the portion of the muscle which contains a trigger area is rolled under the fingers, a localized twitch is usually observed; the muscle contraction may be so vigorous as to cause a perceptible jerk of the part. In addition, fasciculation is often set off and may persist for several seconds afterward. When the examiner sustains the pressure on the tender spot, pain is usually induced in a remote area. The patient points to the region where pain is felt and so delineates the reference zone. When referred pain is not clearly elicited by pressure, contact of a needle will induce it; in this case the stimulus is probably more precisely applied. Thus, a clinically active trigger area is revealed by three things: circumscribed deep hyperalgesia, localized fasciculation, and the capacity to set off referred pain.

In cases of myalgia of the head, there may often be associated neuralgic conditions. It is commonly thought by some investigators that these neuralgic conditions tend to make themselves pronounced and evident over points where the branches of the cranial nerves perforate the skull.

Clinical pattern of myalgia

The clinical pattern is as follows:

1. The pain of myalgia is a deep referred pain which is slow in onset and remission and is nearly always unilateral.
2. It rarely appears before the second or third decade of life and may have been ushered in by infection or severe exposure.
3. Tender areas tend to appear and recur in certain definite muscles.
4. Myalgia of the head and pharynx is not infrequently associated with other conditions thought to be due to physical allergy. These are the vasoatonic (vasodilating) pain syndromes, Meniere's disease, and vasomotor rhinorrhea.
5. Severe exacerbations of headache may be produced by environmental changes, such as approaching storms, damp rainy weather, drafts, air conditioning, and the like or by severe emotional perturbation.
6. "Jelling," as in fibrositis, is not present, and no relief is afforded by mild exercise. Even the slightest use of the involved muscles tends to make the condition worse.
7. The salicylates produce slight to moderate relief of the pain and tenderness.
8. In contrast to fibrositis, no permanent or transient pathologic change can be demonstrated by biopsy.

The average patient with myalgia complains of a severe frontal or temporal headache but on questioning will admit to an additional aching pain in the nuchal region of the homolateral side. Palpation will reveal tender parts in certain muscles. Pressure over these areas will sometimes produce an exacerbation in the frontal or temporal headache. Injection of a strong saline solution into the tender area in muscle will always result in an exacerbation of the pain. Infiltration of the tender portion of the muscle in the nuchal region with 2% procaine hydrochloride will abolish the referred frontal headache temporarily and sometimes more or less permanently. Infiltration of the region of reference with procaine (the area of headache in the frontal region) has no effect on the pain.

DIFFERENTIAL DIAGNOSIS

There are several conditions which may cause some confusion with the differential diagnosis of myalgia of the head. Among the most common conditions are the following.

Sphenopalatine ganglion neuralgia and nerve of the pterygoid canal. The tender regions in the muscles originating from the cranial bones is the determining point in the differentiating.

Sinusitis. In sinusitis referred pain may occur in the same regions as in myalgia, and similar reflex pains of the branches of the fifth cranial nerve are fairly common. This is particularly true in cases of sphenoidal sinusitis due to the vulnerability of the nerve of the pterygoid canal. This, however, is never associated with circumscribed regions of tenderness in the muscles having their origin in the cranial bones, as we have in myalgia of the head. Pressure on these areas will produce the characteristic pain (headache) of myalgia of the head. The absence of symptoms of nasal sinusitis also rules out the presence of sinusitis. This can be ruled out by examination and roentgenographic examination of the sinuses.

Nasal contact headache. The elimination of the headache by cocainization of the contact in the nasal passages is the easiest method of differentiation in these cases.

Psychogenic headache. In psychogenic headache it is characteristic that the symptoms do not fall into any definite clinical pattern. Also, signs of sympathetic disturbances are not found.

Migraine. There are no circumscribed areas of tenderness in the muscle fibers in migraine. In fact, pressure on the head usually feels good in the case of migraine. Migraine tends to occur earlier in life, has a family history in a great percentage of cases, and often has an aura before the actual development of the headache.

Histaminic cephalalgia. This condition has a fulminating onset of the pain, which is not present in myalgia of the head.

Primary fibrositis. In this condition there is a tendency for the tender regions to disappear and reappear in different locations, whereas in myalgia of the head recurrence is in the same region. Referred pain, when present in fibrositis, is in a nerve root distribution. With disuse of the muscles involved, increased subjective stiffness occurs. Also, there is relief of pain on moderate use of the muscles. However, in myalgia of the head, moderate use of the muscles increases the pain.

TREATMENT

Treatment is needed for the patient afflicted with myalgia of the head so that he can perform his daily tasks and resume his social responsibilities at the earliest possible moment. Any treatment that affords relief of an immediate and lasting nature should be rated highly. A factor which is noteworthy in the treatment of myalgia of the head, and one which could conceivably aid in the establishment of a diagnosis, is that acetylsalicylic acid does not produce any definite, significant relief from the pain of the attack.

Myalgia is based on a spasmodic contractive disturbance of the arterial end of the affected capillaries; therefore, if these capillary structures are opened or dilated, there should be some relief from the painful phase of the attack. This may be accomplished by using a vasodilatory substance. During the past several years, various vasodilators have been used to combat myalgia of the head. Among those were neostigmine (Prostigmin), magnesium sulfate, histamine diphosphate, nicotinyl alcohol (Roniacol), and nicotinic acid.

The use of histamine in these conditions was first thought of by Horton and Brown[19] in 1929. Horton made the assertion that since the individual who is found to be sensitive to cold temperatures is also found to be sensitive to a chemical substance formed in the body, autodesensitization would be possible. He advocated the desensitization by the repeated injections of histamine which would be given to the patient over a prolonged period of time. The dosages of these injections of histamine were to be of such a small quantity that they would in turn be of insufficient strength to produce a systemic effect. The dosage was then gradually increased in amount. This work of Horton's led investigators in the field of myalgia of the head to look more in the direction of the vasodilating agents in the treatment of myalgia of the head.

The results obtained with histamine seemed, on the whole, to be of various degrees. Some patients obtain excellent results when given histamine; others experience no relief whatsoever.

A drug which also can be employed as a vasodilator in cases of myalgia of the head is nicotinic acid. Monoethanolamine nicotinate (niacin) has similar reactions to histamine but it shows much less variation and can be used with much less danger of overdosage than histamine. The preparation must be nicotinic acid, not nicotinamide. Nicotinamide does not produce the vasodilation which is needed in these cases and, therefore, will not give the patient his much-desired relief from the attacks.

The injectable form of nicotinic acid which we employ in treating these cases of myalgia of the head is niacin. The initial dose is usually about 25 mg injected intramuscularly. The second injection is increased to 50 mg. The dosage is increased daily until a level is obtained which will produce relief from the symptoms. If this dosage level is exceeded, the injections may well produce the identical symptoms experienced in the patient's typical attack of myalgia of the head. When his optimum dosage level has been reached, the patient should continue to receive the injections daily for at least several weeks. The interval period between the injections should then be increased, and finally the patient can be changed over completely to the oral route of administration of nicotinic acid. At this point the dosage of the oral form should be twice as large as the amount of the nicotinic acid given by the injection method. The oral route of administration of nicotinic acid is naturally not so effective or efficient as the hypodermic route, and in some cases the patient may not obtain as much relief, or even any relief, from the oral administration. In such isolated cases, it will, of course, be necessary to go back to the hypodermic use of the drug. If the oral route of administration does prove to be effective, the patient should continue to take the medication indefinitely, or for at least 6 to 8 months. Then it will be safe to discontinue the medication and observe the patient to see whether the attacks of myalgia return.

As mentioned, the average initial dosage of the nicotinic acid, when taken intramuscularly, is usually about 25 mg. However, some patients cannot tolerate so high a level initially, and it will have to be reduced. The second injection is 50 mg, and the dosage is increased by 25 mg a day until the symptoms are relieved. Usually, a dosage of 100 mg proves to be the average amount required to produce the desired results. If 100 mg is the required intramuscular dosage, the dosage when shifted over to the oral form of medication should be 200 mg. Usually the patient should take the oral medication before meals and twice a day; that is, 100 mg twice a day, once before breakfast and once before the evening meal.

Williams[20] points out that higher dosage levels of nicotinic acid are required for the relief of myalgia attacks when the patient is at a higher altitude. In other words, if the patient is 10,000 feet above sea level, he may need two or three times as much nicotinic acid as he would at sea level.

If, at some future time, as the result of exposure to a preferred stimulus, the symptoms tend to return, treatment may again be instituted by injection of 25 mg; dosage may then be built up to the optimal dosage and continued at that level once daily for a week and then discontinued. Such "booster" shots given now and then at the first reappearance of symptoms will usually maintain relief. Relief is usually obtained for from 3 months to a year. If the condition recurs, it may be found that a larger dose is necessary to reach optimal results. Patients may be instructed in giving themselves the subcutaneous injections.

Nicotinic acid may produce some side effects, but these are usually not serious and are of rather short duration. The most frequently seen side effect is flushing of the skin. This is most commonly seen in the neck and in the head, but it may be seen all over the trunk of the body and in the extremities. This flushing is due to the vasodilation of the superficial skin vessels. It usually persists for 15 to 20 minutes and then fades out. During the flushing stage, the patient feels hot and the skin feels rather itchy. Some patients may get it routinely, whereas others may never get this reaction. Usually, however, the patient will experience it irregularly. The patient, however, should be warned about this side effect so that if it does occur he will not be alarmed or frightened. He should be further told not to be disappointed if it does not occur, as it has no significance so far as the relief from the head pain of the myalgia is concerned.

A much rarer side effect, but one which is sometimes seen when nicotinic acid is administered, is abdominal cramps. This, if it occurs, usually lasts for only 15 to 20 minutes. It is not very frequently seen.

Nicotinyl alcohol (Roniacol) is another vasodilator which may be employed in cases of myalgia of the head. This drug shows vasodilatory action at the level of the small arteries and arterioles. It has a direct relaxing effect on the peripheral blood vessels. It produces less flushing side effects than does nicotinic acid but is not a greater vasodilator. Patients usually do not develop any tolerance to this preparation.

Certain physical therapeutic measures may help to bring about relief in many of these cases of myalgia of the head. Heat, especially wet heat, seems to help many of patients, since it tends to increase the blood circulation of the area to which it is applied. Heat further increases the permeability of the capillary walls to certain cellular and fluid constituents of the blood, which may aid in the treatment of myalgia. Heat will also tend to relax the musculature to which it is applied. Heat increases the alkalinity of the blood, and probably also that of the tissue. Heat also is thought to produce intracellular substances which decrease the resistance of the capillary wall to rupture. Flow of the lymph is increased by heat, which will thus aid in decreasing any edema which might be present. We like the patient to place hot, wet towels over the involved areas. This is a simple form of application of heat and one which can be used by the patient at home. Other forms in which heat may be applied in these cases are the luminous heat lamp or the short-wave diathermy.

Following the application of the heat, there should be some gentle massage applied to the involved areas. Heat and massage work better when used together in these cases than either does when used separately.

If massage is used, a firm, heavy, friction type of massage is more effective than the stroking or kneading type of massage. The most effective local measure begins with stroking massage instituted during the acute stage. Since the parts are more tender at this point, manipulation must be begun gently and in a manner to free the patient from tension. Then gradually much firmer pressure should be used. Since the areas included are small, the usual procedure is to use the fingertips in a circular motion over the area involved. The procedure should start at the periphery of the tender areas and gradually go toward the center of the area. Usually 10 to 15 minutes of massage is sufficient.

In addition to this vasodilatory type of treatment, we have found a very useful electrical instrument called a Medcolator.[21] This machine helps in myalgia of the head in many cases because it plays the part of a muscle stimulator. The stimulation produced by the electrical apparatus proves to be an effective means for increasing the blood flow through the musculature. This is brought about as the Medcolator causes muscular contraction, which produces a vasodilating effect, which in turn increases the blood flow volume.[22] This form of treatment for myalgia of the head is only a supplement, however. Vasodilator drugs are of primary importance. The use of the vasodilator type of drug might fit under the heading of prophylactic treatment, for it is used with the hope of preventing future attacks. However, the Medcolator is used to help bring about relief from an acute attack. It is a form of physical therapy. Before using the Medcolator for this purpose, the application of wet heat packs followed by gentle massage was used. Wet heat and gentle massage help these patients but, in our observations, we find that the Medcolator produces quicker and more pronounced relief.

The Medcolator provides a pulsation output of variable repetition rate. The pulses occur during alternate $1/120$ second periods. The maximum pulse rate with the switch in the high position corresponds to approximately 700 cps; however, only 180 pulses occur during any 1 second because of the rest period between groups of pulses. The corresponding maximum frequency with this switch in the low position is 400 cps, with 120 pulses occurring each second due to the rest period. The tetanizing current of the Medcolator seems to be the one of choice in dealing with cases of myalgia of the head. This provides a constant tetanic contraction of the musculature to which it is applied. The frequency waves of this tetanizing current are approximately 1,000 to 2,000 cps, superimposed on a half-rectified sine wave of 60 cps which are not interrupted.

Most patients seemed to tolerate the tetanizing current with the volume set at about 4 or 4½, when the muscles involved are in the back of the head or the back of the neck. If the painful areas are anterior to this, the volume will have to be considerably smaller. This is applied for periods of 5 to 10 minutes. Patients should then be instructed to apply wet heat and gentle massage to the involved area or areas later on, at home. As mentioned before, these patients should all be placed immediately on vasodilatory therapy in an effort to prevent future attacks.

If used properly, the vasodilatory therapy plus the physical therapy measures of the Medcolator and the wet heat and massage will bring about both relief from future attacks and symptomatic relief from the acute attacks. And, after all, this is what the patient actually desires. He wants his head pain problem to be attacked both prophylactically and symptomatically. If these measures are used, he will find what he seeks.

For many years ethyl chloride spray has been used as a local anesthetic. It has a refrigerant action and acts by freezing the skin. Travell[23,24] believes that ethyl chloride spray is a useful agent in the relief of muscular pain such as we find in myalgia. She points out, however, that this is not so effective in longstanding cases as it is in the acute phase, and therefore, if it is to be successful, it should be employed early in the attack. Travell further points out that to employ the ethyl chloride spray successfully correct technique and a knowledge of the anatomy and function of the musculature involved are necessary, along with a recognition of the pain reference patterns of the musculature and an ability to get the complete relaxation of the patient.

Toxic effects of the use of an ethyl chloride spray, such as increased pain due to the activation of latent trigger areas, allergic skin reactions, skin necrosis due to freezing, and a general necrosis following the inhalation of ethyl chloride, have to be avoided. In using ethyl chloride spray, excessive cooling or frosting of the skin should be avoided.

One must keep in mind the role of somatic trigger areas in hysteria but this is not an explanation of the relief that can be obtained in some cases of myalgia of the head.[25] In other words, the effects of the spray of ethyl chloride are not psychogenic in origin.

Some researchers advocate the injection of a 1% procaine (Novocain) solution into the tender areas involved.[26] They state that this may relax the muscles involved and may be effective for several days or even for a matter of several weeks. We do not employ this type of therapy in the average case of myalgia of the head.

Gonell[27] obtained excellent results with the injection of procaine hydrochloride in muscle pain. He injected procaine into the trigger points. He contends that relief from the pain is immediate or certainly within a few hours.

Roy[28] states that injections into painful areas are sometimes helpful in breaking a vicious cycle of pain-spasm-pain in cases of this type.

This use of muscle relaxants in the symptomatic form of treatment of myalgia of the head has become quite prominent within the past few years.

Diazepam (Valium) was used successfully in cases of myalgia of the head.[29] This drug has use in these cases because of its skeletal muscle–relaxing properties. It relieves skeletal muscle tension and spasticity. The only side effect reported with the use of diazepam in cases of myalgia of the head was drowsiness, but it was not considered to be serious enough to prevent normal activities of the patient in the normal working day.

Hegner[30] also found diazepam to be help

ful in relieving the symptoms of myalgia of the head. He found it to be relatively free from side effects either in the injectable or in the oral forms of administration.

Orphenadrine citrate (Norflex) has been shown to be a good muscle relaxant and desirable in ambulant treatment.[31] Side effects were minor and consisted of mild atropine-like effects such as dryness of the mouth and blurring of vision. Similar results were reported by Finch,[32] using only one tablet twice a day. Finch and Gaillet[31,32] concluded that orphenadrine was a good muscle relaxant.

Blumenthal and Fuchs[33] reported orphenadrine citrate to be a useful drug in affording the patient relief from the pain of muscle spasm. They found gastrointestinal upset, nervousness, drowsiness, and vertigo to be the chief side effects of this drug when used to counteract the pain of muscle spasm.

Methocarbamol (Robaxin) is another drug frequently employed as a muscle relaxant in cases of myalgia of the head.[34] In this study the drug was administered intravenously and orally, and excellent results were obtained with no apparent change in normal reflexes. The quickest and most dramatic results were obtained when the drug was administered by the intravenous drip method. It produced no noticeable side effects other than a mild form of drowsiness.

Park[35] reported excellent results when using methocarbamol in a variety of disorders manifesting an increase in involuntary muscle tone including myalgia.

Carisoprodol (Soma) is another drug employed in the relief of muscle stiffness. It has two primary actions: relief of pain and relaxation of abnormal tension in skeletal muscles. It seems to modify central pain perception without abolishing reflexes.

CASE HISTORY

M.S., a 32-year-old female, complained of a head pain which would originate in the right frontal area, migrate to the right temporal and occipital area, and then go down the back of the neck and occasionally into the shoulder area. The pain would begin gradually and slowly increase until it would reach its maximum intensity and then gradually subside. She experienced her attacks mainly in the damp, cold, wintry, wet season, and her attacks were precipitated by drafts, air conditioning, and any dampness. The pain was not postural but was associated with severe tenderness over the areas involved. It was not a sick headache and there were no associated gastrointestinal or ophthalmic symptoms. Occasionally, she would observe some nasal congestion along with her attacks, with some mucous postnasal discharge; this, however, was never very pronounced. The attacks had no relationship with her menstrual periods or with any element of nervous tension. There was no family history of headaches in her case. She often noticed that she would have an attack if she would go to an air-conditioned movie or dining room. Also an attack would be precipitated if she slept under an electric fan during the summer months. The occurrence of the attacks and the duration of each attack would seem to vary a great deal.

This patient was given intramuscular injections of Nicamin daily, and after receiving 100 mg for about 7 to 10 days, she was completely free from her attacks. She soon was changed over to the oral form of the medication, taking 100 mg two or three times a day and she continued to be free from her attacks.

She applied hot, wet towels to the involved areas at the initial phase of her treatment program and followed this by using massage.

She had previously used, of her own accord, Empirin Compound, Anacin, and aspirin, but received no benefit from any of these. Experimentally, we had her use Fiorinal, which, like the Empirin Compound and aspirin, is an analgesic type of medication, but it failed to produce any relief from the pain of the attacks.

On the whole, we have found Fiorinal to be of little use in treatment of myalgia of the head.[36] However, this preparation was tried in several cases to make sure that it was of no value.

SUMMARY

Symptoms and signs

1. Gradual onset
2. Gradual termination
3. Tenderness to pressure
4. Migratory pain
5. Generalized or localized
6. Patient sensitive to temperature changes
7. No nasal disturbances
8. No ocular disturbances
9. No gastric disturbances

Treatment

1. Nicotinic acid (intramuscularly; later changed to orally), not nicotinamide
2. Wet heat
3. Massage
4. Medcolator
5. Muscle relaxants
6. Ethyl chloride spray
7. Procaine (Novocain) injections

REFERENCES

1. Williams, H. L., and Elkins, E. C.: Myalgia of the head, Arch. Phys. Ther. **23:**14, 1942.
2. Duke, W. W.: Allergy: asthma, hay fever, urticaria, and allied manifestations of reaction, St. Louis, 1925, The C. V. Mosby Co., p. 339.
3. Code, C. F.: The quantitative estimation of histamine in the blood, J. Physiol. **89:**257-268, 1937.
4. Rose, B.: The relation of histamine to anaphylaxis and allergy, McGill Med. J. **10:**5, 1940.
5. Lewis, T., Grant, R. T., and Marvin, H. M.: Vascular reactions of the skin to injury, Heart **14:**139, 1927.
6. Lewis, T., and Grant, R. T.: Vascular reactions of the skin to injury, Heart **13:**219, 1926.
7. Williams, H. L.: A concept of allergy as autonomic dysfunction suggested as an improved working hypothesis, Tr. Am. Acad. Ophthalmol. **55:**123-144, 1951.
8. Lewis, T.: Pain, New York, 1942, The Macmillan Co.
9. Kellgren, J. H.: A preliminary account of referred pains arising from muscles, Br. Med. J. **1:**325, 1938.
10. Kellgren, J. H.: On the distribution of pain arising from deep somatic structures with charts of segmental pain areas, Clin. Sci. **4:**35, 1939.
11. White, J. C., and Smithwick, R. H.: The autonomic nervous system; anatomy, physiology and surgical application, ed. 2, New York, 1941, The Macmillan Co.
12. Selye, H.: Thymus and adrenals in response of the organisms to injuries and intoxications, Br. J. Exp. Pathol. **17:**234, 1934.
13. Williams, H. L.: The intrinsic allergy syndrome, Tr. Am. Acad. Ophthalmol. **48:**379, 1944.
14. Boies, L. R.: Headache and neuralgia of nasal origin, Med. Soc. Bull. **53:**83, 1950.
15. Williams, H. L.: Somatic head pain from the standpoint of the rhinologist, otologist, and laryngologist, Lancet **74:**22, 1954.
16. Pozniak-Patewicz, E.: Cephalgic spasm of head and neck muscles, Headache **15:**261-266, 1976.

17. Robarb, S.: Pain associated with muscle contraction, Headache **10:**105-115, 1970.
18. Williams, H. L.: The syndrome of physical or intrinsic allergy of the head: myalgia of the head, Proc. Staff Meet. Mayo Clin. **20:**177, 1945.
19. Horton, B. T., and Brown, G. E.: Systemic histamine reactions in allergy due to cold, Am. J. Med. Sci. **178:**191, 1929.
20. Williams, H. L.: The treatment of certain common forms of headache confused with sinus headache, Ill. Med. J. **105:**53, 1954.
21. Ryan, R. E.: Myalgia of the head, Med. Times, September 1956.
22. Ryan, R. E.: Treatment of myalgia of the head, J. Mo. Med. Assoc. **51:**735, 1954.
23. Travell, J.: Ethyl chloride spray for painful muscle spasm, Arch. Phys. Med. **33:**291, 1952.
24. Travell, J.: Rapid relief of acute "stiff neck" by ethyl chloride spray, J. Am. Med. Womens Assoc. **4:**89, 1949.
25. Travell, J., and Bigelow, N. H.: Role of somatic trigger areas in the patterns of hysteria, Psychosom. Med. **9:**353, 1947.
26. Ayash, J. J.: Headache and head pain, Lancet **69:**389, 1949.
27. Gonell, R. L.: Procaine injections for musculoskeletal pain, Lancet **75:**32-37, 1955.
28. Roy, J.: The role of muscles in the etiology of headache, Army Med. Corp. **100:**99-106, 1954.
29. Ryan, R. E.: Myalgia of the head and its treatment with diazepam, Headache **3:**63-66, 1963.
30. Hegner, H. L.: Diazepam in the treatment of myalgia, muscle spasm and the anxiety-tension state, Clin. Med. **72:**1980-1989, 1965.
31. Caillet, R.: Clinical value of orphenadrine citrate as a skeletal muscle relaxant, Clin. Med. **7**(8):1581-1588, 1960.
32. Finch, J. W.: Further clinical experiences with orphenadrine citrate: a skeletal muscle relaxant, Am. J. Orth. **2**(8):194-195, 1960.
33. Blumenthal, L. S., and Fuchs, M.: Muscle relaxation in the treatment of headache, Headache **1:**8-20, 1961.
34. Ryan, R. E.: A new agent for the symptomatic relief of myalgia of the head, Clin. Med. **7**(2):323-326, 1960.
35. Park, H. W.: Clinical results with methocarbamol, a new interval blocking agent, J.A.M.A. **167:**168-172, 1958.
36. Ryan, R. E.: Fiorinal—a new agent in the symptomatic treatment of headache, Med. Times **80:**1952.

CHAPTER 18

Depressive headache

Depression is often described as a symptom, as a syndrome, or as a disease. Headache is probably the most common symptom present in the depressed patient. The headache sufferer may often become depressed because of his headaches.

ETIOLOGY

There are numerous things which can bring about depressive headaches. Depression may follow a severe illness or a change in the patient's social or financial status. Loss of someone close to the patient can produce depression. Drugs if improperly employed may produce depression. Depressive headaches may be due to a degenerative disease of the cervical spine which in turn leads to basilar artery insufficiency.

Headache and depression may both exist in the same patient without being causally related.

Depression headache is usually more common in a patient with nonparoxysmal headache than it is in the typical migraine sufferer.

SYMPTOMATOLOGY

Usually depressive headaches will be found to occur at regular intervals in relation to the patient's routine, daily life cycle. These headaches usually have no definite

location, but they are frequently described as being in the occipital area.

The duration of these headaches is a significant factor; they usually are described as being present for years or "all my life."

The pain is usually of a dull nature and more or less generalized, and it usually does not respond to the usual drugs used for symptomatic relief of headache. Patients generally state that their headaches are more severe in the morning than any other time of the day. According to Diamond[1] these headaches occur principally from 4 to 8 P.M. and from 4 to 8 A.M. Diamond also lists associated symptoms of this condition such as sleep disturbance, dyspnea, constipation, weight loss, trouble in getting to sleep, poor appetite, decreased sexual activity, weakness, and fatigue.

It is important for the physician to observe the patient while talking to him. Depressed patients often have a tendency to cry and feel despondent. Many actually have the characteristics of anxiety in their personality. They may appear to be irritable, whereas they actually have a depressive personality.

When depression is associated with a headache problem it is usually in direct proportion to the severity of the headache. These patients also have associated psychogenic symptoms such as poor concentration, lack of interest, poor memory, lack of ambition, and indecisiveness.

TREATMENT

Depression is generally believed to have a better prognosis than most other psychiatric conditions. The depressed patient has a good prognosis for recovery with or without treatment. Most depressions are self-limited, and spontaneous improvement in these cases is of a high level, especially if the case represents a mild reactive depression which occurs suddenly due to a response to untoward life events. After diagnosing the case, the physician should reassure the patient that the case is not hopeless and that he should respond to proper treatment.

The tricyclic antidepressant drugs are useful in these cases. Such drugs as amitriptyline (Elavil), protriptyline (Vivactil), and perphenazine-amitriptyline (Triavil) are examples of this. These drugs seem to interfere with norepinephrine uptake by the brain cells and, thus, indirectly potentiate the effects of catecholamines at adrenergic sites in the brain.[2]

The analgesic group of drugs may be helpful in these patients. Their use must be controlled, however, because, as was pointed out by Barolin,[3] the incidence of addiction to the analgesic type of drug is much greater in the depressive headache group of patients than it is in headache patients who have no element of depression in their case.

Electroshock treatment in these patients may be necessary if the case is a severe one with marked depression. Naturally, this is best suited as a hospital procedure. It is much more inconvenient than taking drugs on an outpatient basis. This is an effective procedure but usually should not be employed in these cases except as a last resort.

Other drugs besides those previously mentioned which may be employed are doxepin (Sinequan), nortriptyline (Aventyl), and imipramine (Tofranil).

Biofeedback is another form of treatment which may be employed in this type of headache problem. It may or may not be of value, but if conservative drug therapy does not bring out the described results, this form of treatment should definitely be tried before considering electroshock treatment.

REFERENCES

1. Diamond, S.: Depressive headaches, Headache **4:**255, 1964.
2. Dalessio, D. J.: Some reflections on the etiologic role of depression in head pain, Headache **8:**23, 1968.
3. Barolin, G. S.: Brief report: headache and depression, Headache **16:**252, 1976.

CHAPTER 19

Headache in children

Headache is a common complaint for the pediatrician to encounter in everyday practice. No particular age group is more prone to this complaint than any other. No age group is free of headache; it is seen even in infancy. Infants experience headache, but they express their pain in a different fashion than an older child. The infant will show signs of irritability and be very fretful at the same time. He shows no interest in his food. The infant cannot tell us what is wrong, so the parent and the physician have a much more difficult job on their hands in diagnosing the case. It is evident that something is wrong, there is pain somewhere but where and how severe—we can merely assume the answer. In infants, unfortunately many cases of headache are associated with increased intracranial pressure or are headaches associated with an infectious disease. In infancy there is little chance that the headaches are of the migraine type or are psychogenic disorders.

As the child gets older vascular headaches, refractory eye headaches, and psychogenic headaches become more frequent. By the time the child is a teen-ager the percentage of various types of headache is the same as for adults.

The successful diagnosis of a headache problem in a child is probably a great deal more difficult than in an adult. As with the adult case, the taking of a careful history is most essential. This, however, is more difficult to do with children because of the age problem. At times the history-taking is made easier by the parents, but at times the parents merely complicate the picture by telling the physician what they think is going on, and they are actually missing the true picture. If this is the case and the child is highly intelligent, the child will frequently interrupt the parent's description and correct the story and tell it as it is. This, of course, can happen only if the child is old enough and smart enough to help out.

The parent will usually give the history, but certain aspects of the problem have to be described by the child, for it is actually the child who is experiencing the headache and he is the *only* one who knows where that pain is, how severe it is, what type of pain it is, what aggravates the pain, and whether it moves from one location to another.

The parent and child should both be questioned about the problem. The frequency, duration, and time of onset should be questioned. Is the onset sudden or gradual? Does the headache terminate suddenly or gradually? Are there any factors which will bring on a headache such as the weather, tension at home or at school, fatigue, foods, or menstrual periods, if they are teen-agers?

Is the headache postural—is it better, is it more severe, or is it not changed by the position of the patient's body? Is there any family history of headace? (This information has to be supplied by the parents.)

What factors will increase the severity of the headache after it starts? Is there anything the child does not like to do when he has a headache because it will make the headache more severe?

Are there any symptoms associated with the headache which are referable to the nose, such as nasal obstruction or nasal discharge? Do any ophthalmologic symptoms enter into the headache picture, such as scotomas, lacrimation, photophobia, conjunctivitis, or visual disturbances?

Inquiry into the evidence of any trauma in the case is also essential.

Does the child have any gastrointestinal symptoms which are associated with the headache problems? Is nausea or vomiting present with the headache attacks?

The condition of the child's teeth should also be inquired about, as should the blood pressure. It is not common to find hypertensive headaches in children, but it does exist.

The onset time is another important question to ask both the parent and the child. Does it begin at any certain time of the day, the week, the month, or the year?

Other questions which should be presented to the parents concerning the child are those pertaining to gait, memory loss, sensory abnormalities, weakness of the limbs, and ataxia.

The physician taking the headache history should observe the behavior of the child and also the behavior of the parents. Is there any hostility between them? Is there any anxiety, insecurity, or depression seen in the child's behavior? This can often be seen from the facial expressions of the child by an observant physician. The facial expressions will often reflect any hidden aspects of the headache problem.

The physician should observe whether one of the parents is the domineering type or is overly strict. Points of disagreements between parents and the child in the history-taking may be observed by the physician; for instance, the child might glare at the parents, indicating hostility.

After the taking of a careful history, a thorough examination of the child is next in order. The nasal sinuses, ears, eyes, blood pressure, and blood and urine examinations are all important. Depending on what might be involved, extra laboratory examinations may be needed or special x-rays, spinal taps, or an electroencephalogram may be needed. Visual fields and funduscopic examinations may also be required.

Many types of headache are found in children. An attempt will be made to discuss the more common types encountered.

MIGRAINE IN CHILDREN

It seems to be frequently taken for granted that migraine is a condition associated only with adulthood. This is definitely not the case. The prevalence of migraine in children is actually much greater than is generally realized by the average individual or the average physician. Many children with migraine never see a physician. It is extremely rare for a child to be hospitalized for headaches of this type, and because of this, the nature of the disease often remains obscure in children. In children abdominal migraine is actually more commonly seen than classic migraine.

All too frequently children suffer with chronic, periodic headaches, and in most of these cases the thought of migraine never occurs. It is overlooked merely because migraine is not thought of when a child presents a chronic headache problem. However, this has often proved to be misleading factor. Migraine does exist in children and should not be overlooked.

The general characteristics of migraine will not be discussed here. These can be obtained from Chapter 4.

During the past several years, there have been many papers, discussions, and studies on the subject of migraine, but most of these have dealt entirely with adult cases. Migraine frequently is found to begin in the first decade of life. It has been estimated that about 2% to 4% of all children manifest symptoms of migraine at some time during their first decade of life. This would mean that approximately 1 million children in the United States under the age of 12 have at one time or another suffered from migraine attacks. From these figures, it is apparent that the detailed study of migraine in children has been neglected, and we feel sure that this subject will progressively become more important as our knowledge of migraine itself becomes greater.

Glaser[1] believes that babies only a few weeks old can have headaches, even the very painful migraine type. If a baby or young child wrinkles his forehead, rubs his head, is restless, or cries, he may have a headache.

Bueke and Peters[2] observed migraine in ninety-two of about 60,000 children examined between the ages of 1½ and 14 years. About half of these had a family history in their case. They observed that nausea and vomiting were more distressing to these children than was any other migraine symptom. They further stated that scotomas and cephalalgia are less common in these cases in children than in adults, but that the gastrointestinal symptoms are more pronounced.

Etiology

As is the case in adult migraine, the etiology of migraine in children is not clearly understood. Many different theories have been advanced, but so far none of these theories has been proved. Many believe that there is a psychogenic factor involved in the child suffering with migraine. Comby[3] pointed out that the migrainous child was extremely nervous, and he recommended that the child be placed in rural surroundings or in a boarding school. Riley[4] noted that many of these children were completely free from their headache attacks during their vacation periods and

this he believes points to a definite psychogenic factor. Friedman and co-workers[5] also believe that there is some psychogenic element in cases of migraine in children, because of the neurotic symptomatology in these cases.

The other theories of the etiology of migraine seen in adults are also voiced in cases of migraine in children. Many of these young patients will observe that their attacks may be brought on by visual fatigue, such as may be produced by too much television or going to the movies. Others often associate their attacks with excessive sunlight or being around brightly lighted areas for any length of time.

Chao and associates[6] believe that etiologic factors of migraine in children could be excitement, school examinations, fatigue, family conflicts, or physical exertion.

Many other theories have been advanced as to the etiology of migraine in children. Among these are allergy, epilepsy, tension, and endocrine disorders. For none of these etiologic theories of migraine is the evidence either consistent or convincing.

There does seem to be a definite relationship between the child's headaches and his emotional upsets. There seems to be an increase in the number of cases of migraine in children in the past several years, and it is possibly due to the manner in which the school systems of the United States have increased the study load of the grade and high school student.[7] This increased load of studies no doubt leads to an increase in tension, fatigue, and emotional upsets. It is typical to find a child to have a migraine attack the night before an examination. However, the majority will have the migraine attack after the examinations are over. This is typical of tension; the actual headache usually comes in the relaxed phase when there is vasodilation, not during the actual tension phase when vasoconstriction occurs. The schools have geared up their programs to such an extent that they are creating many nervous personalities among their students. What is to be gained by rushing these youngsters through various courses in grade school which normally were taken at the high school level is hard to realize.

In general it is safe to say that these children are mentally very alert and rather intelligent. This is also true of the adult patient with migraine. As a rule they do not have any great difficulty with their studies, and they certainly do not use their headache attacks as a defense mechanism for poor marks in school. Most of these children are in the upper level of their classes. However, the excessive pressure exerted by the heavy schedule of classes they carry is the causative factor of their headache attacks. Their will to excel and their heavy schedule of courses are too much for their personalities. This creates emotional upset and tension, which in turn bring about the migraine attacks.

Occasionally we see another example of emotional upset causing migraine when a child is "guided" or "pushed" toward a certain profession or walk of life which the child does not really desire. The child is not given any voice in the decision but is merely told that he should be this or that in life. This will naturally only bring about frustration and a nervous individual. If migraine results in a case of this type, it seems safe to say that the emotional upset was a definite factor in the etiology of this particular case.

Children with migraine are often shy, conscientious, and often strongly attached to their mothers. Not only children with migraine but also their parents tend to be more anxious, tense, and sensitive than the average person. As with migraine in adults, there is a definite family history in these cases of migraine in children.

Contrary to the belief that 80% to 85% of adult patients with migraine are females, it is believed that a slightly greater percentage of children suffering with migraine are males.

Holguin and Fenichel[8] believe that there is no correlation between migraine in children and intelligence. They state that they have actually seen it in the mentally retarded child. They claim that there is a wide variance in the intellectual capacities of the children afflicted with migraine.

Menkes[9] believes that children with migraine usually have the following characteristics: (1) a character structure forbidding the overt expression of aggressive hostile impulses; (2) an above-average feeling of anger; and (3) an incompetent fragile or vulnerable feeling in relation to their families.

Dyken[10] points out that migraine is the most common form of headache seen in children, but that it is unrecognized more than the other forms of headache in childhood.

Symptomatology

In general, the symptoms of migraine in children are the same as those of migraine in adults.

Migraine is seen in the neurotic type of child. The child will often describe the symptomatology in a very dramatic fashion and quite often the symptoms will vary. Many of these children have violent tempers which are easily provoked. It is quite common to see these children go into raving tantrums, during which they may be rather difficult to control.

Ott[11] believes that migraine cases found in children differ from those in adults in that the headache may actually be a minor part of the symptomatology, especially in the very young patient.

Many of these children have certain and definite phobias which quite often are influential in their lives. These young patients frequently complain of vertigo along with the other symptoms of migraine. Nightmares and enuresis are occasionally seen in the youngsters who have been afflicted with migraine difficulties. Many mothers of these patients can actually tell that their child is going to have a migraine attack by the fact that it always follows a restless night's sleep.

As in adults, there is a definite family history in these cases. Migraine is seen in several generations of families and it may be thought of as an expression of some inherited constitutional peculiarity.

In the majority of the cases of migraine which we have seen in children, the gastrointestinal symptoms are quite severe. There is a disturbance in appetite, nausea, vomiting, a generalized abdominal discomfort, and, quite frequently, severe abdominal pain. These children are often found to have a definite disinclination for food. Smith[12] believes that cyclic vomiting and migraine in children have similar symptoms.

The vomiting in migrainous children may appear at the very beginning of the attack. Many children complain of abdominal distention. In complaining of abdominal pain, these children most frequently locate the pain in the epigastrium. Often it is rather localized, but it may be a diffuse abdominal discomfort. The pain in the abdomen may be continuous or it may occur in paroxysms and resemble a colicky type of pain. Emesis may be quite pronounced and may even at times appear to be intractable, only to suddenly stop. The emesis may contain bile and from this the term "bilious migraine" has emerged. The headache in these cases may actually be minor at times, but it generally tends to increase in severity with a corresponding diminution of abdominal symptoms as the child gets older. Because of this excessiveness of the gastrointestinal symptoms, undoubtly many of these cases have been misdiagnosed as cyclic vomiting. Children who actually have cyclic vomiting are often found in migrainous families and they may grow into adulthood and have true migraine.

Visual symptoms of migraine in children are much less constant than the gastrointestinal symptoms. The headaches, when present, are usually seen in the prodromal phase of migraine before the actual headache develops. They tend to leave when the headache develops. These visual symptoms may consist of blurred vision, dimness of vision, or even loss of vision. Transient hemianopia or ocular muscle paralysis may also occur. Scotoma is not a common visual symptom of migraine in children.

Visual hallucinosis is found in the majority of these cases. These symptoms, however, may vary in their severity. In some cases, the physician may be rather surprised to find that the child can actually give him a better description of scotomas than can many adults. Riley[4] believes that this ophthalmic type of migraine is more commonly found in children than it is in adults. In children, however, photophobia is commonly found and some even complain of "double vision."

Gascon and Barlow[13] find that it is not uncommon to find a form of migraine in children in which the most common manifestation is an acute confusional state. They believe this to be not uncommon. These cases usually have no prodrome; they do have sensory symptoms. The headache usually appears after the confusional condition leaves. Neurologic signs are usually present in these cases and may consist of dysphasia, dysconjugate eye movements, dilated pupils, and abnormal electroencephalograms.

In general, in children common migraine is seen more frequently in boys and the classic form of migraine in girls. Also, the common type of migraine is generally seen in younger children while the classic type begins more frequently in the older child.

In the infant under perhaps 3 years of age migraine is less specific, and the positive family history is very essential in the diagnosis. The actual attacks may merely be manifested as cyclic vomiting, periods of head-banging by the child, or only oculomotor signs. The child presents a picture of a crying, irritable patient with vomiting, pallor, and photophobia who sooner or later drifts off to sleep.

Many cases of migraine in children will present a febrile stage in which the temperature may rise as high as 103° or 104° F.

This is not commonly seen in cases of adult migraine. This febrile stage is not, however, a definite requisite for a diagnosis of migraine in children.

It is not unusual to find the migrainous child to have a definite feeding problem.

Cardiac symptoms may be present in these children. Such conditions as pain, palpitation, dyspnea, pallor, cyanosis, and anxiety may be present.

A thickly coated tongue is frequently found on examination of the child. Occasionally, in migrainous children there will be facial edema, especially about the eyes and the eyelids. A periodic skin eruption of a macular type is seen occasionally.

Harry[14] believes that in two-thirds of the cases of migraine in children a bilateral headache is present. In children, there is less likelihood of the headache of migraine being unilateral than it is in an adult patient.

Michael and Williams[15] believe that the outstanding feature differentiating migraine in children from migraine in adults is the greater frequency of attacks in children.

Migrainous children are often found to be hyperactive and will show certain nervous characteristics, such as nail-biting and thumb-sucking. They definitely have an appreciable amount of anxiety-tension in their mental make-up.

L'Hirondel[16] points out that between attacks the migrainous child presents certain stigmas of autonomic instability (emotionalism, anxiety, variation in mood). Importance is attached to the hypersensitivity of certain trigger points (epigastrium, gallbladder area, trapezius muscles, pubic spines).

In some of these children, focal symptoms may initially occur, such as numbness and tingling in the extremities or over the entire body. This may be followed by clonic movements. From this, hemiplegia, which may persist for several hours or even days, may be the next symptom. Transient disturbances in speech may occur. Some of these focal symptoms may become permanent, but this is extremely rare.

Diagnosis

Headache in children may have a variety of causes and migraine must be differentiated from such things as intracranial tumors, nasal sinusitis, refractory errors, hypertension, constipation, and psychogenic headache. However, if the symptomatology of migraine in children is known by the physician, no difficulties should be encountered. The most difficult type of migraine case to be diagnosed in a child is perhaps the one where the symptoms are primarily referable to the abdomen. In such a case, extra tests may be necessary such as an electroencephalogram and radiologic examinations of the digestive, biliary, and urinary tracts. With these tests and diligent observation on the part of the physician, even this type of migraine in a child should be correctly diagnosed.

Prognosis

Migraine attacks in children will frequently cease with a crisis, at which time diarrhea, excessive urinary output, or excessive perspiration may develop. In many cases of migraine in childhood there is a definite tendency for the condition to vanish at the time of puberty, and many of these patients will find that their attacks will recur at the time of their climacteric.

Wadlington[17] believes that migraine in children may disappear before or during puberty; it may develop into adult migraine; or it may appear initially after puberty. The most common course is the first.

Migraine in children which tends to cease with age is most commonly seen in male patients, especially where the onset is at an older age. It is least likely to cease in females when the attacks begin at puberty or beyond.

In general the average case of migraine in a child has a far more favorable outlook than does a case of adult migraine.

Treatment

A mild type of sedative will often help the child. This is especially true if there is any tendency toward convulsive states in the case. Cafergot and Gynergen seem to work as effectively in migraine cases in children as they do in adult cases in regard to aborting the headache attacks. For further information on this, see Chapter 4.

If there are any allergic factors in the background of the patients, these should be eliminated and the parents and the child should be instructed how they should be avoided. If the child is allergic, the antihistamines will help somewhat when these headache attacks appear.

Any predisposing factor or factors should be eliminated, including mental as well as physical factors. Any toxic factors which might be instrumental in bringing on the attacks should be eliminated and avoided completely.

If there is excessive vomiting, the danger of dehydration should be avoided. This may be accomplished simply by forcing fluids, but if the vomiting is excessive and over a prolonged period of time, the intravenous administration of fluids may be needed.

The physician must carefully instruct the parents to guard their child against any contributing factors which might play a role in the child's migraine attacks.

Balyeat and Rinkel[18] believe that if the prodromal symptoms appear, the patient should be given a saline cathartic and should follow a sugar-free and carbohydrate-free diet, so that the child's stomach should be empty by the following morning, when the actual headache would be expected.

Hinrichs and Keith[19] believe that acetylsalicylic acid, rest, and sleep are the best treatment for migraine in children.

Bille[20] believes that maintaining a sound rhythm at work and at play, at meals, and at sleep are the best treatment. Perhaps a mild sedative is also needed.

Sanner[21] obtained good results with migraine in children by using cyproheptadine (Periactin) with few or no side effects.

All sensory disturbances should be eliminated, as well as any other existing disturbance.

If there is any psychogenic element present in these cases, it must be handled in an extremely delicate fashion. With a psychogenic factor present, the child is very "high strung" and emotional, and this type of personality is more often than not quite difficult to handle. It is extremely important, however, that the child and the parents both be reassured that the condition can be controlled and the symptoms and signs can be either greatly reduced or cleared up completely. If there is a psychogenic factor in the background of the case and the physician fails to combat it and check it, the patient and the patient's parents will not be given the desired relief they are seeking from the attacks.

For the relief of persistent nausea and vomiting, phenothiazine drugs may be used. Chlorpromazine, 20 to 40 mg, or dimenhydrinate (Dramamine), 10 to 20 mg, may be given by injection.

If there is excessive vomiting, the danger of dehydration should be avoided. This may be accomplished simply by forcing fluids, but if the vomiting is excessive, intravenous fluids may be necessary.

In general the same type of treatment employed in the treatment of migraine in adults should be used in cases of migraine in children. Naturally, the dosage of the medications used should be reduced. This is true in most other conditions. Vasodilators such as nicotinic acid and histamine are useful in the prophylactic phase of the treatment program of migraine in children.

Attention should be paid to all of the possible causative agents of each case, both physical and emotional. In treating migraine in children, neither diagnosis nor management can be complete without considering the whole child in the context of the family. The physician must carefully instruct the parents of the child to guard against any contributing factors which might play a part in the child's migraine attacks. All sensory disturbances should be eliminated as well as any other existing factors.

How effective is the treatment of this condition in helping these children to be free from their migraine attacks? This is difficult to say because too frequently the treatment is not aimed at the underlying causes and prevention of attacks (prophylactic), but merely at relieving the symptoms (symptomatic). As in cases of any adult migraine patient, the treatment of the symptoms may be a matter of selectivity, as some patients respond to one type of drug while others may respond to a preparation of another type entirely. The outlook for children with migraine is relatively good if the condition is correctly diagnosed and treated. The earlier the treatment, the better the prognosis.

PSYCHOGENIC HEADACHES

Psychogenic headache is not an uncommon form of headache found in children. Frequently poor achievement in school work will be a factor in this type of headache in a child. Divorce, leaving the child living with only one parent, can be a factor, as can poor relationship between the parents and the child or with other children in the family. These headaches may be caused by any uneasy circumstances existing around the home.

This type of headache in children is usually not severe. The symptomatology may be rather bizarre; there is actually no definite set pattern.

Homeyer and Lempp[22] found that about 23.6% of the headaches in children were of this type. So it is not an infrequent type of problem for the physician to confront.

MUSCLE CONTRACTION (TENSION) HEADACHES

This is a common type of headache to find in children. This is often referred to in the European literature as vasomotor headache.

The pain is usually the dull type with a slow, gradual onset. It is usually generalized and may persist for several hours. There may be associated autonomic abnormalities such as palpitation, sleep disturbance, dermographia, sweating, or tremors.

This type of headache is one of the most commonly seen headaches in children. It may be brought on by physical or mental strain. Because of this a strict regimen of rest is instituted in the treatment program with the avoidance of stressful situations. The analgesic drugs are also found to be of benefit in relieving the pain of this condition in children.

Sabbagh[23] reported good results in treating this type of headache with Ergo-Lonarid, which is composed of 0.5 mg dihydroergotamine tartrate, 400 mg acetylaminophenol, 10 mg codeine phosphate, 30 mg amobarbital, and 100 mg caffeine.

Jacobi and associates[24] believe that this type of headache can begin in infancy.

TRAUMA

Naturally trauma can produce headache in children just as in adults. In fact, children "bang" their heads in minor freak accidents much more frequently than adults. Some of these traumatic incidents may cause a concussion, so the physician should be sure to inquire about trauma when taking the headache history. This type of headache is usually accompanied by loss of consciousness at the time of the head injury. Frequently these traumatic headaches have nausea as a symptom.

Mild head trauma may produce prominent but temporary neurologic symptoms in children such as hemiparesis, somnolence, irritability, vomiting, blindness, or brainstem signs.[25] There is usually full recovery from these symptoms should they occur.

In more severe cases of head trauma contusions may occur, manifested by immediate unconsciousness without a latent period between the actual trauma and the onset of the focal signs. Occasionally whiplash injuries to the neck can cause headache.

HYPERTENSION

It is rare to find hypertension in children, but if it is present it may lead to headache. In children hypertension is often associated with nephritis. In these cases the underlying condition should be the primary target in the treatment program. When the etiologic condition is brought under control the headache will usually also be controlled. Alison and co-workers[26] believe that hypertension headaches in children are accompanied by abdominal pain.

INFECTIONS

In children, there are many types of infection which have headache as one of the symptoms. These infections may be in the nasal sinuses, the nasal passages, the teeth, the ear (otitis media), or the throat (pharyngitis).

This type of headache is frequently related to the fever which may accompany these conditions. If present, the headache is a diffuse generalized type of pain.

Other types of more serious infections which have headache as one of the symptoms are meningitis, encephalitis, typhoid fever, and pneumonia.

INTRACRANIAL TUMORS

Intracranial tumors actually produce headache by stretching pain-sensitive structures within the cranium. The severity of this type of headache tends to vary throughout the day, being more severe during the early morning hours, improving throughout the day, and being very mild in the evening hours. These headaches are usually aggravated by coughing.

Other symptoms seen in these cases of intracranial tumors may consist of vomiting (without nausea), increased blood pressure, atoxic gait, papilledema, neck stiffness, or sixth nerve palsies.

Pineda[27] states that infratemporal lesions are twice as common as supratentorial lesions and include cerebellar astrocytomas and medulloblastoma.

Homeyer and Lempp[22] believe that brain tumors in children are not rare. About 50% of them are found in the cerebellum or the fourth ventricle and 40% are benign astrocytomas.

The electroencephalogram is very helpful in the diagnosis of these tumors.

DEPRESSION

Headache in adults is known to be caused by depression. It is also an etiologic factor in children. These problems are seen in children who have a noticeable social withdrawal along with a definite change in mood. The child usually has a poor record in school and may even develop a phobia about school. Sleep disturbances may be present along with energy loss and an aggressive type of behavior which was not present before the onset of the depression. There may also be anorexia and weight loss.

The antidepressant drugs may be used in these cases of childhood headache, but they should be used moderately.

MIGRAINE VARIANTS

Migraine variants can be found in children as well as in adults. In fact, abdominal migraine, complicated migraine, and basilar migraine are more frequently seen in children than in adults. These conditions are discussed fully in Chapter 5.

EYESTRAIN

Eyestrain may be due to refractory errors, astigmatism, muscle imbalance, or inflammation. A rare cause for headache in children is congenital glaucoma.

These cases should all be handled by an ophthalmologist, for when the underlying condition is brought under control, the headache problem is also solved.

SUMMARY

In handling a case of headache in children, the physician should remember that children have a great tendency to mimic their parents. If one parent is subject to headaches, the child may be tempted to complain of headache as an effort to gain attention from or to influence the parent.

The importance of the history in these patients is just as important as in adults. However, because of the age of the patient involved, the taking of the history in the child is much more difficult. This makes observation of the patient and his behavior a very important element in handling such a problem.

The child who is treated as a whole and not merely treated for the headache problem will usually receive the best results.

REFERENCES

1. Claser, J.: Migraine in pediatric practice, Am. J. Dis. Child. **88:**92, 1954.
2. Bueke, E. C., and Peters, G. A.: Migraine in childhood: a preliminary report, Am. J. Dis. Child. **92:**330, 1956.
3. Comby, J.: J.A.M.A. **76:**481, 1921.
4. Riley, H. A.: Migraine in children and the mechanism of the attack, Bull. Neurol. Inst. N.Y. **6:**387, 1937.
5. Friedman, A. J., and others: The psychologic factors of migraine in children, N. Y. State J. Med. **50:**2269, 1950.
6. Chao, D., McGovern, J. P., Haywood, T. J., and Knight, J. A.: Headaches in children: IV. The migraine syndrome, Headache **3:**13, 1963.
7. Ryan, R. E.: Migraine in children, Headache **8:**67, 1968.
8. Holguin, J., and Fenichel, G.: Migraine, J. Pediatr. **70:**290, 1967.
9. Menkes, M. M.: Personality characteristics and family roles of children with migraine, Pediatrics **53:**560, 1974.
10. Dyken, P. R.: Headaches in children, Am. Fam. Phys. **11:**105, 1975.
11. Ott, M. D.: Gastrointestinal allergy and migraine in childhood, J. Iowa Med. Soc. **26:**192, 1936.
12. Smith, P. S.: Cyclic vomiting and migraine in children, Va. Med. Mon. **60:**391, 1934.
13. Gascon, G., and Barlow, C.: Juvenile migraine presenting as an acute confusional state, Pediatrics **45:**628, 1970.
14. Harry, P. A.: Juvenile migraine, Prescriber **34:**243, 1940.
15. Michael, M. I., and Williams, J. M.: Migraine in children, J. Pediatr. **41:**18, 1952.
16. L'Hirondel, J.: Migrainous disease of children with scholastic difficulties, Pediatrics **45:**628, 1970.
17. Wadlington, W. B.: Migraine: not rare in children, Consultant, pp. 142-147, Sept. 1976.
18. Balyeat, R. M., and Rinkel, H. J.: Allergic migraine in children, Am. J. Dis. Child. **42:**1126, 1931.
19. Hinrichs, W. L., and Keith, H. M.: Migraine in childhood: a follow-up report, Mayo Clin. Proc. **40:**593, 1965.
20. Bille, B.: Prophylaxis of migraine in children, Bergen Migraine Symposium, Bergen, Norway, June 1975, p. 18.
21. Sanner, G.: Prophylactic treatment of childhood migraine with cyproheptadine, Bergen Migraine Symposium, Bergen, Norway, June 1975, p. 67.
22. Homeyer, G., and Lempp, R.: Studies on headaches in children, Z. Kinderheilkd. **106**(4):288-297, 1969.
23. Sabbagh, M.: The treatment of vasomotor headache in childhood, Med. Monatsschr. **24**(9):418-420, 1970.
24. Jacobi, G., Emrich, R., Ritz, A., and Herranz-Fernandez, J.: Headaches in childhood: headache and migraine: comparison of clinical and EEG findings, Fortschr. Med. **90**(6):199-204, 1972.
25. Haas, D. C., Pineda, G. S., and Laurie, H.: Juvenile head trauma syndromes and their relationships to migraine, Arch. Neurol. **32:**727-730, 1975.
26. Alison, M., and others: Headaches in children, Rev. Med. Dijon **8**(9):607-618, 1973.
27. Pineda, G.: Headaches in children, Philipp. J. Pediatr. **19**(2):107-111, 1970.

CHAPTER 20

Headache associated with sex

In the past few years there has been a considerable amount of interest in headache associated with sex and actual intercourse. That headache can occur in some people in association with intercourse is a fact. Fortunately, however, this is not a common problem. It may occur during the sexual act or, more commonly, at the conclusion of the act. This is a pathologic problem and is more commonly seen in the male. There is also a psychogenic factor with headache and sex. This is more often seen in the female patient and is more common than the pathologic form.

The psychogenic form of headache associated with sex usually is manifested as an actual headache. Naturally, there is no definite set of symptoms associated with this form of headache; the symptomatology may be quite bizarre. Many people with this type of headache are hypersensitive, excessively irritable, and self-centered. They will often do anything to "get their way" or to "get attention." To put it bluntly, many individuals simply crave attention and use the complaint of headache as a means of obtaining it. An example of this is found in the female partner who can find no better way of getting her husband's attention than by refusing him sex. This may be done very simply by having a severe headache whenever her husband is romantically inclined. Often this is successful and the desired attention is attained.

Frustrated sexuality is usually considered to be the most common cause of headache associated with matters of sex. Anxiety accompanying a headache often focuses on the fear that one's sexual performance is unsatisfactory to one's mate. Impotence and premature ejaculation in males with conscious or near-conscious fantasies of hostility and revenge are relatively easy to treat in therapy. In females, anxiety is more frequently encountered as the underlying difficulty causing sexually related headaches. Many women enter into marriage psychically unprepared for the sexual role they must assume. Orgasm is not as easily achieved by women as it is by men. The women's fear of failure to achieve orgasm is a common cause of avoidance of sexuality. Women frequently present a picture of complaints and rage against their husband's sexuality as a face-saving defense against their deep-rooted anxieties about frigidity. One of the most frequent complaints in cases of this type is chronic headache.

Headaches often accompany depression. In headaches stemming from sexual maladjustment, the greatest number occur in

388

the evening or at the end of the day, because this is the most logical time for sex to occur.

The headache is one of the most frequent psychosomatic symptoms encountered by the physician in situations of marital discord. Some patients bring their marital problems to their physicians all too readily, and physicians may feel they lack the skill to deal with them. Unfortunately some physicians avoid any discussion of marital problems with their patients, while still others cannot avoid it. However, in any case in which sex seems to be in the background of the headache complaint, the physician should investigate the case history very thoroughly or should refer the patient.

As for the actual pathologic headache associated with sex, it may be divided into two separate groups: (1) headache during actual intercourse and (2) headache following intercourse.

PAIN IN THE HEAD DURING INTERCOURSE

Head pain during intercourse is rare, but on occasions some patients will complain of it. These patients usually state that pain occurs without warning at the beginning of orgasm. This pain is usually present for several minutes, but it may last for 24 hours.

The lack of the desire for intercourse does not exist in the few patients of this type we have seen, for the headaches appear even when they are extremely desirous of sexual relationship.

The only plausible basis for this type of abnormality to our knowledge would be that sexual excitement and orgasm will always cause a rise in blood pressure. If these patients have borderline cases of hypertension, the increased blood pressure could result in headache of a hypertensive nature. If this is the case, the headaches should be used as a warning signal, and a full physical examination is indicated, with special attention directed toward the hypertension. Indeed it would be wise to check the blood pressure thoroughly and to inaugurate precautionary measures, if they appear to be needed.

Lundberg and Osterman[1] state that the cardiovascular strain caused by intercourse is modest in middle-aged, long-married men in sexual activity with their wives. However, there is evidence that nonmarried sexual activities and sexual activity with new partners and in unfamiliar environments (hotels) may lead to more profound physiologic cardiovascular changes. Most cases of sudden death during intercourse occur in extramarital relations. This seems to be valid both for coronary patients and for patients with intracranial arterial aneurysms. These facts may serve as a guide for physicians counseling their patients about sexual activities.

Another study on the headache that occurs during intercourse was presented by Martin.[2] In this study, he points out that the susceptible patient is of anxious disposition and likely to be in a phase of physical debility. For example, the patient feels run down and is under some emotional stress. However, in most cases the general health is good. In 50% of the patients there is a history of migraine. Toward the end of intercourse, generally at the moment of orgasm, the patient experiences a headache, usually of abrupt onset. The intensity of the headache varies widely, from moderate to very severe. The pain is situated chiefly at the back of the head but in some cases at the front. In most cases the pain is bilateral. There is no nausea or vomiting nor does the patient look ill. There may be pain in the neck and pain on movements such as stooping, swimming, coughing, and sneezing. There is no neck stiffness of the type seen in meningeal irritation. The patient may become agitated. The duration of the headache may vary from 10 minutes to 30 hours. Physical, neurologic, and radiologic examinations, blood pressure measurements, cerebrospinal fluid studies, and electroencephalographic investigations reveal no abnormalities.

As for the treatment of this form of headache, reassurance and improvement in general health may be the only management required, although the prescription of a tranquilizer or antimigraine drugs may be considered. The experience of some patients suggests that restraint in intercourse is of prophylactic value.

HEADACHE FOLLOWING COITUS

On some rare occasions we find a peculiar type of headache following coitus. This type of headache seems most commonly to make its appearance 24 hours or more following coitus. The description of this type of headache may often resemble a migraine type of headache.

Over 50% of these headache problems seem to occur in people who have had an unsatisfactory sex life, and often emotional problems are found to enter into the picture. In fact, stress and conflicts are frequently found to be the root of the trouble.

Physical examination and laboratory findings are usually normal and will not aid in the diagnosis. These patients usually do not respond to drug therapy. In many cases psychotherapy is of great value.

The pain after intercourse results from a temporary rise in systemic blood pressure. Headache on lifting or strain can occur in similar circumstances and has also been seen with brain tumors, presumably due to temporary venous distention which adds to vascular or tentorial displacement. By a presumably related mechanism, cough which produces localized headache may be indicative of a structural lesion.[3]

Paulson and Klawans[4] believe that two separate pathophysiologic mechanisms are left to be of significance in these patients. Some of the headaches are believed to be related to low cerebrospinal fluid pressure, while others may be migrainous. The benign nature of this syndrome is stressed. The occurrence of headaches precipitated by orgasm is not indicative of a structural or vascular lesion although such a lesion can present in this way. They conclude that though probably most acute, brief, severe headaches which occur immediately after intercourse are vascular and will be innocuous, potential rupture of aneurysm should be considered in each individual patient. The cautious physician may still wish to perform angiography in some of these patients.

Martin[5] states that various form of headache may be accentuated by sexual intercourse, such as migraine, hypertensive headache, intracranial aneurysm, and even muscle contraction headache. So it is apparent that the first step in handling the headache problem associated with sex is to find out whether it is organic or psychologic. If it is psychologic, delicate handling and reassurance are important. If it is organic, the underlying etiologic factors should be discovered and controlled. Then the headaches will usually decrease, if not vanish.

REFERENCES

1. Lundberg, P. O., and Osterman, P. O.: The benign and malignant forms of orgasmic cephalgia, Headache **14:**164-165, 1974.
2. Martin, E. A.: Headache during sexual intercourse (coital cephalalgia): a report on six cases, Irish J. Med. Sci. **148**(6):342-345, 1974.
3. Symonds, C.: Cough headache, Brain **79:**557-568, 1956.
4. Paulson, G. W., and Klawans, H. L.: Benign orgasmic cephalgia, Headache **13:**181-187, 1974.
5. Martin, M. J.: Postcoital headache, Human Sexuality **10:**101-102, 1976.

CHAPTER 21

Generalized vasodilating headache

Vasodilating headache is due to a generalized, diffuse dilation of the cranial vessels. It may be primarily intracranial or extracranial, or both, in origin. To determine the origin of this type of headache, the intravenous administration of epinephrine (Adrenalin) can be employed. If a 1:500,000 solution of epinephrine, injected intravenously, will produce a temporary relief from the headache, it is indicated that the headache is of extracranial origin.

ETIOLOGY

A generalized vasodilation of the intracranial arteries can be due to a variety of conditions. For this reason, the etiology can be very confusing, and to find it may often take considerable time and work.

An anoxemia of any type, such as may be produced by carbon monoxide poisoning, can produce a generalized vasodilating headache. High altitudes and congestive diseases can also produce this type of anoxia. The mechanism in this type of condition is the direct action of the decreased oxygen tension on the vasomotor centers.

If nitrates are absorbed over a long period of time, a generalized vasodilating headache can result. This is seen in industry or in patients receiving nitrites medically. In a person who had been an excessive coffee drinker, we could expect to see this type of headache if there were a sudden withdrawal. A high fever over a prolonged period of time can also produce a generalized vasodilating headache. This is very common.

No organic cause can usually be found for this type of headache. At times the cause of this type of headache can be very difficult to point out. We have seen cases in which the patient complained of this generalized type of headache confused with cases of dysmenorrhea, and, as a result of this, the patients had surgery. The sad result was that after some portions of the female genital tract had been removed, the headaches continued just as they were before.

This type of headache can occur in children. If such is the case, a panicky type of parent will think of such things as encephalitis or meningitis. This, of course, can be ruled out by an examination of the spinal fluid.

Many patients naturally think that they have a brain tumor, but if the physiology of head pain is explained to them they can often obtain some much-needed reassurance from their physician. This, in itself, will be a great psychologic boost to these patients and may often be the initial step in the correct therapy program.

SYMPTOMATOLOGY

The average general physical examination of these patients is negative insofar as any relationship to their headache is concerned. The blood pressure is usually normal; whether it be normal, hypertensive, or hypotensive, it has nothing to do with the etiology of the headache attacks.

The eye ground examination and the general routine neurologic examination are both negative in this type of headache patient. The spinal fluid findings are negative, as are the electroencephalogram and x-rays of both the nasal sinuses and the skull.

There is no prodromal phase to this type of headache, such as we find in the migraine headache attack. This type of head pain is throbbing and generalized throughout the entire head. Very often the pain may occur daily and soon becomes very much diffused and actually pulsating. Some patients describe their head pain as being of a bursting nature. On occasion, we find vertigo in this type of headache pattern, but it is not necessarily a part of the picture.

Sometimes these patients may have an attack which will endure for several weeks or even months without varying in severity. These patients do not have any nasal or ocular symptoms or complaints associated with their attacks. Although some may experience some degree of vertigo, they do not complain of any other symptoms relative to the ear, such as tinnitus or subnormal hearing.

The head pain in this type of patient is usually made more severe when the patient is in a reclining position. This is due to the fact that in the reclining position it is easier for the heart to pump the blood to the head and thus increase the blood supply to the head with less effort. With the cerebrovascular tree in an unbalanced state, this increase in blood flow through these vessels will, in turn, increase the symptoms of pain.

The headache arising from vascular structures is always deep and tends to be referred along the ramifications of the vascular tree.

Headaches in febrile conditions are produced by an increased cardiac activity

without an increased arterial tension. This results in painful impulses against overstretched arterial walls.

It is generally believed in these cases that there is an initial cerebral vasoconstriction of the cranial arteries which is followed by a secondary period in which there is a marked vasodilation and distention of the relaxed cranial arteries. A persistent vasodilation will eventually result in a thickening of the walls of these vessels. Edema of the surrounding tissues may, and usually does, result in a process of this type. The soft collapsible arteries became rigid and pipelike. When this occurs, the pain, which had been of a throbbing or pulsating nature will develop into a diffuse, steady ache. Many factors can initiate this type of cycle. In the vasoconstrictive phase of the cycle there is usually no associated head pain. The pain develops, therefore, during the secondary vasodilation stage.

The severe pain in the cerebral area in a generalized vasodilating headache may be followed by a phase of contraction of the skeletal muscles of the neck and the head. This is, therefore, another component of the picture, and the pain that is produced by these contractions of the skeletal muscles frequently outlasts the original vascular pain.

If it is due to a generalized vasodilation of the intracranial arteries, the headache is temporarily relieved by pressure on the carotid artery, which decreases the blood flow. Also, by exerting pressure on the jugular vein the pain may be temporarily relieved. This is accomplished by the increase in the cerebrospinal fluid pressure, thus supporting the walls of the arteries externally, preventing their maximum dilation, and decreasing the amplitude of the pulsations.

TREATMENT
Prophylactic treatment

Naturally, the removal of the cause will play a part in the prophylactic treatment of this type of headache. In some cases the cause of the trouble may be quite difficult to discover. In other cases removal of the cause may present a problem, especially if it is connected with the patient's occupation.

These headaches frequently respond to vasodilatory therapy such as intravenous histamine and nicotinic acid by mouth (100 mg three times a day before meals). Nicotinic acid is at times a terrific vasodilator of the superficial vessels in the skin. If it acts in this way, it will produce a severe flushing of the skin, especially around the head and neck. Along with this there is a warm, tingling sensation. The patient should be told about this ahead of time so that he may expect this type of reaction and not become alarmed if it does occur, for it will persist for only 15 to 20 minutes and is merely a dilation of the superficial vessels in the skin. He should, on the other hand, be told that he should not be disappointed if this does not occur, because whether or not it occurs will have no effect on the mechanism of the headache. Many patients, if warned of the flushing reaction, figure that the medication is not having effect on them unless they get this reaction. This is definitely not the case, and they should be so informed.

The exact manner in which histamine desensitization is effective in a case of generalized vasodilating headache is not clearly understood, but it does seem to work in a large percentage of cases. However, this is not a universal cureall for the generalized vasodilating type of headache. There are many patients who do not receive the desired results from this type of therapy.

Symptomatic treatment

Symptomatically, these patients obtain relief from the administration of vasoconstrictor drugs. In an attack, the pain occurs only when the affected arteries become dilated. Therefore, it seems reasonable to assume that the sequence of events in an attack could be interrupted if the cerebral arteries were to remain in a state of vasoconstriction.

Ergotamine tartrate has produced results in vascular headache problems for many years when vasoconstriction has been desired. When used in a generalized vasodilating headache, ergotamine tartrate (Gynergen) will abort the headache attack in a large percentage of cases. This is especially true if the preparation is administered during the earlier stages of the headache attack. If it is used after the attack is well established, the results produced are not so pronounced. This preparation seems to restore the cerebrovascular system to its normal tone.

Another such preparation on the drug market is dihydroergotamine (DHE-45). This preparation does not produce the toxic side effects that ergotamine tartrate does and seems to be just as effective. It has a further advantage in that it can be administered during pregnancy.

Because of the many disadvantages of the parenteral form of administration of a drug such as ergotamine tartrate the oral type of drugs available on the drug market may be more suitable. Among these drugs are such products as Cafergot, Cafergot-PB, Migral, Ergomar, Ergostat, and Wygraine. All of these drugs contain ergotamine tartrate. Some have plain ergotamine and others are combined with various other drugs, the most common drug being caffeine. For example, Cafergot is composed of 1 mg of ergotamine tartrate and 100 mg of caffeine. Caffeine, when administered orally, acts as a vasoconstrictor. When caffeine is used in conjunction with ergotamine tartrate, a reduction in the usual dosage level of ergotamine is permissible. By that we mean that a much smaller amount of ergotamine tartrate is required to abort the headache attack when it is used with caffeine than when it is used alone. The side effects of Cafergot are of a gastrointestinal nature, mainly in the form of nausea and stomach cramps but rarely, if ever, vomiting. The proper dosage in the generalized vasodilating type of headache is two tablets to be taken at the immediate onset of the headache attack. If the preparation is not used early enough in the attack, we find it to be of little or no value. In such a case, we have found that the taking of any additional tablets of Cafergot still fails to produce any results whatsoever.

It is generally considered that the vasoconstriction of the cranial vessels through the action of ergotamine tartrate and its derivatives is the most efficient means of aborting the vasodilating type of headache.

Midrin is another preparation which may be helpful in relieving the pain of a generalized vasodilating type of headache. This is the drug of choice if ergotamine tartrate is contraindicated.

Along with the prescribed therapy, there should be an attempt made to correct any abnormalities found in the general physical examination of the patient. In other words, an attempt should be made to improve the general health of the patient whenever possible. If any emotional guidance is needed, it most certainly should be given by the physician. The patient needs reassurance that he does not have anything such as a brain tumor or any other severe pathologic condition which will be difficult to handle.

Of course, the main thing to bring forth in the proper treatment of this type of headache, or any other type of headache, is the correct diagnosis. This, as in any form of headache, will require a thorough case history and examination of the patient.

Another preparation which is of value for symptomatic relief in the generalized vasodilating type of headache is the rectal suppository, Cafergot-PB. It is composed of 2 mg of ergotamine tartrate, 100 mg of caffeine, 0.25 mg of Bellafoline, and 60 mg of pentobarbital sodium. This is discussed thoroughly in Chapter 4.

In some of these cases the employment of one of the analgesic group of drugs may be of benefit in relieving the pain of this type of headache, the choice of drug being a matter of selectivity in each individual case. Various analgesic drugs are mentioned in the chapter dealing with analgesics.

CASE HISTORY

M. A., a 42-year-old female, had as her chief complaint a generalized, throbbing, bursting type of headache. The attack she had on admission for her initial examination had been present for 5 weeks. She had the pain daily and it was more or less constant. Its severity was not too excessive, but very bothersome and always of the same level. The pain would become more severe if she would lie down. There were no ocular symptoms, such as visual disturbances, scotomas, photophobia, lacrimation, or conjunctivitis. There were no nasal symptoms of obstruction, congestion, pus, or any type of nasal discharge. She had an occasional short attack of objective vertigo with accompanying nausea, but no vomiting. There was no association of the headaches with her menstrual periods. She had had these attacks for 10 to 12 years, but they had progressively gotten more severe during the past year. On routine examination, the tests were found to be essentially negative.

She was placed on intravenous histamine therapy and within a week she was entirely free from her headache. After another week of intravenous treatment, she was changed over to the subcutaneous form of administration, and she remained free from attacks for 9 months, at which time she had a slight attack which was easily corrected within a week by the subcutaneous injections. After her injections were stopped, she continued to take 100 mg of nicotinic acid three times a day before meals. This should be carried on over an indefinite period of time.

As previously stated, the exact manner in which histamine will work in such a case is not too clearly understood, but it does work in a great percentage of the cases. However, once again, we must point out that there are many failures encountered in using histamine in the generalized vasodilating type of headache; therefore, the physician should not be disappointed. Sometimes these failures may be due to improper administration or improper diagnosis. Either of these will prevent the patient from receiving the desired results.

SUMMARY

Symptoms and signs

May have vertigo

Pain is:
1. Generalized
2. Throbbing
3. Bursting
4. Often daily
5. More severe in reclining position

Negative

1. Blood pressure
2. Eye grounds
3. Physical examination
4. Neurologic examination
5. Spinal fluid
6. Electroencephalogram

Treatment

Vasodilators

1. Histamine
2. Nicotinic acid

Ergotamine preparations

1. Cafergot
2. Cafergot-PB
3. Migral
4. Ergostat
5. Ergomar
6. Wygraine

Others

1. Midrin
2. Analgesics

CHAPTER 22

Infectious disease headache

There are many infectious diseases which will present headache as part of their usual symptomatology. We shall try to mention the majority of these conditions here. Many of them are seen frequently in the average practice of the physician, but some are quite rare. However, some of these rare pathologic conditions should be mentioned here despite their infrequent occurrence in the United States.

Most headaches seen in infectious diseases are related to fever. They are usually not of a periodic nature unless the fever is periodic. These headaches are generally present during the febrile period of the disease and will abate in most cases with the lowering of the temperature. Most infectious diseases will produce headaches of a throbbing nature, and these are usually generalized or diffuse throughout the head.

The treatment in these cases should be primarily directed toward removal of the cause or treating the infectious disease which is actually causing the headache. The symptomatic relief of this type of headache is usually obtained by use of the analgesics, but sometimes something stronger is required.

INFECTIOUS DISEASES OF BACTERIAL ORIGIN
Pneumonia

Pneumonia frequently presents headache as a part of its picture. Headache is not a major symptom, naturally, but it is present and adds to the patient's discomfort and should be treated symptomatically.

Headache, however, is a common cerebral symptom of pneumonia. It is frequently seen at the onset of the disease or in its very early stages. Headache in pneumonia is even more commonly seen in children, accompanied with vomiting and convulsions at the onset. The "cerebral pneumonia" of children presents headache as one of its more prominent symptoms, along with convulsions, high fever, irritability, delirium, muscular tremor, positive Babinski and positive Kernig's signs, and the usual pulmonary symptoms.

This type of headache is usually a diffuse, generalized, pulsating pain. At times it can become very severe and prolonged until the febrile conditions begin to subside. This headache is due to a generalized vasodilation of the intracranial arteries.

Treatment should be directed primarily toward the pneumonia itself, but symptomatic relief may be obtained by using one of the analgesic drugs. Also, the inhalation of pure oxygen may help both the condition of the lungs and the headaches.

Tonsillitis and adenoiditis

Among the many symptoms of tonsillitis and adenoiditis may be headache; in fact, this is a frequent complaint. In children of school age the headache will frequently in-

396

terfere with their study work, due to the discomfort produced.

The headache in these cases is a generalized, diffuse type felt throughout the entire head. It is the throbbing type of headache and may have various degrees of severity. Relief can be obtained in most cases by correcting the underlying cause —that is, by tonsillectomy and adenoidectomy after all inflammatory processes have been brought under control by using the antibiotics. The analgesics and hydrotherapy are also helpful in these cases.

Scarlet fever

Headache usually is present in the invasive period of scarlet fever. It is pulsating in character and usually diffuse. It is due to a diffuse intracranial arterial vasodilation. These headaches are severe, prolonged, and rather constant. As the temperature increases in cases of scarlet fever, the headache symptoms correspondingly become more pronounced. As the temperature falls, the headaches subside, usually in a gradual manner.

Treatment should be directed toward the cause, which is best accomplished by the use of the antibiotics. Symptomatic relief from the headache produced by scarlet fever may be obtained by using such analgesics as Empirin Compound or aspirin, or either of these in combination with codeine phosphate.

Chorea

Headache may be a symptom of acute chorea, along with certain emotional disturbances, such as fright, crying spells, and terror. Melancholia, dementia, hallucinations, and maniacal delirium are other mental symptoms which may be present.

Typhoid fever

Headache is commonly seen as part of the symptomatology of typhoid fever. Headache usually begins at the onset of the disease and tends to increase in severity gradually during the first week of the disease. In most cases, by the time the second week of

the disease is reached, the headache has either completely subsided or it has greatly diminished. Headache is seldom seen after the third week in the majority of these cases.

The headache of typhoid fever is usually quite severe, generalized throughout the entire head, throbbing, and as a rule constantly present until it subsides completely, which usually occurs about the second week of the disease.

Treatment should be directed primarily toward the typhoid fever, but the headache itself can be symptomatically combated by using one of the analgesic drugs. Cold compresses placed on the head are also helpful. If the headache is extremely severe, lumbar puncture may be required to provide the desired relief. Hydrotherapy and, at times, mild sedatives are helpful in dealing with the headache of typhoid fever. These patients should be watched carefully for the development of delirium or for any other type of cerebral symptoms which may occur.

Paratyphoid fever

Headache may occur at the onset of paratyphoid fever. If so, it is usually found to be accompanied by abdominal pain. The headache is usually characterized by a sudden onset and it is of the throbbing type. Generalized throughout the entire head, these headaches are usually of a constant nature and not the intermittent variety. The higher the fever goes, the more severe the symptom of headache will become.

These headaches are due to a generalized, diffuse dilation of the intracranial arteries. Relief may be temporarily obtained by using the analgesic group of drugs.

Undulant fever (brucellosis)

Frequently we see severe headache associated with cases of undulant fever. These headaches may be of a short duration, but they are prolonged in the majority of cases. The severity of the undulant fever headache is in direct proportion to the fever of the patient, and during the periods of remission the headaches will subside.

These headaches are throbbing and are generalized throughout the entire head. In undulant fever the headache does not help in any way so far as the diagnosis of the condition is concerned, but if the symptoms are all taken into consideration and agglutination tests are run, the diagnosis rarely is difficult. Other agents helpful in establishing a correct diagnosis are positive blood cultures and intradermal skin tests.

Treatment should be directed toward the underlying cause, but, again, the analgesic drugs may be helpful in alleviating the headache of undulant fever.

Tularemia

The symptoms of tularemia ordinarily begin rather abruptly, and during this abrupt onset headache is usually a part of the symptomatology. Other symptoms may consist of chills, fever, vomiting, and a generalized aching. This is followed by weakness, prostration, and weight loss.

The headaches associated with tularemia are the throbbing type of headache, and generalized. If the fever becomes high, the headaches will correspondingly become quite severe. When the febrile conditions subside, the headaches will also subside.

The treatment should be directed toward the cause of the condition, but bed rest, cold compresses, and the analgesics will give temporary relief from this type of headache attack.

INFECTIOUS DISEASES OF VIRAL ORIGIN

There are infectious diseases of viral origin which also produce headache as one of their symptoms, such as acute coryza and influenza. Other viral diseases associated with headache are discussed here.

Poliomyelitis

There are several forms of poliomyelitis. In the meningitic form we find headache as a part of the symptomatology, along with pain and stiffness of the neck, pain and ri-

gidity of the back, vomiting, drowsiness, and, finally, unconsciousness. The meningitic form may begin with paralytic features and show these meningeal features later on.

This headache is usually throbbing and is generalized throughout the entire head, but in some cases it may be more pronounced in the occipital area. It is usually continuous and may or may not reach extreme degrees of severity. The headache is made more severe by any type of straining or movement of the head.

This form of headache may be temporarily relieved by putting the patient to absolute rest, using some form of sedative or analgesic, and, occasionally, using lumbar puncture.

Yellow fever

The onset of yellow fever is usually rather sudden. The patient has a sensation of chills and complains of headaches and pain in the limbs and in the back. Other symptoms consist of the fever, with a slow pulse as the temperature rises, albuminuria, nausea, vomiting, constipation, with clay-colored stools, and certain mental features, such as delirium.

The headache may not play an important part in the symptomatology, but when it is present it is usually a throbbing, generalized, constant type of headache.

Dengue

Due to a generalized dilation of the intracranial vessels, headache is frequently seen in dengue, especially at the onset of the disease. The headache usually begins rather suddenly and gradually increases in severity. It is a throbbing, generalized headache and usually becomes very severe.

This form of headache is temporarily relieved by hydrotherapy, the salicylates, analgesics, or sedatives; the opiates may be required at times.

Rabies

In the so-called premonitory stage of rabies, the patient complains of headache, loss of appetite, depression, and melancholy and is very irritable.

This condition, once it has been diagnosed, should be treated symptomatically. The headaches are a generalized, throbbing type, of various intensities. They may be temporarily relieved by employing such agents as the opiates (morphine or codeine phosphate), analgesics, rest, and quiet.

Smallpox

In this condition the occurrence of extremely severe headaches localized in the frontal region is seen in practically every case. The headaches occur in the so-called invasion period of smallpox and are associated with a severe lumbar pain and vomiting. Headaches are seen in practically all cases of smallpox, regardless of the severity of the condition.

The headache is usually severe and throbbing and will be temporarily relieved by either the analgesic type of medication or a combination of one of the analgesics with codeine phosphate or some other form of opiate. Hydrotherapy is also helpful in obtaining temporary relief.

Psittacosis

Psittacosis is usually conveyed to humans by infected birds. It is characterized in humans by an atypical pneumonia, a generalized weakness, and depression. The onset of the condition is rather sudden and is accompanied by a throbbing type of headache, more or less of a diffuse nature throughout the entire head.

With the growth in the popularity of parakeets as household pets, psittacosis seems to be occurring more frequently. This disease is not difficult to diagnose, but the diagnosis may be missed simply because the possibility is not kept in mind.

The analgesics produce the best results with this form of headache, but the condition itself must be relieved to prevent the headache attacks from continuing. These patients should be isolated and the cough should be treated symptomatically. Chlor-

amphetamine (Chloromycetin) is found to be of great value in combating the causative agent, which is a virus.

Rubella

The onset of central nervous system complications of rubella is usually 3 or 4 days after the rash has appeared. The patient will then complain of headache, apathy, and a stiff neck. This is followed in a few hours by coma which may persist from a few hours to 3 days. If the patient does not die in this stage, he can be expected to recover within a few weeks.

Mitchell and Pampiglione[1] point out that it is uncommon for complete recovery to follow a widespread lesion of the central nervous system due to rubella, and that the brainstem, the spinal cord, or even the frontal lobes may be involved.

An increase in cell count and in protein is found in the cerebrospinal fluid in cases of rubella with neurologic complications.

INFECTIOUS DISEASES OF RICKETTSIAL ORIGIN

Some diseases of rickettsial origin also present headache as one of their chief symptoms. Examples of this are typhus fever and trench fever.

Typhus fever

Typhus fever, which is caused by *Rickettsia prowazeki,* presents headache as a part of its symptomatology in both its epidemic and its endemic forms. In the epidemic form of typhus fever, headache is seen in the invasion period of the disease. The headache comes on rather suddenly with chills, fever, and severe pain in the back and the legs. The headache of typhus fever may be extremely severe and quite prolonged. It is usually a generalized type of headache and is throbbing in character. The fever and the headaches usually fall by crisis, not by lysis. In the endemic form of typhus fever the patients are also distressed by severe headaches, even though the other symptoms are less pronounced than they are in the epidemic form of typhus.

The headache of typhus fever is temporarily relieved by hydrotherapy, the analgesic type of medication, and cold compresses to the head. It is also important to keep the patient's bowels open.

Trench fever

Headache is a prominent symptom of trench fever during the febril periods of the disease. These headaches are associated with tenderness over the areas involved, and the pain frequently migrates, as we see in myalgia of the head. These headaches are frequently found to be more severe at night. The headache symptoms have periods of remission, as do the other symptoms of the disease. These remission periods of the symptoms are helpful in the diagnosis of trench fever.

The analgesic type of drug gives the patient temporary relief from the headache symptoms in cases of trench fever.

INFECTIOUS DISEASE OF PROTOZOAL ORIGIN

Headache may be part of the symptomatology of some diseases which are of protozoal etiology. Such rare conditions as yaws, relapsing fever, Weil's disease, and trypanosomiasis fit into this category. Malaria and syphilis also are diseases of protozoal origin in which headache is a symptom.

Syphilis

Frequently, in the secondary stages of syphilis, headache is found as part of the symptomatology. This headache is often localized in the occipital area of the head and it may migrate up to the vertex area. The headache of syphilis is usually more severe at night, when the patient is reclining.

In cerebrospinal syphilis, headache is often one of the prodromal symptoms. The headaches are usually very severe. Often

the patients go into convulsions or delirium following these acute headaches, or a hemiplegic attack may even occur.

The headaches of neurosyphilis may be generalized throughout the head, or they may be localized in any area of the head. In some cases of syphilis involving the nervous system, headache may be the only symptom present for quite some length of time, perhaps even as long as several years.

In gumma formation in meningovascular cerebral syphilis, headache is one of the most prominent symptoms.

In general paresis, headache may play a part in the early symptomatology, just as it may in the syphilitic form of meningitis. These headaches are always made more severe by any form of straining, sneezing, coughing, or the like.

Malaria

Quite frequently patients with malaria can tell several hours ahead of time that they are going to have a malarial chill by the fact that they have a headache. This is not true in all cases, but it is in more than a few.

The cold stage of malaria is frequently associated with headache, lassitude, fever, and, perhaps, nausea and vomiting; then the chills follow. The headache is usually intense, throbbing, generalized, and, at times, almost unbearable. It persists for 10 to 30 minutes, as a rule.

The so-called hot stage of malaria also has a generalized, diffuse, throbbing headache as part of its symptomatology. This persists for about 1 to 3 hours.

The headache of malaria is temporarily relieved by using one of the analgesic drugs, such as aspirin or Empirin. At times something stronger may be needed, such as codeine phosphate, but this is not usually required. Hydrotherapy is also helpful in affording temporary relief of the headache in malaria, and bed rest is also advisable and indicated. The primary treatment of malaria, however, should be directed toward the causative agent.

REFERENCE

1. Mitchell, W., and Pampiglione, G.: Neurological and mental complications of rubella, Lancet **2:**1250, 1954.

SELECTED READINGS

Craig, C. F.: Malaria, Oxford loose-leaf medicine, vol. 5, chap. 32, New York, 1938, Oxford University Press.

Enders, T. F.: Psittacosis, virus and rickettsial diseases, Cambridge, 1940, Harvard University Press.

Farber, H. K.: Acute poliomyelitis as a primary disease of the nervous system, Medicine **12:**83, 1933.

Goodpasture, E. W.: Herpetic infections with special reference to involvement of the nervous system, Medicine **8:**223, 1929.

Horsfall, F. L., Jr.: Present status of knowledge of influenza, Am. J. Pub. Health **30:**1302, 1940.

Leach, C. N., and Johnson, H. N.: Human rabies, Am. J. Trop. Med. **20:**335, 1940.

Merritt, H. H., Adams, R. D., and Solomon, M. G.: Neurosyphilis, New York, 1946, Oxford University Press.

Mott, F. W.: Syphilis of the nervous system and tabes dorsalis, Oxford loose-leaf medicine, vol. 6, chaps. 19-20, New York, 1939, Oxford University Press.

Netherton, E. W.: Headache of syphilitic origin, Med. Clin. North Am. **24:**349, 1940.

Pinkerton, H.: Diagnosis and classification of rickettsial diseases, Cambridge, 1940, Harvard University Press.

Pinkerton, H., and Weinman, D.: Carrion's disease, Proc. Soc. Exp. Biol. Med. **37:**587, 1937.

Russell, F. F.: Small pox and vaccination, Oxford loose-leaf medicine, vol. 5, chap. 23, New York, 1942, Oxford University Press.

Sawyer, W. A.: Yellow fever, Oxford loose-leaf medicine, vol. 5, chap. 31, New York, 1939, Oxford University Press.

Simmonds, J. S.: Dengue fever, virus and rickettsial diseases, Cambridge, 1940, Harvard University Press.

Strong, R. P.: Trench fever investigations, J.A.M.A. **70:**1597, 1918.

CHAPTER 23

Other conditions with associated headache

ICE CREAM HEADACHE

Some people while eating ice cream on a hot, humid, summer day will experience pain in the frontal temporal area. This follows chilling of the hard palate of the mouth. This is believed to occur in summer more than in winter because the blood vessels of the palate are more easily dilated so as to prevent chilling. In warm, humid weather there may be a generalized vasodilation of superficial vessels to transfer body heat to the outside environment.

This is actually a form of vascular headache and, to our knowledge, was initially described by Smith[1] in 1963.

Raskin and Knittle[2] found this condition to be much more common in patients with migraine than it was in control persons, which they believe to be due to excessive erratic vasomotor regulations. This condition represents a vasodilatory type of pain in one area which is secondary to vasocontriction in another area.

We know that cold will produce symptoms of pain by vasoconstriction, which leads to reduced local circulation. This represents pain of vascular origin. As far back as 1949, Horton[3] described what he called winter headache. This may have been due to the same factors as the so-called ice cream headache.

CHINESE FOOD HEADACHE (CHINESE RESTAURANT SYNDROME)

In many Chinese foods a food flavor enhancer called monosodium glutamate is employed. When this substance is used in sufficient quantities, headache may occur. It may also bring about such symptoms as facial pressure, chest pain, or burning sensations. It has been estimated that as little as 1.5 gm (about ¼ teaspoonful) may produce symptoms in suitable subjects.

Prior ingestion of food delays the absorption of monosodium glutamate and will protect even the most susceptible patient from the Chinese restaurant syndrome.

Glutamic acid, which is an ingredient of monosodium glutamate, is present in large amounts both in the body and in some foods. It is generally regarded as safe, and no limitation is placed on its use as a food additive by the Food and Drug Administration. Naturally, this additive is used more in China and Japan than in the United States.

The Chinese restaurant syndrome is an entity of its own and headache is probably the chief symptom.

HOT DOG HEADACHE (HEADACHE DUE TO NITRITES)

Some individuals are sensitive to sodium nitrite, which is frequently an additive to cured meat such as sausage or frankfurters (hot dogs). This is added to these products to improve the appearance of the meat, though regulations limit the levels of the amount of nitrite which can be used in the treatment of these cured meats.

The headache precipitated by nitrites is usually of a dull aching type, of short duration (1 to 2 hours), and usually not accompanied by any gastrointestinal associated symptoms. Henderson and Raskin[4] did some interesting research involving nitrites and headache.

BENIGN EXERTIONAL HEADACHE

A headache that transiently interrupts complete comfort in response to exertion is an exertional headache. This type of headache may occur with coughing, sneezing, straining, bending, etc. It is of short duration—only a few moments—and occurs immediately with the etiologic factor involved.

Naturally, patients with this type of headache should have headache of a more serious nature ruled out before this diagnosis is made. This is a relatively rare condition but it does exist. It is seen more in males than females and in older patients and it usually improves or vanishes after time has passed. The management of these cases is conservative.

Rooke[5] points out that care should be taken in all of these cases to rule out such lesions as Arnold-Chiari deformity and other foramen magnum conditions.

PAGET'S DISEASE

Paget's disease of the skull may produce headache. This headache may at times resemble migraine. The pain is of a throbbing type with a rather sudden onset, occurring at irregular intervals. These headaches may persist for several days. Usually this type of headache gradually increases in frequency. Treatment is often extremely difficult, but some of these cases respond (headachewise) to the ergotamine tartrate preparations, analgesics, or sedatives. Still other headaches do not respond to any medication.

Fortunately, headache is not found in all patients with Paget's disease, but it is one of the most frequent symptoms. If seen, it is usually at an early stage of the disease.

MULTIPLE SCLEROSIS

Pain may be one of the symptoms of multiple sclerosis, and one of these painful symptoms may be headache. Actually, headache is one of the common symptoms of this disease.

The headache of this condition is recurrent and of a throbbing unilateral type. Many patients have been found to be migraine sufferers. There is a higher incidence of migraine in patients with multiple sclerosis than in the non–multiple sclerosis population. The reason for this is not clear.

Besides the migraine possibility in these cases, there is also the possibility of a tension type of headache occurring due to the emotional pressures which may occur when the condition becomes severe.

INFECTIOUS MONONUCLEOSIS

Infectious mononucleosis is frequently seen in the practice of otolaryngology. One of its symptoms is a dull, throbbing, constant, generalized type of headache. The symptomatology of infectious mononucleosis varies with each individual case. There may be malaise, anorexia, lymph node enlargement, abdominal pain, throat pain, enlarged spleen, gastrointestinal symptoms (such as nausea and vomiting), and a generalized weakness. There is usually a leukocytosis and a positive heterophil antibody reaction. Optic neuritis has also been seen in cases of infectious mononucleosis.

The type of headache seen in cases of infectious mononucleosis is usually relieved by the analgesic type of drug, such as Empirin Compound or aspirin. We have obtained excellent results with Fiorinal in treating this headache. Usually, two tablets of Fiorinal will give these patients temporary relief from their headaches. Cold compresses to the head are also helpful, as are rest and proper elimination.

In infectious mononucleosis, if meningeal irritation occurs, cytologic changes may be present in the spinal fluid in the absence of a meningeal syndrome. Also, the clinical syndrome may exist in the presence of a normal spinal fluid. The Paul-Bunnel reaction is only weakly positive in the spinal fluid.

In the encephalitic forms of infectious mononucleosis there may be no meningeal reaction, or there may be meningoencephalitis or meningoencephalomyelitis.

FIBROSITIS

Fibrositis is an inflammation of the fibrous tissue which may occur in many parts of the body. It involves such structures as ligaments, tendons, muscle sheaths, fascia, nerve sheaths, periosteum, or any place where fibrous tissue might be found.

Fibrositis may be due to focal infections, trauma, muscular strain, or overexposure to the elements. It is commonly seen in cold and damp weather and frequently follows chilling of the body parts.

The form of fibrositis associated with the head and the neck at first causes a swelling and a puffiness and later on is followed by an indurative stage. These areas are found primarily in the back of the neck and in the musculature of the scalp. An indurative headache occurs in these cases. At times the headaches may actually simulate the migrainous type of headache.

The pain in typical cases of fibrositis is usually bilateral and most commonly is found to occur in the muscular attachments in the nuchal line. These areas of attachment are often found to be extremely tender to pressure.

We frequently see patients with fibrositis who obtain relief from mild forms of exercise. However, if this exercise is continued and is overdone, the pain may actually be increased.

These painful areas are usually localized, are of a burning nature, and are very sensitive to the slightest amount of pressure or palpation. These patients show a considerable amount of stiffness with disuse, and relief is frequently obtained by exercising the areas involved in a mild manner. Severe exercise is likely to increase the pain. If this should occur, it will be relieved by rest of the part or parts involved.

Treatment consists in the removal of any focus of infection which might be present, rest of the musculature involved, wet heat applications, the analgesic type of drugs, and massage. Sometimes the injection of such preparations as procaine hydrochloride (Novocain) or cocaine locally to the area involved will be needed to relieve the pain.

EPIDEMIC MYALGIA

Epidemic myalgia is most prominent in the Scandinavian countries, Iceland, Norway, and Denmark. Its etiology has not been proved, but it is believed to be a filtrable virus.

Frontal headaches are a pronounced feature of this disease. These headaches are throbbing, dull, localized, of sudden onset, and of short duration. The primary symptoms of this disease are diaphragmatic pain and tenderness.

Temporary relief is obtained by the use of hydrotherapy and the analgesic group of drugs.

GOUT

In the irregular or atypical types of gout we may find, along with the other symptoms, that there are certain manifestations of nervous system involvement present.

Among these are neuralgia, sciatica, paresthesias, and headache. These are not among the most prominent symptoms of gout, naturally, but they can and do occur in some cases. They are not characteristically seen in the ordinary case of gout, but are seen in what is often called gouty diathesis or irregular cases of gout. In this type of gout there may be cutaneous, cardiovascular, gastrointestinal, urinary, ophthalmologic, pulmonary, and nervous system manifestations.

CHRONIC POSTHERPETIC NEURALGIA

Postherpetic neuralgia is confined to patients past middle age. It is seldom helped by medical treatment, and it seldom improves. Often it has been present for several years when it is initially encountered by the physician. It is more often seen in elderly patients.

The pathophysiology is not definitely known, but it is known that virus infection causes extensive and persistent inflammatory changes along the neural pathways from the spinal cord to the terminal ramifications in the skin.

Medical attention should be focused on the preventive aspect of postherpetic neuralgia by perfecting measures to reduce the severity of the acute attack. Many procedures that fail to relieve postherpetic pain are quite effective in treating the discomfort of acute herpes zoster.

Analgesic blocking is often successful in breaking up the vicious pain cycle and in preventing the process from spreading. The earlier this is used, the better the chance of relief. Chlorprothixene, a psychotherapeutic agent used to treat emotional disorders, may help in these cases. It works as an analgesic.

PLUMMER-VINSON SYNDROME

Plummer-Vinson syndrome is associated with severe headaches located just above or deep in the root of the nose. Generalized weakness and fatigue are also present,

along with a mild dysphagia and a sensation of nasal stuffiness and obstruction. Patients always show an iron deficiency, and prolonged course of iron administration always causes a disappearance of the symptoms.

This condition is often seen in patients with profuse menstrual flow, severe menorrhagia during menopause, a total gastrectomy, and chronic malaria.

ARNOLD'S NEURALGIA

Arnold's neuralgia is characterized by suboccipital pain that shifts to the vertex or, less frequently, to the shoulder. It is usually paroxysmal and stabbing or burning in nature. During remissions, tenderness and such paresthesias as tightness, oppression, and formications are present. Cough, friction from clothing, changes in temperature, and other minor stimuli are capable of inducing the painful paroxysms. Usually emotional tension, restlessness, neurovegetative dystonias, and mild stiffness of the nucha are associated with the condition.

Because of the varied anastomoses of the auricular branch of the vagus, the condition may stimulate cervicofacial neuralgia and even atypical trigeminal neuralgia.

If the disease is caused by organic processes involving the bone or vertebral ligaments, it is accompanied by limitation of the motion of the neck, crepitation, and constant pain which is aggravated by moving the head and which is relieved by rest and immobility.

HEADACHE FOLLOWING PNEUMOENCEPHALOGRAPHY

The pneumoencephalogram is generally recognized as an important tool when used as a diagnostic agent in the study of intracerebral lesions. In using the pneumoencephalogram, the risk is very low, but there are some hazards. Usually these consist of severe throbbing, persistent headaches which may be associated with nausea and vomiting. These headaches are frequently aggravated by body or head movement. The duration of this type of headache may be from 1 to 6 days after the procedure. It has been estimated that only 8.4% of these patients were free from headache following pneumoencephalography.

Because of the lack of unanimity of opinion regarding the cause of these postencephalographic symptoms, it has been difficult to develop any satisfactory method of active treatment or prophylaxis. The difficulty is indicated by the fact that there is such a large variety of treatment found in the literature. Cortisone sometimes helps these patients. One group of patients was given 50 mg of cortisone orally every 6 hours for a total of 400 mg following pneumoencephalography. A placebo was given to a second group of patients. The cortisone produced relief from the headaches in severity, incidence, and duration of the attack. This was especially true in the patients whose symptoms were organic rather than psychogenic.

Intrathecal injections of methylprednisolone acetate are also used to prevent the occurrence of this type of headache. The mechanism of action is unknown.

MYOFASCIAL PAIN SYNDROMES

Although patients with the myofascial syndrome may present a wide variety of clinical symptoms, including pain, stiffness, limitation of motion, tremors, weakness, and manifestations of autonomic nervous system dysfunction, the chief complaint is usually pain, which may vary in quality and intensity from a low-grade discomfort to a type of pain that is severe and incapacitating and frequently associated with a deep, burning, aching sensation. The trigger points can occur in any muscle. Several of the more common trigger points in the upper trunk are in the levator muscle of the scapula and the infraspinous muscles, and in the lower trunk in the quadratus lumborum, tensor fasciae latae, and anterior tibial muscles. Myofascial pain syndromes are so common that they should not be overlooked

when one is faced with a pain problem that does not fit familiar clinical patterns.

VERTEBRAL ARTERY CONSTRICTION

Pain in the upper cervical region and head can in some cases be produced by a constriction or an occlusion of the vertebral artery in different positions of the neck. This occlusion can be either complete or partial. The symptoms produced by this condition are pain in the upper cervical and suboccipital region. This pain radiates superiorly behind the ear or ears to the retroorbital region. When the pain is severe, there may be a blurring of vision or diplopia. Associated unsteadiness on the feet is frequently mentioned in the patient's history. In some cases a typical vertigo may occur, as may nausea and vomiting.

A feeling of stiffness of the neck is usually present in these cases. Faulty neck posture seems to be present in most cases, and trauma may or may not be a factor. Tension and anxiety can also help to bring about an attack.

On examination, cervical spine tenderness is noticed, especially over the transverse process of the atlas on the side involved. Neck extension against resistance is very painful. Hypoesthesia and hypalgesia in the occipital area are common and may be present as far anteriorly as the forehead. Lateral nystagmus is often produced following a rotation of the neck with the head in a forward position or when the neck is extended for a few seconds.

Prolonged neck extension may produce a feeling of faintness, and this may also initiate an attack of the pain.

HEADACHE FOLLOWING ELECTROSHOCK

Headache following electroshock is a common occurrence and may be prevented by premedication with meprobamate. This also decreases the pretreatment anxiety. Dosage is 400 mg about 1 hour before treatment. This will diminish the intensity of the tonic and the clonic phases of the seizure. When this premedication is used the patients seem to regain consciousness much more rapidly.

OCCIPITAL NEURALGIA

Occipital neuralgia produces headache in the occipital areas. It is usually seen in the tense and anxious type of patient. There is also scalp pain associated with the condition, along with tenderness and paresthesia along the distribution of the second cervical dermatome. Other characteristics are loss of cervical lordosis and mild neurologic signs.

The etiology of this condition is usually a malformation or instability of the joint space between the first and second cervical segments, with intermittent subluxation or root compression resulting in pain in the distribution of the greater auricular, greater occipital, and lesser occipital nerves. There is a reflex spasm of the posterior neck muscles which reduces the mobility of the neck and produces pain and occipital tension.

Treatment consists of a Thomas collar or surgical fixation.

CAROTID ARTERITIS

Carotid arteritis is a common cause of neck pain and tenderness. It often simulates painful cervical lymphadenopathy. The etiology of this condition is unknown, but it may be related to some abnormal dysfunction of the autonomic nervous system.

Headache in these cases often is similar to the vascular type of headache. The headache will be located in the area in front of the ear, radiating into the adjacent temporal area.

The cardinal symptoms of carotid arteritis are neck pain and severe tenderness which usually extends along the entire course of the carotid artery. Many patients complain of a sore throat but on examination, pharyngitis, tonsillitis, or laryngitis is never found to be present.

At the bifurcation the artery will actually seem to pulsate. Swelling of the neck may be noticeable.

Treatment with the corticosteroids is as useful as any type of treatment; however, it is not always successful. Some stubborn cases may require psychotherapy, as many of these patients have chronic anxiety. The analgesics may be helpful.

ACUTE YELLOW ATROPHY OF THE LIVER

Acute yellow atrophy of the liver may occur in certain infections, such as typhoid fever, septicemia, diphtheria, and syphilis. It may also be due to certain poisons from such substances as the sulfonamides, phosphorus, mercury, and chloroform. It has also been found during pregnancy.

This condition usually has an initial stage which lasts from a few days to 2 or 3 weeks, during which times there is a catarrhal jaundice present. Following this, abrupt symptoms set in, which may include convulsions, delirium, trembling of the musculature, vomiting, jaundice, and headache.

The headache in this condition may resemble the headache of meningitis. It comes on abruptly and is rather severe. The headache is more or less diffuse throughout the entire head, and it is of a constant nature. Often these headaches may seem to be more intense in the occipital area. They are throbbing, and often they are made more severe by such acts as straining, stooping, coughing, or sneezing.

Treatment should be directed toward eliminating the toxic substances causing the condition. Intravenous saline injections or the subcutaneous administration of saline is helpful. Intravenous glucose, sedatives, and hydrotherapy are also helpful in relieving the headache phase of this disease.

HEADACHE ASSOCIATED WITH GASTROINTESTINAL DISTURBANCES

The causes of headache associated with gastrointestinal disorders may be multiple, such as alkalosis associated with obstruction; splanchnoptosis; typhoid fever; duodenal stasis; vagal irritation; toxemias due to disease of the liver and kidney; cecal stasis which may be due to atony, adhesions, or congenital bands; fatigue; exposure to intoxicants such as carbon monoxide, arsenic, or lead; a low blood sugar; or any emotional conflict.

The most frequent gastrointestinal symptoms accompanying headache are abdominal distress, pain, nausea, vomiting, anorexia, epigastric fullness, diarrhea, constipation, and pyrosis.

The treatment program for relief of the headache should be directed against the causative factor.

EPHEMERAL FEVER

Ephemeral fever is a disease of unknown etiology characterized by an abrupt fever, malaise, loss of appetite, a flushed skin, herpes of the lips, and headache. The headache begins suddenly and tends to terminate in like manner. It is generalized, dull, and usually throbbing. The headache is most frequently present for only a short period of time.

Temporary relief of the headache of ephemeral fever can be obtained by using the analgesic type of drug, hydrotherapy, and bed rest.

BASILAR ARTERY AND CAROTID ARTERY INSUFFICIENCY

Basilar artery and carotid artery insufficiency may produce headache accompanied by both sensory and motor disturbances. This type of headache is throbbing and is thought to be secondary to the dilation of the extracranial arteries. Collateral circulation is produced by the increased blood flow.

If the occlusion or stenosis is vertebrobasilar, headache is more commonly seen as a symptom. Headache is less commonly seen if the occlusion is in the middle cerebral or the internal carotid artery. If the occlusion or stenosis is in the subclavian or

innominate arteries, headache is rarer. When stroke occurs, headache may disappear.

This type of headache is usually in the occipital area and the back of the neck. It may be in the frontal area; however, it may be bilateral if the vertebrobasilar vessels are affected.

Treatment is directed toward removing the cause, which may require surgical intervention.

POSTTHYROIDECTOMY HEADACHE

Postthyroidectomy headaches are actually much more common than one would believe. They are usually due to prolonged contraction of the cervical muscles, which is actually due to the surgery. The patient has a tendency to hold his neck muscles rather rigidly following surgery. He is fearful of moving this head because this might aggravate the incision area. This positioning produces the headaches. These headaches and neck aches are quite severe and are usually located in the frontal or occipital areas. Their duration may be up to 1 week or so.

These headaches usually respond to the analgesic drugs. Massage and heat to the back of the neck are also helpful, along with active neck exercise.

ALTITUDE HEADACHE

Appenzeller[6] describes this type of headache. It is one of the prominent symptoms of acute mountain sickness. It occurs when individuals are in altitudes of 8,000 feet or higher. Altitude headache may be due to brain edema, hypoxia, vasodilation, or increased intracranial pressure. It is usually generalized throughout the head or in the frontal area. The pain is aggravated by such things as straining, coughing, exertion, and lying down.

Altitude headache is usually found in people who are not accustomed to high altitudes. Relief from this type of headache may be obtained by using the analgesics potassium chloride and ammonium chloride; furosemide and acetazolamide may also be of benefit.

GREATER OCCIPITAL NEURALGIA

The greater occipital nerve is actually a continuation of the second cervical nerve root, which receives branches from the spinal accessory nerve, the superior cervical sympathetic ganglion, the fifth (trigeminal) cranial nerve, and the vestibular and acoustic nerves. The greater occipital nerve supplies the scalp, shoulders, side of the neck, and portions of the face in a sensory fashion.

The headache associated with this condition is usually present on arising in the morning. It is a constant, dull aching. The pain may vary in duration from days to weeks, and the frequency may also vary from a few weeks to a few months. The pain does not occur at regular intervals and is not periodic.

The headache of this pathologic entity is usually bilateral and located in the occipital temporofrontal areas of the head. There may be associated scalp and neck tenderness. This condition is more commonly seen in women than in men, and it usually occurs in persons between the age of 20 to 60.

There are no prodromal symptoms or trigger areas.

Associated manifestations may consist of blurred vision, stuffiness of the nose, toothache, tinnitus, or vertigo.

As for treatment, Chouret[7] advocates injection of 2 ml of 1% lidocaine (Xylocaine) with 3 ml of 0.6% aqueous solution of ammonium chloride immediately below the occipital bone protuberance.

RAEDER'S SYNDROME

Raeder's syndrome is a rare condition which has head pain as one of its characteristic symptoms. The pain is usually associated with the distribution of the ophthalmic division of the fifth cranial nerve (trigeminal nerve). Other symptoms associated with this condition are ptosis of the eyelid without enophthalmos, meiosis, and no sweating abnormalities over the face. There may, however, be a limited area of anhidrosis in the supraorbital area.

This condition seems to be more prevalent in males than in females.

The etiology of this condition is rather obscure. However, it does seem to be definitely associated with hypertensive cardiovascular disease, with migraine, with inflammatory conditions such as nasal sinusitis, and with head trauma of a minor nature. Still some cases of Raeder's syndrome have been reported having no apparent etiologic factor.

When the etiology is known, the treatment of this form of headache should be directed to correcting the etiologic factor.

TRANSIENT ISCHEMIC ATTACK HEADACHE

Headache is frequently associated with transient ischemic attacks. In these cases, headache may be one of two types: episodic or late onset vascular. One or both forms may be present in the same patient.

The episodic headaches occur during, immediately before, or after the transient ischemic attacks. These headaches usually have a short duration (up to 2 hours or so), but they may persist for several days. The pain is usually of a moderate severity and of the pressure type, or it may be throbbing in nature, in the frontal area, and unilateral.

The late onset vascular type of headache in these patients occurs independently of the transient ischemic attacks. The headache has general characteristics identical with the episodic type of headache.

The pathophysiology of both of these types of headache appears to be quite similar.

It is sometimes thought that these headaches might be a warning sign of an approaching transient ischemic attack or even a warning of a possible complete stroke.

MECHANICAL HEADACHE

Travell[8] describes a headache problem which she calls mechanical headache. She defines this as a headache due to a repetitive mechanical derangement of the musculoskeletal system which results in faulty body mechanics, which in turn results in headache. The muscles most commonly involved are the sternomastoid, the trapezius, the muscles of mastication, and the temporal.

This type of headache is a deep ache, pulsating, and unilateral or bilateral, depending on the muscle or muscles involved in the process.

The etiology of this condition can be gross trauma to the muscles or constant muscular strain.

The pain may be relieved by the use of analgesics. However, for complete relief, the muscles affected must receive local treatment along with correction and elimination of the mechanical cause.

INFLAMMATORY HEADACHE

Inflammatory headaches may be due to any chronic low-grade inflammation of the meninges, the basal periosteum, or the dura mater.

Any exogenous factor, infectious in nature, causing either direct or indirect irritation of the intracranial structure may produce this form of headache.

These headaches are characteristically seen in younger patients, primarily in females. They are often severe and may be preceded by a serous or a lymphocytic form of foci of infection.

This condition is frequently associated with a low-grade fever, generalized disability, and, in the female patient, menstrual disorders.

The etiologic factors are frequently found to be infectious diseases of the nose, sinuses, or pharynx, rheumatic disease, exogenous allergy, tuberculin hyperergia, or infection anywhere in the body.

Treatment consists of removal of the foci and the cause. Antibiotics, antihistaminics (if allergic etiology is present), or steroids may be of benefit. Each case is an individual entity and has to be handled as such.

SYSTEMIC LUPUS ERYTHEMATOSUS

Headache may occur in systemic lupus erythematosus in cases with or without central nervous system lupus. Therefore, headache in this pathologic entity where other neurologic symptoms and signs are absent is not an indication of central nervous system involvement.

Neurologic signs of central nervous system involvement in cases of systemic lupus erythematosus consist of tinnitus, vertigo, loss of balance, poor memory, slurred speech, hemiparesis, upper extremity palsy, chorea, and pseudobulbar palsy.

Psychiatric symptoms indicating central nervous system involvement in systemic lupus include hallucinations, delusions, behavior problems, depression, schizoid reactions, psychotic reactions, and emotional instability.

TOLUSA HUNT SYNDROME

The etiology of Tolusa Hunt syndrome may be neoplasm, infection, specific granulomas, or trauma. Any of these conditions involve the orbital apex, the superior orbital fissure, or the anterior cavernous sinus.

This syndrome presents the symptoms of orbital pain, extraocular muscle palsies, and frontal numbness. There is a steady retroorbital pain that may or may not precede the ophthalmoplegia. There may be neurologic involvement of either the third, fourth, fifth (ophthalmic division), or the sixth cranial nerves or all of them. The symptoms may persist for days or weeks, and there may be spontaneous remissions.

The condition is quite rare and responds to steroid therapy. Prompt diagnosis and treatment result in a minimal amount of permanent damage.

REFERENCES

1. Smith, R. O.: Ice cream headache, Va. Med. Mon. **90:**562, 1963.
2. Raskin, N. H., and Knittle, S. C.: Ice cream headache and orthostatic symptoms in patients with migraine, Headache **16:**222, 1976.
3. Horton, B. T.: Clinical varieties and therapeutic suggestions, Med. Clin. N. Am. **33:**995-996, 1949.
4. Henderson, W. R., and Raskin, N. H.: "Hot-dog" headache; individual susceptibility to nitrite, Lancet **2:**1162-1163, 1962.
5. Rooke, E. D.: Benign exertional headache, Med. Clin. North Am. **52:**801-808, 1968.
6. Appenzeller, O.: Altitude headache (editorial), Headache **12:**126-129, 1972.
7. Chouret, E. E.: The greater occipital neuralgia headache, Headache **7:**33-34, 1967.
8. Travell, J.: Mechanical headache, Headache **7:** 23-29, 1967.

SUGGESTED READINGS

Atkinson, R. A., and Appenzeller, O.: Headache in small vessel disease of the brain, a study of patients with systemic lupus erythematosus, Headache **15:** 198-201, 1975.

DeWitt, D., and Thompson, S. W.: Raeder's syndrome: a case with maxillary sinusitis, Headache **15:**91-95, 1975.

Greppi, E.: Inflammatory headache, Headache **3:**138-142, 1964.

Medina, J. L., Diamond, S., and Rubino, F. A.: Headaches in patients with transient ischemic attacks, Headache **15:**194-197, 1975.

Peters, G. A.: Post-thyroidectomy headache, Headache **2:**88-89, 1962.

Index

412